IMMUNOLOGY:
Essential and Fundamental

SECOND EDITION

IMMUNOLOGY:
Essential and Fundamental

SECOND EDITION

Sulabha Pathak, PhD

Department of Biological Sciences
Tata Institute of Fundamental Research
Mumbai, India

Urmi Palan, MPhil

Department of Microbiology
R Ruia College
Mumbai, India

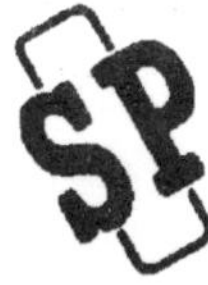

Science Publishers, Inc.

Enfield, New Hampshire, USA

SCIENCE PUBLISHERS, INC.,
Post Office Box 699
Enfield, New Hampshire 03748
United States of America

http://www.scipub.net

sales@scipub.net (marketing department)
editor@scipub.net (editorial department)
info@scipub.net (for all other enquiries)

CIP DATA WILL BE PROVIDED ON REQUEST

ISBN: 1-57808-378-8 (Paperback)
     1-57808-379-6 (Hardcover)

Content Editors:	Scott Cameron
	Claire Dunn
Language Editor:	Gauri Pathak
Illustrations:	Abhishek Chakravorty
Cover illustration:	Scanning electron micrograph of a lymphocyte migrating into the high endothelial venule in the lymph node (1000x), a kind gift of Dr. W. van Ewijk, Leiden University, The Netherlands

Published by Science Publishers Inc., Enfield, NH, USA
Printed in India

To
Our parents

Icons

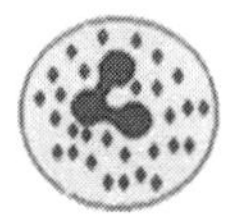

neutrophil rested

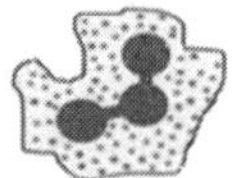

neutrophil activated

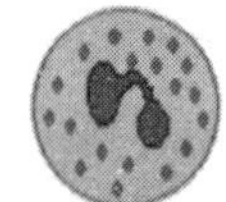

eosinophil

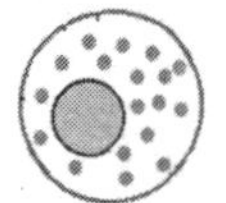

mast cells/ basophils

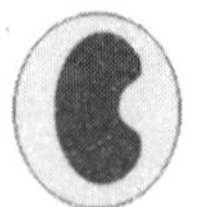

monocytes

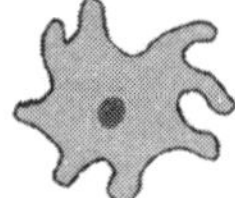

immature DC

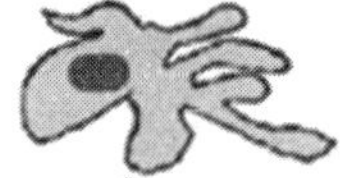

mature DC

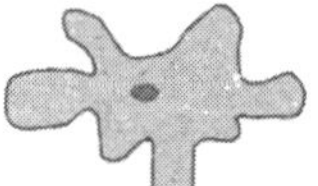

macrophage

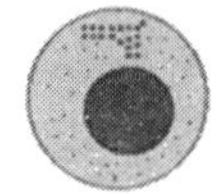

NK cells

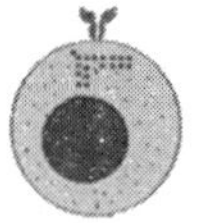

NKT cells

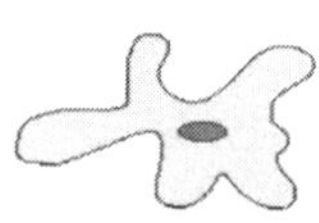

FDC

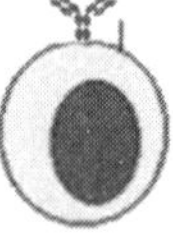

B cell

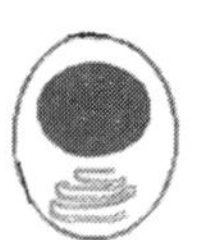

Plasma cell

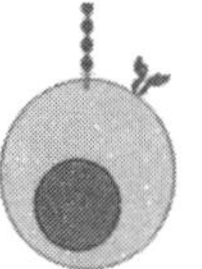

TH cell

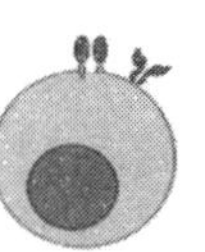

CTL

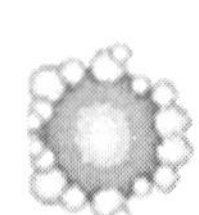

apoptotic cell

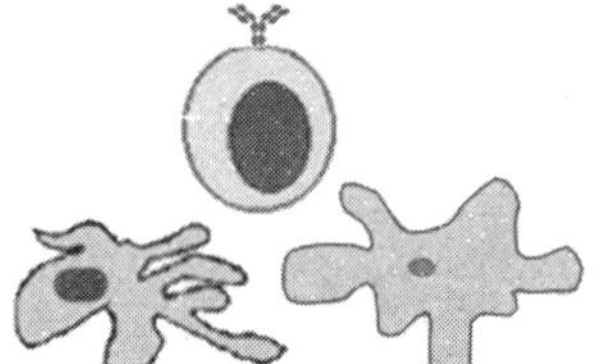

donor cells

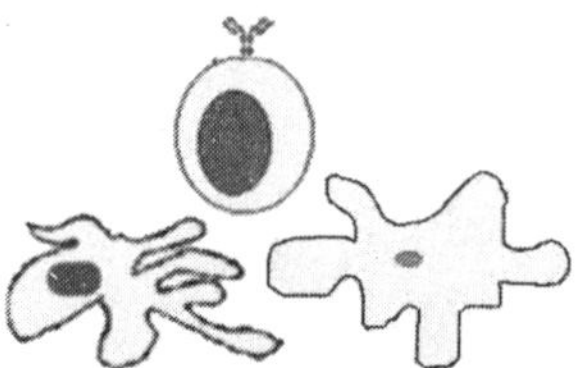

recipient cells

Ig domain

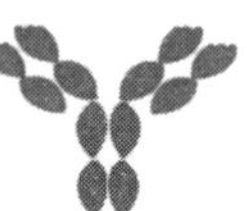

IgA/IgD/IgG

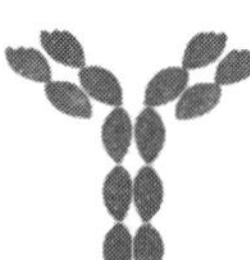

IgM/IgE

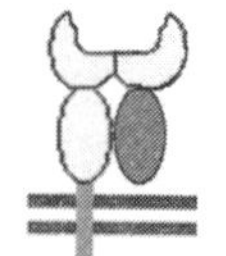

MHC class I molecules

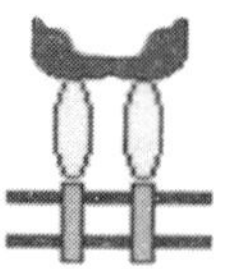

MHC class II molecules

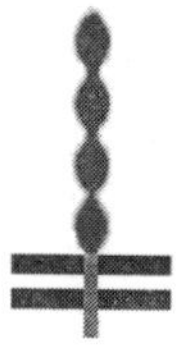

CD4

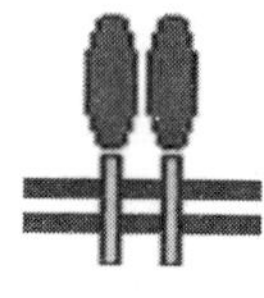

CD8

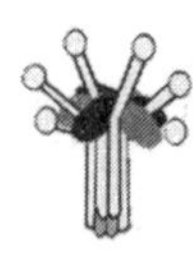

C1qrs

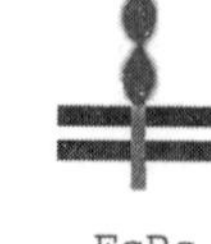

FcRs

Foreword

When Dr Pathak, then still Ms Pathak, was a doctoral student in my lab in the 1980s, we would often hear her talk of Immunology textbooks — of the need to make these books relevant to the students' lives and the need for such quality books to be made easily available to the average students. When the first edition of Immunology: Essential and Fundamental *was published in 1997, I knew the book to be the culmination of this dream.*

In this second edition, Dr Pathak, with her international research exposure, and Ms Palan, with her extensive experience of teaching, collaborate once again to bring to students the latest in the field of Immunology in a format that is comprehensible and non-intimidating. This book views Immunology in the context of everyday human life. It challenges scientific imagination by bringing the interested reader sidetracks, digressions as they may seem, that add a different dimension to the subject being discussed. Immunology: Essential and Fundamental *constantly reminds the reader that the subject that it gets its name from, although being an extensively specialized field, must be viewed in the context of the human body, the individual, and the society s/he inhabits. It helps us appreciate that Immunology goes beyond being a compartmentalized and specialized field and enriches our understanding of the big picture.*

It is with pleasure that I welcome the reader to this book — not only a textbook, but a map for the individual's discovery and exploration of the body's system of defense, its organization, and its functioning.

Prof. Rob Benner
Head, Department of Immunology
Erasmus MC
University Medical Center, Rotterdam
The Netherlands

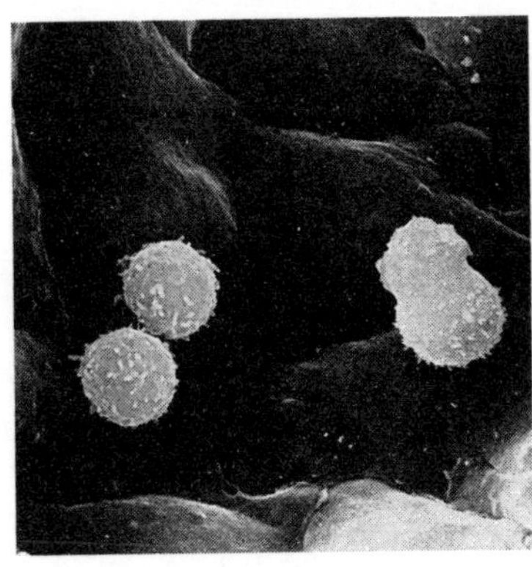

Preface to the Second Edition

It is with great pleasure that we release the second edition of this book. This version, almost completely rewritten, reflects the developments that Immunology as a subject and we as authors have undergone in the years since the publication of the first edition. Although retaining popular features such as section summaries, the book's layout, illustrations, and contents have been considerably altered, and the subject matter has been restructured for easy comprehension. Sidebars (called sidetracks) of extra information presenting real-life applications, clinical use, or research implications have been added to the chapters to spark students' interests and imaginations. Logos that epitomize the essence of each chapter and metaphors that link the subject matter to popular culture have been worked into the chapters to aid retention. This edition also features an expanded, extensive glossary and the liberal use of footnotes to facilitate learning. Immunological acronyms have increased almost exponentially in the past few years. Undoubtedly, these terms make reading immunology a daunting task for the uninitiated. In order to make reading easier for the learner, acronyms that occur in a chapter have been placed in the left margin at the beginning of that chapter for ready reference.

It is now well appreciated that components of the immune system (whether tissues, cells or their products, signalling molecules, or proteins like complement) may have roles other than in host defence. Conversely, factors that affect the well-being of the individual, whether physiological or psychological, are known to affect the immune system. These facts have been included in the appropriate chapters to encourage a more holistic approach to the subject.

The introductory chapter discusses the major players of the host immune system. The major events of an immune response are explained by following the fate of a pathogen that tries to gain entry into the body. The current hypotheses about what triggers an immune response and why have been included in the sidetrack. Thus, information is available to the interested without overwhelming those new to the field.

Great strides have been made in our understanding and appreciation of the innate component of the host defence in the last decade, and consequently, chapters dealing with this subject have been expanded upon in this edition. Some sidetracks touch upon how life-style choices affect components of the immune system. The structures of the antigen-receptors, antigen-activated signalling pathways, and proteins involved in these pathways have been described in a separate chapter. We hope that this will give students an appreciation of the commonality in design.

The essentials of the pathways have been summarized in bullet points, and details appear as sub-bullets. A similar layout has been adapted for the chapter dealing with genetic mechanisms that are responsible for the observed diversity of the immune response. We believe this layout aids easier assimilation. A chapter dealing with cancer and how the immune system deals with it has been added in this edition. The section describing newer approaches to cancer immunotherapy should help ignite student's imagination.

A careful reading of this book ought to prepare the student to understand immunological research papers. Various techniques used in research and diagnosis have been compiled into Appendix III, and this appendix should serve as a ready reference.

We are grateful to many people who have contributed directly and indirectly to bringing this project to fruition. First and foremost, we thank Dr. Rob Benner, Erasmus MC, University Medical Centre, Rotterdam, the Netherlands for his foreword. For the wonderful scanning electron micrographs, we are grateful to Dr. Willem van Ewijk, Leiden University, the Netherlands. Thanks are also due to Dr. Neill Harris for kind permission to use his unusual depiction of B cell development. For their critical reading of the manuscript, we thank Dr. Claire Dunn and Dr Scott Cameron — Scott's medical background made his feedback all the more relevant to us non-medicos. We must also thank Sulabha's daughter, Gauri, whose diligence and enthusiasm in editing the language were infectious. It was her almost encyclopaedic knowledge of modern music that helped identify the lyrics quoted before each chapter. Thanks to Abhishek Chakraborty, we have managed to improve upon the illustrations in this edition. We deeply appreciate technical support from the members of 'The Source,' particularly Ms. Smita Rao, and the Microbiology Department of R Ruia College, Mumbai. We would also like to mention the direct and indirect contributions of our many students who enthusiastically supported the idea of a new edition. And ultimately, we must also acknowledge our family and friends. Endeavours such as this tend to become obsessions that can be difficult to live with. Without the support and understanding of our spouses and extended families, this project would have been impossible to complete.

S. Pathak, PhD
U. Palan, MPhil

December, 2004

Contents

Introduction

We shall defend our Island, whatever the cost may be, we shall fight on the beaches, we shall fight on the landing grounds, we shall fight in the fields and in the streets, we shall fight in the hills; we shall never surrender.

— Winston Churchill, 1940

1.1 Introduction

A multicellular organism, with its warmth, moisture, and easy supply of nutrition, is an attractive target for pathogens and parasites. With the evolution of multi-cellularity, there has therefore been a parallel evolution in a system of defence. The ability to defend against infectious agents is 'immunity'. 'Immunology' is the study of all aspects of host defence (including its adverse consequences). The terms 'immune response' or 'immune reactions' refer to the production of cells and soluble factors that defend the body against potentially dangerous biological and chemical agents, which in turn are referred to as 'immunogens' or 'antigens'.

Immunology, like most other sciences, has its own lexicon (jargon, if you will). This terminology has developed to convey scientific principles and definitions in their proper context. Although essential to the study of immunology, these terms can be discouraging to a new learner. Trying to figure out where to start studying (and understanding) immunology is a bit like trying to figure out the age-old chicken or egg dilemma. To understand immunology, you need to know the terminology, and to understand the terminology, you need some basic knowledge of immunology. In this introductory chapter, we have attempted to introduce some terms and immunological concepts simplistically — necessitating over-simplification. This over-simplification will be rectified in later chapters.

An immune response is the result of a perceived threat to an animal's well-being[1]. The immune system has a two-pronged strategy to defend the human body 'fortress'. A similar strategy is used in homes of the rich and famous. In the medieval ages, a peripheral area stocked with predators discouraged intruders; now a walled fence and watchdogs serve the same purpose. Armed guards — often issued with photographs of known criminals or stalkers — are deployed around the house to take care of any unlawful entrants.

1.2 The First Line of Defence

The innate immune system is the body's watchdog and is discussed in chapters 2 and 3. What the immune system considers a potential threat is outlined in chapter 4 (see sidetrack 'Us and Them'). The innate immune system consists of multiple layers of security measures. First are the physical and chemical barriers designed to keep out intruders. Second are the antimicrobial substances (present in the blood and body secretions) that try to eliminate, before they gain a foothold in the body, any pathogens that may breach the barriers (fig. 1.1). Chief amongst these is a family of proteins called complement, described in chapter 3. Complement gets activated (amongst other things) by the outer coat of the intruder and can result in lysis of the intruding cell. Even as the pathogen tries to escape the chemical attack, other innate immune mechanisms swing into action. Chemical signals released as a result of the pathogen's metabolic activities and/or tissue trauma cause an influx of fluids and leukocytes to the site. Some of these leukocytes are scavenger cells that normally phagocytose (internalize and degrade) the dead and dying cells of the body. When the phagocytic cells sense intruders, they get activated and phagocytose the aggressor as well. Activated phagocytes also liberate a large number of enzymes and chemicals that are capable of killing the pathogen. Other cells, such as natural killer cells, are lymphocytes, belonging to the innate immune system, that contain cytotoxic granules filled with poisons. They get activated by chemical signals released by phagocytes. The natural killer cells can recognize infected body cells. These infected cells are like spies working for the enemy, and they must be eliminated. Activated natural killer cells release the cytotoxins directly at the infected cells, thereby killing them and the pathogen inside them. Thus, the innate defence mechanisms collectively try to overwhelm and kill the pathogen.

[1] This is a classic example of circular logic in immunology. An immunogen is defined as that which elicits an immune response in a healthy individual, whereas an immune response is the result of introduction of the immunogen. The immune system responds to immunogenic challenge by the production of cells and soluble proteins capable of specifically recognizing and reacting with the immunogen.

1.3 Specific Defence

In case these measures fail and the pathogen establishes a focus of infection, the adaptive immune system is recruited to the battle by cells of the innate immune system. This arm of immunity is also called 'specific immunity', since it seems to track specific threats and responds to repeated assaults with greater ferocity, ie, it appears to have a memory of past encounters. Chapters 5 through 12 describe aspects of the adaptive immune system.

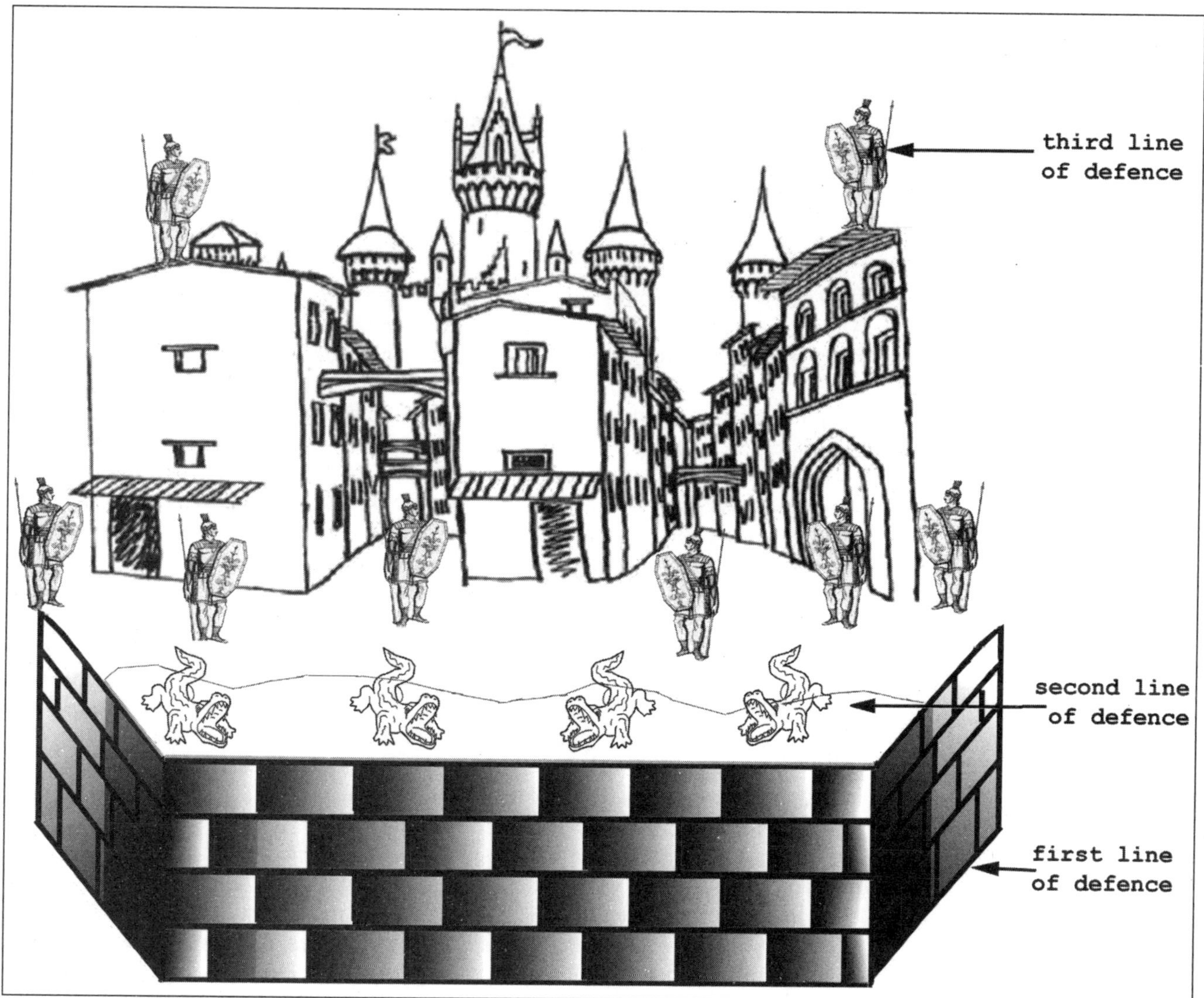

Figure 1.1 The human body is a well defended fortress with different components having designated defensive functions. The physical and chemical barriers consisting of intact skin, moist mucous membranes, complement, and antimicrobial substances in the blood and secretions act as the first line of defence. Together, they act as a bulwark against the entry and establishment of pathogens. In case this outer wall is breached, the phagocytic cells and cytotoxic cells, called NK cells, form the second line of defence. The phagocytes rapidly engulf and ingest any pathogens that have entered the fortress, while NK cells release cytotoxins that cause the death of the intruder. Lymphocytes of the adaptive immunity are the third line of defence. They specifically recognize and destroy intruders. This specific defence is a two-pronged strategy consisting of free-roaming antibodies and cells that defeat the microbe in one-on-one combat.

1.3.1 Organization of the Adaptive Immune System

The tissues and cells of the adaptive immune system are collectively called the lymphoid system. This system consists of organs such as the thymus, bone marrow, spleen, and lymph nodes, as well as loose patches of tissues distributed throughout the body. The lymphoid system is described in chapter 5. The adaptive immune system, like any defensive organization, has a hierarchical structure. At the helm of this hierarchy are the thymus and bone marrow. They are involved in producing lymphocytes — the immune system's armed guards — and the effectors and executors of adaptive immunity. The local branches of the adaptive immune system — the lymph nodes — are distributed throughout the body; the spleen could be regarded as the regional military headquarters that deals with all blood-borne threats. The thymus and bone marrow are also training camps for the lymphocytes. Those that get trained in the bone marrow are called the B lymphocytes, while those that get trained in the thymus are the T lymphocytes. During the training process, lymphocytes get equipped with images that help them to recognize criminals and become licensed to kill, maim, or otherwise damage anything that dares to enter the fortress without permission. The lymphocytes are thus equipped with the wherewithal necessary to respond to immunogenic challenges (described in chapter 8).

1.3.2 The Recognition Molecules

Cells of the adaptive immune system are equipped with special recognition molecules. Any recognition system implies two parts — an identity tag and a detector for that tag. All body cells sport the identity tags and cells of the adaptive immune system, ie, the lymphocytes, are equipped with detectors. These detectors allow the lymphocytes to recognize intruders that do not display the correct identity tags. The two classes of lymphocytes differ in their detectors. T and B cells' detectors (called antigen receptors) are described in chapter 6. Genetic mechanisms of their development are explained in chapter 10. We like to think of the lymphocyte, with its antigen receptor, as Cinderella's prince with his glass shoe. The lymphocyte tries to find cells with the appropriate fit. In this search, receptors on the lymphocytes briefly engage with a prospective counterpart. If there is a fit, cells enter a prolonged relationship. There is an exchange of chemical messages, resulting in lymphocyte activation. If the fit is not good enough, the lymphocyte moves on.

B lymphocytes have receptors that directly recognize and bind antigens, ie, intruders or their metabolic products. Thus, B cell antigen recognition is similar to a soldier recognizing invaders by the colour of their uniforms. Antigen detection by T cells is more complicated than that by B cells. T cell detectors cannot recognize antigens by themselves; the antigens have to be loaded on special molecules called MHC molecules. Thus, in contrast to B cells, T cells recognize invaders based on the badges they wear or the flags they carry. The MHC molecules are the identity tags and are described in chapter 7. Cells that do not express MHC molecules or those that express a different MHC molecule are immediately attacked by the immune system. MHC molecules can be thought of as flagpoles. Depending upon the fabric available in the cell, different flags are mounted upon them. Self-cells load fragments derived from self-proteins, thereby declaring to the T cells that they are part of the system, and escaping immune attack. In contrast, infected cells load fragments of proteins derived from the infecting pathogen, and recognition of such MHC:peptide complexes by T cell detectors triggers an immune response. MHC molecules come in two different varieties. MHC class I molecules are present on all nucleated cells of the body and help announce them as cells belonging to the body, ie, self-cells. MHC class II molecules have a more restricted distribution — they are usually expressed by cells of the immune system, and other cells start expressing them only when the system senses danger. Two types of T cells have been recognized on the basis of the MHC molecules they interact with. Those recognizing antigen loaded on MHC class I molecules express CD8 molecules and are called CD8$^+$ T lymphocytes. These are killer T cells (called cytotoxic T lymphocytes) that kill target cells by releasing toxins. T cells that recognize antigen loaded on MHC class II molecules express the CD4 molecule, ie, they are CD4$^+$ T cells. These cells help B cells, phagocytic cells, and CD8$^+$ T cells mount an immune response. Consequently, CD4$^+$ T cells are usually referred to as 'T helper cells'. CD4$^+$ T cells are also involved in regulating immune responses and ensuring that they are not deleterious to the individual. T lymphocytes are thus multifunctional cells involved in assisting B cells, regulating immune responses, and killing infected self-cells.

1.3.3 The Weaponry

The immune system's destructive weaponry is described in chapters 9 and 11. Using these weapons, an adaptive immune response can damage unwelcome guests. The first arsenal in its repertoire is the production of antibodies (or immunoglobulins) that can specifically bind and neutralize the pathogen (eg, virus or bacteria) or its products. Immunoglobulins are comparable to free-roaming pre-programmed guided missiles that can combine with and destroy specific targets. Five classes of immunoglobulins are recognized in humans, based on their structure and function. Binding of some classes of antibodies to a pathogen can activate complement, and result in the lysis of the target cell. Alternatively, the antibodies can prevent the binding of the pathogen to self-cells. Since viruses have to bind to host cells before infection can occur, the coating of viral particles with antibodies can prevent further infection of host cells. Immunoglobulins are also important in neutralizing toxins and enzymes of the pathogen; they combine with the active site of the toxin or enzyme, thereby interfering with its activity. Additionally, antibody-coated target cells are more easily phagocytosed by phagocytic cells, helping in their removal and destruction.

If the pathogen is inside an infected cell immunoglobulins cannot reach it, and the best way to eliminate the pathogen is to kill the infected cell. Hence, activation of the immune system also results in the formation of CD8$^+$ cytotoxic T lymphocytes that can specifically recognize and kill infected cells. These cells have toxin-filled granules that can cause lysis of target cells. Toxins liberated by cytotoxic T lymphocytes cause the formation of pores in the target cell's plasma membrane, resulting in its death. This is not the only way that the cytotoxic T cell kills the target cell. It can also induce target cell death by inducing it to commit suicide.

1.4 The Immune Response

The players and the principles of the immune system are most easily understood by following the fate of an intruder that tries to gain entry into the body. When a pathogen falls on intact skin, it will be unable to cross this barrier and will eventually be shed along with an outer layer of skin cells. A pathogen trying to gain entry via the respiratory system will likely suffer the same fate — reflexes such as coughing or sneezing will throw the pathogen out. If, on the other hand, these barriers have already been breached (eg, due to a cut or wound), the pathogen may enter. Once inside, the pathogen will try its best to settle into its niche and proliferate, ie, establish a focus of infection. This will be made difficult by a plethora of antimicrobial substances in the blood and tissue fluids that the pathogen will encounter. The phagocytic cells get activated by the chemical signals released by the pathogen and the damaged tissue cells. Activated phagocytic cells are potent killing machines. They also activate the natural killer cells. Together, these cells try to kill the pathogen as well as infected tissue cells in an attempt to prevent the spread of the pathogen. Meanwhile, the immune system cannot wait idly for the conclusion of the pathogen-innate immune system tussle, lest it lose. Hence, the adaptive arm of the immune system is recruited by some innate immune system cells that also act as messengers for the adaptive immune system. These messenger cells are called antigen-presenting cells. Prominent amongst these are the dendritic cells distributed throughout the body.

Dendritic cells and phagocytic cells capture the pathogen or its products and carry it to the nearest local branch of the adaptive immune system, the lymph node. *En route*, they digest the pathogen and load peptide fragments derived from the pathogen onto MHC molecules and display them on their cell surfaces. The actual recognition of the MHC:peptide complex by T cells occurs in the lymph node. T cell recognition of the intruding pathogen-derived protein fragments loaded on MHC class I and class II molecules is the first in a chain of events that results in specific action against the pathogen.

As mentioned before, the immune system uses a multi-pronged approach to neutralize invaders — a humoral response that consists of specific proteinic missiles that bind target cells and a cytotoxic cell-mediated response that kills infected cells.

- ❑ **Humoral immune response.** Lymphocytes that have never seen their antigens are called naïve or virgin cells. Recognition of MHC class II:peptide complexes by naïve $CD4^+$ T cells activates them. The activated T cells start proliferating immediately and slowly metamorphose into T cells capable of helping other lymphocytes in fighting the intruder (ie, they become 'T helper cells'). B cells also join this developing response. Unlike T cells, B cells need not wait for messenger cells to deliver news of an intrusion. Their receptors directly recognize strange molecules (or antigens). Thus, not only the pathogen, but also enzymes, toxins, etc, produced by the pathogen are recognized by B cells. They get stimulated by an encounter with the antigen, but mere recognition of the pathogen (or its product) is often not sufficient to activate them. They need signals from activated T helper cells and start proliferating only after receiving appropriate T cell help. The proliferating B cells eventually differentiate and give rise to two types of cells — memory cells and plasma cells.
  - **Memory cells** are long-lived cells essentially similar to the mother cell, ie, they are capable of proliferating and differentiating in response to that particular antigen. Their major feature is that they are more sensitive to their specific antigen, and their response is much more rapid.
  - **Plasma cells**, in contrast, are virtual weapon factories. They produce and secrete large amounts of immunoglobulins. These antibodies find their way into tissue fluids and the blood. Since these immunity-conferring molecules are found in the blood, tissue fluids, and secretions, this form of immunity is called humoral immunity.

- ❑ **Cell-mediated immune response.** Cytotoxic $CD8^+$ T cell receptors can recognize pathogen-derived peptides loaded on MHC class I molecules expressed on the surface of messenger cells. Recognition of class I MHC:peptide complexes is the first step in $CD8^+$ T lymphocyte activation. Just like B cells, recognition alone is not enough to activate $CD8^+$ T cells. They too require T helper cell signals to get activated[2]. Once activated, cytotoxic T lymphocytes also proliferate and differentiate; they produce daughter cells similar to the mother cell (memory cells) and effector cells capable of killing their targets. These effector cells have cytotoxins-filled granules. They recognize infected cells because of the expression of MHC class I molecules loaded with pathogen-derived peptides. Once their receptor is engaged by the appropriate MHC class I:peptide complex, cytotoxic T cells direct their cytotoxic cargo at the infected cell, causing its lysis.

[2] This two-signal system is similar to having two separate keys, with two different persons, that need to be operated together to unlock a bank vault. It is a common feature of immunology and is thought to be a mechanism that attempts to avert accidental activation of the immune system.

Thus, the immunoglobulin molecules and cytotoxic T lymphocytes (ably assisted by T helper cells) cause the death of the pathogen. The tissue debris resulting from all this activity is mopped up by phagocytic cells, and the body is then free to repair wounds caused by the infection and the battle that followed. Some daughter T helper cells, B cells, and cytotoxic T lymphocytes survive. Since they have already encountered antigen, they are no longer 'naïve'. Additionally, since these cells have undergone proliferation in the course of the immune response, their numbers are higher. Moreover, in the course of this antigen-induced proliferation, their genetic make-up and antigen receptors change subtly. Hence, if they encounter a similar pathogen again, their response is much faster, and is called a 'memory response'. The progeny of activated lymphocytes are therefore called memory cells.

1.5 Controls and Failures

Considering that our environment is full of chemical and biological agents that can harm us, one can't help but marvel at the number of battles that are being fought daily in the human body. It is obvious that the immune system, armed with potent instruments capable of causing death and destruction, has to be well regulated. Therefore, the immune system has evolved mechanisms that allow it to discriminate between intruders and its own cells (self-cells). They allow the immune system to concentrate its destructive powers on the former while being tolerant of the latter. The mechanisms of immune tolerance are discussed in chapter 12. Application of these principles in organ and tissue transplantation is discussed in chapter 13. The last four chapters discuss failures of the defence mechanisms. When the immune system starts attacking self-cells, it results in a spectrum of disorders called 'autoimmune diseases'. The mechanisms and possible causes of autoimmune disorders are discussed in chapter 14. The immune system may become hypersensitive and start reacting to innocuous substances in the environment. Chapter 15 describes such hypersensitive disorders and their effects. The last two chapters (16 and 17) are devoted to cancer and AIDS — scourges directly linked to the failure of the defensive functions of the immune system.

This book attempts to introduce the fundamental principles and all aspects of immunology. Some of the latest concepts and ideas in the field essential to the understanding of the subject are also included. A careful reading of this book will introduce students to the world of immunology and also familiarize them with the terms and concepts necessary to refer to current research papers on the subject.

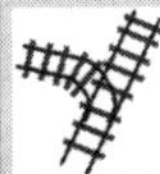

Us and Them

The immune system has a difficult mandate. It must destroy pathogens and infected cells, but at the same time, it must spare healthy self-cells. *Per definition* then, the immune system must have discriminatory powers, ie, it must distinguish self from non-self. A model was needed to explain how the immune system decides when, how, and by what means to respond. Until recently, an explanatory theory based on Burnet's clonal deletion hypothesis was generally accepted. This self-non-self theory of immune recognition postulates that the immune system defines 'self' as that which is present early in life; anything that comes later is deemed 'non-self'. The immune system is trained to tolerate the self while identifying and attacking the non-self. The theory proposes that lymphocytes capable of responding to self-antigens are deleted in the primary lymphoid organs (ie, the thymus and the bone marrow) during the process of lymphocyte maturation. There is ample experimental evidence to show that such deletional mechanisms are indeed active in both the thymus and the bone marrow. Since B cells require T cell help to respond to most antigens, the thymus is thought to be more important in the deletional process. Thus, according to this theory, the body is populated with mature lymphocytes that only react to foreign antigens. Self-cells are spared by the immune system since the surviving lymphocytes are incapable of reacting to antigens expressed on self-cells. Although a simple and elegant model, this theory takes a very simplistic view of immunology. The basic assumption of the self-non-self theory is that the thymus has a sampling of all the antigens expressed in the body. Yet, it is well established that many new proteins are expressed during puberty and maturation. The theory fails to explain how self-reactive cells to these proteins can be eliminated during early development. It also fails to explain the observed presence of autoreactive antibodies and cells in healthy adult mice and humans that fail to cause autoimmune diseases. There is also no explanation for the foetus not being rejected by its mother or the lack of her immune response to her lactating breasts or her milk.

The last decade has seen the emergence of two theories that help explain what the immune system considers dangerous and why. The first is the INS (for **I**nfectious **N**on-**S**elf) theory of the late Charles Janeway, the second, the danger hypothesis of Paula Matzinger. Both rely on the foundation of the self-non-self theory; they accept the need and use of deletional mechanisms that eliminate most self-reactive cells. Both these theories differ from the self-non-self theory in that they shift the emphasis on self-non-self discrimination away from the adaptive immune system. The INS theory lays a greater emphasis on the role of the innate immune system in initiating an immune response. It proposes that the innate immune systems of vertebrate animals recognize pathogens (the infectious non-self) by virtue of the host's ability to recognize conserved products of microbial metabolism that are unique to the microbe (and not expressed by host cells). Thus, the recognition strategy is based on invariant structures unique to and produced by all micro-organisms. It suggests that recognition of these pathogen-associated molecular patterns allows the innate immune system to discriminate between the infectious non-self and the non-infectious self. In the absence of pathogens, antigen-presenting cells remain quiescent (not activated), and fail to activate T cells even if the MHC:peptide complexes they display are recognized by T cells. The recognition of pathogen-associated molecular patterns activates antigen-presenting cells. Such activated cells can efficiently stimulate T cells and trigger an immune response. The discovery of a number of receptors that recognize pathogen-associated molecular patterns (chapter 2) has helped strengthen the INS hypothesis.

The Danger Hypothesis suggests that the immune system is more concerned with damage than with foreignness and is called into action by alarm signals from injured tissues rather than by recognition of non-self molecules. It postulates that antigen-presenting cells are activated by danger/alarm signals from injured cells exposed to pathogens, toxins, mechanical injury, etc. Antigen presentation by such activated cells results in an immune response, while antigen presentation in the absence of danger signals results in tolerance. The discovery of endogenous non-foreign alarm signals such as mammalian double stranded DNA, heat shock proteins, and interferon-α has lent support to the Danger Model. The Danger Model shifts the focus of triggering the immune response away from the immune system (whether adaptive or innate) altogether. Instead, it seems to believe in tissue power. It assumes that when healthy, tissues induce tolerance; when distressed, they trigger an immune response. Thus, the last decade has witnessed a shift of emphasis regarding when to respond and how much to respond away from the adaptive immune system. Whether it is the innate immune system or a cross-talk between tissues and cells of the immune system that triggers the immune response is still under debate.

Innate or Non-adaptive Immunity

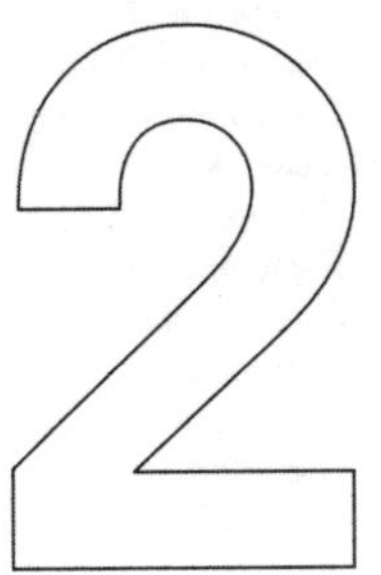

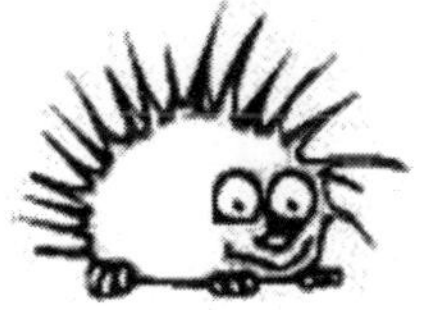

In order to protect its vulnerable northeastern border, the French government began construction of the 'Great Wall of France' in 1929. The Maginot Line was a state-of-the-art network of hardened fortifications, heavy gun emplacements, underground transportation networks, and soldiers' quarters designed to utterly smash any conceivable German invasion. It was built to give the French army enough time to mobilize and deploy troops.

— Adam Hamilton

ADCC:	Antibody-dependent cell-mediated cytotoxicity
ANCA:	Anti-neutrophil cytoplasmic antibodies
APCs:	Antigen-presenting cells
BPP:	Bacterial permeability-increasing protein
CNS:	Central nervous system
CR3 & 4:	Complement receptors 3&4
DCs:	Dendritic cells
ECF-A:	Eosinophil chemotactic factor-A
ECP:	Eosinophil cationic protein
EDN:	Eosinophil-derived neurotoxin
EPO:	Eosinophil peroxidase
FcRs:	Fc receptors
G-CSF:	Granulocyte-colony stimulating factor
GM-CSF:	Granulocyte macrophage-colony stimulating factor
HPA:	Hypothalamus-pituitary adrenal
ICAM:	Intracellular adhesion molecule
IFN:	Interferon
Ig:	Immunoglobulin
IL:	Interleukin
ITIMs:	Immunoreceptor tyrosine-based inhibitory motifs
ITAMs:	Immunoreceptor tyrosine-based activating motifs
KIR:	Killer cell Ig-like receptor
LAK:	Lymphokine-activated killer

2.1 Introduction

Immunity, simplistically defined, is the recognition and elimination of infectious organisms. Two systems have been evolved to achieve this goal — the innate and the adaptive. Innate immunity, also referred to as non-specific[1] or non-adaptive immunity, is developmentally the older of the two. An animal's first exposure to an invader results in a complex and interrelated series of events which, only after four to seven days, culminates in an effective specific response. During this time, protection is primarily limited to the largely non-adaptive component of immunity. It is the first and immediate response to an infectious challenge. In the past, the innate immune system was naïvely assumed to be simple, like a coat of armour that helped hold pathogens at bay. We should have known better... evolution has ensured that *nothing* in human biology is simple! Innate immunity is now known to be involved in the triggering and regulation of adaptive immunity besides being the first and second line of defence. It is thus critical to the well-being of the individual. Physical and emotional stress, chronic diseases, old age, malnutrition, etc. can affect the innate immune system, predisposing a person to ill health (see sidetrack 'Staying Fighting Fit'). To summarize, innate immunity

❑ is the most primitive form of defence, present in almost all vertebrates
❑ is specific
❑ consists of molecules and cells that recognize specific conserved constituents on micro-organisms, ie, it is directed against any potential threat to the body
❑ the receptors involved in threat recognition are germ-line encoded; their specificity is genetically determined; unlike the antigen receptors of adaptive immunity, these receptors are not clonally distributed; identical receptors are present on all clones of a given cell type
❑ can be mobilized within hours of contact with a potential pathogen
❑ does not bestow lasting protection, and the degree of resistance conferred remains unchanged even after repeated challenges by the same agent

2.2 The Main Players

Innate immunity is the combined effect of a number of factors which can be divided into two main groups — the physiological and chemical barriers that prevent entry and establishment of pathogens and cells that are actively involved in pathogen elimination. The two are, of course, intimately linked.

2.2.1 Physiological and Chemical Barriers

These are the relatively passive players of innate immunity.

❑ **Epithelial surfaces[2].** A large part of the body surface is in constant contact with the outside environment and is covered by the epithelium. Intact healthy skin, consisting of an outer layer of keratinized dead cells covering the epidermis, is virtually impenetrable to most organisms. The repeated shedding of cells also helps dislodge organisms from the body surface. Mucous membranes present in areas not covered by skin have a damp, wet surface that acts as an efficient trapping agent. Ciliated cells present at some sites (eg, in the respiratory tract) help sweep away any foreign particles that may gain entry. Apart from acting as a physical barrier, epithelial cells lining the skin, gastrointestinal tract, and bronchi express antimicrobial peptides. These peptides prevent pathogens from adhering to epithelial surfaces. Peptides with a significant role in innate defence include the following.
  • **Defensins and cathelicidins** are widely distributed antimicrobial peptides conserved throughout phylogeny. They are expressed either constitutively or

[1] Given the fact that the recognition systems involved are actually very specific to certain pathogens, it is time we dropped the 'non-specific' designation!

[2] The epithelium is a diverse group of tissues that covers or lines nearly all body surfaces, cavities, and tubes. It functions as an interface between different biological compartments. The epithelium is separated from the underlying supporting tissue by a basement membrane consisting of myriad glycoproteins. Epithelial layers provide physical protection and containment. They are also involved in organ-specific transport. Often, one surface of the epithelial cell (called the apical surface) comes in contact with a non-sterile environment. Hence, these cells have special junctions called tight junctions that join them and do not allow movement of fluids across the cells. Various epithelia are classified according to the arrangement and shapes of cells present. The endothelium, in contrast, is the inner layer of capillaries, blood vessels, etc and is an essentially sterile environment.

can be induced by the action of pro-inflammatory cytokines[3]. Two major families are recognized in humans — cathelicidins and defensins (the murine counterpart of defensins is cryptidins). Apart from their antimicrobial action, both defensins and cathelicidins have been shown to possess chemotactic properties for various phagocytic leukocytes, immature **Dendritic Cells (DCs)**, and lymphocytes. They seem to have a role in alerting, mobilizing, and amplifying innate and adaptive antimicrobial immunity.

- **Dermicidin** is a protein specifically and constitutively expressed in sweat glands. It is secreted into the sweat and transported to the epidermal surface, where it undergoes proteolysis to generate a broad spectrum antimicrobial peptide. This peptide remains active over a broad pH range and in high salt concentrations, and it may help limit infection by potential pathogens.
- **Melanin** is the pigment responsible for skin colour and protects against damage caused by exposure to UV rays, found in sunlight. Recent research shows that melanin is also a potent antibacterial and antifungal agent[4].

❑ **Adverse conditions in the digestive tract.** The digestive tract is constantly exposed to a wide variety of micro-organisms; therefore, a number of protective factors operate here. The pH of the stomach (pH 1–2) helps eliminate a large fraction of organisms entering the digestive tract. A reversal of pH (acid to alkaline) due to the presence of bile in the gut helps eliminate many of the acidophilic organisms that survive the stomach. The surfactant property of bile also aids in microbial destruction.

❑ **Normal flora.** All exposed surfaces of the body are colonized by microbes, and the body has learned to live in semi-peaceful co-existence with them. To protect its ecological niche, normal flora produces many antimicrobial factors such as colicin (gastrointestinal tract), long chain fatty acids (skin), and acidity (vagina). Normal flora thus unintentionally helps in the defence of the body. Moreover, because of the sheer unavailability of space, potential pathogens are prevented from colonizing areas occupied by the normal flora, whom they must compete with for nutrients.

❑ **Microbicidal factors in tissues and in blood** try to eliminate any microbes that may have breached the physical barriers.

- A variety of **basic proteins** (spermine, spermidine, histones, protamine, etc) derived from damaged tissue cells and blood cells are bactericidal.
- **Lysozyme** present in secretions of the nose, tissues, tears, etc is effective against Gram-negative organisms.
- **Lactoferrin**, an ubiquitous and abundant constituent of human external secretions, chelates iron, making it unavailable to bacteria.
- **Haeme compounds** such as haematein and mes-haematein derived from erythrocytes are inhibitory to a variety of Gram-positive bacteria.
- **Complement** consists of a complex group of heat labile proteins found in the blood. It is important in inflammation, opsonization[5], activation of macrophages, etc. Complement components aid phagocytosis by immobilizing the organism on the macrophage surface and activating the process of ingestion and degradation of the internalized organism (chapter 3). The opsonic activity is especially important in clearing pathogens from the blood stream. Activation of complement also starts a cascade of events involving many components of this group of proteins, and it ultimately leads to lysis of target cells. This activation can occur by three different pathways — classical, lectin-binding, and alternative pathways. Two components of the cascade — C3a and C5a — are chemotactic and help recruit phagocytes to the site of invasion. Complement deficiency can lead to increased susceptibility to infections by Gram-negative organisms as well as to autoimmune[6] diseases.
- **Properdin**, a γ globulin that can activate complement, is found to exert haemolytic, bactericidal, and virucidal action (section 3.4).

LBP:	Lipopolysaccharide-binding protein
LDL:	Low density lipids
LFA:	Leukocyte function associated antigen
LPS:	Lipopolysaccharide
LT:	Lymphotoxin
MBL:	Mannose binding lectin
MBP:	Major basic protein
MCP:	Macrophage chemotactic protein
M-CSF:	Macrophage colony stimulating factor
MIP:	Macrophage inhibitory protein
MPO:	Myeloperoxidase
NCR:	Natural cytotoxicity receptor
NK:	Natural killer
NO:	Nitric oxide
NOS:	NO synthases
PAF:	Platelet activating factor
PAMPs:	Pathogen-associated molecular patterns
PDGF:	Platelet-derived growth factor
PECAM-1:	Platelet endothelial cell adhesion molecule-1
PG:	Prostaglandins
PMNs:	Polymorphonuclear leukocytes
PRRs:	Pattern recognition receptors
PUFA:	Polyunsaturated fatty acids
RNI:	Reactive nitrogen intermediates
ROI:	Reactive oxygen intermediates
SERPIN:	Serine protease inhibitor
SP-A and SP-D:	Surfactant proteins A and D
SRS-A:	Slow-reacting substance of anaphylaxis
TLRs:	Toll-like receptors
TNF:	Tumour necrosis factor
VIP:	Vasointestinal peptide

[3] Cytokines are soluble glycoproteins produced by a variety of cells. They are multipotent (ie, have multiple effects) and play a major role in the initiation, regulation, and course of the immune response. Cytokines also affect a variety of other processes. Those that promote inflammation include Tumour Necrosis Factor-α (TNF-α) and interleukins like IL-1 and Interferon-γ (IFN-γ). Cytokines are discussed in chapter 8.

[4] Anti-perspirants and 'fairness creams' do not seem to be such good ideas after all!

[5] Certain proteins such as acute phase proteins, antibodies, and complement components can interact with and coat target cells. These proteins are called opsonins. Specific receptors on the cell surface of phagocytes recognize opsonins. The opsonin coated particle gets bound to the cell surface. Opsonins enhance engulfment and digestion of target particles by the phagocytes; the process is called opsonization.

[6] Autoimmune diseases are caused when the immune system attacks self-tissues and organs.

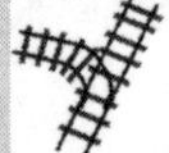

Staying Fighting Fit:
Nutrition, Exercise, Stress and Immunity

It makes intuitive sense that lifestyle choices directly influence immunity — both innate and adaptive. Recent studies now provide scientific evidence for this instinctive wisdom.

Diet and immunity have for centuries been considered intertwined by ancient medical traditions and popular wisdom. Systematic studies have now shown that nutrient deficiencies impair the immune response and can lead to frequent and severe infections, especially in children. Protein-energy malnutrition results in a reduction in numbers and functions of T cells and phagocytic cells. Secretory IgA response is also impaired. Additionally, levels of many complement components are reduced. Other nutritional factors — especially vitamins A, B_6, C, E, and trace elements such as Cu, Fe, Se, and Zn have been found to be important to optimal immune function. Their mode of action is, unfortunately, not well understood.

❏ **Vitamin A** deficiency impairs innate immunity by impeding the normal regeneration of mucosal barriers damaged by infection and by diminishing the function of neutrophils, macrophages, and NK cells. Vitamin A is also required for adaptive immunity and plays a role in the development of both **T H**elper (T_H) cells and B cells. In particular, vitamin A deficiency diminishes antibody-mediated responses directed by T_{H2} cells.

❏ **Vitamin D** is important in suppressing autoimmune disorders. It is thought to suppress inflammatory T cell activity by stimulating TGF-β and IL-4 production.

❏ **Vitamin E** is a potent anti-oxidant with the ability to modulate immune functions. Deficiency of this vitamin leads to a downward trend in most immune parameters. Vitamin E plays an important role in the differentiation of immature T cells in the thymus. Its deficiency leads to decreased differentiation of immature T cells, resulting in an early decrease of cellular immunity with aging in spontaneously hypertensive rats. In contrast, vitamin E supplementation has various beneficial effects on the host immune system. Decreased cellular immunity due to aging or during the development of AIDS is markedly improved by a diet high in vitamin E. Furthermore, in animals, vitamin E supplementation induces the early recovery of thymic atrophy following X-ray irradiation. These results suggest that vitamin E is important to effective maintenance of the immune system, especially, in the sick and aged.

❏ **Zn** deficiency is associated with profound impairment of cell-mediated immunity in terms of the number of $CD4^+$:$CD8^+$ T cells and decreased chemotaxis of phagocytes. In addition, thymic function is also affected, since the levels of Zn-dependent hormones such as thymulin are markedly decreased in Zn deficiency.

❏ **Cu** is also critical to the proper functioning of the innate and adaptive arms of the immune system. Recent research has shown that even marginal Cu deficiency is linked to IL-2 deficiency and is likely to be the cause of reduced T cell proliferation. The number of neutrophils in human peripheral blood also reduces in the case of severe Cu deficiency. Their ability to generate the superoxide anion and kill ingested micro-organisms is reduced in both overt and marginal Cu deficiency.

❏ **Arachidonic-acid-derived eicosanoids**[7] modulate the production of pro-inflammatory and immunoregulatory cytokines. Over-production of these cytokines is associated with septic shock and chronic inflammatory diseases such as arthritis and Multiple Sclerosis. The n-3 **P**oly**u**nsaturated **F**atty **A**cids (PUFAs), eicosapentaenoic acid, and docosahexaenoic acid, all found in fish oils, suppress production of arachidonic-acid-derived eicosanoids. Thus, dietary fats rich in n-3 PUFAs have the potential to alter cytokine production. Several human studies have shown that supplementing the diet of healthy volunteers with n-3 PUFAs results in reduced *ex vivo* production of IL-1, IL-6, TNF-α, and IL-2 by peripheral blood mononuclear cells. Animal studies indicate that dietary fish oil reduces response to endotoxins and pro-inflammatory cytokines, resulting in increased survival; such diets have been beneficial in some models of bacterial challenge, chronic inflammation, and autoimmunity.

Exercise. Experimental evidence has failed to support the intuition that exercise increases immunity. Generally speaking, moderate exercise seems to increase resistance to upper respiratory tract infections, irrespective of age. Most studies have reported that immune systems of athletes and non-athletes in the resting state are more or less similar, with the exception of NK cell activity,

---

[7] Eicosanoids derive their name from the Greek *eicosa*, meaning twenty. They are a class of lipid mediators having twenty carbon fatty acid derivatives with a wide variety of biological activities. Four main classes of eicosanoids are recognized — prostaglandins, prostacyclanes, thromboxanes, and leukotrienes.

which tends to be elevated in athletes. Repeated strenuous exercise, on the other hand, has been found to suppress immune function. After intense long-term exercise, the immune system is characterized by concomitant impairment of the cellular immune system and increased inflammation. Strenuous exercise seems to decrease both the number of circulating lymphocytes and their proliferation, and it suppresses innate immunity. The levels of secretory IgA in saliva are lowered simultaneously with high levels of circulating pro-inflammatory and anti-inflammatory cytokines. Conversely, exercise has been found to attenuate changes in the immune system related to aging, provided the exercise is long-term and of a sufficient volume to induce changes in body weight and fitness. Only such exercise can improve immunity, especially in the old.

Stress is known to affect immunity in different ways. It is established that there is bi-directional interaction between cytokines and neurotransmitters with cells of the central and peripheral nervous system and immune system respectively. There is continuous direct and indirect chemical communication between the neuroendocrine and immune systems. Although growth hormones are involved in the priming of phagocytic cells, glucocorticoids severely impair the phagocytic and cytotoxic activities of neutrophils and macrophages. Their capacity to produce ROI, induce NOS, and secrete lysosomal enzymes in response to activation is substantially reduced. The oxidative burst of phagocytes is also inhibited by both epinephrine and β-endorphins. Thus, stressed individuals are likely to have impaired innate immune responses and be more susceptible to infections.

Aging is associated with a generalized reduction in immunity and increased inflammatory activity which is reflected by increased levels of circulating levels of TNF-α, IL-6, cytokine antagonists, and acute phase proteins *in vivo*. Epidemiological studies suggest that chronic low-grade inflammation in aging promotes an atherogenic profile and is related to age-associated disorders (eg, Alzheimer's disease, atherosclerosis, and type 2 diabetes) and enhanced mortality risk. It is therefore suggested that dysregulated production of inflammatory cytokines is important to the aging process. *In vivo* infectious models show delayed termination of inflammatory activity and a prolonged fever response in elderly people, suggesting that the acute phase response is also altered in aging.

- **Interferons**[8] (IFN-α, IFN-β, and IFN-γ) are potent immunomodulatory cytokines that also act as links between adaptive and innate immunity. They are especially important in host defence against viral infections.
  - IFN-α and IFN-β, also called type I IFNs, are produced by leukocytes, fibroblasts, etc upon exposure to viruses. A type of DC, called plasmocytoid DC, is the major source of these IFNs. IFN-α, though called by a single name, is a family of closely related proteins; IFN-β is a single protein. The binding of these IFNs to receptors on infected cells induces the formation of a number of molecules that interfere with viral replication. Type I IFNs also activate **Natural Killer** (NK) cells. In certain viral infections they also potentiate the production of IFN-γ, itself a potent immune stimulator. Additionally, they induce MHC[9] class I expression on uninfected cells, making them resistant to the action of NK cells (section 2.2.2.2).
  - IFN-γ (type II IFN) is produced by T lymphocytes and NK cells. Recent reports suggest that it may also be produced by IL-12 activated macrophages and DCs, but this is still controversial. It enhances macrophage activity and triggers the maturation of DCs. DCs are crucial in triggering an adaptive response. IFN-γ also increases expression of MHC molecules by all types of cells and augments the activation of the adaptive immune response. Apart from its role in inflammation and the potentiation of NK cell activity, IFN-γ also plays a crucial role in the development and functioning of a subset of helper T cells called T$_{\mathrm{H1}}$ cells (section 8.3.5.1).
- **Other physiological non-specific defence mechanisms.** While often diagnosed and treated as deleterious reactions, diarrhoea, vomiting, and sneezing are all designed to dislodge micro-organisms and constitute a part of the innate defence mechanism. If uncontrolled, these physiological processes may prove harmful. IL-l, IL-6, **Tumour Necrosis Factor-α** (TNF-α), and lymphotoxin produced by damaged tissue cells, activated macrophages, lymphocytes, and brain cells affect the hypothalamus — the centre of temperature control — resulting in pyrexia

[8] These cytokines are called interferons because they interfere with the replication of viral RNA or DNA.

[9] MHC stands for **Major Histocompatibility Complex** proteins. They are crucial in triggering the adaptive immune response and are discussed in chapter 7.

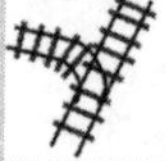

Iron Politics: Fe and Innate Immunity

In the febrile response, most bacteria have a decreased ability to synthesize their own Fe chelators (called siderophores) and are therefore in greater need of an iron source. Since iron is needed for the bacterial electron transport chain, its lack inhibits the growth of most bacteria. During infection, the body makes considerable metabolic adjustments to make iron unavailable to micro-organisms. Much of this is through the production of a defence chemical called leukocyte-endogenous mediator. Consequently, during infection, there is decreased intestinal absorption of iron. The amount of Fe in plasma declines with a concomitant increase in Fe storage in the form of ferritin. There is an increased synthesis of Fe chelators such as lactoferrin and transferrin which trap Fe for use by human cells while making it unavailable to most microbes. A further decrease in available Fe is affected by transporting lactoferrin to common sites of microbial invasion such as the mucous membranes. Recent evidence indicates that the chelating activity of lactoferrin causes a characteristic twitching in the underlying cells, dislodging bacteria and preventing them from forming biofilms at the environmental interface. In contrast, transferrin gains entry into tissues during inflammation, causing a local decline in iron concentrations. Some bacteria such as *Neisseria gonorrhoeae*, *Neisseria meningitidis*, and *Hemophilus influenzae*, however, have receptors for human lactoferrin and transferrin, and they can utilize iron bound to these compounds.

(fever). Increase in body temperature is also a defence mechanism, since many pathogens are sensitive to or grow poorly at higher temperatures[10]. Moreover, phagocytosis, enzyme activity, etc are also enhanced at elevated temperatures. Thus, fever can be a beneficial response provided, of course, that it does not rise above a certain limit (104°F, 40°C) and is of a short duration.

❑ **Pattern Recognition Receptors or molecules (PRRs).** Molecules present on the cell envelope of micro-organisms form a unique geometric pattern and are often referred to as PAMPs (**P**athogen-**A**ssociated **M**olecular **P**atterns). Such PAMPs that are indispensable to microbial survival, are unique to the microbes, are found on a large group of microbes, and become excellent targets for the host system. LPS (**Lipopolysaccharide** of Gram-negative bacteria) is one of the best examples of PAMP. Host molecules capable of recognizing and reacting with these molecular patterns (*leit motifs*) are termed **P**attern **R**ecognition **R**eceptors. Thus, the innate immune system seems to be designed to focus on a few highly conserved structures in a large group of potential pathogens rather than on recognizing individual organisms. In contrast to the antigen receptors of adaptive immunity (discussed in chapter 6), PRRs are expressed on effector and non-effector cells of innate immunity. Their expression, unlike immunoglobulins, is not clonal — each type of PRR expressed by a particular cell type has identical specificity. Moreover, their engagement by a molecular pattern on the pathogen triggers the effector cell to perform its function immediately, rather than after proliferation. The concentration of some of these receptors increases dramatically in the acute phase reaction (section 2.3.2). Three broad functional classes of PRRs are recognized: secreted, endocytic, and signalling (Table 2.1).

● **Secreted PRRs** function as opsonins; the binding of these molecules to microbial cell walls tags them for phagocytosis and results in their lysis by the complement cascade.

♦ **C-reactive protein**, so named because it was found to bind the C-protein (a phosphorylcholine moiety) of pneumococci, can recognize and bind to molecular groups found on the cell walls of a wide variety of bacteria and fungi (eg, phosphocholine residues present on bacterial cell membranes and lipoproteins, monophosphate esters, and histones). It can also activate the complement cascade. It is thought to be a prototype pattern recognition molecule. Historically, the presence of this protein in serum was recognized to be an indicator of pathological activity and is used as such even today.

[10] In 1927, Wagner-Jauregg was awarded the Nobel Prize for having discovered malariotherapy for curing neurosyphilis. It consisted of inoculating patients of neurosyphilis with Plasmodium vivax. The resultant high temperatures (caused by malaria) was thought to cause the death of the spirochete that caused syphilis. The patients were eventually treated with quinine to get rid of the malaria!

- **LBP.** LPS is the major outer surface membrane component of Gram-negative bacteria. It is an extremely strong stimulator of innate immunity in diverse species, ranging from insects to humans. **LPS Binding Protein** (LBP) is an acute phase protein with the ability to bind and transfer bacterial LPS. LBP binds LPS and then transfers the complex to cell surface CD14[11], a receptor on macrophages and B cells. Engagement of CD14 triggers the inflammatory response through the engagement of **Toll-Like Receptors** (TLRs), described later in this section. LBP is also postulated to be involved in alcohol-induced liver injury.
- **Mindin** is a secretory protein expressed in several tissues. It binds bacteria by sugar entities found in bacterial cell walls and leads to their agglutination and opsonization. Mindin seems to have two separate but essential functions in host defence — phagocytosis and promotion of pro-inflammatory cytokine production by macrophages. The specific sugar residues recognized by mindin are yet to be determined.
- **Collectins** are a group of PRRs structurally similar to the complement component C1q. They derive their name from the fact that they have a collagen domain connected to a lectin[12]-binding domain. They recognize distinct but overlapping carbohydrate ligands such as mannose, N-acetyl glucosamine, and L-fucose found on the microbial cell walls. They do not bind galactose and sialic acid, two carbohydrates commonly found on mammalian cell walls. The binding specificity of these proteins is due to the shape of their respective binding pockets that distinguish subtle alterations in topology. The collectins include the following.
  - **Mannose Binding Lectin or Protein** (MBL/MBP[13]) is a serum protein that selectively recognizes and binds to mannose or N-acetylglucosamine on pathogens. In humans, MBL can recognize Gram-negative enteric organisms, group B streptococci, and certain strains of the influenza virus. MBL can opsonize bacteria, enhance their clearing by phagocytes, and activate complement by cleaving C3 (chapter 3).
  - **Surfactant Proteins A and D** (SP-A and SP-D) are associated with phospholipids of lung surfactants and have an important role in the host defence of alveoli. They protect the lung through their interaction with a variety of potential pathogens, including viruses, bacteria, and fungi. They recognize and bind mannose and N-acetylglucosamine residues on microbial cell walls, resulting in enhanced killing and/or clearance by phagocytes. Although most extensively studied in the lungs, both SP-A and SP-D or proteins closely resembling them are found in a number of other sites in the body, eg, the respiratory tract, the gastrointestinal tract, the middle ear, and the peritoneal cavity.
  - **Ficolins** are characterized by the presence of a collagen-like domain and a fibrinogen-like domain. They activate complement by the alternative pathway.
  - **Conglutinin** is a pattern recognition molecule of ruminants; it helps in defence against *Salmonella typhimurium* and inhibits the haemaglutinin activity of the influenza virus.
- **Endocytic PRRs** occur on the surfaces of phagocytes. On recognizing molecular patterns on a microbial cell, these receptors mediate the uptake and delivery of pathogens into lysosomes.
  - **The mannose receptor** is a member of the Ca-dependent lectin family. It specifically recognizes carbohydrates with a large number of mannoses or fucoses. Engagement of this receptor has been shown to initiate phagocytosis and generate pro-inflammatory signals that lead to the eventual secretion of cytokines like TNF-α, IL-1, IL-6, and IL-12.

---

[11] The term CD stands for **Cluster of Differentiation** — a historical term used to define cell surface molecules recognized by a given set of antibodies of a single specificity. As each new molecule was discovered and defined by scientists, it was given a number reflecting the order of discovery. Thus, CD14 implies that it was the 14th molecule so defined and has no bearing on its function. Determining the function was a different task altogether. It is still on in the case of some molecules. A complete list of CDs used in this book is given in Appendix I.

[12] Lectins are a group of proteins that specifically bind or cross-link carbohydrates; C-type lectins are Ca-dependent lectins, ie, require Ca^{2+} for binding activity.

[13] MBL is the preferred name, as it helps avoid confusion between the mannose binding protein and the major basic protein of eosinopohils.

Table 2.1 Common human PRRs

PRR	Type of PRR	PAMPs recognized	Function
C-reactive protein	Secreted	Molecular groups found on the cell walls of a wide variety of bacteria and fungi, including phosphocholine moieties, lipoproteins, monophosphate esters, and histones.	Promotes opsonization and activates the complement cascade
LBP	Secreted	LPS	Binds LPS and transfers the complex to cell surface CD14
Mindin	Secreted	Recognizes sugar moieties	Opsonizes bacteria and promotes their phagocytosis; promotes secretion of pro-inflammatory cytokines by macrophages
Collectins	Secreted	Bind glucose, L-fucose, mannose, N-acetyl mannosamine, and N-acetyl glucosamine residues on microbial cell walls.	
		1. MBL, and SP-A and SP-D recognize mannose or N-acetylglucosamine residues	Opsonize bacteria and enhance their clearance; MBL can also activate complement by cleaving C3
		2. Ficolins recognize N-acetyl glucosamine, N-acetyl galactose, and L-fucose	Activate complement by the alternative pathway
Mannose receptor	Endocytic	Recognizes carbohydrates with a large number of mannoses or fucoses	Initiates phagocytosis; promotes secretion of pro-inflammatory cytokines by macrophages
Scavenger receptors	Endocytic	Bind micro-organisms and their products including lipoteichoic acids, LPS, CpG DNA and low-density lipoproteins.	Initiate internalization of the bound entity
CD14	Signalling receptor	Binds LPS and other cell wall constituents of Gram-positive and Gram-negative bacteria	Together with TLRs results in activation of a number of genes involved in innate and adaptive immune responses
TLRs	Signalling receptors	Recognize conserved products of microbial metabolism such as LPS, peptidoglycan, and lipoteichoic acids.	Activation induces the expression of a variety of cytokines and costimulatory molecules crucial to the initiation of adaptive immune responses

♦ **Scavenger receptors** are a broad group of receptors expressed by myeloid cells (macrophages and DCs) and certain endothelial cells. They bind and internalize micro-organisms and their products, including lipoteichoic acids of Gram-positive bacteria, LPS of Gram-negative bacteria, intracellular bacteria, and CpG DNA[14]. They are involved in lipid metabolism and bind modified low-density lipoproteins. These receptors can alter cell morphology, and their expression is affected by various cytokines.

● **Signalling receptors** recognize PAMPs and activate signal-transduction pathways (ie, they transmit the signal generated by the binding of the ligand to the receptor across the cell membrane, and thus activate a series of reactions; see chapter 6 for a better understanding of signal transduction).

♦ **CD14** is expressed on phagocytic cells; a soluble form is also found in serum. It recognizes LPS and other cell wall components of Gram-negative and Gram-positive bacteria[15]. CD14 does not have a cytoplasmic domain; hence, it requires TLRs (see next section) for signal transduction. Binding of LPS or other bacterial constituents to CD14 starts a signalling cascade through

[14] Unmethylated CpG dinucleotides are very common in bacteria. Conversely, they are highly under-represented in vertebrates. PRRs that can recognize these oligonucleotides found in bacteria have evolved in vertebrates. CpG DNA is thus a very potent immune stimulator.

[15] LBP is required for the binding and transfer of LPS to CD14.

TLRs, resulting in the activation of a number of genes involved in innate and adaptive immune responses.

- ♦ **Toll receptors.** The first toll receptor was identified in *Drosophila* and was shown to be involved in embryonic development. It was later found to be involved in immune responses of adult flies. Homologues of Toll were also identified in humans and are referred to as **T**oll-**L**ike **R**eceptors (TLRs). To date, ten members of the TLR family have been reported. They play a key role in the induction of immune and inflammatory responses to pathogens. TLRs recognize conserved products of microbial metabolism such as LPS, peptidoglycan and lipoteichoic acids (fig. 2.1). They are expressed by a variety of cells, including macrophages, immature DCs, vascular endothelial cells, and intestinal epithelial cells. Activation of TLRs induces the expression of a variety of cytokines and costimulatory molecules[16] that are also crucial to the initiation of adaptive responses.

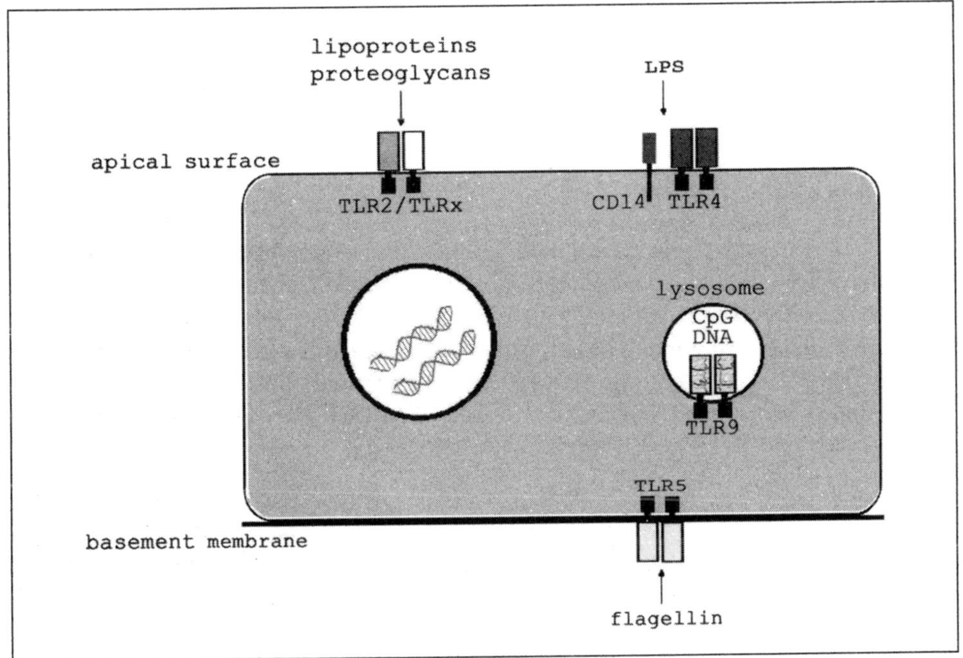

Figure 2.1 Toll-like receptors play a key role in the induction of immune and inflammatory responses to pathogens. These leucine-rich receptors recognize a variety of products of microbial and host origin. Some, like TLR2, associate with other TLRs (eg, TLR1 or TLR 6; represented as TLRx) and are expressed on the surface of the cell. TLR2 heterodimers can specifically bind products of microbial cell walls (LPS, peptidoglycan, yeast cell walls, etc). CD14 also expressed on the cell surface recognizes and binds LPS, but it cannot communicate this message to the interior of the cell, and TLR4 is necessary for this signal transduction. By contrast, TLR5 is expressed on the basolateral surfaces of intestinal epithelial cells that are not exposed to the outside environment. These receptors are therefore engaged only when flagellated bacteria penetrate the epithelial surface. Engagement of TLR5 activates pro-inflammatory gene expression. TLR9, essential for responses to bacterial or viral DNA and CpG DNA, is not expressed on the surface but is present in the cytoplasm of the host cells. Microbial DNA has to be internalized to trigger immune activation via TLR9.

- ♦ **Integrin family members.** Although members of the integrin family are known to be adhesion molecules that act as a sort of glue for bonding cells, some can also function as PRRs. CD11b/CD18 (Mac-1; CR3) and CD11c/CD18, present on macrophages and neutrophils, can recognize LPS, lipophosphoglycans, β-glucans, etc and lead to activation of the phagocyte.

[16] Costimulatory molecules are expressed on cells of the immune system. Engagement of these molecules is a pre-requisite for the initiation of adaptive responses. See chapters 6 and 8 for more information.

THE FIRST LINE OF DEFENCE

Physiological and chemical barriers to the entry/establishment of microbes constitute the first line of defence and include:

❑ Epithelial surfaces such as the skin and mucous membranes and antimicrobials produced by them
- defensins and cathelicidins
- dermicidin
- melanin

❑ Adverse conditions in the digestive tract

❑ Normal flora

❑ Microbicidal factors in tissues and blood
- lysozyme
- complement and properdin
- IFNs
- basic proteins, haeme-containing compounds, etc

❑ Pattern recognition molecules
- secreted PRRs — C-reactive protein, LBP, collectins, mindin
- endocytic PRRs — mannose receptor, scavenger receptor
- signalling PRRs — CD14, TLRs, integrin family members

2.2.2 The Cellular Players

Several cells are actively involved in the elimination of pathogens that have entered the body. These include phagocytic cells that internalize and kill microbes and cytolytic cells that bring about their lysis. Also included are some lymphocytic cells. Although originally thought to be solely involved in adaptive immunity, three subsets of lymphocytes are now recognized to participate in innate immune responses. DCs, a large and diverse family of leukocytes, are also considered a part of the innate immune response. Their sole function is to trigger the adaptive immune response.

2.2.2.1 The Phagocytic Cells

Although multiple cell types such as epithelial cells and endothelial cells have limited phagocytic capacity, they are inefficient in phagocytosis, and that is not their principle function. Truly phagocytic cells are extremely efficient at internalization and degradation, and scavenging is one of their main functions. These are the cells considered here. Phagocytes are found in almost all tissues of the body and are located in strategic positions to maximize the chances of encountering and trapping foreign particles. Although originally thought to be merely scavengers that mop up after the lymphocytes, phagocytic cells have now been established to play a key role in host defence and the maintenance of normal tissue structure and function. Their major functions are given below.

❑ To engulf, internalize, and finally destroy foreign particles — especially large particles (>0.5 μm). Apart from clearing infectious agents, phagocytes also clear senescent (old) cells and cellular debris from tissues. Activated phagocytes have potent microbicidal activity and are important in cell-mediated immunity (chapter 11).

❑ To secrete a variety of biologically active compounds. Phagocytes secrete a number of hydrolytic enzymes, complement components of the classical (Cl - C5) as well as the alternative pathway, plasma proteins, coagulation factors, oxygen metabolites, metabolites of the archidonic pathway, etc. Thus, they are crucial not only in host defence, but also in tissue regeneration (Table 2.2). Moreover, macrophages secrete TNF-α, IL-l, and IL-6 — cytokines involved in the inflammatory response. These cytokines are called 'endogenous pyrogens', since

Table 2.2 Overview of macrophage products and their functions

Function	Product
Microbicidal	
1. ROI	Superoxide anion, H_2O_2, hydroxyl radicals, singlet oxygen, chloramines
2. RNI	NO, nitrates, nitrites
3. Bioactive peptides	Defensins, cathelicidins, glutathione
4. Enzymes	Neutral proteases, acid hydrolases, lysozyme
Tissue acting	
1. Tissue damaging	ROI, RNI, TNF-α, neutral proteases
2. Tissue remodelling	Elastase, collagenase, hyaluronidase, growth factors (fibroblast growth factor, angiogenesis factor, TGF-α, TGF-β[*])
Pyrogenic	Cytokines (IL-1, TNF-α, IL-6)
Inflammation regulators	Bioactive lipids such as metabolites of the archidonic pathway: prostaglandins (PGE2, PGE2α), prostacyclin, thromboxane A2, leukotrienes (LTB4, LTC4, LTD4, LTE4)
	Bioactive peptides like glutathione
	Coagulation factors including tissue thromboplastin, Factors V, VII, IX, prothrombin, plasminogen activator and its inhibitor
	Components of the complement pathway (C1, C2, C3, C4, C5, Properdin, Factors B, D, I, P, H)
	Proteinases such as plasminogen activator, and neutral proteases (collagenase, elastase, angiotensin convertase, stromlysin)
	Acid hydrolases which include acid proteases (cathepsin D, L) and other hydrolytic enzymes (lysozyme, lipases, glycosidases, ribonucleases, phosphatases)
	Cytokines including IL-1, IL-6, IL-8, TNF-α, IFN-γ, erythropoietin, MIP-1[*], MIP-2, MIP-3, GM-CSF[*], M-CSF[*], G-CSF[*], PDGF[*]
	Protease inhibitors (α2-macroglobulin, α-antitrypsin, plasmin, and collagenase inhibitor, plaminogen activator inhibitor)
	Stress proteins, most importantly heat shock proteins

[*] G-CSF — Granulocyte-Colony Stimulating Factor, GM-CSF — Granulocyte Macrophage-Colony Stimulating Factor; M-CSF Macrophage-Colony Stimulating Factor, MIP — Macrophage Inhibitory Proteins, PDGF — Platelet-Derived Growth Factor, TGF-α and TGF-β — Transforming Growth Factor-α and -β

they are responsible for the elevation of body temperature. TNF-α, IL-l, and IL-6 also induce synthesis of acute phase proteins by liver hepatocytes (section 2.3.2).

❑ To present antigen (ie, act as **Antigen-Presenting Cells; APCs**). Macrophages internalize pathogens or other antigens, break them down to small peptide fragments, and then load and display the fragments on MHC molecules (chapter 7). Recognition of the peptide:MHC complex by specific antigen-sensitive lymphocytes (T lymphocytes) results in their activation. This activation culminates in an adaptive immune response.

❑ To retain the antigen for a prolonged period of time, thereby avoiding overwhelming the adaptive immune system. The phagocytes thus have a major role in augmenting and/or controlling the adaptive immune response.

i. Macrophages and related cells. Macrophages are actively phagocytic cells that arise from bone marrow stem cells or circulating monocytes. Mature macrophages localize in different tissues and display considerable heterogeneity. They exhibit unique characteristics and are relatively long-lived (average life of 6–16 days) phagocytic cells. They are found in connective tissues or at other sites of possible pathogenic challenge such as the gastrointestinal tract, the lungs and in organs like the liver and spleen, which take care of old and dying cells (Table 2.3). These tissue macrophages (called resident macrophages) proliferate locally but can also be augmented by the influx of blood monocytes. Normal tissue macrophages are immunologically quiescent. They have low O_2 consumption and do not secrete cytokines. Cytokines like IFN-γ or TNF-α produced in response to invasion, activate them. Activated macrophages express a variety of cell receptors and secrete an array of antimicrobial agents and cytokines, turning them into potent mediators of innate immunity.

Table 2.3 Macrophages and related cells

Site	Type
Brain	Microglial cells
Lungs	Alveolar macrophages
Spleen	Splenic macrophages
Liver	Kupffer cells
Kidney	Mesangial macrophages
Lymph nodes	Resident and recirculating macrophages
Bone marrow	Promonocytes and monocytes
Synovial cavity	Synovial cells
Blood	Monocytes
Serous fluids	Pleural and peritoneal macrophages

Macrophages and monocytes express a number of specialized receptors and markers on their cell surfaces. The number and type of receptors expressed at any point in time depends upon the state of activation (quiescent versus activated), location, life cycle, local milieu, etc. They include PRRs, FcRs[17], receptors for complement components, receptors for various cytokines, chemokines,[18] and growth factors. Like all nucleated cells of the body, they express MHC class I molecules. They also express MHC class II molecules that are involved in antigen recognition by T cells. The expression of these molecules is upregulated by activation or exposure to cytokines like TNF-α and IFN-γ or microbial products like LPS. Important types of macrophages include:

❑ **Monocytes.** Promonocytes in the bone marrow give rise to blood monocytes. These form a circulating pool from where they migrate to various organs and tissue systems to give rise to macrophages. In addition, monocytes can also differentiate into immature DCs. It is thought that there is a regular migration of monocytes from the blood into tissues where they can differentiate into immature DCs or macrophages, depending upon the cytokine environment (fig. 2.2). Monocytes that enter a site of inflammation have variable fates. They may become resident macrophages, transform into epitheloid cells, fuse with other macrophages to become multinucleated giant cells, or simply die.

❑ **Kupffer cells**[19]. The largest concentrations of macrophages in the body are in the lungs and liver. Both organs contain a heterogeneous population of macrophages. The Kupffer cells are the liver's resident macrophages, situated at locations that expose them to any foreign material entering the liver via the blood stream. They are among the first phagocytic cells to encounter the antigen after it is absorbed from the intestinal lumen. These cells have lysosomes rich in acid hydrolases needed for digestion of internalized matter. The Kupffer cells digest not only foreign matter but also a large number of dead self-cells and could therefore trigger an autoimmune response. Luckily, Kupffer cells express low levels of the MHC class II molecules needed to activate T lymphocytes and are situated such that they are not easily accessible to naïve T cells (ie, T cells that have never encountered antigen). On infection or inflammation, however, MHC class II expression is upregulated, allowing the Kupffer cells to present antigen to T cells. The Kupffer cells are activated by various bacterial stimuli including LPS and

[17] Antibodies (immunoglobulins) are Y-shaped structures that bind specifically to antigens by the two arms of the Y. The stem of the Y is called the Fc region. Many cell types express receptors for this region. These receptors are collectively called FcRs. The outcome of the binding of antigen-antibody complexes to the FcR is dictated by the type of cell and the type of FcR and is discussed in chapter 9.

[18] Chemokines are kind of cytokines that attract phagocytic cells to the site of inflammation. Apart from directing the migration of leukocytes along a concentration gradient, they are also important in their activation (see sidetrack Instant chemistry, chapter 8).

[19] They were first identified by German scientist von Kupffer. Thank God this system of naming cells or molecules after scientists has now been abandoned!

superantigens[20]. Activated Kupffer cells secrete IL-12 and IL-18. These cytokines in turn activate liver NK cells and eventually T$_{H1}$ cells. The liver leukocytes and the adaptive immune responses they induce play a crucial role in defence against bacterial infections and haematogenous tumour metastases.

❑ **Alveolar macrophages.** The lungs represent the largest epithelial surface area of the body in contact with the external environment. As a consequence, the airways need an active and elaborate defence system. Alveolar macrophages along with interstitial macrophages are a part of this defence. Alveolar macrophages line the alveoli of the lungs. Inhaled particulates such as pollutant particles, allergens, and micro-organisms are rapidly cleared by these macrophages. Apart from other receptors, these macrophages also express receptors for IgA, an antibody involved in mucosal immunity.

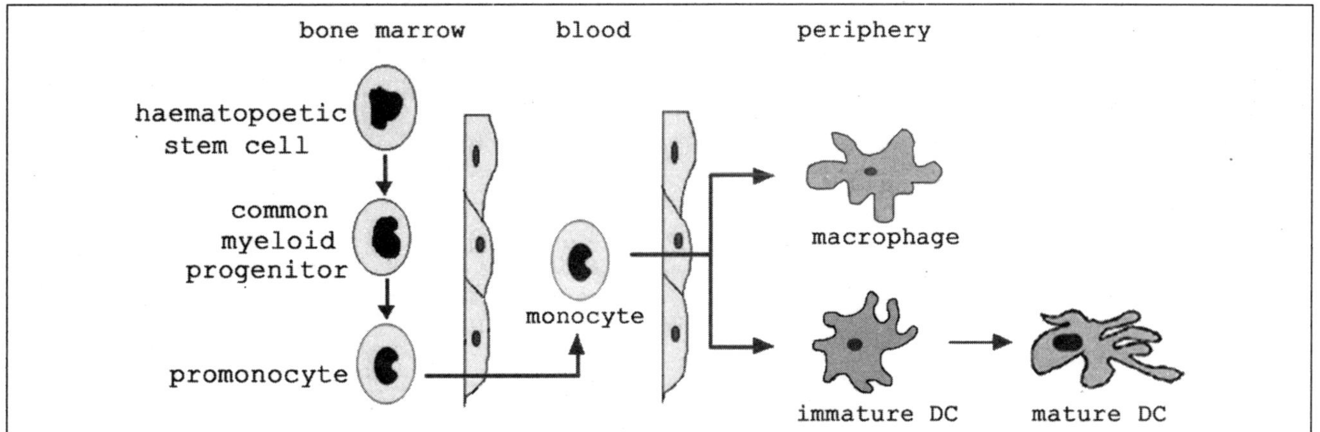

Figure 2.2 Monocytes arise from haematopoietic stem cells and can differentiate into macrophages or DCs. Haematopoietic stem cells in the bone marrow give rise to CD34$^+$ common myeloid progenitor cells that further give rise to promonocytes. Promonocytes give rise to monocytes that circulate in blood. Monocytes can further differentiate into macrophages or DCs depending upon the cytokine milieu. Cytokines such as GM-CSF promote differentiation to DC lineage, whereas exposure to cytokines like M-CSF promotes differentiation to macrophages.

ii. PolyMorphoNuclear granulocytes (PMNs) are produced in the bone marrow. They are short-lived cells that do not differentiate further. These granulocytes make up to 70% of the leukocytes in normal blood. The mature granulocyte contains a multi-lobed nucleus and many cytoplasmic granules. PMNs have an important role in acute inflammation. They accumulate rapidly at the site of inflammation. Acting in concert with complement and antibodies, PMNs are the major defence against micro-organisms. Based on their morphology and staining reactions, PMNs are divided into neutrophils, eosinophils, basophils, and mast cells.

❑ **Neutrophils.** Human neutrophils have a multi-lobed nucleus and a highly granular neutrophilic cytoplasm. These represent about 90% of circulating granulocytes and 60–65% of blood leukocytes. They are derived from the bone marrow[21]. When released from the bone marrow into circulation, these cells are in a non-activated state and have a half-life of only four to ten hours before they marginate and enter tissue pools where they survive for one to two days. Cells of the circulating and marginated pools can interchange. Senescent neutrophils are thought to undergo apoptosis, or programmed cell death[22], prior to their removal by macrophages. Being a highly mobile cell type responding to various stimuli, neutrophils have a major role in inflammation and are one of the first cells to be recruited at the site of tissue damage. **The main function of these cells is phagocytosis**. Unlike macrophages though, neutrophils do not actively produce

[20] Superantigens are powerful B and T cell mitogens discussed in chapter 4.

[21] The bone marrow of a normal adult produces 10^{11} neutrophils per day, and this number can increase to 10^{12} during infection.

[22] Cell death is one of two types — necrosis and apoptosis. Necrosis occurs when cells die from severe injuries (physical/chemical trauma). Generally the cell membrane is damaged in necrosis. There are early changes in mitochondrial shape and function. The cell swells and ruptures, spilling its contents into the surrounding tissue spaces and provoking an inflammatory response. Apoptosis is a more subtle form of cell death often seen when cell death is physiologically determined or acceptable, ie, when a few cells are to be sacrificed for the general well-being of the body. Examples include elimination of self-reactive clones, cells with short half-lives, involution of cells deprived of essential growth factors, and the morphogenetic death of cells during embryonic development. In apoptosis, the cell membrane becomes ruffled and blebbed (resembling bubbles). The cell shrinks. Generally, the nucleus also shrinks, becomes dense, and the DNA undergoes fragmentation. Intracellular contents are not released, so inflammation is not provoked. Apoptosis and its induction by lymphocytes is described in chapter 11.

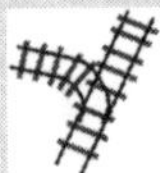

The Neutrophil Paradox

Although neutrophils are essential to host defence, they have also been implicated in the pathology of many chronic inflammatory conditions. A large influx of neutrophils in the blood of people with an acute bacterial infection or in the lungs of patients with the adult respiratory distress syndrome causes widespread tissue damage. The tissue damage is due to the oxidants and hydrolytic enzymes released from activated neutrophils and may eventually lead to death as the body tries to switch off the immune response in an attempt to prevent further damage. Activation of neutrophils by immune complexes in synovial fluid contributes to the pathology of rheumatoid arthritis. Chronic activation of neutrophils may also initiate tumour development; ROI generated by neutrophils damage the DNA, and the released proteases can promote tumour cell migration. Oxidants of neutrophil origin have also been shown to oxidize **L**ow-**D**ensity **L**ipoproteins (LDL) which are then more effectively bound to the plasma membrane of macrophages through specific scavenger receptors. Uptake of these oxidized LDL by macrophages is thought to initiate atherosclerosis. Cytoplasmic constituents of neutrophils are known to give rise to specific **A**nti-**N**eutrophil **C**ytoplasmic **A**ntibodies (ANCA) in susceptible individuals. ANCA are antibodies directed against enzymes that are found mainly within the azurophil granules of neutrophils. These antibodies are closely related to the development of systemic vasculitis and glomerulonephritis. Neutrophils release a large number of hydrolases besides ROI. Under normal conditions hydrolytic damage to host tissue, and therefore chronic inflammatory conditions, are kept at bay by the presence of antioxidants and protease inhibitors in the blood. Many of these protease inhibitors are members of the **Ser**ine **P**rotease **In**hibitor (SERPIN) family. If the antioxidants and anti-proteases are overwhelmed or excluded from tissue, severe damage can occur. Oxidative stress may initiate tissue damage by reducing the concentration of extracellular protease inhibitors to below the level required to inhibit released proteases. Anti-protease deficiency is thought to be responsible for the pathology of emphysema. High levels of primed neutrophils have been found in people with essential hypertension, Hodgkin's disease, inflammatory bowel disease, psoriasis, sarcoidosis, and septicaemia. Priming of the neutrophils in all these cases correlates with high concentrations of circulating TNF-α.

pseudopods, but they phagocytose only those cells that have adhered to their cell surface via receptors.

Neutrophil granules are like storage depots for mediators of innate host defence. These granules are generated during cell differentiation, and their contents are available on demand as soon as a pathogen is encountered. On the basis of function and enzyme content, human neutrophil granules can be divided into three main types — azurophil granules, specific granules, and small storage granules. Individual granule populations can also be characterized morphologically (eg, azurophil granules are larger and contain more electron-dense material than specific granules) or biochemically. Their function is not just to provide enzymes for hydrolytic substrate degradation but also to kill ingested bacteria and to secrete contents extracellularly so as to regulate various physiological and pathological processes, including inflammation.

Neutrophil granules contain antimicrobial or cytotoxic substances, neutral and acid proteases, acid hydrolases, and a pool of membrane receptors (Table 2.4). **M**yelo**pero**xidase (MPO), present in azurophil granules, is a critical enzyme in the conversion of hydrogen peroxide (H_2O_2) to hypochlorous acid. Along with H_2O_2 and a halide cofactor, it forms the most effective microbicidal and cytotoxic mechanism of leukocytes — the myeloperoxidase system[23]. Azurophil granules function predominantly in the intracellular milieu (in the phagolysosomal vacuole) where they are involved in the killing and degradation of micro-organisms[24]. Conversely, neutrophil specific granules are particularly susceptible to releasing their contents extracellularly and appear to have an important role in initiating inflammation. Specific granules represent an intracellular reservoir of various

[23] MPO is responsible for the characteristic green colour of pus.

[24] Latest research indicates that the human neutrophil elastase may be a key host defense protein that targets bacterial virulence proteins. It may be especially important in immunity to enteric pathogens like *Shigella* spp.

Table 2.4 Neutrophil granules

Function		Azurophil granules	Specific granules	Small storage granules
Antimicrobial		Myeloperoxidase Lysozyme BPP* Defensins Cathelicidins Azurocidin	Lysozyme Lactoferrin	–
Proteolysis:	Neutral proteases	Elastase Cathepsin G Proteinase 3	Collagenase Complement activator	Gelatinase Plasminogen activator
	Acid proteases	Cathepsin B Cathepsin D	–	Cathepsin B Cathepsin D
Hydrolysis		β-D-glucoronidase α-mannosidase Phospholipase-A2	Phospholipase-A2	β-D-glucoronidase α-mannosidase
Membrane receptors		–	Complement receptor 3 and 4 Laminin receptor N-form-met-peptide receptor$	– –
Miscellaneous		Chondroitinsulphate	Cytochrome $b558$ Monocyte chemotactic factor Histaminase Vitamin B_{12} binding protein	Cytochrome $b558$

*Bacterial **P**ermeability-increasing **P**rotein (BPP) is a member of the perforin family (see section on NK cells) and is highly toxic to Gram-negative bacteria.

$ N-formylmethionine is an amino acid exclusive to bacterial protein synthesis; the receptor is thus a detector of bacterial protein synthesis.

plasma membrane components, including cytochrome $b558$ (a component of NADPH oxidase, the enzyme responsible for the production of superoxide), receptors for complement fragment iC3b (CR3, CR4), laminin, and formyl-methionyl-peptides. Newly discovered functions for individual granule proteins suggest that granule constituents may also participate in adaptive immune responses. In this respect, defensins and cathelicidins seem to be particularly important. Apart from mobilizing various types of phagocytic leukocytes, immature DCs, and lymphocytes, they can also stimulate IL-8 production and mast cell degranulation. Thus, neutrophils are critical in alerting, mobilizing, and amplifying the innate and adaptive antimicrobial immunity of the host.

❏ **Eosinophils** take up the acidic component (eosine) of compound stains used in blood staining. They account for 2–5% of leukocytes in healthy non-allergic individuals. Only a small fraction of the total eosinophil population is in circulation. Most eosinophils are present in connective tissues immediately underneath the respiratory, gut, and urinogenital epithelium. Their numbers may shoot up dramatically in allergic states or worm infestations. Human eosinophils usually have a bi-lobed nucleus and many cytoplasmic vesicles. Apart from the usual receptors (for complement components, adhesion molecules, cytokines, chemokines, etc), eosinophils also express FcεRI (the high affinity receptor for Fc region of IgE antibodies; section 9.8) and a low affinity receptor for IgG. Eosinophils have also been shown to express MHC class II proteins under the influence of certain cytokines and can act as APCs under those conditions.

The large granules (vesicles) in the mature eosinophil are membrane bound organelles having a 'core' that differs in electron density from the surrounding matrix. They contain four distinct cationic proteins that exert a range of biological effects on host cells and microbial targets. The **M**ajor **B**asic **P**rotein (MBP; not to be confused with MBL) is thought to be responsible for the cytotoxicity of eosinophils to parasites. It is even demonstrable in the blood and sputum of patients with hypereosinophilia. Other cationic proteins found in the large granules are **E**osinophil **C**ationic **P**rotein (ECP), **E**osinophil-**D**erived **N**eurotoxin (EDN), and **E**osinophil **P**er**o**xidase (EPO). These cationic proteins are important not only in host defence against helminthic parasites, but also in tissue dysfunction and damage in eosinophil-related inflammatory and allergic diseases. Additionally, the large granules contain histaminase, arylsulphatase, and large amounts of peroxides. Like neutrophils, eosinophils also possess small granules that house enzymes like arylsulphatase, acid phosphatase, and gelatinase. Upon degranulation, they also synthesize and release prostaglandins, leukotrienes, and cytokines that augment the inflammatory response, activate epithelial cells, and help recruit more phagocytes and leukocytes. The cytokines secreted by eosinophils include IL-3, IL-5, IL-6, IL-8, GM-CSF, TNF-α, and both TGF-α and TGF-β. They also synthesize IL-4 when stimulated with chemokines.

Eosinophils are capable of phagocytosing, but only to a limited degree as that is not their primary function. Whereas the neutrophil lysosomal enzymes act primarily on material engulfed in phagolysosomes, the contents of the eosinophil granule act mainly on extracellular targets such as parasites. **Eosinophils degranulate when triggered by an appropriate stimulus**. Resting eosinophils do not express FcϵRI. Upon activation by cytokines and chemokines, they start expressing this receptor and become primed for their protective function. Cross-linking of the FcϵRI receptors by the IgE-antigen complexes leads to activation of the cell membrane and finally, degranulation of the cell (fig. 2.3). During degranulation, the vesicles (of the granules) fuse with the cell membrane, and their contents are released outside the cell. Through this simple strategy, eosinophils use antimicrobial substances in granules on large targets that could not otherwise be phagocytosed. **This degranulation mechanism may be important in defence against helminth infestations**; infected tissues show degranulated eosinophils adhering to helminths. Perhaps due to the eosinophils' role in allergic reactions, doubts regarding their exact role in such protection continue to persist.

Eosinophils also participate in hypersensitivity reactions, especially through two lipid inflammatory mediators, LTC4 and **P**latelet **A**ctivating **F**actor (PAF). Both mediators contract airway smooth muscles, promote mucus secretion, alter vascular permeability, and elicit eosinophil and neutrophil infiltration. In addition to the direct activities of these eosinophil-derived mediators, MBP can stimulate the release of histamine from basophils and mast cells by a non-cytotoxic mechanism. It also stimulates the release of EPO from mast cells. In this way, once stimulated, eosinophils can serve as a local source of specific lipid mediators and induce the release of mediators from mast cells and basophils. The cationic proteins of eosinophils by themselves can also contribute to acute manifestations of allergy and inflammation. Paradoxically, like many cells of the immune system, eosinophils can also negatively regulate their effector function, and some of the granular contents can actually lead to inactivation of mediators of anaphylaxis. Thus, for example, arylsulphatase B can inactivate the **S**low-**R**eacting **S**ubstance of **A**naphylaxis (SRS-A, a mixture of LTC4, LTD4, and LTE4; see table 15.2), phospholipase D destroys the platelet lytic factor, and histaminase degrades the histamine released by mast cell degranulation.

❑ **Basophils and mast cells** possess many similar properties. Although introduced in this section, these cells will be discussed in greater detail in the chapter on hypersensitivity. Basophils, like other PMNs, circulate in the blood and account for 0.5–1.0% of blood leukocytes. Mast cells, on the other hand, are exclusively sessile, ie, tissue dwelling, and are associated with mucosal epithelial cells and connective tissues. They are seen in abundant numbers in organs such as the skin, lungs, and gastrointestinal tract, which are exposed to the external environment, enabling the mast cells to rapidly respond to foreign stimuli. Both these cells

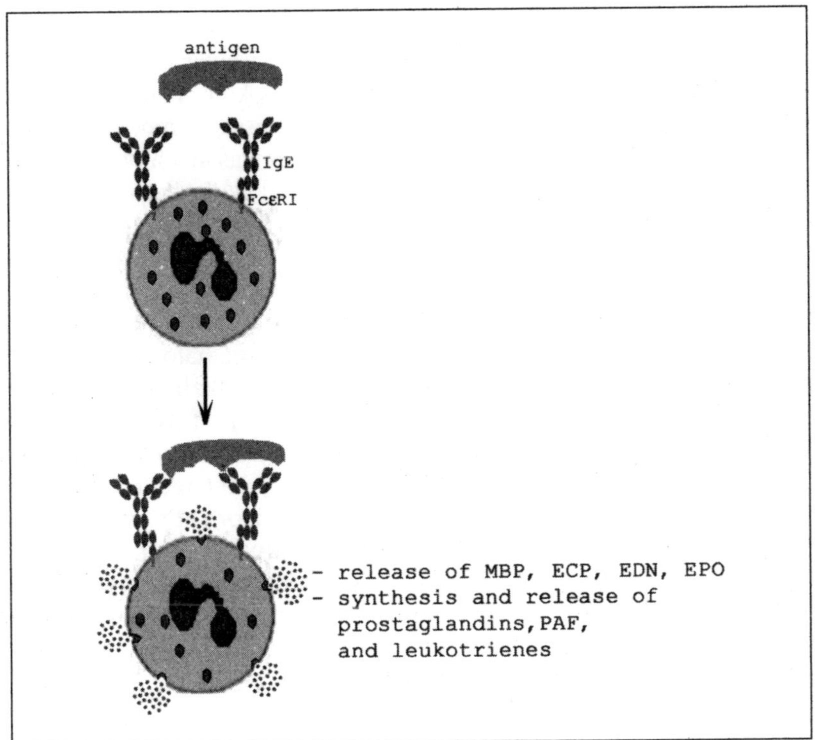

Figure 2.3 Cross-linking of FcεRI bound IgE by multivalent antigen results in eosinophil degranulation. *Eosinophils are considered important in defence against helminth infestations. Cross-linking of IgE bound to the high affinity IgE receptors (FcεRI) expressed on the eosinophils by epitopes on parasites starts a signalling cascade that results in the fusion of the granule membranes with the cell membrane. There is a rapid release of granular contents to the external milieu. Eosinophil granules are a rich depository of toxic metabolites such as Major Basic Protein (MBP), Eosinophil Chemotactic Protein (ECP), Eosinophil-Derived Neurotoxin (EDN), and Eosinophil Peroxidase (EPO). MBP causes the release of histamine from basophils and mast cells. Degranulation also results in the synthesis and release of pro-inflammatory mediators such as prostaglandins, PAF (platelet activating factor), and leukotrienes. Together, these mediators result in contraction of smooth muscles and mucus secretion — physiological responses important in ridding the body of the parasite. In hypersensitive persons, however, these same mediators are responsible for the unpleasant manifestations of allergies.*

contain granules that stain prominently with basic dyes because of the presence of large amounts of acidic proteoglycans. These membrane-bound granules are storehouses for mediators such as histamine, heparin, **E**osinophil **C**hemotactic **F**actor-**A** (ECF-A), and neutral proteases. However, basophils contain only about one fourth as much MBP as eosinophils and merely detectable amounts of EDN, ECP, and EPO. Additionally, these cells are capable of synthesizing mediators upon receiving appropriate signals (see below). Hence, the mediators contained in these granules are called 'preformed' while those synthesized just before release are referred to as 'newly synthesized'. Both cell types express FcεRI and receptors for complement components (C3a and C5a). Mast cells also express a low affinity receptor for IgG (FcγRIII). Similar to what happens in the eosinophils, **cross-linking of FcεRI (or FcγRIII in the case of mast cells) by antibody-antigen complexes leads to the degranulation of these cells**[25]. Membranes of the granules fuse with the cell membrane and release the preformed mediators to the external milieu. Antibody-mediated degranulation also results in the release of newly synthesized mediators such as LTC4, PGD2, cytokines (TNF-α, TGF-β, IL-1, IL-4, IL-5, IL-6), and chemokines. In addition, mast cells (but not basophils) secrete PAF. Thus, IgE mediated degranulation leads to the release of a host of

[25] Although it is the most studied, FcεRI cross-linking is by no means the only mode of inducing degranulation. Other factors that induce degranulation include tissue injury caused by high temperature, irradiation, trauma, chemicals like toxins and venoms, and proteases or cationic mediators released by eosinophils or neutrophils.

pharmacologically active mediators. These mediators cause the adverse symptoms of allergy (inflammation, vasodilation, increased vascular permeability, smooth muscle contraction, etc), while cytokines and chemokines play an important role in inflammation, adaptive immune responses, and tissue remodelling (fig. 2.4).

For years the function of mast cells and basophils was in doubt. The persistence of mast cells throughout evolution (they are found as far back in phylogeny as insects) and their presence at most portals of entry suggested a protective role. It has now been established that mast cells can actively phagocytose opsonized bacteria via either complement receptors or IgG receptors. In addition, cytokines like TNF-α secreted by these cells help in the control of pathogens by augmenting the neutrophil/macrophage response. Chemotactic mediators released by mast cells and basophils recruit phagocytes to the site of challenge and thus aid in pathogen clearance. ECF-A, in particular, is important in recruiting eosinophils to the site of response and augmenting the antiparasite response. Mast cells also promote the flow of lymph from the site of antigen interaction to the regional lymph node, the site of lymphocyte activation. Importantly, mast cells trigger muscular contraction that can contribute to the expulsion of the pathogen from the body. Mast cells and basophils may be involved in immunity against parasites, since animals deficient in these cells show impaired parasite clearance. Therefore, it is now accepted that mast cells and basophils have an important role in innate immunity.

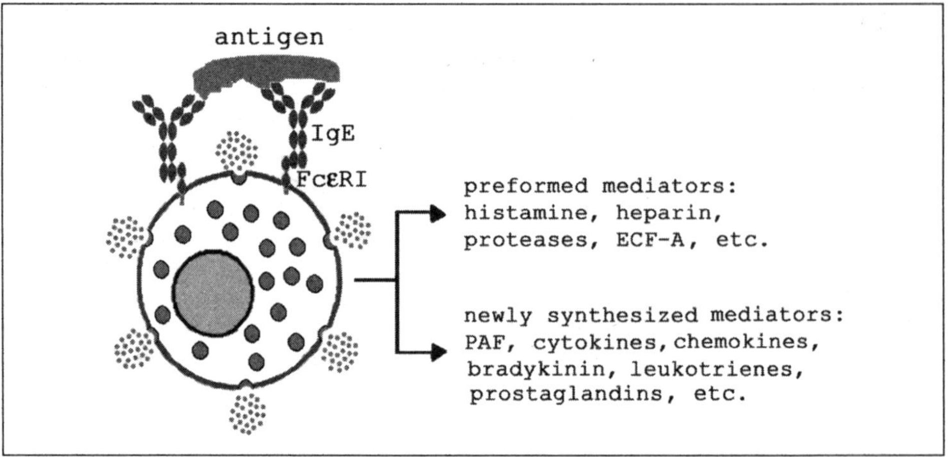

Figure 2.4 Mast cell degranulation results in the release of pharmacological mediators responsible for a number of physiological manifestations. Mast cells express high affinity receptors for IgE (FcεRI), low affinity receptor for IgG (FcγRIII), and receptors for complement components, toxins, etc. Cross-linking of these receptors causes rapid degranulation of the cells and the release of bioactive compounds such as histamine, chemotactic factors for eosinophils and neutrophils, and proteases. Additionally, the cells rapidly synthesize and release PAF, leukotrienes, cytokines, and prostaglandins. Together, these compounds cause vasodilation, increased vascular permeability, smooth muscle contraction, and mucus secretion. They also recruit and activate other cells (eosinophils, neutrophils) to the site of antigen challenge, thus helping in host defence. This protective mechanism can become deleterious to the host if the host has IgE against innocuous substances such as pollens or peanuts.

iii. Movement of phagocytic cells. Cells of the immune system circulate as non-adherent cells in the blood and lymph, and when necessary, they migrate as adherent cells in tissues. Rapid transition between adherent and non-adherent states is crucial to their functions of immune surveillance and responsiveness. This capability allows them to efficiently protect the body from infectious agents. Although only the migration of phagocytic cells in and out of blood vessels is described below, other

PHAGOCYTIC CELLS

☐ Phagocytic cells are crucial to both innate and adaptive immune responses.
- These are scavenger cells involved in clearance of self old, dead, or dying cells.
- They phagocytose intruders that have breached the first line of defence and gained entry.
- Phagocytes produce and secrete several enzymes, cytokines, and other microbicidal factors of innate immune response.
- They promote inflammation.
- Phagocytic cells link innate and adaptive immunity by presenting antigen to T lymphocytes.
- They help regulate the adaptive immune response.

☐ Macrophage and related cells phagocytose by actively producing pseudopods and are involved in tissue remodelling and wound healing. They are a major source of
- ROI, RNI,
- pro-inflammatory cytokines,
- antimicrobial peptides,
- components of the classical (C1-C5) and alternative complement pathway,
- a variety of bioactive lipids, enzymes, and coagulation factors.

☐ PMNS comprise neutrophils, eosinophils, and basophils.
- Neutrophils accumulate rapidly at site of inflammation.
  - ♦ They phagocytose cells that are immobilized to cell via receptors.
  - ♦ Their granules act as storage depots for bioactive moleucles; three types recognized — azurophil, specific, and storage granules.
  - ♦ They are a major source of azuricidin, defensins, cathelicidins, MPO, lysozyme and lactoferrin.
- Eosinophils are thought to be important in defence against parasites and helminths.
  - ♦ They have large granules rich in cationic proteins (MBP, ECP, EDN, EPO), arylsulphatase, histamine, and peroxides.
  - ♦ They have small granules rich in enzymes like gelatinase, acid phosphatase, arylsulphatase, etc.
  - ♦ They express receptors for IgE (FcεRI).
  - ♦ Eosinophils are responsible for some of the manifestations of allergies and immediate hypersensitivities.
- Basophils stain with basic dyes.
  - ♦ They have granules containing preformed mediators such as heparin, histamine, ECF-A, and MBP.
  - ♦ Basophils degranulate upon cross-linking of surface FcεR by antigen-IgE complexes.
  - ♦ They can synthesize and release LTC4, PGD2, cytokines, and chemokines upon IgE-linked degranulation.
  - ♦ They play a role in allergic responses and may be involved in anti-parasite immunity.

☐ DCs are a diverse family of leukocytes that are efficient sentinels of the immune system.
- They are a major source of IFNs; they help in augmenting innate responses.
- They act as a link between innate and adaptive immune responses.
  - ♦ Immature DCs are highly endocytic cells.
  - ♦ They capture antigen and transport it to lymphoid tissue.
- They process and present captured antigen to T cells.

cells of the immune system (eg, DCs, lymphocytes) also move in an essentially similar fashion through blood vessels or tissues.

Phagocytes are capable of chemotactic movement and move towards the source of chemotaxin by cytoplasmic streaming. Common chemoattractants include LTB4, LPS, histamine, PAF, peptides having N-formylmethionine, chemokines (eg, IL-8), complement component C5a, and to a much lesser degree, C3a. In order to enter various tissues, circulating monocytes and neutrophils must first adhere to and then cross the endothelial lining of blood vessels. Thus, migration in host tissues consists of three key steps — rolling, adhesion, and extravasation.

☐ **Rolling.** Under normal circumstances, leukocytes are transported by the blood stream and collide with the endothelial cells lining the blood vessels. These collisions are weak interactions that allow the phagocytes to probe the endothelial surface. Firmer interaction is required for emigration. Blood flow rate is slowest in post-capillary venules, and it is here that this interaction takes place. At sites of

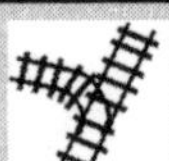

The Inner Lining: Endothelium

The cells lining the body surfaces and blood vessels are not passive observers in protection and immunity. Endothelial cells, by virtue of their capacity to express adhesion molecules and cytokines, are intricately involved in inflammatory processes. During immune injury, activation of endothelial cells by inflammatory cytokines stimulates leukocyte adhesion to the endothelium. This transforms the endothelium from an anti-coagulant surface to one that is frankly pro-coagulant and results in the release of vasoactive mediators, cytokines, and growth factors. Endothelial cells have been shown to express cytokines like IL-1, IL-5, IL-6, IL-8, IL-11, IL-15, several colony-stimulating factors (G-CSF, M-CSF, and GM-CSF), the chemokines **M**acrophage **C**hemotactic **P**rotein-**1** (MCP-1) and RANTES, and growth-related oncogene protein-α. Diverse processes such as hypoxia and bacterial infection can induce the expression of these cytokines. IL-1 and TNF-α, produced by infiltrating inflammatory cells, can induce endothelial cells to express several of these cytokines and adhesion molecules. There seems to be a cross-talk between inflammatory cells and the endothelium, and this may be critical to the development of chronic inflammatory states.

The escalating inflammatory processes that are set off by the entry of the pathogen must also be diffused. Otherwise, the pro-coagulant endothelium will allow the adhesion of cells indiscriminately, leading to the blocking of blood vessels. Endothelial cells have a role to play in this process as well. Cytokine activation of endothelial cells in the later stages of the immune response results in increased synthesis of TGF-β. This cytokine is known to be immunosuppressive and is found to inhibit E-selectin expression, hindering leukocyte adhesion, and transmigration. TGF-β also influences the mechanisms of vascular remodelling and tissue healing. Thus, endothelial-derived cytokines may be involved in a variety of process such as haematopoiesis, cellular chemotaxis and recruitment, bone resorption, coagulation, acute phase protein synthesis, and regulation of the inflammatory response.

inflammation, blood flow rate is further reduced because of dilation of vessels, increasing chances of collision between the leukocyte and the endothelium. A set of adhesion molecules called selectins initiate the first transient contact of the leukocyte with the endothelium. L-selectin expressed by leukocytes transiently interacts with carbohydrates on the endothelial cells in the initial interaction. Normally, endothelial cells do not express selectins but store them in granules. Exposure to LTB4, C5a, or histamine released by local trauma leads to the release of P-selectin — a member of the selectin family — to the cell surface. The next to appear is E-selectin. Together, these molecules allow a loose attachment between the endothelium and the phagocytic cell surface glycoproteins. Coupled with the force of the bloodstream, this leads to rolling (also called margination) of leukocytes along the endothelium.

❑ **Adhesion.** Under the influence of chemotaxins like IL-8 and PAF released by platelets, phagocytes upregulate the expression of integrins. These are a family of adhesion molecules such as LFA-1 (**L**eukocyte **F**unction associated **A**ntigen-**1**; a heterodimer of CD11a/CD18), and Mac-1 (CD11b/CD18) that orchestrate critical steps in leukocyte trafficking. LFA-1 and Mac-1 bind to other integrin members ICAM-1 (**I**ntra**c**ellular **A**dhesion **M**olecule-**1**) and ICAM-2 expressed on endothelial cells. The resting endothelium does not express ICAM-1, and it expresses only low levels of ICAM-2. Exposure to TNF-α induces the expression of ICAM-1 and upregulates the expression of ICAM-2. These adhesion molecules act like glue and arrest the rolling leukocytes, allowing them to stick to the endothelium. New adhesion contacts are formed in the direction of movement while adhesion is reduced at the trailing end.

❑ **Extravasation.** The phagocytes move towards endothelial cell-cell junctions because of the integrin-mediated adhesive interactions. An immunoglobulin-like molecule, PECAM-1[26] — expressed both by the leukocytes and the intracellular junctions of the endothelial cells — helps the phagocyte squeeze through the

[26] PECAM-1 (Platelet Endothelial Cell Adhesion Molecule-1; CD31) acts as homophilic glue, ie, its ligand is also CD31.

junction and cross the endothelial wall (the crossing of the endothelial wall is called extravasation, and movement through the wall is called diapedesis). The phagocytes initially extend a pseudopod between the endothelial cells while maintaining the nuclei and granules on the lumenal side. Eventually, the whole cell migrates across the endothelial boundary. Transmigration across the endothelium to the basal membrane of the endothelium is rapid (within minutes of attachment) and one-way. The phagocytes accumulate briefly between the basement membrane and the endothelial cells before entering the connective tissue. Proteases secreted by phagocytes help in digestion of the proteins of the basement membrane (fig. 2.5).

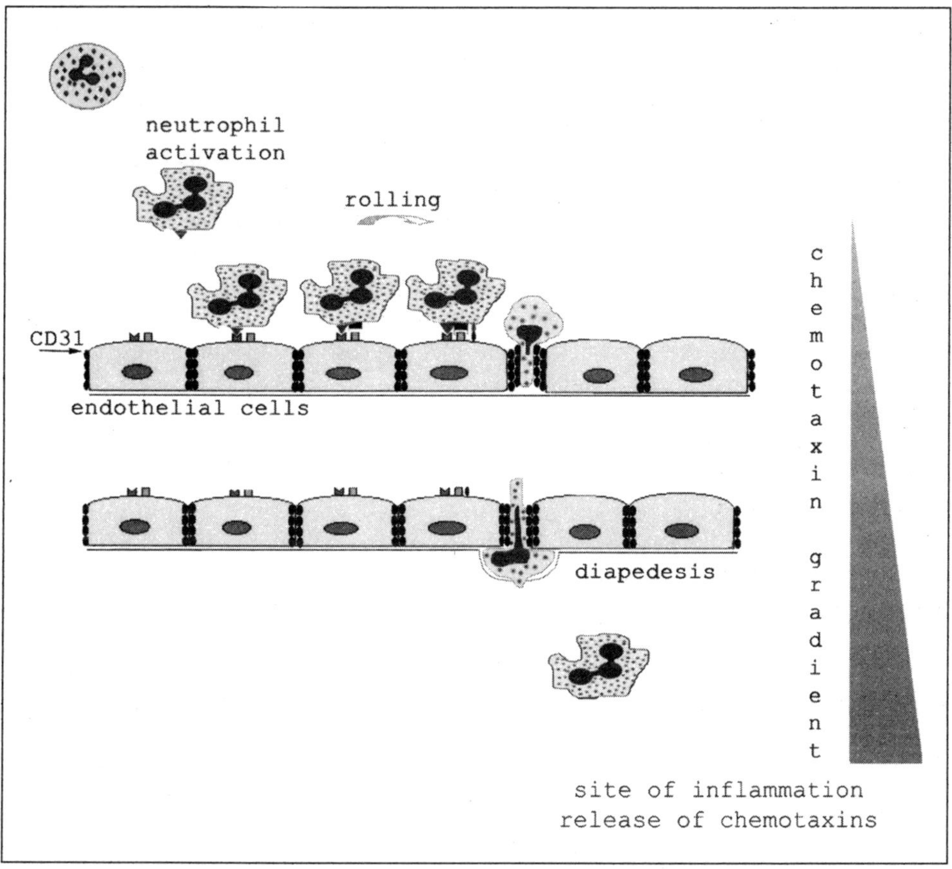

Figure 2.5 Phagocytes cross the endothelium and enter the site of infection by a multi-step process initiated by adhesion molecules expressed by activated endothelial cells. The normal endothelium is non-adhesive and interacts fleetingly with the leukocytes as they are transported across the endothelium by the blood flow. Tissue injury induces the expression of selectins on endothelial cells, allowing a firmer interaction with glycoproteins on the phagocytic cell surface. This interaction is not firm enough to anchor the phagocyte to the endothelium but slows it down and causes it to roll across the endothelial surface. New adhesion contacts are formed in the direction of movement while adhesion is reduced at the trailing end. Expression of ICAM-1 on the endothelium and expression of its ligands such as LFA-1 (or Mac-1) on the phagocytes allows stronger interaction. It causes the phagocyte to adhere to the endothelium and move towards the intracellular junctions. CD31 expressed by both the endothelial cells and the phagocytes helps the cells squeeze through the junction towards the basement membrane and is called diapedesis. Matrix metalloproteases, expressed by the phagocyte, help in digesting the proteins of the basement membrane. Once outside the blood vessel, the leukocyte migrates in response to a concentration gradient of chemokines. Such chemokines are released by interaction of tissue cells or macrophages upon initial encounter with the pathogen, and they bind to proteoglycans in the extracellular matrix of the tissue. `Chemokines thus form a matrix-associated concentration gradient along which the leukocytes migrate to the focus of infection.

[27] Several intracellular pathogens such as *M. tuberculosis* or *Chlamydia* spp. subvert the system and survive by interfering with phagolysosome formation.

iv. Phagocytosis was first discovered by Metchenikoff in 1884. It can be defined as a process by which particulate substances are ingested and destroyed by a cell. Phagocytosis by macrophages is crucial for the uptake and degradation of not only pathogens but also senescent, apoptotic, and damaged tissue cells. Phagocytosis is an integral part of development, tissue remodelling and wound healing, innate and adaptive immune responses, and inflammatory processes. It can be divided into three distinct phases:

- ❑ **Attachment.** The first step in phagocytosis is the attachment of the micro-organism to the phagocyte. By virtue of their receptors, phagocytes can attach themselves to a variety of organisms. Apart from PRRs, two other receptors expressed by phagocytes are important to attachment — FcRs and receptors for complement components. Opsonization of an organism by complement components, antibodies, fibronectin, etc or expression of adhesion molecules on the phagocytic cell membrane, greatly enhance attachment.

- ❑ **Pseudopod formation.** The membrane of the phagocyte is activated by this attachment and leads to the formation of pseudopods and eventual engulfment of the organism. The formation and fusion of pseudopods involves proteins such as actin and myosin (the same proteins that are involved in muscle movement). When the pseudopods fuse, the micro-organism is internalized into a phagosome. The phagosome then matures via a series of fusion and fission events. Finally, lysosomes fuse with the mature phagosome to form a phagolysosome[27].

- ❑ **Digestion.** Within the confines of the phagolysosome, the micro-organism is subjected to a battery of bactericidal factors and is killed by two different mechanisms.
  - **The oxygen-dependent mode** of intracellular killing is dependent upon cellular glycosis and is a by-product of a marked increase in metabolic activity, called the metabolic or respiratory burst, that accompanies phagocytosis (fig. 2.6). The cells in the metabolic burst consume a large amount of oxygen and

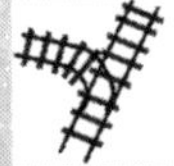

NO Laughing Matter: NO and RNI

NO and RNI, formed by **NO S**ynthases (NOS), are one of the most enigmatic molecules in immunology. They are produced by cells of the immune system (DCs, NK cells, mast cells, and phagocytic cells) as well as other cells involved in the immune reaction (such as endothelial cells, epithelial cells, vascular smooth muscle cells, fibroblasts, keratinocytes, and hepatocytes). NO is derived from the amino acid L-arginine by the enzymatic activity of NOS. It is known to have multiple roles in the immune and other organ systems. Although some of its effects, such as its antimicrobial activity, are well documented, others such as its immunosuppressive effect are very poorly understood. NO and RNI seem to be potent molecules that can have local effects at the site of synthesis and, due to rapid and unhampered diffusion, effects at sites farther away as well. The most obvious function of NO or RNI is antimicrobial action; they can kill or reduce the replication of a variety of pathogens such as bacteria, fungi, and viruses. NO or RNI combine with DNA, causing mutations. Additionally, they inhibit synthesis and repair of nucleic acids of the pathogen, cause alterations in proteins because of S-nirtosylation or tyrosine nitration, and disrupt enzymes by disrupting S-Fe clusters or haeme groups or by peroxidation of membrane lipids. NO may combine with O_2^- to form peroxynitrite ($ONOO^-$), a potent antibacterial molecule. Local arginine depletion caused by NO synthesis in host tissues can also lead to growth inhibition and parasite death. NO is found to inhibit tumour cell growth and may also induce their death; however, many tumours seem to express NOS, and NO seems to actually help their survival. NO can influence leukocyte chemotaxis by modulating the production of chemokines and/or functioning as an intracellular messenger in chemokine signalling pathways. NO has been shown to downregulate endothelial expression of adhesion molecules and hence can significantly affect the rolling and transmigration of leukocytes. Thus, NO seems to govern a broad spectrum of processes. These include the differentiation, proliferation, and apoptosis of immune cells; production of cytokines and adhesion molecules; and the synthesis and deposition of extracellular matrix components.

as a result, H_2O_2 production increases. Other bactericidal oxidizing agents such as the superoxide anion (molecular oxygen having an extra electron; O_2^-), singlet oxygen ($^1O_2^*$, molecules with high energy electron), and hydroxyl radicals (OH^* together called **R**eactive **O**xygen **I**ntermediates or ROI) are also produced. The enzyme MPO, also present in neutrophils, increases damage by catalyzing the toxic peroxidation of a variety of surface molecules on micro-organisms in the presence of toxic oxygen metabolites.

- **The oxygen-independent mechanism** of killing includes:
  - ♦ **A progressive decrease in pH, in concert with hydrolytic enzymes** such as cathepsins, phosphatases, phospholipases, glycosidase, lysozyme, and arylsulphatase, bring about digestion of cell walls or the outer covering of the pathogen. Ribonucleases, lipases, and proteases further digest the intracellular contents.
  - ♦ **Nitric Oxide (NO)**, which may be one of the most important weapons in the macrophage arsenal, is effective in both the immediate vicinity of the phagocytes as well as a considerable distance from it, since it diffuses easily across cellular barriers. The antimicrobial activity of NO is thought to be due to its mutagenic activity. Moreover, RNI (**R**eactive **N**itrogen **I**ntermediates) formed during NO synthesis are also bactericidal.
  - ♦ **peptides** such as defensins, cathelicidins, and cationic peptides that are microbicidal.
  - ♦ **lactoferrin** that binds Fe^{2+}, making it unavailable to the microbe.

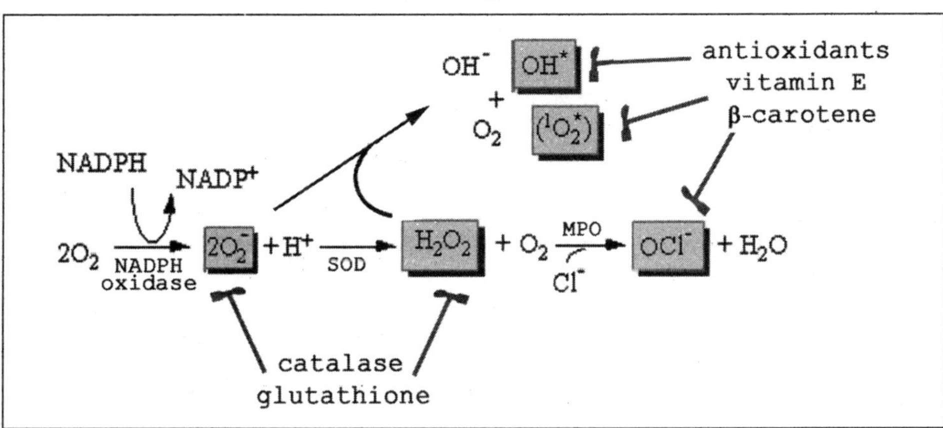

Figure 2.6 Phagocytosis causes a respiratory burst that is accompanied by a transient increase in oxygen consumption and results in the production of superoxide anions (O_2^-), hydrogen peroxide, singlet oxygen ($^1O_2^*$), hydroxyl radical (OH^*), and hypohalite (OCl^-) by macrophages and neutrophils. The respiratory burst is a part of the oxygen-dependent mechanism of killing that allows the formation of highly toxic but short-lived metabolites and free radicals. They are generated by NADPH oxidases and other enzymes present in the lysosomes of the phagocytes. The critical intermediate is the highly reactive superoxide which can be converted to the equally damaging H_2O_2 by the action of Superoxide Dismutase (SOD). In the presence of chlorides, this can lead to the formation of hypochlorite because of the presence of Myeloperoxidase (MPO) in neutrophils. The toxic metabolites can, however, also cause extensive host tissue damage and need to be rapidly neutralized. Antioxidants such as β-carotene, vitamins C, and E help in scavenging the free radicals, whereas catalase and glutathione help convert H_2O_2 and superoxide anions to water.

Eventually, the micro-organism is digested (fig. 2.7). Portions of the microbial cell are displayed on the surface of the phagocyte in the context of MHC molecules, setting the stage for T cell stimulation. If the ingested particle is too large, the phagocyte is frustrated in its attempt to digest the particle. The whole particle-containing lysosome is then thrown out of the cell by exocytosis. Such liberation of the particle along with the corrosive lysosomal brew is damaging to bystander tissue cells. Some of the harmful effects of hypersensitivity are attributed to such exocytosis.

When antigens or micro-organisms effectively resist the microbicidal activity of macrophages, the resulting chronic inflammation leads to the formation of a characteristic tumour called granuloma (section 2.3.1).

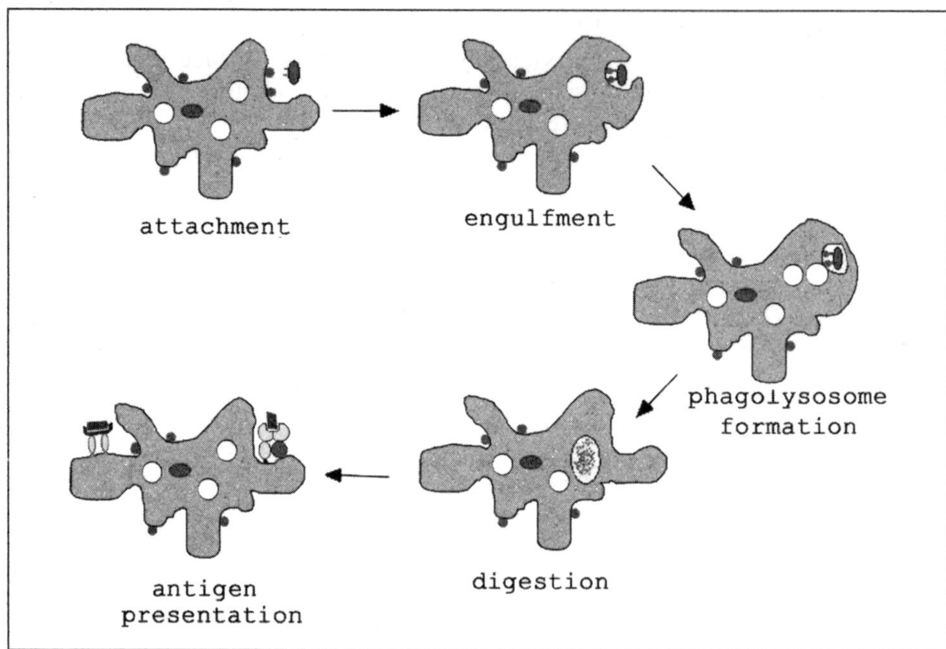

Figure 2.7 Engagement of receptors on phagocyte surface by ligands on the microbe results in phagocytosis and the eventual destruction of the pathogen besides triggering the adaptive immune response. Resident macrophages are one of the first cells to encounter pathogens. They are soon reinforced by recruitment of neutrophils and macrophages from the blood. The first step in phagocytosis is the attachment of the micro-organism to the phagocyte, brought about by the ligation of cell surface receptors on the phagocytes by molecules on the outer cover of the pathogen. The activated phagocytic cell membrane rapidly forms pseudopodia and engulfs the pathogen. The pathogen is internalized in a membrane-bound vesicle called the phagosome. The phagosome is then fused with highly acidic internal vesicles called lysosomes that are rich in enzymes and toxic metabolites required for the destruction of the microbe. The pathogen is eventually digested in the phagolysosome. Fragments derived from the pathogen are loaded on MHC molecules and displayed on the cell surface, helping trigger the adaptive immune response.

2.2.2.2 The Lymphocytic Cells

Most immunological research was originally focused on antibodies produced by B cells and the effector functions of T cells, resulting in the general perception that lymphocytes were the instruments of adaptive immune responses only. In recent years, it has been shown that some lymphocytes are also involved in innate responses. Of these, the NK cells are relatively better understood. Two other types of lymphocytes — γδ T cells and B1 cells — are more enigmatic, and their precise function is still a hot topic of research.

i. NK cells have an instrumental role in innate immune responses against bacterial, viral, and parasitic pathogens. They have been shown to play a crucial role in suppressing tumour metastasis and outgrowth. They are called 'natural killer' cells because they are naturally present and demonstrate their cytolytic activity even in normal animals not exposed to an infectious agent. They constitute about 15% of peripheral blood lymphocytes. These are a heterogeneous group of cells arising from the bone marrow and characterized by their large granular morphology and the ability to lyse target cells. They do not express immunoglobulins and T cell receptors and hence are distinct from both B and T lymphocytes. NK cells can mature in the absence

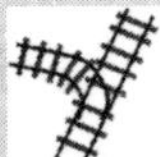

Up in Smoke and Down the Drain: Cigarette Smoke and Innate Immunity

Tobacco contains more than 4500 compounds in particulate and vapour phases. These compounds contain at least five known human carcinogens and many toxic agents including CO, NH_3, acrolein, acetone, benzopyrenes, nicotine, hydroquinone, and NO. Since a cigarette burns at much higher temperatures during inhalation, many of these compounds are at much higher concentrations in sidestream smoke (that is released in the air during burning) than in mainstream smoke (which is inhaled by the smoker). The carcinogenic action of many of these compounds has been linked to DNA damage and/or increased cellular proliferation.

The lung is equipped with non-specific and specific defence mechanisms to protect it against the large number of environmental pathogens it is exposed to. Alveolar macrophages and other monocytes are the most important for the innate immune response of the lung. Cigarette smoking increases by several folds the number of alveolar macrophages. These cells express increased levels of lysosomal enzymes and elastase which are thought to damage connective tissue and parenchymal cells of the lung, greatly increasing the risk of bronchitis and emphysema. Alveolar macrophages from smokers are functionally impaired and show a decreased ability to phagocytose and kill pathogens. They are also found to secrete considerably lower levels of pro-inflammatory cytokines. These cytokines are crucial for early responses to immunological challenges and upregulation of local host defences. NK cells of smokers also show reduced activity against tumour cells. Chronic exposure to cigarette smoke increases the frequency of spontaneous tumours in laboratory animals, which could be partially attributed to the impaired NK cell function. To summarize, smoking produces various morphological, physiological, biochemical, and enzymatic changes in macrophages and NK cells, which might impair antibacterial defences, regulatory activity, and inflammatory responses in the lungs, leading to lung pathogenesis.

of the thymus, unlike T cells, and can be found even in animals lacking this organ. Many NK cells originate from precursors in the foetal liver (6–8 weeks), although they may also develop from immature thymocytes. A special subset of these cells, the NKT cells, express T cell receptors and are discussed in chapter 8.

A large body of work on NK cells has been conducted in rodents and mice, and therefore, the grouping and nomenclature can be confusing. For the sake of simplicity, only human NK cells will be considered here. Human NK cells can be divided into two subsets on the basis of CD56 expression, CD56^{bright} and CD56^{dim}. The functional significance of CD56 expression is not understood, and a murine homologue of CD56 has not yet been discovered. Generally speaking, CD56^{dim} cells are more cytotoxic than CD56^{bright} cells and are consequently more granular. NK cells express a number of other receptors and markers on their cell surface, though all the markers need not be present simultaneously on the same cell. Thus, different clones of NK cells express a different subset of markers. These include CD16 (a kind of FcR; FcγRIII), cytokine receptors (IL-1, IL-2, IL-10, IL-12, IL-15, IL-18, and IFN-γ), and chemokine receptors. NK cells expressing CD16 can target antibody-coated pathogens and participate in ADCC (**A**ntibody-**D**ependent **C**ell-mediated **C**ytotoxicity). This subset of NK cells, called K cells, will be dealt with later in the chapter on cell-mediated immunity.

The mechanisms by which NK cells recognize target cells are not entirely understood. NK cells express both activatory and inhibitory receptors (fig. 2.8). **Engagement of the activating receptors triggers killing by NK cells, while coligation of the inhibitory receptors spares the target cell from NK cell-mediated killing.** Inhibitory receptors have Immunoreceptor Tyrosine-based *Inhibitory* Motifs (ITIM[28]) in their cytoplasmic domains. Signals delivered by the inhibitory receptors are often dominant over signals emanating from activating receptors with ITAMs (Immunoreceptor Tyrosine-based *Activating* Motifs) and prevent NK cell effector functions. A balance of signals generated by these inhibitory and activatory receptors, along with engagement of various adhesion (ICAM-1,

[28] ITIMs and ITAMs are universal motifs found in the cytoplasmic domains of molecules involved in signal transduction and are discussed in chapter 6.

LYMPHOCYTES OF INNATE IMMUNE RESPONSE

❑ NK cells are heterogeneous cells characterized by large granular morphology and ability to lyse target cells.
- They do not express immunoglobulins or the T cell specific CD3 molecule.
- Human NK cells are grouped on the basis of
  - ◆ CD56 expression
  - ◆ T cell receptor expression (NKT cells)
  - ◆ CD16 expression (K cells)
- NK cells express activating receptors and inhibitory receptors; a balance of signals generated by the activatory and inhibitory receptors dictates activation of NK cells.
- Activated NK cells bring about the death of target cells by
  - ◆ inducing apoptosis,
  - ◆ releasing cytotoxic granules containing perforin and granzymes.
- These cells are major source of IFN-γ.
  - ◆ IFN-γ activates macrophages; augments ROI and RNI production
  - ◆ causes DC maturation
❑ $\gamma\delta$ T lymphocytes are found in intraepithelial sites.
- They do not express CD4 or CD8 molecules.
- They do not recognize antigen in context of MHC molecules.
❑ B1 B lymphocytes express the T cell specific CD5 marker.
- They do not require T cell help in mounting an immune response.
- They are important in the initial stages of immune response.
- B1 B cells produce mainly IgM antibodies.

LFA-3, etc) and costimulatory molecules, governs the activation of NK cell cytotoxicity. Superfamilies of NK receptors include:

❑ **K**iller cell **Ig**-like **R**eceptor (KIR) which primarily recognizes MHC class I molecules (HLA-A, -B, and -C)
❑ C-type lectin superfamily heterodimers of NKG2 and CD94 that recognize HLA-E
❑ **N**atural **C**ytotoxicity **R**eceptors (NCRs), a family of receptors identified in humans with their ligands yet to be established. These receptors have very short cytoplasmic domains but associate with other molecules such as DAP12, FcϵRIγ, and CD3ζ (pronounced zeta) that have ITAMs. Engagement of NCRs therefore results in the activation of NK cells and lysis of the target cells.

NK cells can be visualized as constantly being in a tug of war regulated by opposing signals from receptors that can either activate or inhibit their effector functions. Inhibitory receptors, including those belonging to KIR family and NKG2/CD94 family, recognize MHC class I molecules. Their murine equivalents are the Ly49 C-type lectin family. Their engagement cancels any activating signal the cell may have obtained from other receptors. All nucleated cells of the body express MHC class I molecules. These inhibitory receptors are therefore critical in ensuring that self-cells are protected from the destructive potential of NK cells. Downregulation of either MHC class I synthesis or their export to the surface is a mechanism used by many viruses to escape recognition by cytotoxic T cells (eg, cytomegalovirus). Activating receptors recognize carbohydrates, sulphated proteoglycans, or glycoproteins expressed on cell surfaces. Viral infection often results in an alteration in the glycosylation pattern of cellular proteins, and these receptors therefore allow NK cells to detect such changes. Activating signals, in the absence of inhibitory receptor engagement, allow the NK cell activity to be targeted at infected and/or transformed cells that may otherwise escape the specific killing mechanisms of the body.

Engagement of activatory receptors along with exposure to cytokines such as IFN-α, IFN-β, and IL-12 activates NK cells. IFNs not only activate the cells but also enhance cytolytic capacity of these activated cells. Activated NK cells bring about the lysis of target cells by cell-to-cell interaction through the release of granzymes and perforin contained in the lysosomes or by inducing the cell to apoptose (chapter 11). Perforin inserts itself in the target cell membrane and polymerizes to form transmembrane channels. These channels lead to the leakage of low molecular weight cellular contents while allowing an influx of water. Granzymes are a family of enzymes that promote DNA fragmentation and cell death (chapter 11). Apart from direct cytolytic activity, NK cells secrete IFN-γ and other cytokines in significant amounts following stimulation. IFN-γ production is an important function of NK cells. It induces NO synthase and promotes the production of ROI and RNI. It is also known to activate macrophages and cause the maturation of DCs, thus triggering adaptive immune responses. NK cells can also secrete TNF-α which has antiviral and immunoregulatory properties. It has been suggested that cytolytic functions of NK cells may be used uniquely in particular compartments. In the case of cytomegalovirus infection, for instance, perforin dependent NK cell effects may be more important in the spleen, whereas IFN-γ production may be more important for defence of the liver.

One more class of lymphocytic cells — the **L**ymphokine-**A**ctivated **K**iller (LAK) cells — derived from NK cells, specialize in the lysis of tumour cells. These cells have the capacity to induce apoptosis, and their cytotoxic potency is enhanced by IL-1, IL-2, IL-6, IL-15, IFNs, TNF-α, etc. Although LAK cells represent a very minor subset, they are important in tumour immunity because of their ability to

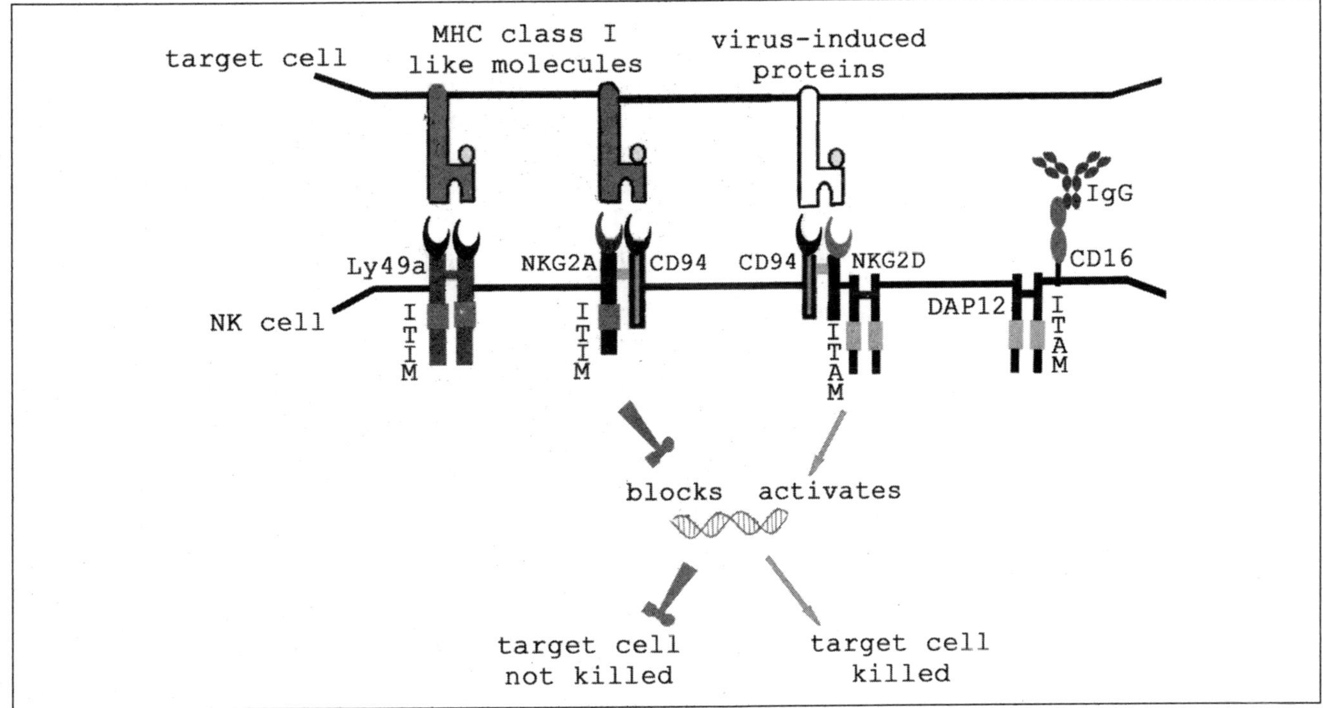

Figure 2.8 A balance of signals generated by the inhibitory and activatory receptors governs NK cell cytotoxicity. *NK cells express a variety of receptors for ligands on target cells. Activatory receptors have ITAMs in their cytoplasmic tails and result in NK cell activation. Inhibitory receptors have ITIMs in their cytoplasmic tail, and signals generated by their recognition are dominant over any activatory signal. Recognition of MHC class I or MHC class I-like molecules expressed on self-cells by inhibitory receptors such as heterodimers of NKG2A-CD94 (in humans) or the homodimeric Ly49a (in mice) therefore allows the target cell to escape. Activating receptors such as NKG2D recognize ligands induced by viral infection. Viral infections often result in downregulation of MHC class I molecule expression. This results in the lack of an inhibitory signal and therefore allows NK cell-mediated lysis of the virally infected cell. Some activating receptors do not have a cytoplasmic tail and transmit the activating signal via bridging molecules (called adaptor molecules) such as DAP12. Many NK cells also express CD16, a low affinity IgG receptor, that is also dependent upon DAP12 for signalling. Cross-linking of CD16-bound IgG by an antigen transmits an activating signal and may result in the lysis of the target cell.*

stimulate T cell and eosinophil activity. LAK-cell therapy has been shown to induce partial and complete remissions in up to 20% of patients of malignant melanoma and renal cell carcinoma.

ii. γδ T lymphocytes are a special subset of T cells that express a receptor different from the T cells of the adaptive immune response. **They are considered important in conferring immunity against infections in the intraepithelial sites**. The precise role of these cells in immune defence is unclear. These cells differ from other T cell types in two respects — they do not express CD8 or CD4 surface molecules (hence referred to as double negative cells), and they do not recognize peptide:MHC complexes. They express receptors of a very limited diversity which seem to recognize target antigens directly and can potentially recognize and respond to molecules expressed by different cell types. γδ T cells are proposed to recognize ligands that are expressed by tissue cells only in response to infection such as heat shock proteins. If true, this makes γδ T cells unique, in that they are activated by self-molecules expressed as a consequence of infection rather than pathogen-associated molecules. Mice deficient in γδ T cells have been shown to have exaggerated responses to pathogens and self-tissues, leading to the suggestion that they may play a role in modulating immune responses. γδ T cells have been shown to secrete cytokines upon activation and may modulate immune responses via these molecules.

iii. B1 cells are a distinct set of B lymphocytes (< 5%) that develop in the foetal/neonatal animal and express CD5 molecule. The B lymphocytes that develop in adult bone marrow are, by this system of nomenclature, of the B2 type. B1 cells are thought to contribute to the production of serum immunoglobulins and 'natural antibodies'. Typically, these cells do not need the help of T lymphocytes in mounting an immune response. In adult animals, B1 cells proliferate in the peritoneal and pleural cavities and seem to interact with self-antigens and bacterial antigens found in the gut flora. They differentiate to antibody-producing plasma cells rapidly in the first stages of immune response. By contrast, it is almost a week before conventional B cells differentiate and start producing antibodies. Antibodies produced by these cells are predominantly of the IgM type and have been demonstrated to play a role in defence against bacteria and viruses. They are thought to be especially important in mucosal immunity and are often regarded to be a part of a primitive mechanism bridging innate and adaptive immunity.

2.2.2.3 DCs

DCs is a collective term used to describe a heterogeneous group of cells that reside in most areas of the body. They derive their name from their peculiar morphology — immature and mature DCs show the presence of dendrites or veils (ie, long processes). Immature DCs may be formed directly from haematopoietic stem cells of the bone marrow or from other cell types such as monocytes which can differentiate to immature DCs upon cytokine stimulation. Such cells that can differentiate to DCs are often called 'pre-DCs'. DCs (whether pre- or immature) are efficient sentinels of the immune system. Immature DCs are a highly mobile cell type that colonizes lymphoid and non-lymphoid tissue extensively (chapter 5). They have a role in both the innate and adaptive immune responses besides being a major source of type I IFNs. They are therefore important in antiviral defence and NK cell activation. TNF-α and NO produced by DCs are thought to be important in antimicrobial defence, especially in the early hours after infection. Immature DCs also double up as 'lookouts' of the immune system that continuously scout the body for signals of potential danger and trigger adaptive immune responses in response to such signals. Accordingly, **immature DCs are highly endocytic cells that capture and internalize intruders that have breached the innate barriers and gained entry**. The array of PRRs expressed by immature DCs allows them to recognize and capture such intruders. They efficiently trap and transport the captured antigen to lymphoid

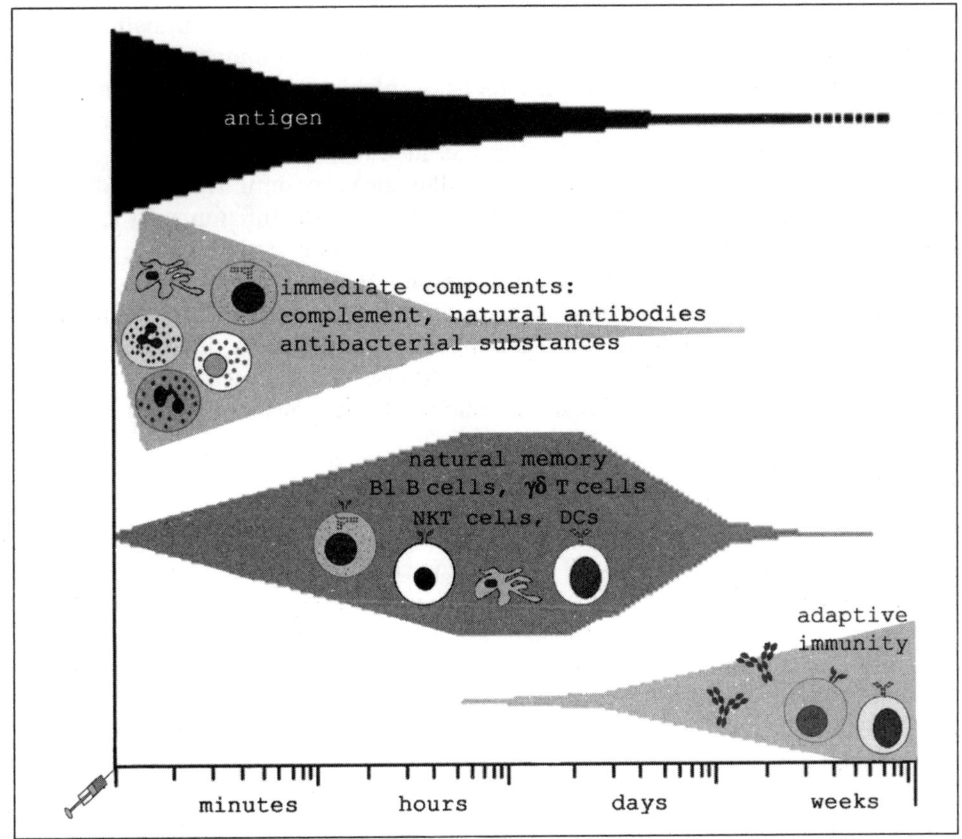

Figure 2.9 Different components of the innate immune system act at different stages of the innate immune response to effectively meet the antigenic challenge and remove majority of the antigen before the adaptive immune system swings into action. Complement, 'natural antibodies', and antimicrobial factors of the innate immune system act within minutes of microbial invasion to try to restrict the invader. The cellular component of the innate system is the next to join the battle. Neutrophils are one of the first cells to enter the site of infection. Together with mast cells and eosinophils, they rapidly recruit macrophages and DCs into the developing response. The actively phagocytic cells try to limit spread of the infection while killing the infectious agent by releasing antimicrobial substances. Meanwhile, lymphocytic (or natural memory) component of innate immunity (B1 cells, γδ T cells, and NKT cells) also join the developing response. Days to weeks elapse before the development of the adaptive response, since it is triggered only after the capture and transport of the antigen to the lymphoid organs. The lymphocytic compartment of innate immunity bridges this gap, ensuring an optimal transition, while aiding antigen removal (Adapted from Current Opinion in Immunology (2001), 13:195).*

tissue. Contact with microbes or their products triggers DC maturation. **Mature DCs interact with T lymphocytes in the lymphoid tissue and activate them.**

DCs thus function as the link between innate and adaptive immune responses. DCs and their role in triggering adaptive immune responses is discussed in chapter 5.

2.3 The Innate Immune Response

Cells and cellular processes involved in the innate immune response have been discussed so far. To give a better perspective, the events following an encounter with a pathogen are described here. The epithelial barriers act as a first line of defence and try their best to keep the microbe out. If the pathogen succeeds in breaching these barriers, it is immediately recognized by phagocytes in the subepithelial connective tissues. These cells bind and phagocytose the pathogen. The pathogen is then subjected to an arsenal of antimicrobial substances in the phagolysosome, resulting in its destruction. If only a few microbes have crossed the epithelial barrier this proves to be the end of the encounter. If the innate immune system fails in overcoming the microbial challenge, a focus of infection is established, and both, innate and adaptive immune responses need to be brought into action. As a result of interaction with the pathogen, phagocytes recruited to the site of infection secrete a number of cytokines. The combined effect of the release of antimicrobial molecules and cytokines in turn starts a series of events culminating in an inflammatory response. This response occurs within hours of microbial intrusion. Some phagocytic cells (DCs, macrophages, eosinophils) load fragments of the ingested pathogens onto MHC class II molecules and display them on their cell surfaces. Recognition of these peptide:MHC complexes by T lymphocytes triggers the adaptive immune response. The primary adaptive immune response takes between 4–7 days for generation, but later encounters result in much faster responses.

2.3.1 Inflammation

Inflammation can be defined as a localized, protective event elicited by injury which serves to destroy, dilute, or wall off both the injurious agents and the injured tissue. The inflammatory response is triggered by chemical signals released upon tissue intrusion by a microbe. Appropriate cells are immediately recruited and dispatched to the site to kill the microbes and host cells infected by them. Inflammatory mediators stimulate endothelial cells to express proteins that trigger blood clotting in local small vessels. This helps prevent the spread of the pathogen. The tissue surrounding the intrusion is liquefied to halt the spread of the microbe. In the final phase of the response, tissues damaged by either the microbe or by the host response are repaired. The inflammatory response is analogous to a quick central government response wherein paramilitary and military forces are rushed to the area of disturbance to avoid further unrest and begin damage control. The inflammatory response is a well-orchestrated event caused by the interaction of several inflammatory mediators. The process of inflammation is initiated in response to a traumatic, infectious, post-ischaemic, toxic, or autoimmune injury[29] (fig. 2.10). Bioactive peptides released by neurons and heat shock proteins or mitochondrial proteins released by dying cells trigger cytokine production by tissue cells. Pharmacological mediators released by mast cells and chemokines and cytokines released by macrophages cause the endothelium to express adhesion molecules resulting in an influx of PMNs. The endothelium also becomes leaky, leading to the influx of fluids to the site of inflammation. The released cytokines and pro-inflammatory mediators also cause the activation of macrophages and neutrophils, turning them into virtual killing machines. Thus, there are three major components of acute inflammatory response — vascular changes resulting in increased flow and adhesion; increased vascular permeability; and increased leukocyte margination, migration, and activation. The inflammatory mediators include:

❏ **Chemokines**. These are a superfamily of polypeptides that cause chemotaxis, increased cellular adhesion, and leukocyte activation. Chemokines are thus important in controlling the movement of phagocytic cells. As described in the preceding sections, multiple cell types involved in the innate response secrete chemokines.

❏ **Cytokines**. Cells of the innate immune system (especially phagocytes) secrete a number of cytokines in response to infection. These cytokines promote inflammation and are therefore called pro-inflammatory cytokines (examples include IFN-γ, TNF-α, IL-1, and IL-6). They have local effects (recruitment of cells to the site of infection and their activation, chemotaxis, activation of the endothelium, increased vascular permeability, etc) and systemic effects (pyrexia, induction of the acute phase response, increased metabolism, etc). One interesting

---

[29] The easiest way to demonstrate an inflammatory response is to slap hard on the inner forearm with your three fingers. The area immediately turns red in response to the trauma. It also feels warmer and is painful enough to dissuade repetitions.

INFLAMMATION

- ❑ It is a localized, protective event elicited by injury.
- ❑ Inflammation serves to destroy or wall off both the injurious agents and the injured tissue.
- ❑ The inflammatory process includes:
  - tissue based response triggered by recognition of microbial penetration,
  - recruitment of macrophages, PMNs, and DCs, and unleashing their molecular arsenal to kill the invading microbe,
  - dispatching of APCs to the draining lymph node,
  - liquefaction of surrounding tissues to prevent microbial spread, and
  - healing of tissue damaged by the infectious agent or the host response.
- ❑ Inflammation is characterized by:
  - rubor (redness) due to increased blood supply,
  - calor (heat) caused partly by the influx of blood and partly by the release of cytokines and chemotaxins,
  - tumor (swelling) due to increased capillary permeability and fluid influx,
  - dolor (pain) due to release of bioactive peptides by neuronal cells, and
  - loss of function of the affected organ or part.
- ❑ It is induced by pro-inflammatory mediators such as:
  - chemokines (IL-8, monocyte chemotactic protein, RANTES),
  - cytokines (TNF-α, IL-1, IL-6, IFN-γ, TGF-β),
  - components of the complement cascade (C3a, C5a),
  - plasma mediators (bradykinin, fibrinopeptides), and
  - lipid mediators (metabolites of the archidonic pathway).
- ❑ The resolution of inflammation is promoted by:
  - serine protease inhibitor released by macrophages,
  - endogenous anti-inflammatory mediators such as adrenaline and noradrenaline,
  - cAMP,
  - annexin-1,
  - lipoxins and cyclopentones, and
  - TGF-β.

---

systemic effect of these pro-inflammatory cytokines is an increase in the number of leukocytes in circulation (the extra leukocytes are called in from the bone marrow) and the recruitment of immature DCs to the site of infection. DCs are potent APCs, and they help prepare for the next phase of defence — the adaptive immune response.

❑ **Components of the complement cascade.** C3a and C5a released as a result of activation of complement are potent mediators of inflammation. Binding of these molecules to receptors on mast cells degranulates them, releasing histamine and other pharmacologically active mediators. These mediators cause an increase in the capillary diameter (vasodilation), increased motility of phagocytes, and an increased influx of fluids to the site of infection. This influx allows antibodies, enzymes, and phagocytes to enter the site of inflammation.

❑ **Plasma mediators.** Endothelial damage starts a cascade of events in the kinin enzyme system that leads to the formation of bradykinin. This is a potent vasoactive peptide that increases vascular permeability, causes smooth muscle contraction, and induces pain. Similarly, damage to blood vessels starts the fibrinogen cascade to help form a clot, minimize loss of blood, and isolate the damaged area. One of the by-products of this cascade is the formation of fibrinopeptides that act as chemoattractants and further increase vascular permeablilty.

❑ **Lipid inflammatory mediators.** Phagocytes release a variety of molecules in response to infectious challenge, including metobolites of the archidonic pathway such as leukotrienes, prostaglandins, PAF, and thromboxane. Leukotrienes cause smooth muscle contraction and are potent chemoattractants, whereas prostaglandins induce chemotaxis and vasodilation. Thromboxane causes platelet aggregation and blood vessel constriction.

Thus, a characteristic inflammatory response results in

- ❑ **Increased blood supply** to and resultant reddening of the affected area (this reddening is also referred to as erythema).
- ❑ **Increased capillary permeability** that causes swelling, ie, oedema, which is partially a result of the retraction of endothelial cells that normally line blood vessels. The increased permeability allows larger molecules normally incapable of penetrating the endothelium to reach the site of infection/injury. This enables various soluble mediators of immunity to reach the affected site.
- ❑ **Migration of leukocytes** to the affected area. It is facilitated by newly expressed adhesion molecules on the endothelial cells lining the blood vessels.
- ❑ **Local increase in temperature and pain**. The increase in temperature is partly due to increased blood supply and in part due to the effect of the different chemicals (cytokines, chemotaxins, etc) released in the area. Together, the inflammatory response may result in the **loss of function** of the affected body part.

This achieves a two-fold objective.

- ❑ It limits the exposure of tissue to the external environment (therefore limiting entry of potentially harmful agents).
- ❑ It walls off the damaged area so that any harmful agent that may gain entry cannot easily spread to other parts of the body.

Acute inflammation (ie, inflammation that lasts from a few hours to a few days) is generally associated with a systemic response known as the acute phase reaction, and is normally self-limiting. Chronic inflammation (ie, inflammation that persists beyond 10–14 days) develops because of pathogen persistence or chronic activation of the immune system, eg, infection with *M. tuberculosis* that is resistant to digestion by phagocytes, autoimmune disorders, or some cancers. Chronic inflammation leads to an accumulation and activation of macrophages. This chronic activation also results in the activation of fibroblasts and production collagen, leading to fibrosis at the inflamed site. Formation of such scar tissue (eg, in the joints) can interfere with normal function and precipitate diseases. Chronic inflammation can also lead to granuloma formation (chapter 15). Granuloma is a characteristic nodular mass consisting of a central area of activated macrophages surrounded by activated lymphocytes. Multi-nucleated giant cells consisting of fused macrophages form the centre of these nodules. They are surrounded by large macrophages, that because of their resemblance to epithelial cells, are called epitheloid cells. In a way, this is a protective response, since the damaging pathogen is effectively isolated from the rest of the tissue. In the case of tuberculosis, cells in the centre of the granulomas die, giving a characteristic cheesy appearance of diagnostic significance.

Prolonged inflammation ceases to be beneficial and instead has deleterious effects. Dysregulated production of pro-inflammatory cytokines such as TNF-α and IL-1 can lead to acute systemic shock, resulting in capillary leakage, lowering of blood pressure, and organ failure. It is often fatal. Hence in the later stages of the inflammatory response, counter-regulatory molecules are produced to restore the immunological equilibrium. The resolution of inflammation is a highly controlled and coordinated process that suppresses pro-inflammatory gene expression, leukocyte activation and migration, and is followed by enhanced clearance of cell debris and apoptotic cells by phagocytes. The molecules and signals involved in this process are still being elucidated. The process of resolution begins with the death and removal of microbes and their products by the macrophages. Neutrophils initiate the process by triggering the production of anti-inflammatory lipoxins by tissue cells.

- ❑ **Lipoxins** are extremely potent endogenous lipid anti-inflammatory mediators. They seem to act early in the process of resolution.
  - • They inhibit neutrophil and eosinophil activation and migration.
  - • Lipoxins suppress the release of superoxide anions by neutrophils.

- They dampen genes involved in adhesion molecule expression and activation.
- They inhibit secretion of chemotactic IL-8.

❏ Macrophages secrete a **serine protease inhibitor** that is expressed late after exposure to microbial products or cytokines. It suppresses ROI production and elastase secretion by neutrophils. It also promotes tissue healing.

❏ Systemic production of **endogenous anti-inflammatory molecules** such as

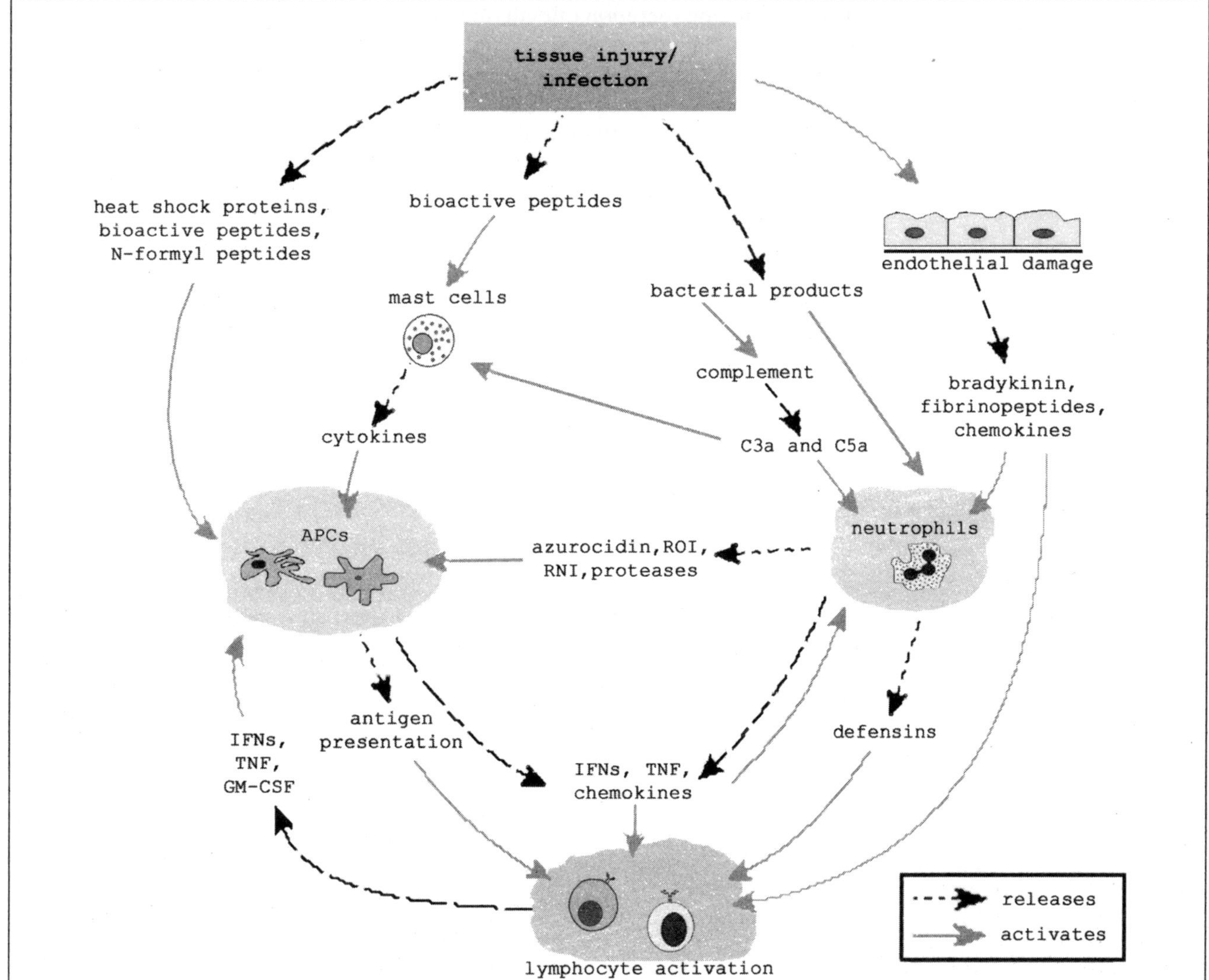

Figure 2.10 A complex interplay of factors is responsible for the initiation of the inflammatory response. *The inflammatory response is a well-orchestrated protective event involving multiple cell types. Each cell type gets activated by chemical signals released by other cell types and in turn releases factors that activate/recruit still other cell types. Chemical signals released by tissues injured either by physical trauma or bacterial invasion trigger the inflammatory response. Infection results in the activation of the complement cascade and release of chemotactic C3a and C5a. Release of bradykinins and fibrinopeptides by the damaged endothelial cells along with chemokines released at the site of injury results in the recruitment of neutrophils, the first cells to arrive at site of injury. Neutrophils express PAMPs and are activated by the bacterial infection. Bioactive peptides released as a result of tissue injury also activate mast cells in the vicinity, causing their degranulation. Pharmacological mediators released by the mast cells result in the further recruitment of neutrophils, immature DCs, and macrophages. Heat shock proteins, neuropeptides, and intracellular contents released by dead or dying tissue cells or N-formyl peptides that are the signature molecules of bacterial metabolism activate the immature DCs and phagocytic cells through the engagement of PRRs. ROI, RNI, azurocidin, etc produced by neutrophils enhance the activities of the macrophages and immature DCs. Antigen capture, transport, and presentation by the DCs activates naïve T cells, while defensins liberated by neutrophils recruit memory T lymphocytes to the developing response. Both the phagocytic cells and lymphocytes cross-regulate each other's activation via cytokines. Thus, through a well-coordinated response the body rids itself of the challenging agent and, at the same time, arms the adaptive immune system for future challenges (Adapted from Nature (2002) 420:346).*

adrenaline, noradrenaline, and 5-hydroxytryptamine reduce vascular leakage. This helps reduce inflammation since reduced vascular leakage stops fresh neutrophils from entering the site.

❑ **cAMP**, induced by several hormones, inflammatory mediators, and cytokines, has a central role in dampening the inflammatory response. It has multiple functions.
- It suppresses the release of histamine and leukotrienes from mast cells, monocytes, and neutrophils.
- It inhibits the secretion of cytokines and NO from macrophages.
- It inhibits the release of lysosomal enzymes and ROI from neutrophils.

❑ **Glucocorticoids**, produced by the adrenals, further help by inducing the expression of anti-inflammatory proteins like annexin-1.

❑ **Cyclopentenone** prostaglandins are anti-inflammatory prostaglandins with multiple functions found in the resolution phase of inflammation.
- Cyclopentenone prostaglandins decrease expression of adhesion molecules by endothelial cells.
- They inhibit macrophage/monocyte activation and migration.
- They decrease expression of NO synthase by the macrophages.
- Cyclopentenone prostaglandins increase myeloid cell apoptosis.
- Along with lipoxins, cyclopentone promote leukocyte apoptosis and their uptake and clearance by phagocytic cells.

❑ Uptake of apoptotic cells by phagocytes induces them to release the immunosuppressive cytokine TGF-β, promoting tissue repair.

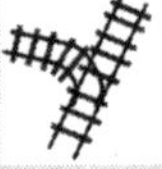

Mind your Immunity

The two major 'adaptive systems' of the body — the brain and the immune system — are involved in bi-directional communication (or cross-talk) that allows homeostasis (the maintenance of status quo). Neuroendocrine regulation of immune function is also essential for survival during stress or infection and to modulate immune responses in inflammatory diseases. The brain, or more specifically the **C**entral **N**ervous **S**ystem (CNS), regulates the immune system through two major pathways — the HPA axis and the sympathetic nervous system. CNS can also regulate the immune system via peripheral nerves with release of neuropeptides and locally produced corticotrophin-releasing hormone.

The main components of the HPA axis are the paraventricular nucleus in the hypothalamus, the anterior pituitary gland, and the adrenal glands. Corticotrophin-releasing hormone secreted by the paraventricular nucleus stimulates release of adrenocorticotropin hormone (ACTH) by the anterior pituitary gland, which induces the adrenal glands to produce and secrete glucocorticoids in plasma. Cells of the immune system express receptors for glucocorticoids. Binding of the glucocorticoid to its receptor leads to the translocation of this receptor to the nucleus, where it can modulate gene expression by binding to various transcription factors. Glucocorticoids have an anti-inflammatory effect on the immune system.

❑ They suppress the expression of pro-inflammatory cytokines such as IL-1, IL-2, IL-6, IL-8, IL-11, IL-12, TNF-α, IFN-γ, and GM-CSF.

❑ Glucocorticoids upregulate expression of anti-inflammatory cytokines like IL-10 and IL-4.

❑ They decrease neutrophil and macrophage migration by
- repressing the expression of adhesion molecules such as ICAM-1 and E-selectin on endothelial cells.
- decreasing expression of chemokines like IL-8, RANTES, and MCPs.

❑ Glucocorticoids suppress synthesis of pro-inflammatory mediators like prostaglandins and NO at the site of inflammation.

❑ They promote the rapid transport of the anti-inflammatory molecule annexin-1 from the cytoplasm to the surface of cells and also upregulate its synthesis.

The catecholamines norepinephrine (also called noradrenaline) and epinephrine are the principal end products of the sympathetic nervous system. The sympathetic nervous system modulates local immune responses via these neurotransmitters. Noradrenergic sympathetic nerve fibres run from the CNS to primary and secondary lymphoid organs. These nerve terminals make synaptic-like connections with neighbouring immune cells by releasing norepinephrine. B cells, T cells, NK cells, neutrophils, and macrophages have been shown to express adrenoreceptors that bind norepinephrine. Locally released norepinephrine or circulating epinephrine released by the sympathetic nervous system can affect lymphocyte trafficking, circulation, and proliferation. They also modulate cytokine production and the functional activity of different lymphoid cells. Both B and T cell differentiation and proliferation has been shown to be influenced by norepinephrine. Microbes, or their products like LPS, can influence the turnover of norepinephrine in lymphoid organs. Both epinephrine and norepinephrine were originally thought to have immunosuppressive effects. Recent data suggests that they may be immunostimulatory or immunosuppressive, depending upon the location and the stage of development of the target cells.

The immune system in turn signals the CNS through cytokines. Cytokine receptors are expressed on cells of the CNS, peripheral nerves, and ganglia and can influence neuronal survival, growth, and differentiation. Through their receptors, cytokines can also influence peripheral nerve activity and neurotransmitter release. Thus, neuronal cells respond to IL-2 treatment by enhanced neurite growth *in vitro*. IL-1, IL-2, IL-6, and TNF-α have all been shown to influence norepinephrine release. They signal the brain to trigger the activation of HPA axis and sympathetic nervous system (fig. 2.S1).

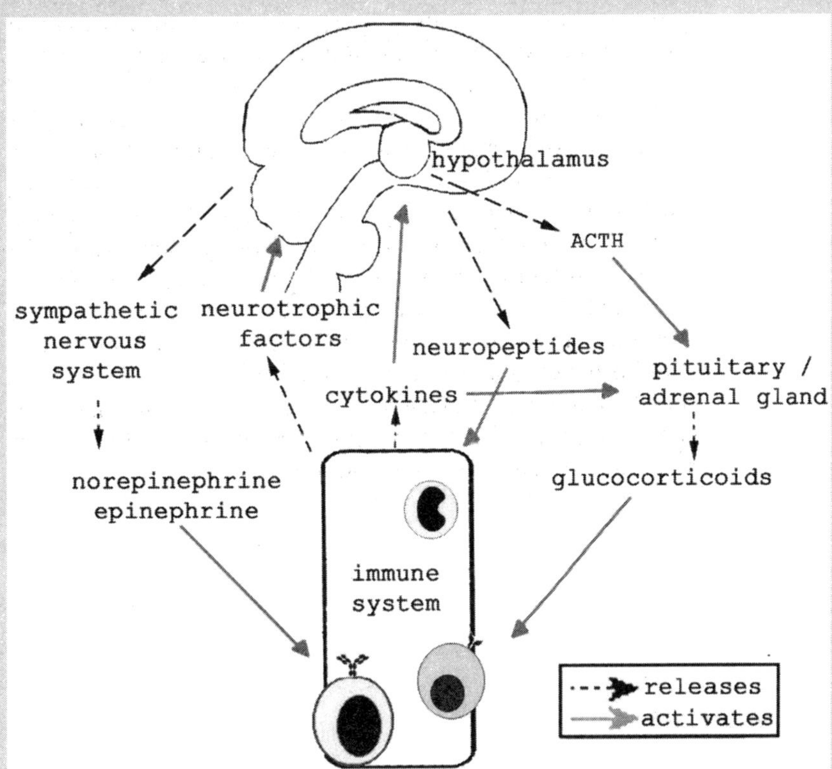

Figure 2.S.1 The CNS — through the HPA axis and sympathetic nervous system — and the immune system can communicate and influence each other. The neuroendocrine system regulates the functioning of the immune system through the release of ACTH (adrenocorticotropin hormone) glucocorticoids, epinephrine, and norepinephrine. Cytokines and neurotrophic factors secreted by the immune system, on the other hand, influence neuroendocrine functioning.

2.3.2 Acute Phase Reaction

Acute phase reaction is the set of immediate inflammatory responses initiated by PRRs. Recognition and engagement of PRRs by PAMPs induce host responses that localize the spread of infection and enhance systemic resistance to infection. **The acute phase response is a systemic response initiated by a sudden rise in circulating cytokines such as IL-1, IL-6, and TNF-α.** These cytokines act on the brain, the neuroendocrine system, and on other tissues and organs, leading to fever and profound hormonal and metabolic changes. The **H**ypothalamus-**P**ituitary **A**drenal (HPA) axis is then activated and serves as the primary regulator of immune and inflammatory reactions. Insulin, glucagon, and catecholeamine levels rise. Activation of HPA also leads to the release of glucocorticoids by adrenal glands. Bone marrow activity and leukocyte function are high, so the number of circulatory leukocytes increases dramatically. The liver initiates rapid production of acute phase proteins with a parallel decrease in the production of other proteins such as albumin and transerythrin[30]. These are a group of about 20 proteins which include $\alpha 1$ acid-glycoprotein, serum amyloid A and P, $\alpha 2$ macroglobulin, PRRs (C-reactive protein, LBP, MBL, SP-A and -D), fibrinogen, some complement components, enzyme inhibitors, and anti-inflammatory proteins whose serum concentration increases several hundred- to thousand-fold within 24–48 hours. Many of the acute phase proteins can bind a broad range of pathogens, and hence, they equip the body for antimicrobial defence. They also cause increased synthesis of pro-inflammatory cytokines (IL-1, IL-6, TNF-α) in the brain, resulting in pyrexia. Others are serine/cysteine protease inhibitors responsible for inactivating the proteolytic enzymes secreted during the inflammatory response, and with anti-inflammatory proteins, help in limiting inflammation.

The thymus is dramatically affected by the acute phase response, which is accompanied by profound neuroendocrine and metabolic changes. The most striking effect of the glucocorticoids on the immune system is the induction of apoptosis in the thymus. In concert with glucocorticoids, elevated catecholamine levels selectively suppress immune responses. This temporary suppression of specific immunity might serve to protect the body from adverse immune reactions that could be otherwise generated. The acute phase reaction may be regarded as an emergency response that represents a switch of the host defence from the adaptive immune response, which is slow to develop and is commanded by the thymus and T lymphocytes, to a less specific but more rapid and intense reaction. Acute phase proteins, therefore, provide enhanced protection against micro-organisms and modify inflammatory responses by affecting cell trafficking and mediator release.

[30] The acute phase response is an expensive, energy consuming event, which explains the drained feeling that a bout of fever can leave.

Complement

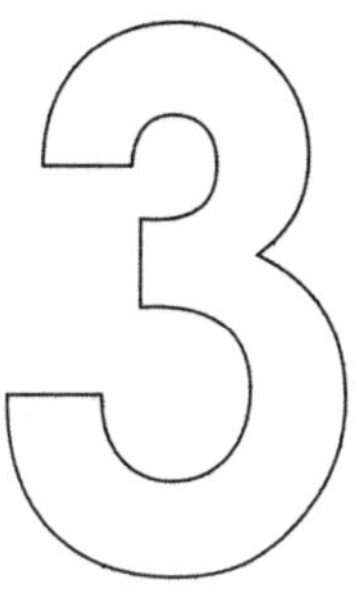

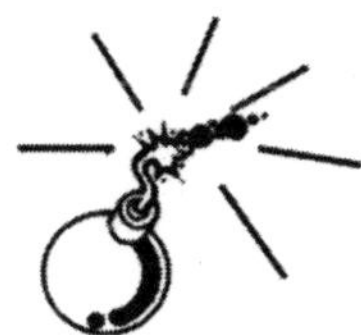

All it took was one kiss one touch
Like a long line of dominoes
I'm fallin' in love
It's a physical, spiritual, chemical strong attraction
Girl, you've started an unstoppable chain reaction

       — Paul Brandt, *Chain Reaction*

C1EI: C1 esterase inhibitor
C1INH: C1 inhibitor
C4bp: C4 binding protein
CR1:   Complement receptor 1
CR2:   Complement receptor 2
DAF: Decay accelerating factor
FDCs: Follicular dendritic cells
FHL-1:   Factor H-like protein-1
HRF: Homologous restriction factor
Ig: Immunoglobulin
KO: Knock out
MAC: Membrane attack complex
MA-p19:   MBL-associated protein of 19 KD
MASPs: Mannose-binding lectin-associated serine proteases
MBL: Mannose-binding lectin
MCP: Membrane cofactor protein
MCP-1:   Macrophage chemoattractant protein-1
RCA: Regulation of complement activation
SCID: Severe combined immunodeficiency
Serpins: Serine protease inhibitors
SLE: Systemic lupus erythematosus
sMAP: Small MBL-associated protein

3.1 Introduction

The term 'complement' is used to describe a complex group of thirty or so heat labile, sequentially interacting proteins and glycoproteins found in the blood, plasma, and cell surfaces of all vertebrates. Complement was originally thought to be a single component that *complemented* an antibody's antibacterial activity. Immunology has come a long way since; it is now well established that complement components and their receptors are important in a variety of interrelated physiological activities such as augmentation of innate and adaptive immune responses and aiding in apoptotic cell clearance (section 3.6).

Complement activation is a cascading[1] and sequential process. Each protein in the cascade activates the next one. Many components exist as proenzymes, ie, the inactive or nearly inactive precursors of enzymes, and they require conversion to the active form by proteolytic cleavage. When activated, several become serine proteases that cleave and activate the next component in the cascade. **The key event in complement activation is the formation of the enzyme C3-convertase which cleaves C3.** This activation can occur through three different pathways (fig. 3.1). The downstream events following C3 cleavage — called the terminal pathway — can result in the lysis of the target cell[2]. The three different pathways that can activate C3 are:

- the classical pathway,
- the MBL (**M**annose-**B**inding **L**ectin) pathway, and
- the alternative pathway.

The nomenclature of complement proteins is far from logical. The letter C followed by a number designates all classical pathway proteins. Unfortunately, numerical insanity reigns supreme, since the numbering has been in the order of discovery, not reaction. Native molecules are labelled C1 to C9, and the products formed are named by adding lower case letters (C4a, C3b, etc). The smaller fraction is generally labelled 'a' while the larger is designated 'b', although C2 is an exception. C2a is the larger fragment, C2b is the smaller. Proteins of the alternative pathway are named factors, followed by a letter. The proteins of the MBL pathway are MASPs (for **M**annose-binding lectin-**A**ssociated **S**erine **P**roteases) followed by a number.

Complement components, except C1, are primarily synthesized by liver cells, although other cells such as tissue macrophages, monocytes, fibroblasts, epithelial and endothelial cells, adipocytes, and astrocytes also synthesize them. Interestingly, even neurons are involved in their synthesis. C1 is primarily synthesized by the epithelium of the gastrointestinal and urinogenital tracts. Inflammation increases the synthesis of complement components, probably as a result of the IL-1 and IFN-γ produced during inflammation. Complement proteins appear in the blood during foetal development, before circulating antibodies put in their appearance. This probably reflects complement's evolutionary history — phagocytic cells and complement were major defence mechanisms of vertebrates before they developed the capacity for antibody production.

3.2 The Classical Pathway

The first step in the classical pathway is the binding and activation of C1. The prototypical activator of C1 is an antibody bound to its homologous antigen. All Immunoglobulin (Ig) isotypes, however, are not capable of binding C1. Only **IgG1, IgG2, IgG3, and IgM antibodies can activate the classical complement cascade.**

3.2.1 Binding and Activation of C1

C1 consists of three subunits — C1q, C1r, and C1s — that are held together by Ca^{2+} ions. C1q is a 400 KD protein itself made of six subunits, each subunit consisting

---

[1] That is it is like a waterfall – increasing in strength as the reaction proceeds; this is achieved by built-in activation where each activated component has the potential to activate many molecules of the next component.

[2] Erythrocyte lysis was one of the first observed effects of complement. It is still used in evaluating and/or demonstrating its effect.

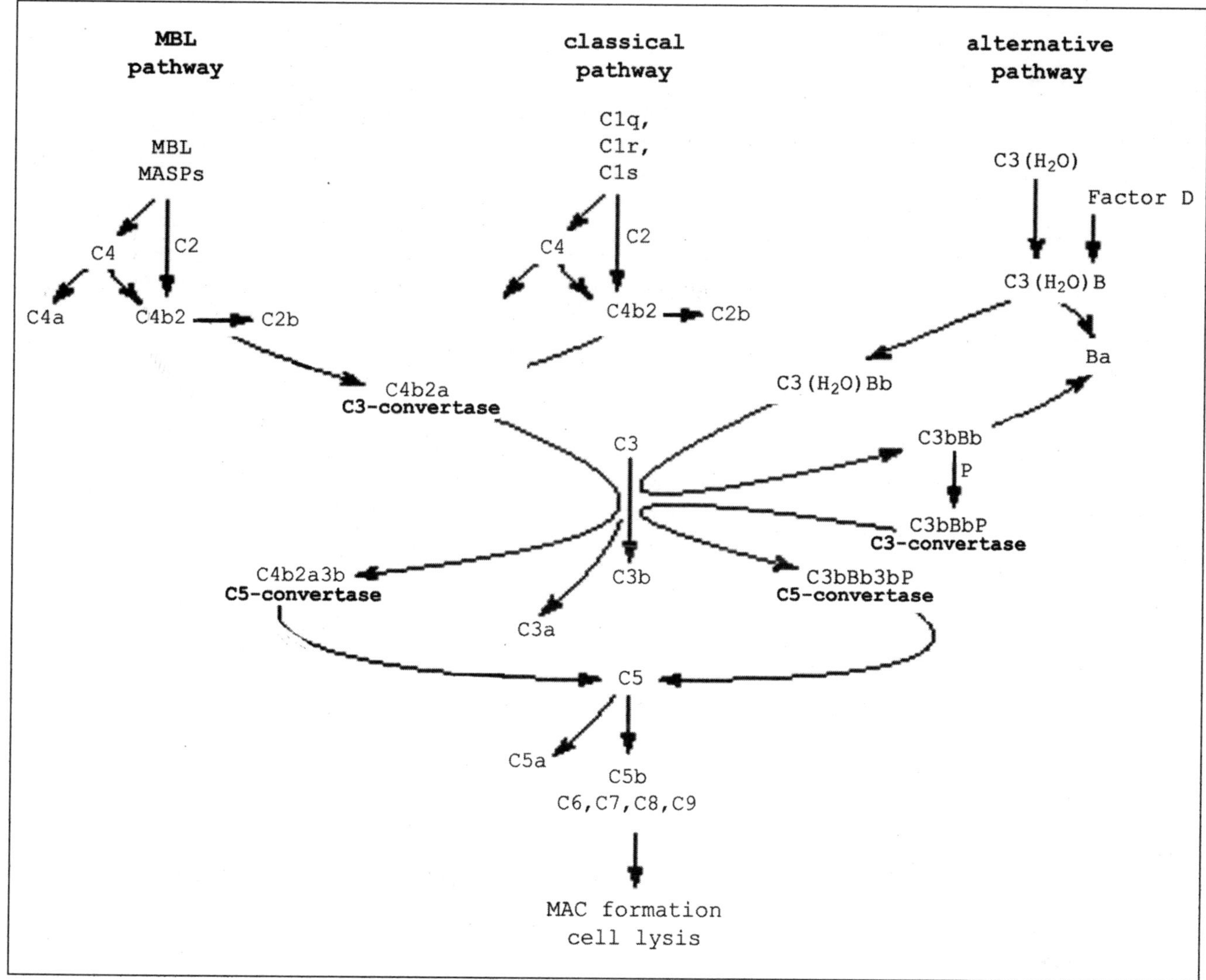

Figure 3.1 *Three different pathways can result in complement activation; C3 activation is the central event common to these pathways, and they share some of the downstream events that can lead to lysis of the target cell. Binding of C1q, a subunit of C1, to antigen-bound antibody results in the activation of the classical pathway. Activated C1q activates C1r, and later, C1s. Activated C1s cleaves C4 and C2 to yield C4b2a — the classical C3-convertase. C4b2a cleaves a molecule of C3 to yield C4b2a3b, the classical pathway C5-convertase. The second pathway of complement activation, the MBL pathway, is activated by binding of MBL or ficolins to structures on microbial surfaces. This binding activates MASPs and results in C4 cleavage. The resultant C4b binds C2 and is also cleaved by MASPs to yield the classical C3-convertase C4b2a. The classical and MBL pathways merge beyond this point. The alternative pathway of complement activation is initiated by microbial cell wall constituents such as LPS. Cell-bound or fluid phase hydrolyzed C3, C3(H₂O), binds Factor B and results in the formation of a few molecules of C3b. The hydrolyzed C3 binds Factor B and makes it susceptible to the action of Factor D. Cleavage of C3b-bound Factor B yields C3bBb — the alternative C3-convertase. This complex is unstable; properdin stabilizes the complex. C3bBb3bP — the C5-convertase of the alternative pathway — is formed when one more molecule of C3b binds to C3-convertase. Irrespective of the initial pathway of activation, the terminal pathway begins with the cleavage of C5 to yield C5a and C5b. C5b combines sequentially with C6, C7, and C8. The C5b678 complex causes polymerization of C9 and formation of the Membrane Attack Complex (MAC). Insertion of MAC into the target cell membrane allows free exchange of electrolytes and water through its channel, destroying the osmotic stability of the cell and resulting in lysis.*

of three polypeptide chains. When assembled, the polyprotein resembles a bunch of six tulips or pods (fig. 3.2). C1r and C1s are smaller (83 KD) proteins that have catalytic domains which allow them to act as serine proteases and interacting domains that facilitate their interaction with each other or with C1q. They exist in serum as 'S' shaped C1r2s2 tetramers. Binding to C1q changes the 'S' configuration to that of the figure '8' and yields the C1qr2s2 complex.

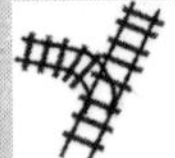

Wasted by Waste: C1q and Autoimmunity

C1q had been shown to bind to monocytes, PMNs, B lymphocytes, platelets, endothelial cells, and fibroblasts, suggesting the existence of protein receptors. Identifying these receptors (C1qRs) was difficult because of the sticky nature of C1q; however, a number of receptors have now been identified.

❑ Two intracellular proteins that may be found on the cell surfaces of damaged or apoptotic cells have been shown to be C1qRs. One is calreticulin, a chaperone protein, and the other, a mitochondrial matrix protein. They have been shown to bind both C1q and MBL. These proteins bind C1q, and the complex then associates with CD91, a signalling molecule that drives apoptotic cell phagocytosis.

❑ Another C1q binding molecule has recently been found to be expressed on phagocytic cells and is called C1qRp (C1qR of phagocytosis).

❑ CR1 (Complement Receptor 1; CD35) has also been shown to bind C1q.

C1q helps remove damaged or apoptotic cells by tagging them for removal by phagocytes or erythrocytes. These damaged tissue cells are thought to be the major source of autoantigens. C1q deficiency has been shown to be a greater risk factor for developing autoimmune diseases than the deficiency of any other complement components. C1q seems to be especially important in the development of SLE (**S**ystemic **L**upus **E**rythematosus), an autoimmune disease with severe and multiple manifestations. There is an almost 100% correlation between C1q deficiency and the development of SLE, although a lack of C4 can also cause the disease. The role of complement components, especially C1q, in mediating the clearance of apoptotic cells has led to the hypothesis that SLE is a result of an antibody response to self-antigens, driven by the non-clearance of necrotic and apoptotic cells.

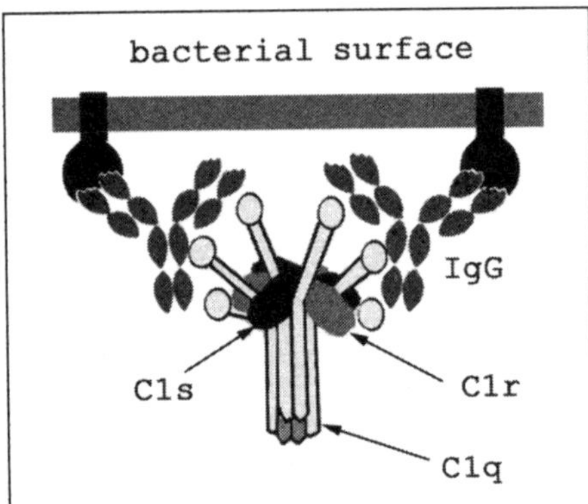

Figure 3.2 C1, the first component of the classical pathway, can bind antigen-bound immunoglobulin molecules. It consists of three subunits — C1q, C1r and C1s — that are held together by Ca²⁺ ions. C1q consists of six subunits that are associated together and resembles a bunch of tulips. One unit of C1q associates with two units each of C1r and C1s. The C1q binding site is not exposed on the native Ig; antigen binding causes a conformational change in the Ig molecule that exposes this binding site. At least two subunits of C1q have to be engaged for C1q activation. Activated C1q activates C1r, and later, C1s and converts them to serine proteases. C1s cleaves C2 to trigger the classical complement pathway.

❑ C1q binds to the C_H2 domain[3] of IgG or the C_H4 domain of IgM molecule via the tulip heads. Native Ig molecules have a relaxed conformation, and hence, the binding site is not accessible to C1q. Antigen binding causes a conformational change in the Ig molecule that exposes the binding site. C1q recognition and binding is stabilized mainly by electrostatic charges and hydrophobic interactions. Since binding of each individual pod is dependent on intrinsically weak interactions, multiple pods must be engaged for activation. A doublet of antigen-bound IgG molecules (two molecules lying side by side) is therefore necessary for C1q activation. A single molecule of IgM can activate C1q, provided that more than one subunit of the pentamer binds the antigen. C1q activation is not exclusively dependent upon antigen-antibody interaction. A variety of non-Ig molecules can activate C1. These include acute phase proteins (eg, C-reactive protein), certain bacterial glycolipids, monosodium urate crystals, LPS, nucleic acids, and chromatin.

[3] Ig molecules are made of two chains — light and heavy; each of these chains has different domains with differing functions, as explained in section 9.5.2.

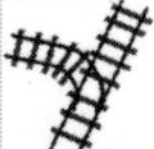

Serine Breakdown: Serine Proteases in the Complement Family

Many enzymes involved in physiological reactions such as digestive enzymes (trypsin, chymptrypsin, elastase), blood clotting enzymes (thrombin, plasmin), and several complement components belong to the trypsin family of serine proteases. The complement system consists of a number of proteases, nine of which are serine proteases[4]. These enzymes are modular proteins consisting of multiple independently folding domains. The nine serine proteases of the complement system are C1s, C1r, and the closely related MASP-1, -2, and -3, C3/C5-convertases, Factors B, D, and I. They have a very restricted specificity and low enzymatic activity. C1r, C1s, and MASPs are synthesized as inactive proenzymes or zymogens and are activated at the site of action. The activation process usually involves proteolytic cleavage of the proenzyme. The activity of C1r, C1s, and MASPs is regulated by the serpin C1INH (**C1 Inh**ibitor, see below). C2 and Factor B are also synthesized in an inactive form and are regulated by a group of complement proteins called the RCA (**R**egulation of **C**omplement **A**ctivation) proteins. In contrast, Factors D and I circulate in the active form and have no natural inhibitors.

Serpins are a class of **Ser**ine **P**roteases **In**hibitors that control the action of serine proteases. They mimic the three-dimensional structure of the normal substrate of the protease so that the enzyme binds the inhibitor instead of the substrate. The serine protease therefore cleaves the serpin, resulting in the formation of a covalent bond between the two molecules. The serpin then undergoes a massive allosteric change in its tertiary structure. The altered inhibitor now acts as a chaperone and targets the serpin:protease complex for degradation. The importance of serpins can be gauged from the fact that almost 20% of blood plasma proteins are serpins. C1INH, which controls C1 activity, is a serpin. Deficiency of C1INH causes hereditary angioedema. Apart from inactivating C1r and C1s, it also inactivates other serine proteases such as kallikrein of the kinin system and activated factor XI and XII of the coagulation system.

☐ Conformational change caused by the binding of C1q to a receptive surface leads to the autoactivation of C1r and its conversion to a serine protease; activated C1r cleaves C1s and converts it to a serinc csterase.

3.2.2 Formation of C4b2a Enzyme

Both C4 and C2 are substrates of activated C1s. C4 and C2 can also be cleaved by the MBL pathway. Thus, the classical and the MBL pathway converge at this point.

☐ Activated C1s cleaves C4 to form a larger C4b and smaller C4a[5] fragment; C4a is released to the fluid while C4b binds to a site in the vicinity of the molecule.

- Several C4 molecules can be cleaved by one molecule of activated C1s — this is the first amplification step in the cascade.
- C4 cleavage exposes a highly reactive thioester bond on the C4b molecule. This bond allows covalent binding of C4b to a site in the immediate vicinity of the molecule, eg, a cell membrane near the site of activation or to the C1qrs complex itself. If C4b is not rapidly and covalently bound, the thioester bond is hydrolyzed irreversibly, inactivating the molecule. This mechanism ensures that complement action remains localized to the surface of target cells.

☐ C2 binds to C4b in the presence of Mg^{2+}; C1s cleaves the bound C2[6] to yield a small C2b fragment and a larger C2a one.

- Free C2 is only weakly susceptible to the proteolytic action of C1s; the free C2a formed by this cleavage cannot bind C4b and hence has no role in the complement cascade.
- C2b released to the fluid is a prokinin that becomes biologically active upon enzymatic alteration by plasmin.
- Activated C2b leads to accumulation of fluids, and hence oedema, at the site of complement activation.

[4] Serine proteases are thus called because of the presence of a serine (often called super-reactive serine) in their active site.

[5] Although initially thought to be bioactive, no known function has been observed for C4a; research has also failed to identify a receptor for it.

[6] Naming of C2 fragments is a classic case of confusion. The large active fragment of C2 was originally designated C2a. It was later proposed that the nomenclature be reversed and brought in line with the other components (ie, rename the old C2a to C2b). In a recent meeting, however, the proposal has been laid to rest and it has (finally) been decided to continue with the old nomenclature.

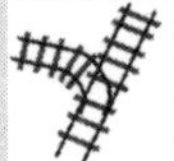

More than Just the Sum of its Parts: Multiple Functions of Complement Components

It is now well established that complement

❑ acts as an effector system in host defence against invading pathogens and a vital link between innate and adaptive immunity,
❑ contributes to inflammation through the release of pro-inflammatory mediators,
❑ may cause tissue injury at sites of inflammation, and
❑ is implicated in the pathogenesis of several autoimmune, ischaemic, and vascular diseases.

The existence of distinct expression profiles for various complement components in different tissues and at varying developmental stages led to studies that provided evidence for alternative functions of complement components, other than their traditionally assigned roles in inflammation and immunity.

Complement components have recently been implicated in bone development. C3 has been shown to be secreted by bone marrow derived stromal cells and primary osteoblastic cells *in vitro*. It has also been shown to promote differentiation of mononuclear progenitors to osteoclasts. The distribution pattern of C3, Factor B, Factor H, C5, C9, and properdin has suggested a potential role for these components in cartilage-bone transformation, matrix degradation and bone remodelling, and vascularization. Additionally, C1q has been recently suggested to be a possible marker for the differentiation of mesenchymal cells into chondrocytes during skeletal development.

The presence of almost all complement components and membrane regulators has been documented in the epithelial and vascular tissues lining the entire female reproductive tract. This prominent expression of DAF, MCP, CR1, and CD59 in reproductive epithelia and the sperm surface was thought to protect these tissues from autologous complement activation. It is now proposed that these regulators have a role in maintaining foeto-maternal tolerance during early pregnancy. There is also increasing evidence that the biosynthesis of several complement components and receptors in the reproductive tract is subject to fine hormonal regulation; it follows stage-specific expression patterns during the menstrual cycle, suggesting a role in the normal reproductive processes. Some tantalizing evidence points to a role of complement components in fertilization, but further research is needed to clarify this.

C3 has been known to be involved in limb regeneration in urodeles (amphibians such as axolots and newts). In mammals, the liver is one of the few organs capable of regeneration. TNF-α and IL-6 have been shown to be crucial in regulating the early stages of liver regeneration. Recent findings add C5a and its receptor C5aR to the list. Research further suggests a novel role for C5 in liver regeneration and implicates the complement system as an important immunoregulatory component of hepatic growth and homeostasis. C1q and its phagocytic receptor C1qp have been implicated in early haematopoietic development. Taken together, these results clearly show that a lot still remains to be discovered about complement and its components.

❑ C2a binds to C4b to form the classical pathway C3-convertase — C4b2a (fig. 3.3).
  • The C4b2a complex is unstable and dissociates with a half-life of less than five minutes.
  • Two plasma proteins, Factor H and **D**ecay **A**ccelerating **F**actor (DAF), interact with this complex to accelerate dissociation; the dissociated C4b is then cleaved to a biologically inactive form by Factor I (section 3.7).

3.2.3 C3 Cleavage

C3 is the most abundant of all complement components (1.2 gms/litre in blood) and has a pivotal role in complement-mediated immune functions. It is a 185 KD glycoprotein composed of two polypeptides linked by a disulphide bond.

❑ The classical pathway C3-convertase — C4b2a — cleaves C3 into a small C3a and a larger C3b fragment. Over 200 C3 molecules are split by a single molecule of C3-convertase, representing a major amplification loop.

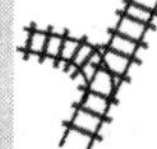

The Heart of the Matter:
Complement and Heart Disease

Complement is implicated in both atherosclerosis and ischaemic heart disease. 'Atherosclerosis' is derived from the Greek words *athero,* meaning gruel or paste, and *sclerosis,* meaning hardness. The narrowing and hardening of the coronary arteries that nourish the heart muscles restricts blood flow to the heart muscle. As a consequence, oxygen supply to the heart is inadequate, and this can result in cardiac arrest. Atherosclerosis seems to be a consequence of a chronic inflammatory process induced by the activation of macrophages, complement, and T lymphocytes. Current research indicates that complement may have an important role in both the initiation and progression of atherosclerosis.

❏ Continuous activation of complement seems to be an active part of the atherosclerotic process.
- There is evidence that autoantibodies against lipoproteins are deposited in the arterial walls and can lead to complement activation.
- Cholesterol, especially enzymatically modified LDL cholesterol, can activate complement by the alternative pathway.
- Cellular debris and subcellular particles of the arterial walls can also activate complement.

❏ Chronic complement activation has multiple effects on arterial walls.
- It acts as a proinflammatory stimulus.
- Its activation releases chemoattractants like C5a and MCP-1 (**M**acrophage **C**hemoattractant **P**rotein-**1**) which recruit monocytes to the site of activation.
- It induces cell injury and lysis, which further potentiate the inflammatory response.
- Sublytic assembly of MAC on smooth muscle cells and endothelial cells can induce their activation and proliferation, thus contributing to fibrosis of the arterial wall.

The narrowing of arteries caused by atherosclerosis can lead to ischaemia. Ischaemia is defined as an insufficient supply of blood to an organ, usually caused by a blocked artery. Tissues and organs deprived of oxygen are often severely damaged when revascularized. This phenomenon is known as ischaemia/reperfusion injury. Part of the damage is due to exposure of the hypoxic (ischaemic) tissue to oxygen when reperfused — the sudden increase in oxygen results in the formation of reactive oxygen radicals. A considerable body of evidence suggests that complement plays a key role in causing further damage during reperfusion and therefore contributes to the pathophysiology of ischaemic heart disease. Experimental models of acute myocardial infarction and autopsy specimens taken from acute myocardial infarction patients demonstrate that complement is selectively deposited in areas of infarction. Furthermore, inhibition of complement activation or depletion of complement components prior to myocardial reperfusion has been shown to reduce complement-mediated tissue injury in numerous animal models. The exact pathway of complement activation in ischaemia is unclear. There is evidence suggesting naturally occurring IgM antibodies may have a role in causing this damage. Therapeutic approaches to prevent ischaemic injury include:

❏ administration of C1INH (a naturally occurring inhibitor of classical and MBL pathways of complement activation),
❏ use of anti-MBL antibodies to control the lectin pathway, and
❏ administration of recombinant soluble CR1, or peptides derived from it, to mop up C3b, C4b, and C1q released during ischaemic injury.

❏ The smaller C3a, a multipotent molecule, is released in the fluid phase. It is called an anaphylatoxin, since it can mimic some effects of anaphylactic shock (chapter 15).
❏ The C3b fragment closest to the complex binds to C4b2a to form the final proteolytic complex, C5-convertase of the classical cascade — C4b2a3b; however, not all C3b molecules produced by C3 cleavage bind C4b2a, and they all end up with different fates.
- C3 is structurally and functionally homologous to C4.
- C3, like C4, has a reactive thioester bond that is exposed on cleavage and allows C3b to be covalently bound to appropriate surfaces; cleavage of covalently bound C3b by serum enzymes results in the formation of a number

of products (iC3b, C3c, C3d(g), etc) that are bio-active. These bioactive products exert their effect via receptors found on a variety of cells.

- Some C3b molecules may be deposited on membrane surfaces in the vicinity of the reaction and may be inactivated or further cleaved; the carbohydrate environment and the nature of the surface to which C3b is attached largely dictate whether inactivation or further amplification of the reaction occur.
- Some C3b molecules are released in the fluid phase and bind to and opsonize microbes in their vicinity.
- Some C3b molecules may bind Factor B and thus activate the alternative pathway. In contrast, C3b molecules that bind to Factor H become susceptible to Factor I which catabolizes them to inactive products.
- Unbound C3b molecules are rapidly inactivated by hydrolysis.

❑ The formation of C5-convertase results in the cascade entering the terminal pathway. C4b2a3b complex binds C5 and makes it susceptible to the activity of C2a; this C5-convertase of the classical pathway can hydrolyse both C3 and C5. Binding of additional molecules of C3b increases its affinity for C5.

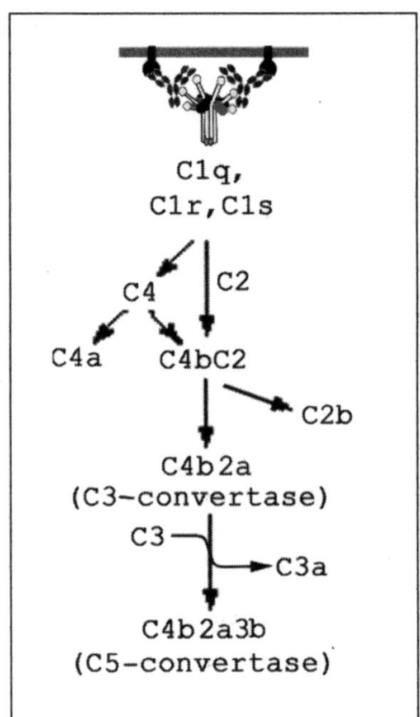

Figure 3.3 The classical pathway of complement activation is triggered when two subunits of C1q bind adjacent antigen-bound immunoglobulin molecules. Activation of C1q results in sequential activation of C1r and C1s. Activated C1s cleaves C4; C4a is released in the fluid phase while C4b binds C2. C1s also cleaves C4b-bound C2. C2b, a bioactive molecule, is released to the fluid phase while C2a remains bound to C4 to yield C4b2a — the classical pathway C3-convertase. The enzyme can rapidly cleave many molecules of C3. The bioactive C3a is released to the fluid phase. C3b binds the C4b2a complex to yield C4b2a3b — the classical pathway C5-convertase. With the formation of this final proteolytic complex the cascade enters the terminal pathway.

3.3 The Lectin Pathway of Complement Activation[7]

This is a relatively newly discovered pathway of complement activation. Mounting evidence supports the importance of this pathway in innate immunity. MBL deficiency has been shown to be associated with repeated and severe infections in some individuals.

[7] The nomenclature of this pathway is still to be settled. Although it is referred to as the lectin-binding pathway, this is not the best name. The term 'lectin-binding' can be presumed to imply that any lectin can activate complement. It would be more appropriate to call it the MBL pathway.

Tri n 'C':
The Key Complement Component

C3 is a key molecule of the complement cascade. It is central to all three pathways of complement activation and is probably the most versatile protein of this system. The molecule's structural features allow it to react with 25 different proteins. It arose early in evolution, about 700 million years ago, long before Igs put in their appearance. The recent development of C3 KO (**K**nock **O**ut) mice has greatly helped in understanding its importance in health and disease.

Human C3 is a heterodimer consisting of α and β chains held together by a single disulphide bond and non-covalent forces. Cleaving of C3 represents a major amplification step in the cascade. It is also the key event leading to target cell lysis. C3 is cleaved to C3a and C3b. Both these products of C3 cleavage are multifunctional molecules. C3a is a potent anaphylatoxin (see sidetrack 'Shock and Awe'), while C3b is associated with many complement functions. Native C3 has an internal thioester bond that is hidden inside a hydrophobic pocket and exposed only in the C3b fragment. This thioester bond has a half-life of 100 µs and can transiently participate in transacylation reactions with hydroxyl groups in its neighbourhood. Unlike native C3, C3b expresses multiple binding sites for various complement components, including C5, properdin, Factors B, H, and I, and **M**embrane **C**ofactor **P**rotein (MCP — no relation whatsoever of Macrophage Chemotactic Protein; CD46). Binding of these proteins leads to either the amplification (and formation of membrane attack complex) or inactivation of C3b (fig. 3.S1).

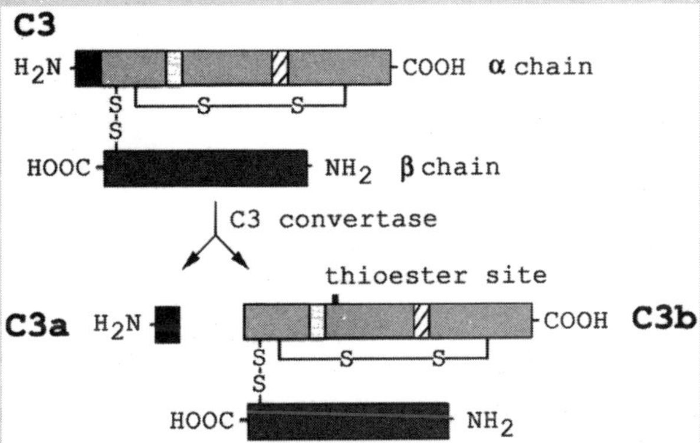

Figure 3.S1 Human C3 is a heterodimer consisting of an α and a β chain held together by a single disulphide bond and non-covalent forces. Cleavage of the molecule results in a large fragment, C3b, consisting of a fragment of the α chain and the whole β chain. The smaller fragment, C3a, is a powerful anaphylatoxin. C3 has an intramolecular thioester bond that is exposed only upon cleavage of the molecule and is present on the C3b fragment. This thioester bond can transiently participate in transacylation reactions with hydroxyl groups in its neighbourhood. C3b also has sites for binding to C5, properdin, Factors B, H, I, etc and can be cleaved further. These properties make the molecule highly versatile and central to the complement activation pathway.

The role of C3b or its fragments in immune responses is outlined below and summarized in fig. 3.S2.

❑ C3b[8] promotes opsonization, immune adherence, and phagocytosis.
- Binding of C3b or iC3b to receptors on phagocytic cells (CR1, CR3, or CR4) delivers the activation signal required for the phagocytosis of complement-coated bacteria.
- Aggregation of complement receptors via C3b or its split products is often associated with the early stages of phagocytosis and can trigger the oxidative burst and upregulation of FcγR-mediated phagocytic activity.
- Heterodimers of FcRs and CR1 or CR2 (cross-linked via their ligands IgG and C3b respectively) are much more effective than monomers in inducing phagocytosis.

❑ C3b can promote the interaction of APCs with T cells; binding of C3b or its fragments to their receptors forms a non-antigen-specific *second* bridge between the two cells.

❑ iC3b, a by-product of C3b cleavage, promotes killing by NK and K cells by holding the target cell in close proximity to these cells. It is especially important in ADCC.

---

[8] Not only C3b, but some of its fragments such as iC3b and iC3dg, can also bind complement receptors, and hence, they exert a similar effect.

❑ C3b has a critical role in normal immune complex catabolism. CR1, the C3b receptors on erythrocytes, bind complement-coated immune complexes; the bound complexes are subsequently removed by macrophages from the RBC surface without any damage to the erythrocytes as the RBCs pass through the spleen or liver sinusoids.

❑ C3b can enhance or inhibit B cell activation.
- Coligation of B cell antigen receptor and CR1/CR2 on B cells reduces the antigen threshold required for B cell activation.
- C3b-coated antigen is efficiently internalized and processed by B cells, resulting in enhanced and prolonged stimulation of T cells.
- Coligation of CR2 and FcγRII (the low affinity receptor for IgG) or cross-linking of CR2 on the surface of B cells enhances expression of costimulatory molecules by these cells.
- Monomeric C3b and iC3b are found to inhibit B cell activation by an unknown mechanism.
- When cross-linked to the B cell antigen receptor via immune complexes containing IgG antibodies, FcγRIIB downregulates antigen-mediated stimulation through a variety of mechanisms.

❑ C3b may have a role in the localization of immune complexes in germinal centres. Trapping of antigen in the follicles is found to be complement-dependent. It is therefore postulated that non-recirculating marginal zone B cells bind antigen-antibody-complement complexes via CR1, CR2, and FcRs, and transport these to FDCs in germinal centres (chapter 5).

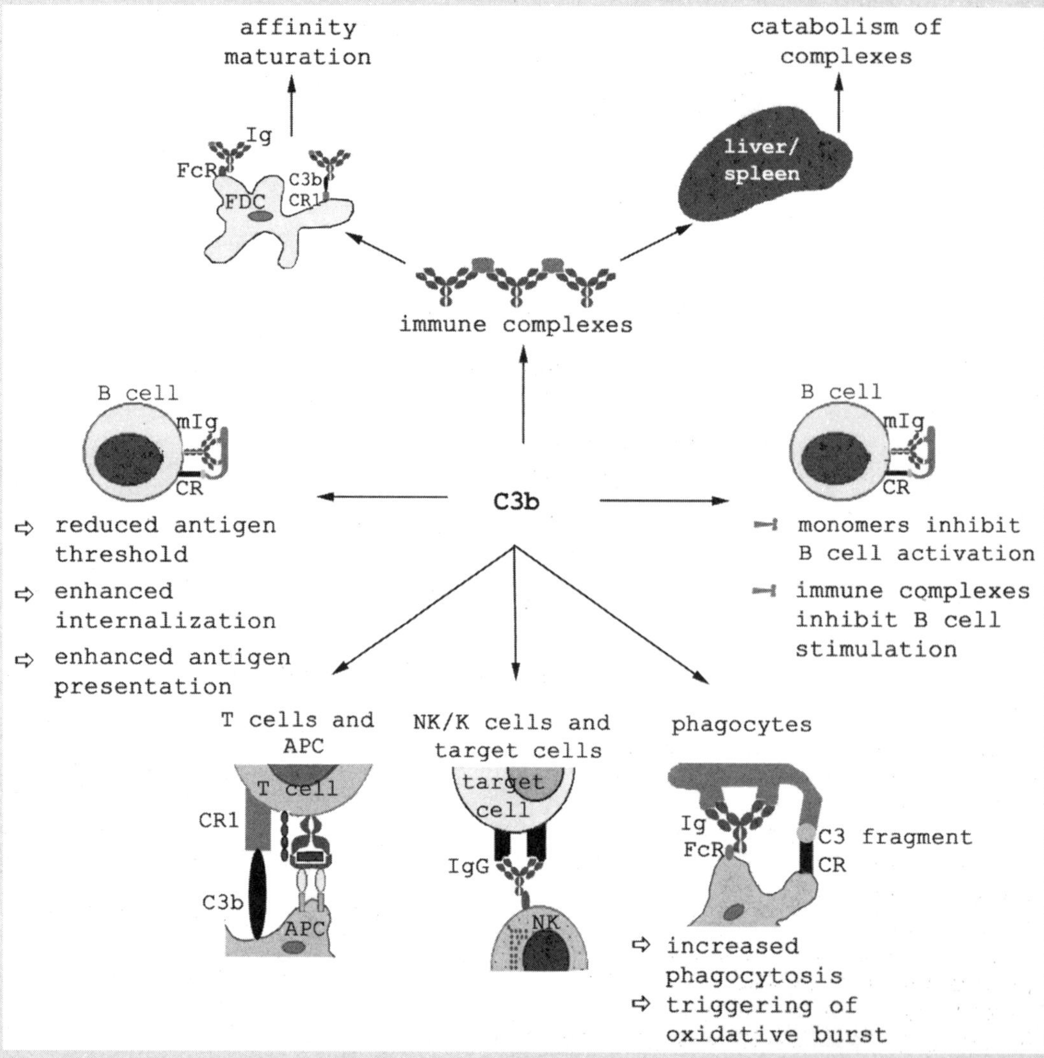

Figure 3.S2 Receptors for C3b or its cleavage products are expressed on multiple cell types and hence can affect their functioning.

3.3.1 *MBL Pathway Proteins*

The proteins of this pathway are essentially homologues of classical pathway components. The pathway is initiated by binding of a lectin — MBL — to carbohydrates.

❑ **MBL** is a C-type lectin, ie, it requires Ca^{2+} for binding to carbohydrates. It is a member of the collectin family of proteins, which includes C1q, MBL, surfactant proteins A and D, and the liver protein CL-1. The members of the collectin family have a collagen-like region and a carbohydrate recognition domain. **MBL can bind to an array of carbohydrate structures on the surfaces of microbes** (yeasts, bacteria, viruses, and parasitic protozoa). It is effective in recognizing microbial patterns formed by repetitive mannose or N-acetylglucoseamine residues. Hence, MBL preferentially recognizes glucans, lipophosphoglycans, or glycoinositol phospholipids with mannose, glucose, fucose, or N-acetylglucosamine as terminal hexoses. Such patterns are either absent or present in limited amounts in mammalian cell walls. Instead, mammalian cell walls have structures that terminate with sialic acid and are hence protected from MBL damage.

❑ **MASPs.** Three serine proteases are found to be associated with MBL and are called MASPs (MBL-Associated Serine Proteases-1, -2, and -3). The association between MBL and MASPs is Ca^{2+} dependent. MASP-1 and -2 are homologous to C1r and C1s. These serine proteases normally exist as zymogens and have to be converted to the active form. MASP-3 is an alternatively spliced version of MASP-1.

❑ **MA-p19** (**MBL-A**ssociated **p**rotein of **19** KD) or **sMAP** (**s**mall **MBL-A**ssociated **P**rotein) is a non-protease protein found associated with the MBL pathway. It is a truncated form of MASP-2. The exact role of this protein in the MBL pathway is yet to be elucidated.

❑ **Ficolins** are lectins that contain a collagen-like structure but recognize carbohydrates (N-acetyl glucosamine) via a fibrinogen-like structure. Complexes of ficolin and MASPs can also activate the MBL pathway.

3.3.2 *Activation and Progress of the MBL Pathway*

Since MBL and MASPs are homologues of C1q, C1r, and C1s, the MBL and classical pathways are very similar and result in the generation of C3-convertase of the classical pathway.

❑ Binding of MBL or ficolins to microbial surfaces activates the serine protease MASP-2; it cleaves C4 to C4a and C4b.

MBL PATHWAY OF COMPLEMENT ACTIVATION

MBL	Binding of MBL to microbial surfaces activates MASP-2
MASP-2	Cleaves C4 to C4a and C4b
C2	Binds to C4a
MASP-1/ -2	Cleave C4a bound C2 to C2a and C2b; C2b remains with C4a to form the classical pathway C3-convertase C4b2a

ALTERNATIVE PATHWAY OF COMPLEMENT ACTIVATION

C3	Spontaneously assumes a C3b-like conformation C3 (H_2O)
Factor B	Attaches to C3b-like C3 to yield C3bB
Factor D	C3bB is cleaved by Factor D to release the biologically inactive Ba, while Bb remains attached to C3b to form the alternative pathway C3-convertase C3bBb
Properdin	Attaches and stabilizes the convertase to yield C3bBbP
C3bBbP	Further cleaves molecules of C3 to release C3a; C3b attaches to the complex to form C3bBb3bP — alternative pathway C5-convertase
C3bBb3b	C5 cleavage and membrane attack follows the classical pathway route

❑ C2 binds to C4b and is cleaved by MASP-1 or MASP-2, resulting in the formation of the classical C3-convertase C4b2a.

❑ Further cleavage of C3 and formation of C5-convertase occurs by the classical pathway and sets the terminal pathway in motion.

❑ MASP-1 by itself has been shown to cleave C3; thus, the low levels of cleaved C3 required for the alternative pathway may be formed through the binding of MBL to receptive surfaces.

3.4 The Alternative Pathway of Complement Activation

The components of the alternative pathway bypass the initial sequences of the classical pathway and directly cleave C3.

3.4.1 Alternative Pathway Proteins[9]

The alternative pathway can function in the absence of IgM or IgG, and it is basically spontaneous[10]. It thus provides a means of non-specific resistance against infection without the participation of antibodies; hence, like the MBL pathway, the alternative pathway provides a true first line of defence against several infectious agents. The alternative pathway is thought to be a prototype of the classical pathway; the classical pathway may have developed later in evolution through gene duplication after or along with the development of antibodies. **LPS, teichoic acids of Gram-positive bacteria, zymosan of yeast cell walls[11], and the surface components of some animal parasites are capable of activating complement by the alternative pathway.** Igs that cannot fix complement by the classical pathway (IgE, IgA) can also activate the alternative pathway.

Serum proteins important in the initiation and progress of the alternative pathway are:

- **Factor B** (C3 proactivator) is a β globulin zymogen serine protease very similar to C2. It is even produced by a gene closely linked to the *C2* gene (fig. 7.7). Factor B is cleaved into Ba and Bb. Ba has no known biological activity, but Bb combines with and cleaves C3.
- **Factor D**, a γ globulin glycoproteinic enzyme found in serum in trace amounts, is a serine protease resembling activated C1s. An active enzyme, it can cleave Factor B only after it has combined with C3b. It is ineffective on free Factor B.
- **Properdin** is the protein that led to the discovery of the alternative pathway. The name is derived from the Latin word *perdere* — to destroy. Properdin is a γ globulin quatromer. It stabilizes the alternative pathway C3-convertase.
- **Factor H** is a regulator of the alternative pathway.

3.4.2 Activation and Progress of the Alternative Pathway

The first step in the alternative pathway is the formation of a few molecules of C3b. Native C3 has a thioester bond that tends to hydrolyse spontaneously at a very slow rate. Trace amounts of C3b can thus be found in normal serum and can activate the alternative pathway under appropriate conditions.

❑ The cell-bound or fluid phase hydrolyzed C3 (C3(H_2O)[12]) binds Factor B in the presence of Mg^{2+} ions; binding of B to C3b/C3(H_2O) exposes a site on Factor B recognized by Factor D.
- If C3b or C3(H_2O) attach to the surface of host cells, the molecules are quickly inactivated by sialic acids present on the surface of most mammalian cells.
- Microbial cell walls generally lack sialic acids, and deposition of C3b or C3(H_2O) can result in the 'switching on' of the alternative pathway.

[9] In a way, the name alternative pathway is now a misnomer, a hangover from the era when only two pathways were known to activate complement — the classical and the non-classical (ie, alternative).

[10] Although the alternative pathway can function in the absence of antibodies, it can also be activated by antigen-antibody complexes. Recent reports suggest that the joint inflammation observed in rheumatoid arthritis could be due to the activation of the alternative pathway by antibodies to the enzyme glucose phosphate isomerase.

[11] Zymosan is an insoluble preparation from yeast cell wall. It is a mixture of glucans, mannans, proteins, chitins, and lipids. Several key functional effects related to zymosan can be ascribed to its major component ß-glucan. A zymogen, by contrast, is a pro-enzyme.

[12] C3(H_2O) is also referred to as C3i.

- C3b formed by the classical or MBL pathway may act as the focus for the formation of alternative pathway convertase.
- ❑ Factor B is cleaved by Factor D to Ba and Bb. Ba is released, leaving behind the C3bBb/C3b(H$_2$O)Bb complex — the C3-convertase of the alternative pathway.
  - The complex is inherently unstable and is stabilized by properdin.
  - C3bBbP is an efficient C3-convertase that cleaves many molecules of C3; this step represents an amplification loop.
- ❑ An additional molecule of C3b associates with C3bBbP to form the C5-convertase of the alternative pathway (C3bBb3bP) (fig. 3.4). Once the C5-convertase is formed, the two pathways converge into the terminal pathway. C5 cleavage and membrane attack stage are set into motion, ultimately resulting in cell lysis.

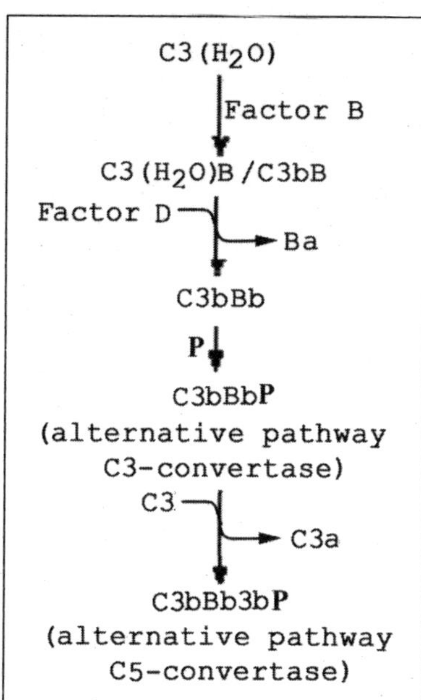

Figure 3.4 Multiple proteins are involved in the initiation and progress of the alternative pathway of complement activation. Native C3 has a thioester bond that tends to hydrolyse spontaneously at a very slow rate. C3b or C3(H$_2$O) formed as a result of this hydrolysis binds Factor B and makes it susceptible to the action of Factor D. Factor D cleaves Factor B to release Ba and yield C3bBb, the alternative pathway C3-convertase. Binding of properdin stabilizes the enzyme and allows the formation of further molecules of C3b. Association of an additional molecule of C3b with this complex yields the alternative pathway C5-convertase. The classical and alternative pathways merge beyond this point and share the terminal pathway.

3.5 The Terminal Pathway

Whatever the mode of formation of C5-convertase, its formation sets the terminal pathway in motion. Complement components C5 to C9 involved in the terminal pathway are called the MAC (**M**embrane **A**ttack **C**omplex) components. Except for C5, which is a structural homologue of C3 and C4, the remaining components of the terminal pathway are non-enzymatic, hydrophilic proteins that display a hydrophobic conformation on binding. C6, C7, the α and β subunits of C8, and C9 are all structurally and genetically related proteins.

- ❑ C5-convertase (whether C4b2a3b or C3bBb3bP) binds C5 and cleaves it to smaller C5a and larger C5b fragments; C5b binds C6.
  - C5a, an extremely potent anaphylatoxin (see sidetrack 'Shock and Awe'), is released in the fluid phase.
  - C5b is highly unstable and is inactivated within two minutes unless bound by C6.

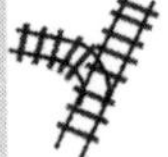

Shock and Awe: Anaphylatoxins

C3a and C5a are bioactive molecules formed by the cleavage of C3 and C5. C3a is a 77 amino acid non-glycosylated protein; C5a is a 74 amino acid protein bearing a complex oligosaccharide. Both C3a and C5a mimic some of the symptoms of anaphylactic shock (smooth muscle contraction, vasodilation, mast cell degranulation, etc) and are therefore called anaphylatoxins. Of the two, C5a is the more potent molecule; it is effective at concentrations of 10^{-12} M. Receptors for C3a and C5a (C3aR and C5aR) are expressed on mast cells, neutrophils, eosinophils, basophils, and monocytes. Anaphylatoxins regulate vasodilation, increase the permeability of small blood vessels, and can induce smooth muscle contraction. In macrophages, eosinophils, and neutrophils, they can trigger an oxidative burst. Both these molecules can also profoundly affect eosinophils. They regulate the synthesis of eosinophil cationic protein, increase eosinophil adhesion to endothelial cells, and influence eosinophil chemotactic migration. Both C3a and C5a can cause basophil and mast cells degranulation, leading to histamine release by these cells. C3a can stimulate serotonin release from platelets in guinea pigs and modulate the synthesis of IL-6 and TNF-α by B lymphocytes and monocytes. C3a can also induce mucus secretions by tracheal goblet cells[13] *in vitro*. C5a is a powerful chemoattractant for macrophages, neutrophils, basophils, mast cells, and activated B and T lymphocytes. It induces the production and secretion of leukotrienes[14] and IL-1 by macrophages.

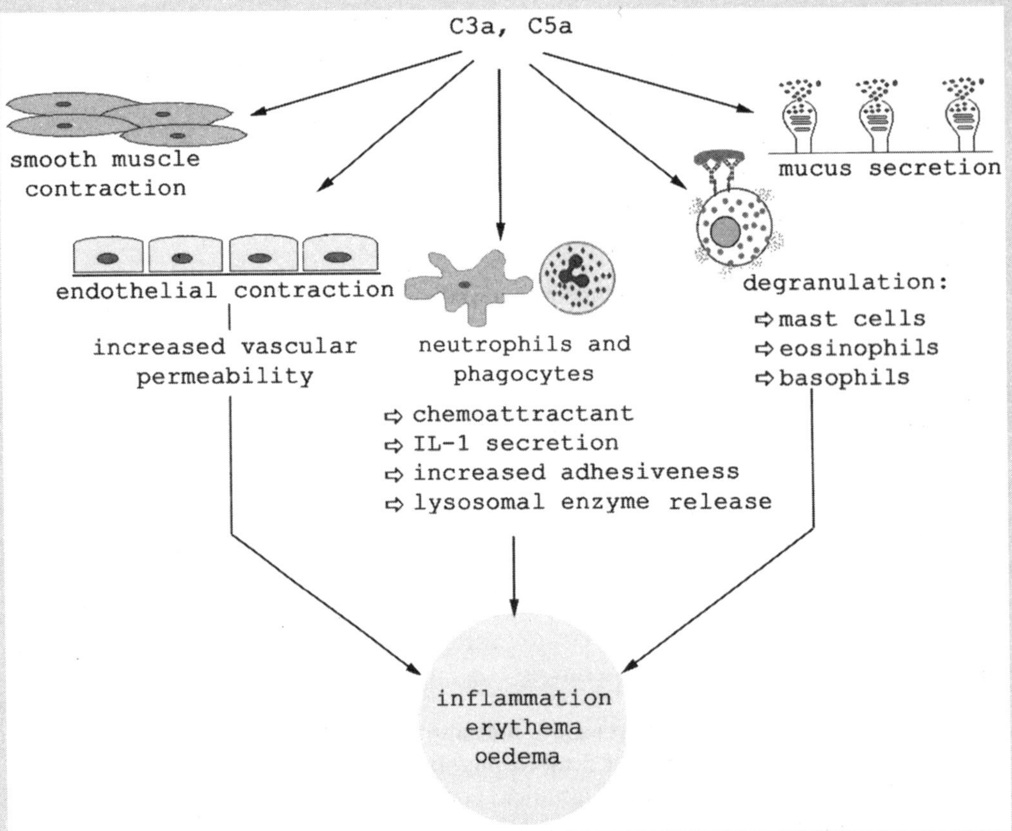

Figure 3.S3 C3a and C5a formed by the cleavage of C3 and C5 respectively are bioactive molecules that can augment the inflammatory response. They can also mimic some of the symptoms of allergies.

C3 and C5 cleavage results in a terminal arginine at the Carboxy– end. The properties of both C3a and C5a are critically dependent on this terminal arginine, and the active site lies in a short octapeptide sequence at this end. Carboxypeptidase N, present in serum, can remove the terminal

---

[13] Tracheal goblet cells are cells lining the trachea; they are responsible for mucus secretions. When you have a bad cold, these cells are working over-time!

[14] Leukotrienes are by-products of the arachidonate pathways. Those induced by complement components include prostaglandin E_2, leukotriene B4, and thromboxane. They have a range of effects similar to histamine.

arginine from these molecules and seems to be especially important in inactivating C3a. Recent evidence shows that another enzyme, carboxypeptidase R (also called carboxypeptidase U), is the key enzyme in the inactivation of C5a. C3adesarg, formed by removal of the terminal arginine, cannot bind to C3aR and is devoid of biological activity. C5adesarg can, however, bind to C5aR, and hence, it is capable of exerting considerable functional activity. Loss of the arginine leads to a loss of spasmogenic activity of C5a, even though chemotactic and other neutrophil-stimulating effects are retained, albeit at a reduced level. Being such potent molecules, the anaphylatoxins are implicated in a number of diseases, including septic shock, asthma, immune complex disease, and delayed-type of hypersensitivity.

CLASSICAL COMPLEMENT PATHWAY

C1	Consists of three subunits — C1q, C1r, and C1s; binding of two subunits of C1q triggers the classical pathway
C4	Activated C1s cleaves C4
C2	C2 binds to C4b; C1s cleaves C2 to form the classical pathway C3-convertase — C4b2a
C3	C3-convertase cleaves C3; C3b binds to C4b2a to yield the classical pathway C5-convertase — C4b2a3b
C5	C5 is cleaved by C5-convertase
C6 and C7	C5b gets sequentially attached by C6 and C7; C5b67 gets inserted into the lipid bilayer
C8	Consists of α, β, and γ subunits; C8β binds to C5b67, and both C8α and C8β get inserted into the lipid bilayer
C9	The amphophilic complex causes polymerization of C9 and formation of MAC; MAC lesions allow the outward passage of small molecules and inward passage of water, leading to cell lysis

❑ C5b6 binds one molecule of C7, causing a conformational change and transiently exposing a hydrophobic lipid-binding site; the C5b67 complex gets inserted in a membrane.
  - Up to this point, the reaction occurs in the fluid phase because of its hydrophilic nature; binding of C7 causes the complex to become hydrophobic.
  - In the absence of a membrane to insert into (as would happen on the surface of an immune complex), the C5b67 complex dissociates from the surface.
  - Under rare circumstances (in autoimmune disorders, for example), the dislodged complex attaches to neighbouring cells, causing the lysis of these 'innocent bystander' cells.
❑ The next step in MAC formation is the binding of C8 to the complex. C8 binds to C5b67 via its β subunit; C8α and C8β get inserted in the lipid bilayer (fig. 3.5).
  - C8 is an oligomeric protein consisting of three subunits — C8α, β and γ encoded by different genes; C8α and γ form a disulphide-linked dimer and C8β is non-covalently associated with that dimer.
  - The α subunit of C8 has multiple binding sites. It has sites for binding C8β and γ. A third site binds C9 and directs the incorporation of this component in MAC. It also has a site for the regulatory protein CD59 which inhibits the formation of MAC. A lipid-binding site is exposed upon binding of C8α to the complex.
  - C8β has a binding site for C5b67 and one or more sites that can bind to the target cell membrane.
  - The role of C8γ in MAC formation remains unclear.
  - The complex C5b678 can cause moderate membrane damage, especially in non-nucleated cells such as RBCs. Serum high density lipoproteins, as well as polyanionic agents such as heparin, block the interaction of the complex with the cell membrane; histones and protamines enhance its lytic activity.

❑ C5b678 facilitates the binding and polymerization of multiple molecules of C9 and the formation of MAC — an annular ring structure of 12–18 molecules of C9.

- Binding of one molecule of C9 initiates the process of C9 oligomerization.
- After at least 12 molecules are incorporated in the complex, a discrete channel is formed; the size of the channel varies according to the number of C9 molecules incorporated into the structure.
- During polymerization, C9 undergoes a hydrophilic-amphophilic transition so that the polymerized C9 is hydrophobic and can insert itself into the lipid bilayer.
- The completed MAC has a hydrophobic external surface and a hydrophilic internal channel of about 7–10 nm diameter.
- MAC allows free exchange of electrolytes and water through its channel, destroying the osmotic stability of the cell and causing its lysis.
- MAC damage is restricted to cells on which initial events of the cascade have occurred; bystander cells escape because of the instability of MAC (it quickly loses its cytotoxicity).
- Nucleated cells try to limit complement damage by exocytosing or endocytosing the area of the membrane that has MAC complexes.

❑ Suboptimal concentration of MAC on the cell membrane of nucleated cells is not lytic. Instead, it induces proto-oncogenes, activates the cell cycle, and enhances cell survival. It also inhibits apoptosis.

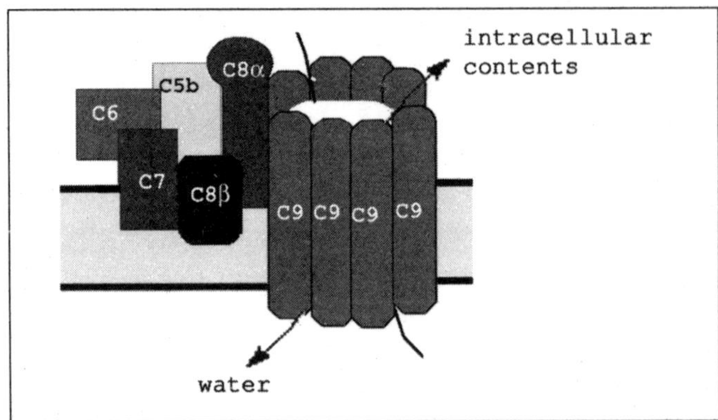

Figure 3.5 The Membrane attack complex is formed by the polymerization of C9, and this is facilitated by C5b678. As the complement cascade enters the terminal pathway, the C5-convertase cleaves C5; the bioactive C5a is released to the fluid phase. C5b binds C6 and C7. Binding of C5b6 complex to C7 causes a conformational change in the molecule and exposes a hydrophobic site that allows it to be inserted in the cell membrane. C8 binds to C5b67; the α and β subunits of C8 also get inserted in the lipid bilayer. The C5b678 complex promotes the polymerization of C9 and results in the formation of an annular structure consisting of 12–18 molecules of C9. MAC allows free exchange of electrolytes and water through its channel, destroying the osmotic stability of the cell and causing its lysis.

3.6 Complement in Health and Disease

Complement plays a major role in innate and adaptive immune responses. The role of complement is not limited only to immune responses (see sidetrack 'More than Just the Sum of its Parts'). Not surprisingly, deficiencies in any of the components or regulators of complement can lead to a number of diseases (Table 3.1).

❑ **Complement components are integral to innate immune defence.** Complement promotes

- Opsonization. Binding of complement coated target cells to complement receptors expressed on phagocytic cells promotes their phagocytosis and destruction. Interestingly, complement component C5a dramatically increases the number of such receptors on phagocytic cells.

Table 3.1 Diseases associated with complement deficiencies

Deficiency	Associated diseases
C1	Hypogammaglobulinaemia Severe Combined Immunodeficiency (SCID) Systemic Lupus Erythematosus (SLE) Glomerulonephritis
C2 and C4	Recurrent bacterial infections Organ non-specific autoimmune diseases
C3	Severe infections; susceptibility to pyogenic infections Decreased antibody repertoire Immune complex disease (glomerulonephritis, vasculitis, etc)
C5	Increased susceptibility to infection
C6, C7, and C8	Increased susceptibility to *Neisseria* infections
Properdin	Meningococcal infections
Factor D	Respiratory infections
C1INH	Hereditary angioedema Autoimmune diseases
DAF and CD59	Haemolysis and thrombosis, resulting in paroxysmal nocturnal haemoglobinuria
Factor I	Recurrent bacterial infections
CR1	Immune complex disease
CR3	Recurrent infections
MBL	Recurrent pyogenic infections and a failure to thrive in young children

- Macrophage activation and chemotaxis. C3a and C5a, released as a result of complement activation, can enhance macrophage activity.
- Lysis of the target cell. Gram-negative bacteria and many enveloped viruses are susceptible to complement-mediated lysis. Gram-positive bacteria and nucleated cells, on the other hand, are resistant to complement-mediated damage.
- Virus neutralization. Complement aids in the process of virus neutralization in multiple ways, independent of the neutralizing effect of antiviral antibodies.
    - Complement causes the lysis of many enveloped viruses.
    - Complement components coat virus particles and physically interfere with their attachment to host cells.
    - Complement component C3b facilitates the aggregation of viruses and their eventual phagocytosis.
- Augmentation of inflammatory responses. Complement has a pro-inflammatory effect.
    - Complement components C3a and C5a are vasodilators and cause an influx of fluids to the site of complement activation; C2b increases fluid accumulation.
    - C3a, C5a, and the complex C5b67 increase the adhesion of monocytes and neutrophils to vascular endothelial cells and their extravasation and migration towards the site of complement activation.

❑ Augmenting adaptive immune responses

- Complement aids in antigen processing and presentation. Coating of the antigen by complement allows it to be more efficiently internalized by the APCs.

- It enhances B cell activation. Coligation of the **C**omplement **R**eceptor **2** (CR2; CD21) and B cell antigen receptor by complement coated antigen-antibody complexes reduces by 100 to 1000 fold the amount of antigen required for B cell activation.
- Complement components are necessary for the localization of antigen-antibody complexes on **F**ollicular **D**endritic **C**ells (FDCs) in germinal centres[15]. Such localization is essential for memory B cell development.

❏ **Aiding waste disposal.** Complement opsonizes apoptotic cells, hastening their clearance by phagocytes.
  - C1q, the first component of the classical cascade, and MBL of the lectin pathway bind to blebs on apoptotic cells and aid in their clearance.
  - Erythrocytes bind opsonized cells/pathogens/immune complexes via CR1 and target them to the spleen and liver for disposal.

3.7 Regulation of the Complement Cascade

Complement activation has a tremendous potential for self-amplification. For example, approximately 1200 C3b molecules can be deposited on the cell membrane near a single IgM molecule by C3-convertase. C5-convertase is equally efficient in cleaving C5. Once switched on, the cascade has tremendous destructive potential. This is extremely dangerous, since the system is non-specific and does not discriminate between host cells and microbes. It is essential that activation of complement is focused on the surface of the invading pathogen and its deposition on normal cells or tissues is limited. This, and the fact that complement has multiple functions, necessitates its strict regulation. If this regulation goes awry, the complement system can be injurious to health. The complement pathway is, therefore, subject to dual regulation — the intrinsic level and the extrinsic level. Intrinsic regulation ensures that each activated component has a short half-life; it gets inactivated if it fails to attach to a cell membrane or activate the next component. Extrinsic regulation provides for inhibitory molecules that can inactivate or degrade activated components. Thus, a number of proteins and regulatory mechanisms are actively involved in controlling excess complement activation[16]. Many pathogens subvert the defensive action of complement by expressing ligands that bind the regulatory components/receptors and use them to gain entry into cells (Table 3.2).

❏ **Inactivation of C1 and MASPs. C1** Esterase Inhibitor (**C1EI** also called **C1INH**) inhibits initiation of the classical pathway by forming a complex with C1r and C1s causing them to dissociate from C1q. It also controls MASPs.

❏ **Inactivation of the C3-convertases and C5-convertase.** C3- or C5-convertases of the human complement system are controlled by fluid-phase and membrane proteins belonging to the RCA (**R**egulators of **C**omplement **A**ctivation) family. Closely linked genes on human chromosome 1 encode these RCA family proteins. They inhibit convertases of both the classical and the alternative pathways by causing their decay and/or by acting as cofactors for their degradation by Factor I — a serine protease that can cleave C4b and C3b.
  - Three different proteins, C4bp (**C4b b**inding **p**rotein), DAF (CD55) and CR1 (CD35), cause the decay of C3-convertase of the classical pathway by binding and displacing C2a from the C4b2a complex. C4bp is a soluble protein, and both DAF and CR1 are membrane bound proteins. The released C4b is cleaved by Factor I into two fragments — the larger C4c is released and the smaller C4d remains attached to the activated surface. Apart from disrupting the already formed C3-convertase, these proteins can also block its formation by binding C4b and allowing its cleavage by Factor I. CR1 and C4bp act as cofactors in this cleavage. Another member of the RCA family, **M**embrane **C**ofactor **P**rotein

[15] Germinal centres are structures found in secondary lymphoid organs, and are described in chapter 5. FDCs are specialized cells present in these structures. They express receptors for complement components and Ig and trap antigen-antibody complexes on their cell surface for prolonged periods (chapter 10).

[16] The one exception is properdin. It is the only regulatory protein that actually stabilizes alternative pathway C3-convertase.

(MCP; CD46), also acts as a cofactor for cleavage of C4b by Factor I, but it cannot cause the decay of C3-convertase (fig. 3.6). Both DAF and MCP are expressed on a wide variety of cells and are thought to protect these cells from complement attack.

- CR1, DAF, and a homologue of C4bp (called Factor H) cause the decay and degradation of alternative pathway C3-convertase (C3bBb). Factor H competes with Bb for the binding site on C3b. The surface to which C3b is attached determines which of the two ultimately combines with C3b. Certain surfaces, like those containing polysaccharides, are called activator surfaces, since they favour the binding of Factor B to C3b. Others, like heparin, favour the binding of Factor H, even when the C3b is bound to an activator surface. The inactivation of C3b by Factor I also requires Factor H, CR1, or MCP. An additional member of the RCA family has recently been discovered. Named FHL-1 (**Factor H-Like protein-1**), it is capable of causing the decay of the alternative

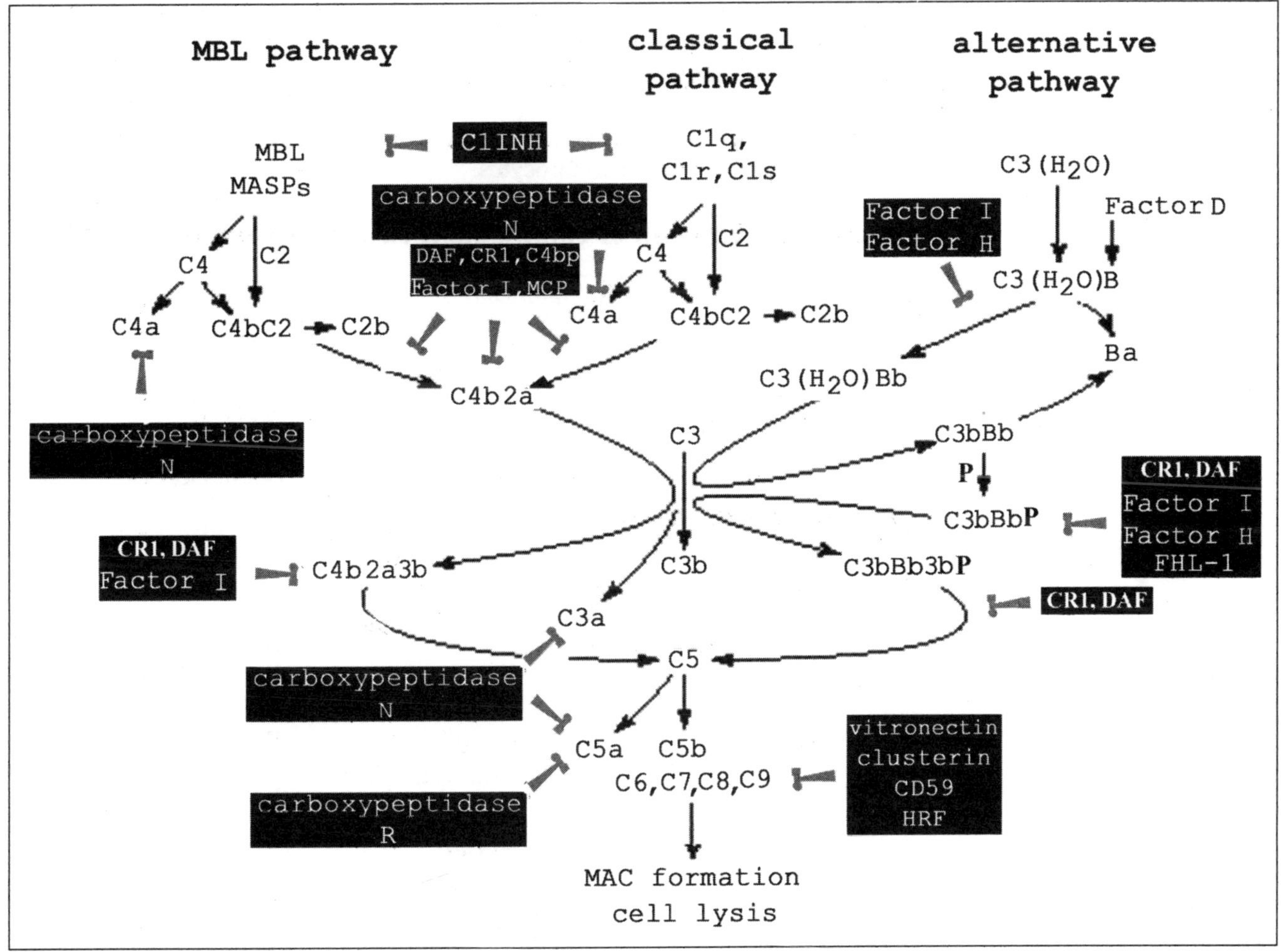

Figure 3.6 The complement cascade is regulated at almost every step by multiple regulatory proteins. *The fluid phase C1 inhibitor (C1INH) regulates the activation of the MBL and classical pathways by regulating MASPs and C1. It thereby controls the triggering of these two pathways. Two homologous proteins, C4bp and Factor H, inactivate C3-convertase of the classical pathway and alternative pathways respectively. Factor I, CR1, DAF (Decay Activating Factor), and MCP (Membrane Cofactor Protein) aid this inactivation. Additionally, FHL-1 (Factor H-Like protein-1) inactivates the alternative pathway C3-convertase. Apart from regulating the C3-convertases, CR1 and DAF can also accelerate the inactivation of both classical and alternative pathway C5-convertase. The progress of the terminal pathway is inhibited by vitronectin and clusterin that bind the C5b67 complex; C9 polymerization is inhibited by CD59 and HRF (Homologous Restriction Factor). The complement cascade also liberates multipotent molecules, C3a and C5a. Carboxypeptidase N inactivates them and the non-reactive but homologous C4a and helps preventing a runaway response. Together, these members of Regulators of Complement Activation prevent the damage that could result from excess complement activation.*

C3-convertase besides being able to act as a cofactor in its degradation. It is an alternatively spliced variant of Factor H.

- C5-convertase of the classical and alternative pathway can similarly be disrupted by CR1 or DAF. These regulators bind C3b in these enzyme complexes; the bound C3b is then susceptible to cleavage by Factor I. Another trypsin-like enzyme in the serum then cleaves C3b (called C3bi) to form a larger C3c that is released and a smaller C3d that remains attached to the cell surface.

❑ **Inactivation of the terminal pathway.**

- S protein (vitronectin) and clusterin (also called Apolipoprotein J) which are both found in serum are fluid phase inhibitors of the terminal pathway. They compete with membrane lipids for the metastable binding sites on C5b67. They bind the complex in the fluid phase and prevent it from binding to cell membranes. S protein allows the binding of C8 and C9 to Cb567 but prevents C9 polymerization. The bound complex retains its hydrophilic character and is therefore unable to insert into membranes.

- CD59 (originally called by the tongue-twisting name 'membrane inhibitor of reactive lysis'), a protein anchored in the cell membrane, can bind C8 and prevent C9 polymerization.

- Another membrane-anchored protein, HRF (**H**omologous **R**estriction **F**actor), can prevent channel formation and C9 polymerization. It is a 65 KD protein isolated from human erythrocytes.

Table 3.2 Evasion of complement cascade by micro-organisms

Protein	Micro-organism	Ligand in Microbe
C1q	*Escherichia coli*	C1q binding protein
Properdin	Herpes simplex virus	gC-1
CR2 (CD21)	Epstein-Barr virus	gp350/220
CR3	*Mycobacterium tuberculosis* West Nile virus (Flavi virus)	C3 fragments deposited on cell surface
Members of the RCA family		
CR1	*Candida albicans*	Not known
MCP (CD46)	*Neisseria gonorrhoeae* *Neisseria meningitides* *Helicobacter pylori* Measles virus Human Herpes virus 6	Pili Pili BabA protein Haemagglutinin Not known
DAF (CD55)	*Escherichia coli* *Trypanosoma cruzi* HIV-1 ***Picorna viruses:*** Echovirus 7 Coxsackie virus A21	Dr-like antigens, X adhesin gp 160 trypomastigote-DAF Acquires host DAF Capsid Capsid
C4bp	*Streptococcus pyogenes* *Bordetella pertussis* *Neisseria gonorrhoeae* Vaccinia virus	Some M proteins Not known Porin VCP
Factor H	*Streptococcus pyogenes* *Neisseria gonorrhoeae* *Streptococcus pneumoniae* HIV-1	Some M proteins Lipooligosaccharides, Porin Not known gp41, gp120
Factor H like-protein-1	*Streptococcus pyogenes*	Some M proteins
CD59	HIV-1	Acquires host CD59

3.8 Complement Receptors

Effector molecules combine with specific receptors on the target cell surface and exert their action. These receptors are involved in ligand recognition, signal transduction, and induction of cellular responses. Receptors that bind split-products of complement components are expressed on a variety of cell types. Complement receptors exist in the intracellular pool and cycle to the cell surface. Expression of some of these receptors increases upon the activation of cells or by stimulatory signals. The variety of cells that express these receptors can to some extent help us gauge the wide range of effects complement components can induce (Table 3.3).

Table 3.3 Receptors for complement components

Receptor (Ligand)	Characteristics
CR1 or CD35 (*C3b, iC3b, C4b*)	Found on erythrocytes, neutrophils, eosinophils, mononuclear phagocytes, mast cells, FDCs, B cells, and some T cells Promotes opsonization, stimulates phagocytosis, helps in the clearance of apoptotic cells and immune complexes, and promotes immune adherence Blocks/promotes cleavage of C3/C5-convertase by Factor I
CR2 or CD21 (*major ligand: C3b; can bind iC3b, C3c, C3dg*)	Expressed by B cells, thymocytes, and FDCs Part of B cell antigen co-receptor; engaging this receptor makes the B cell 100 times more sensitive to the antigen Is a receptor for the Epstein-Barr virus
CR3 or CD11b/CD18 (*iC3b*)	Found on monocytes, macrophages, neutrophils, eosinophils, FDCs, NK cells, and K cells Facilitates extravasation of neutrophils Stimulates phagocytosis
CR4 or CD11c/CD18 (*iC3b*)	Expressed by monocytes and macrophages — especially tissue macrophages, neutrophils, NK cells, and K cells Closely related to CR3
CR5 (*C3d*)	Expressed by neutrophils and platelets
C1qR (*C1q*)	Expressed on B cells, macrophages, monocytes, platelets, and endothelial cells Helps bind immune complexes to phagocytes Helps in the clearance of apoptotic cells
C3aR and C5aR (*C3a and C5a respectively*)	Expressed on mast cells, monocytes, macrophages, neutrophils, basophils, and T cells Small G protein coupled receptors Responsible for biological manifestations of anaphylatoxins

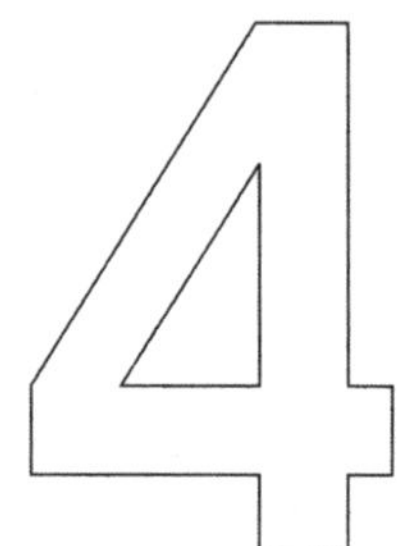

4 Entities of the Adaptive Immune Response: Immunogens

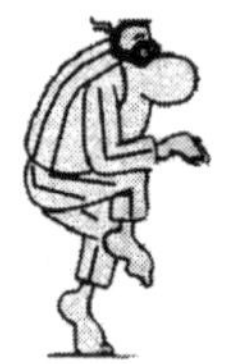

We're gonna find out where you folks really stand.
Are there any queers in the theatre tonight?
Get them up against the wall!
There's one in the spotlight, he don't look right to me,
Get him up against the wall!
That one looks Jewish!
And that one's a coon!
Who let all of this riff-raff into the room?
There's one smoking a joint,
And another with spots!
If I had my way,
I'd have all of you shot!

— Pink Floyd, *In the Flesh*

4.1 Introduction

A perceived threat to the well-being of an immunocompetent host results in an immune response. In this chapter and the next we will try to understand the two entities involved in this adaptive immune response — what triggers an immune response and which organs of the animal are involved in that response.

4.2 Immunogens and Antigens

Immunogens are substances capable of stimulating the immune system (that is, eliciting a B or T cell response) **and reacting with the product of such stimulation** (antibodies and/or cells expressing specific receptors). The term 'immunogen' is often confused with the term 'antigen[1]'. An antigen reacts specifically and observably with a lymphoid cell or cell product formed specifically in response to immunogenic challenge. Specific reactivity is the only criterion for defining an antigen and the definition does not include the capability of immune stimulation. Put differently, all immunogens are antigens, but not all antigens are immunogens. The terms antigen and immunogen have been used interchangeably, creating ambiguity. Regrettably, this continues and except for academic discussion the two terms remain synonymous.

BcR:	B cell antigen receptor
CFA:	Complete Freund's adjuvant
im:	Intramuscular
ip:	Intraperitoneal
iv:	Intravenous
ISCOM:	Immune stimulatory complexes
MDP:	Muramyl-di-peptide
sc:	Subcutaneous
TcR:	T cell antigen receptor
TD antigens:	T-dependent antigens
TI antigens:	T-independent antigens
TSST-1:	Toxic shock syndrome toxin-1

People involved in writing and developing computer software are known to borrow biological terms, with the result that words such as 'virus' and 'worms' have become commonplace in computer jargon. What is not so well known is that the way computer security specialists define and detect intrusions is eerily similar to the way our immune systems seem to define and detect intrusions. Computer security systems define the act of an intrusion as 'someone attempting to break into or misuse your system'. The definition of *someone* and *break into* or *misuse* is left to the organization's individual management. Two major models are used to detect intrusions. The Anomaly Detection Model detects intrusions by looking for activity different from a user's or system's normal behavior, and the Misuse Detection Model detects intrusions by looking for activity that corresponds to known intrusion techniques (signatures) or system vulnerabilities.

As explained in chapter 1, specific immune responses are mounted by T and/or B lymphocytes. T cells themselves are of two types — $\alpha\beta$ and $\gamma\delta$ — depending upon their antigen receptor. The manner in which these cells are stimulated differs.

❑ To stimulate $\alpha\beta$ T cells, the immunogen has to be processed and presented to the T lymphocytes in the context of MHC molecules. $\alpha\beta$ **T c**ell antigen **R**eceptors (TcRs) cannot bind or recognize the antigen in its native form. $\alpha\beta$TcR only recognizes antigen-derived peptides that have been loaded on appropriate MHC molecules.

❑ $\gamma\delta$ T cells are not constrained by the need for MHC molecules in antigen recognition.

❑ **B c**ell antigen **R**eceptors (BcRs), being membrane forms of Ig, can recognize and bind native (ie, unprocessed and free) antigen. This recognition alone though is not sufficient for B cell activation. B cells can be activated only when they receive T cell help in conjunction with antigen recognition[2].

To elicit a sustained immune response, the immunogen should ideally stimulate both T and B cells. The portion of the immunogen that binds specifically with membrane receptors on T or B cells is called its antigenic determinant or epitope. An epitope can be defined as a discrete site on a macromolecule which is recognized by and binds to a lymphocyte receptor. An immunogen may have more than one such epitope. The number of epitopes on a given immunogen is referred to as its valency. Some epitopes (whether B or T cell) are called immunodominant, because the immune response seems to be preferentially (or disproportionately) directed against these epitopes rather than other (called sub-dominant) epitopes of the

[1] Both the terms were perhaps derived similarly. Antigen = **anti**body **gen**erator or immunogen = **immuno**globulin **gen**erator. It is important to note that antigens/immunogens give rise to both B and T cell responses, ie, are **immun**e response **gen**erators.

[2] The exception being T-independent antigens (these should really be called T-independent immunogens, but old nomenclature is hard to get rid of!), which can stimulate B cells independent of T cell help (see section 4.3); however, these antigens do not elicit a sustained, all out, humoral and cell-mediated immune response.

immunogen. Although TcR and BcR belong to the same structural family (the immunoglobulin superfamily discussed in chapter 6), the natures of their epitopes differ.

4.2.1 B Cell Epitope

The BcR is an Ig molecule expressed on the surface of B cells (chapter 6). Since Igs recognize and bind soluble antigens, B cells have similar recognition capabilities. The nature of the B cell epitope is determined by the antigen-combining site (also called the paratope) of the Ig. Major characteristics of the B cell epitope are listed below.

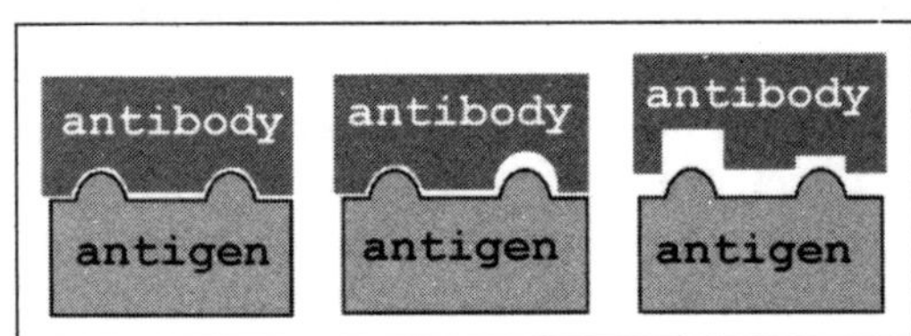

Figure 4.1 *In order to interact, conformations of the B cell epitope and the antigen-binding pocket of antibody molecules (paratope) must be complimentary, like the fitting contours of a jigsaw puzzle.* Antigen-antibody binding takes place by the formation of multiple non-covalent bonds such as Van der Waal's bond, H-bonds, and hydrophobic interactions. A large number of such bonds are required to hold the two molecules together and suitable atomic groups must be present on the corresponding parts of the molecules to allow for simultaneous formation of these bonds (left panel). If the epitopes and paratopes are not complimentary, the intermolecular attractive forces are not strong enough, and repulsive forces will drive the reactants apart (middle panel). If the conformations of the epitopes and paratopes are completely different, the repulsive forces will far exceed the attractive forces and the reactants will fail to interact (right panel).

- ❑ **It forms a binary complex with the BcR.** Since the BcR is an Ig molecule, the interaction between the BcR and its epitope is an antigen-antibody interaction, ie, one epitope reacts with one antigen-binding site of the BcR.
- ❑ **The B cell epitope is generally hydrophilic in nature.** When assuming its three-dimensional conformation, hydrophobic amino acids of the proteins get buried deeply in the structure, away from the water molecules of the surrounding medium. In contrast, hydrophilic portions of the molecule are exposed to the water molecules. Since B cell epitopes are located on the surface of the molecule, they tend to be hydrophilic.
- ❑ **It is conformational.** The antigen-antibody reaction can be viewed as a lock and key arrangement (the epitope acting as the key to the antibody's lock), or more appropriately, it is like the fitting contours of a jigsaw puzzle (fig. 4.1). For a proper antigen-antibody fit, the molecules must have complementary shapes. Antigen-antibody binding takes place by the formation of multiple non-covalent bonds such as Van der Waal's bond, H-bonds, and hydrophobic interactions (Table 4.1). Owing to the weak nature of such bonds, a large number of these bonds are needed to hold the interactants together. Suitable atomic groups must be present on the corresponding parts of the molecules to allow for simultaneous formation of these bonds. Water molecules may help in the process by filling gaps and increasing binding. Proteins and polysaccharides have a peculiar three-dimensional structure; the surface of these molecules is not smooth but consists of projections and contusions. These conformational structures behave as B cell epitopes. Thus, the B cell epitope is often found on bends on the molecule or in areas of high segmental mobility[3]. Even a single change in the amino acid sequence of a protein or carbohydrate in a glycoprotein/polysaccharide can change the three-dimensional conformation of that molecule, leading to altered antigenicity. Similarly, if a molecule unfolds or is partially denatured (eg, by

[3] Proteins are not static objects. They undergo a range of motions from simple side chain rotations to entire domain movements, all of which can play important functional roles. A large scale molecular motion occurs when two parts of the molecule move rigidly relative to each other and can be traced to a small segment of the molecule that acts as a hinge. B cell epitopes are often located in such areas of segmental flexibility.

heating or chemical modification), the conformation of the molecule changes; the original epitopes may be destroyed or rendered inaccessible, while normally hidden epitopes will be exposed (fig. 4.2). The denatured protein will therefore be antigenically different from the native protein and give rise to antibodies against the newly exposed epitopes. Moreover, antibodies produced against the original molecule may not react with the denatured molecule. For the same reason, antibodies produced against a linear polypeptide will not react with a α-helical polypeptide and vice versa.

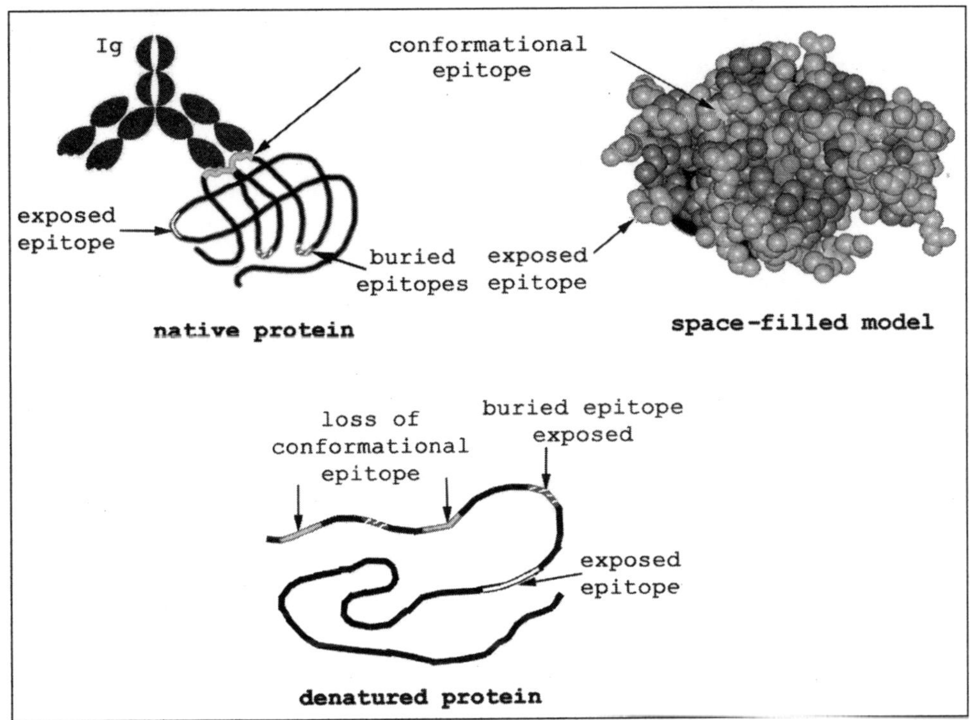

Figure 4.2 The B cell epitope can be sequential or non-sequential but has to be accessible. The three-dimensional conformation of epitope is important for antigen-antibody interaction. It therefore does not matter if the residues that form the epitope are continuous or not, as long as they are brought together by the folding of the molecule (top panels). Denaturation of the protein results in the linearization of the protein molecule and hence destroys the non-sequential epitope while the sequential epitope may not be affected. Denaturation also exposes hidden epitopes that were formerly inaccessible to the BcR (bottom panel).

Karl Landsteiner used a protein carrier coupled to various haptens[4] via the NH_2^- group of azo-benzene to demonstrate this conformational specificity of BcR. This was a simple but elegant approach to the problem, since the haptens behaved as the dominant antigenic determinants of the carrier molecule, and by changing the chemical nature and/or position of the hapten, he could alter the conformation of the carrier-hapten complex. The results of his experiments are summarized in fig. 4.3. When animals were injected with various hapten-conjugates, antibodies produced against the administered conjugate (*m*-sulphonyl derivative) readily reacted with it. Slight changes in the position of hapten (from *meta*- to *para*- or *ortho*-) led to a complete or partial loss of reactivity, showing that the position and nature of epitopes is extremely important in immune recognition, and therefore, immunogenicity. Similarly, changes in a single chemical group (SO_3^- to AsO_3^{2-}, or COO^-) also led to loss of reactivity (fig. 4.3). When α-D-glucose was substituted with β-D-glucose, anti-α-D-glucoside antibodies reacted with β-D-glucoside but with reduced reactivity. In contrast, antisera raised against α-D-glucoside failed to react with α-D-galactoside, confirming the importance of three-dimensional conformation of BcR recognition.

[4] Haptens are small molecules that are too small to be immunogenic when administered by themselves but can elicit an immune response when conjugated to a large carrier molecule (the term hapten is derived from Greek *haptein* — to fasten). However, haptens can react specifically with Igs formed in response to hapten-carrier stimulation. Thus, haptens are partial immunogens, ie, they have the property of antigenicity but not immunogenicity. Generally, the carrier activates T cells and the hapten reacts with the BcR. Hence, hapten-carrier conjugates elicit predominantly anti-hapten Igs. Large proteins are excellent carriers. The large number of peptides generated from such protein allow the activation of several TH cells, thereby enhancing the speed and efficiency of the resultant immune response.

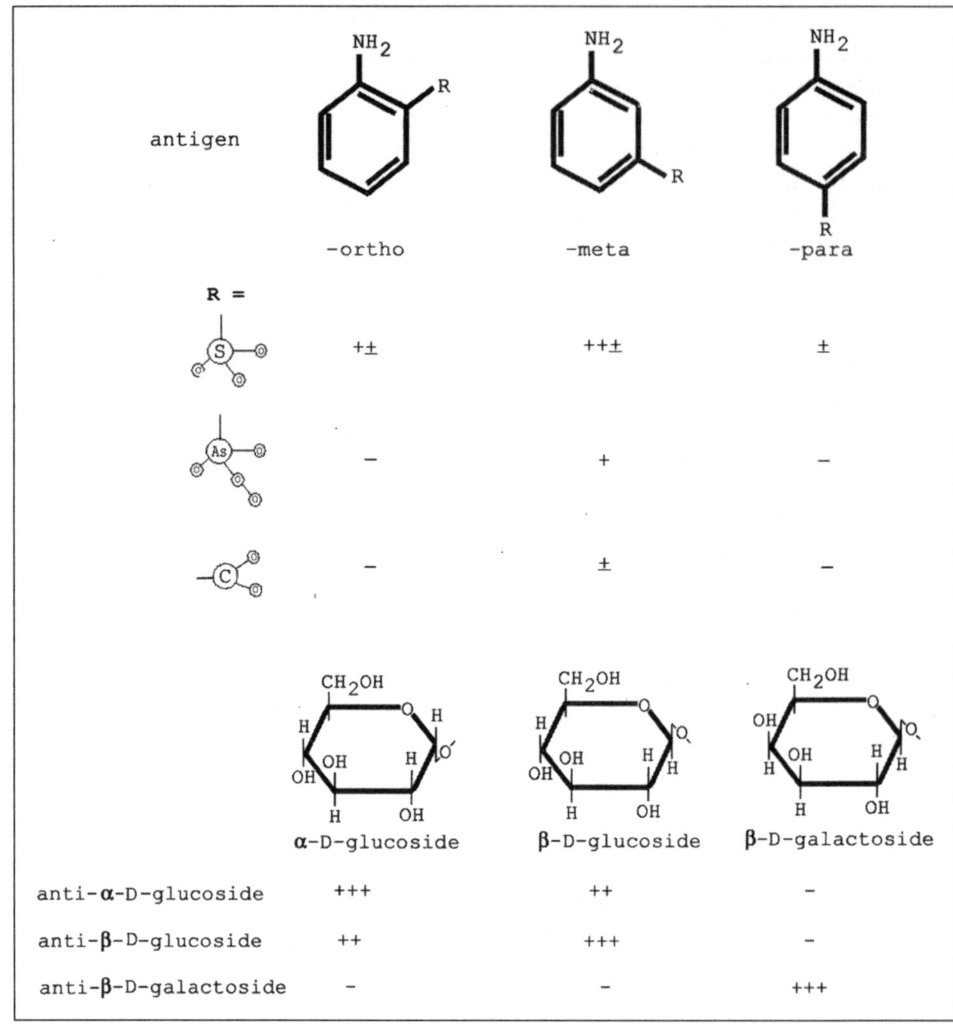

Figure 4.3 Landsteiner's experiments demonstrated the importance of three-dimensional conformation in antibody recognition. *Antibodies raised against a particular antigen readily bind that antigen. Changes in the position or the chemical nature of the epitopes can result in reduced or complete loss of binding. Thus, antibodies raised against the tetrahedral m-isomer of aminobenzene sulphonate react strongly with it but weakly with the p-isomer, and negligibly with the o-isomer. They can also weakly recognize another tetrahedral hapten, aminobenzene arsonate, at the m- position but not in the o- or p- positions. Only negligible recognition is observed in the case of the planar hapten aminobenzene carboxylate, and that too only in the m- position. If the antigens are chemically related, their conformations may be close enough for antibodies raised against one to bind the other (eg, α-D-glucose and β-D-glucose). If they are conformationally different (eg, α-D-glucose and α-D-galactose), however, antibodies raised against one fail to recognize the other.*

❑ **It can be sequential (continuous) or non sequential (discontinuous).** A sequential epitope is a stretch of amino acids on the surface of a protein that assumes a specific conformation and thus allows antibody binding. Since the three-dimensional conformation of the molecule is important in BcR recognition, B cell epitopes need not be restricted to continuous stretches of amino acids. Amino acids or carbohydrates located on different segments of the primary structure may contribute to epitope formation if they are brought together by folding of the molecule.

❑ **The B cell epitope is small.** The size of the B cell epitope is dictated by the size of the antigen-binding site of the antibody. The epitope cannot be larger than its binding pocket. The shape of the epitope, however, is entirely dependent upon

Table 4.1 Non-covalent forces involved in antigen-antibody interaction

Non-covalent force	Nature of the force	Example
Electrostatic force	• Is the result of the attraction between oppositely charged ionic groups on protein side chains such as $R\text{-}NH_3^+$ and $R\text{-}COO^-$	carboxyl group · · · amino group
Hydrogen bond	• Is a reversible bond formed between hydrogen attached to strongly electronegative atoms (N, O); results in the hydrogen acquiring a partial positive charge and a pair of negatively charged electron pairs on the electronegative atom • May be formed between charges located on different molecules or on different parts of one large molecule • In proteins the normal hydrogen bond donors are –O-H and N-H and the lone pair acceptors are =O, –O–, and –N	(electron pair) · · · hydrogen bond
Salt bridges	• Ionic interactions in proteins are often called salt bridges and occur between carboxylate groups and amino- groups of lysines and arginines; these often occur whenever the arginine or lysine residues are buried in the interior of proteins	
Van der Waal's forces	• Are the attraction between induced oscillating dipoles in two electron clouds • Induced oscillating dipoles are caused by the 'sloshing' of electrons in a molecule; such sloshing causes the molecule to temporarily become slightly negative at one end and hence temporarily slightly positive at the other end; a molecule approaching this temporarily polar molecule will be 'induced' to become polar — when the original dipole reverses charges, the charges on the induced dipole will also change • Decline rapidly with increasing distance	original dipole · · · temporarily induced dipole
Hydrophobic forces	• Combination of Van der Waal's forces and the tendency of hydrophobic groups to pack together to exclude water • Strength of the hydrophobic interaction is proportional to the surface area hidden from water	

the tertiary structure of the protein. Smaller ligands such as oligonucleotides, peptides, and haptens consisting of 4–8 hydrophilic residues can form compact structures and often bind deep within the antibody-binding pocket. With large globular proteins, the interacting face between the antibody and the antigen can be a flat or undulating surface in which the protrusions on the protein surface complement the depression in the antibody-binding site. In such cases, upto 15–20 amino acids on the protein surface may make contact with a similar number of amino acids on the antibody molecule.

❑ **It must be accessible.** In 1969, Sela demonstrated the importance of accessibility for immunogenicity. He used a non-immunogenic synthetic peptide of repeated units of a single amino acid (a poly amino acid) and attached the aromatic amino acid tyrosine at the branched chains. He found that when the amino acid was at the outer end of the branched chains, ie, accessible to BcR, the molecule was immunogenic. If the tyrosine was attached to the inner ends of the poly amino acid backbone, where it was inaccessible, the molecule was non-immunogenic. For proteins, this means that a native protein will elicit antibodies only to the exposed determinants on its cell surface. The antibodies elicited will fail to react with epitopes that are buried deep in the molecule (fig. 4.2).

4.2.2 αβ T Cell Epitope

About 95% of circulating T cells express the αβTcR, and it is this T cell epitope that we consider here.

❑ **The αβ T cell epitope is recognized only in the context of a MHC molecule.** The T cell epitope has to be loaded on a MHC molecule (either class I, class II, or CD1[5]) for TcR recognition and binding. Consequently,
  - T cells do not recognize either native or soluble antigens,
  - only proteinic (and in some instances lipid) antigens can stimulate T cells; they do not recognize polysaccharides or nucleic acids, and
  - the three-dimensional conformation of the protein is not important in T cell recognition; a similar T cell response will be generated whether a native or denatured protein is used in immunization.

❑ **It forms trimolecular complexes with TcR and MHC molecules.** Two distinct interaction sites on the peptide are involved in antigen recognition — the site that binds to the TcR (ie, the epitope) and the site that reacts with the MHC molecule (called agretope; fig. 4.4)

❑ **The T cell epitope is generated by APCs.** APCs internalize and digest native proteins. Peptides generated in this process are loaded onto the MHC molecules and exported to the cell surface; the MHC:peptide complex together binds TcR. Small linear peptides may be loaded onto MHC molecules at or near the cell surface, but such loading is inefficient. Thus,
  - viable, functional APCs are generally required for T cell epitope generation,
  - the epitopes are generally internal, ie, they need not be accessible, and
  - the haplotype of the MHC dictates the kind of epitope presented; MHC molecules are highly polymorphic and different individuals express different MHC molecules (chapter 7). Of the number of peptides generated from an antigen during processing, only those peptides that can bind to the particular MHC molecules expressed by the individual will be presented to T cells.

❑ **It is sequential (ie, continuous).** Since peptides generated by digestion of the native antigen are loaded onto MHC molecules, the epitope consists of a primary sequence of amino acids in the protein.

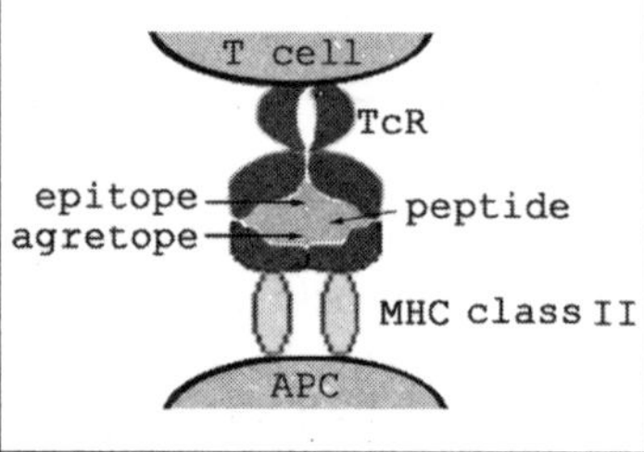

Figure 4.4 The αβ T cell epitope forms a tri-molecular complex with TcR and MHC. αβ T cell epitope is recognized only in the context of MHC molecules. APCs internalize and degrade protein antigens. Peptides derived from these antigens are loaded on MHC molecules. αβ TcR recognizes this peptide:MHC complex. The TcR must recognize both the MHC and the peptide. The site on the peptide that is recognized by the MHC is called the agretope; the site that binds the TcR is the epitope.

[5] Until recently, T cells were thought to recognize only peptides loaded on MHC molecules. It is now established that a type of T cell — the NKT cell — has a receptor that can recognize lipids or glycolipids loaded on CD1 molecules. These molecules are similar in structure to MHC class I molecules. Although this discussion focuses on proteinic antigens, it applies equally to lipid antigens.

❑ **αβ T cell epitope is between 8–20 amino acids in length.** The MHC molecule that binds the peptide dictates the length of the T cell epitope. MHC class I molecules have a closed groove that can bind peptides of 8–11 amino acids in length. The binding groove of the class II molecules is open at both ends and can bind longer peptides. Generally, class II peptides are 13–20 amino acids long, although sometimes peptides of 25 amino acids or longer can also be bound.

❑ **It is generally amphipathic.** Amphipathic peptides contain both a hydrophilic and hydrophobic region. The peptide-binding groove on MHC molecules has hydrophobic regions. To fit into this groove, the T cell epitope needs hydrophobic amino acids; hydrophilic regions are needed for interaction with TcR.

<table>
<tr><td>

B CELL EPITOPE

❑ It forms a binary complex with BcR.

❑ B cell epitope is conformational.

❑ It can be continuous or discontinuous.

❑ It consists of small 4–8 hydrophilic residues that are accessible to BcR.

❑ B cell epitope can be derived from proteins, carbohydrates, nucleic acids, etc.

</td><td>

αβ T CELL EPITOPE

❑ αβ T cell epitope forms a trinary complex with TcR and MHC molecules.

❑ It has to be processed and loaded on MHC molecules by APC.

❑ It is sequential.

❑ The αβ T cell epitope is derived from proteins or lipids.

❑ It consists of 8–20 amphipathic residues.

</td><td>

γδ T CELL EPITOPE

❑ γδ T cell epitope can be proteinic or non-proteinic in nature.

❑ It forms a binary complex with γδTcR.

❑ It is not processed and loaded on MHC; γδTcR recognizes native molecules independent of MHC.

</td></tr>
</table>

4.2.3 γδ T Cell Epitope

The γδ T cells comprise less than 5% of total T cells. Not much is known about these T cells, their mode of antigen recognition, signaling pathways, their role in health and disease, etc. Their unique features are listed below.

❑ γδ T cell epitope is similar to B cell epitope, ie, is recognized independent of MHC molecules.

❑ It need not undergo processing and presentation by APCs.

❑ It may be either proteinic or non-proteinic. Intact proteins or glycoproteins (eg, glycoproteins from herpes simplex virus) or small non-proteinic molecules such as phosphates (eg, pyrophosphomonoesters from *M. tuberculosis*) or amine-containing molecules (eg, alkylamines from several natural sources) are recognized by the γδTcR (fig. 4.5).

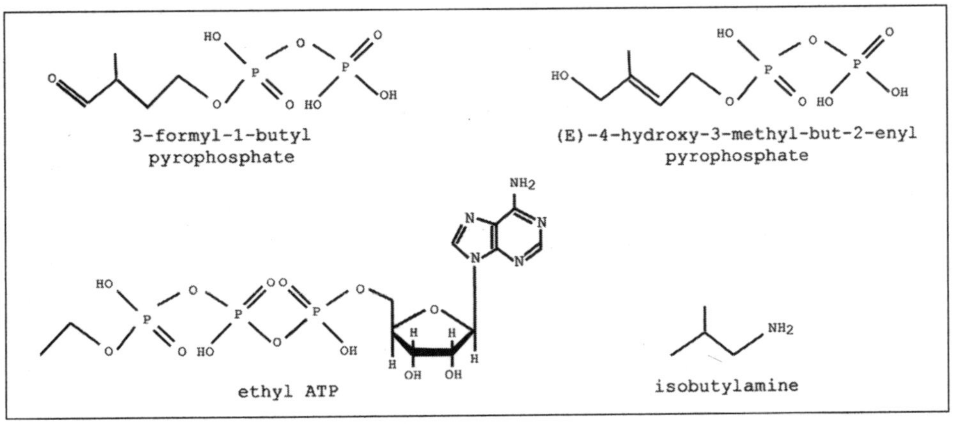

Figure 4.5 Proteinic or non-proteinic epitopes are recognized by the γδTcR. *The γδTcR epitope is recognized independent of MHC molecules. The diverse spectrum of molecules recognized includes intact proteins, small molecules like ethylamine or isobutyl amine, ethyl ATP, and pyrophosphates.*

4.3 Types of Antigens

❑ **Heterophile antigens.** Antigens or epitopes shared by unrelated (widely divergent) species are called heterophile antigens. Forsmann discovered these antigens. He found that antiserum raised by injecting guinea pig tissues (liver, kidney, brain, etc) in rabbits was capable of reacting with **S**heep **R**ed **B**lood **C**ells (SRBC), ie, antibodies produced against the guinea pig tissue recognized epitopes on SRBC. The antigen was called Forsmann antigen, and the resultant antibodies were called heterophile antibodies. Human B group RBCs and *E. coli* also share heterophile epitopes. Another example of a heterophile antigen is the one shared by Epstein-Barr virus and SRBC; antibodies in the serum of patients suffering from infectious mononucleosis (caused by the virus) lyse SRBC and bovine RBC in the presence of complement. The Weil-Felix test used in the diagnosis of rickettsial fevers exploits this phenomenon. Sera of patients suffering from some rickettsial infections have antibodies that can cross-react with certain *Proteus* strains (Table 4.2).

Table 4.2 Weil-Felix test

Infection (causative agent)	*Proteus strains*		
	OX19	*OXK*	*OX2*
Epidemic typhus (*R. prowazeki*)	++	-	-
Endemic typhus (*R. typhi*)	++	-	-
Scrub typhus (*R. tsutsugamushi*)	-	++	-
Rocky Mountain spotted fever (*R. rickettsii*)	++	-	++
Indian tick typhus (*R. conori*)	++	-	++

Legend: ++ – pronounced agglutination; + – agglutination, – – no agglutination;
Diagnostic titre: 1:80

❑ **Isophile antigens** are antigens found in some individuals of a species that are capable of eliciting an immune response in other, genetically distinct members of the same species. Blood group antigens are the best-known example of isophile antigens (chapter 13). Different alleles of the same genes code for these proteins. Thus, isophile antigens reflect allotypic variation in the genetic makeup of an individual.

❑ **Sequestered antigens.** 'Sequestered' means secluded, isolated, or set apart. Certain tissue antigens such as eye lens proteins or sperm antigens are sequestered from circulation and are not accessible to the cells of the immune system. It is thought that these antigens are not expressed in the thymus when the immune system 'learns' self and non-self discrimination (chapter 8). Hence, sequestered antigens can elicit an immune response if the cells of the immune system gain access to these sites, especially after trauma or infection. For example, the barrier membrane that protects sperm-forming tissue is damaged in mumps allowing cells of the immune system to access the tissue. The resulting orchitis (inflammation of the testicle) can damage the sperm-forming tissue and may result in impotency. Similarly, trauma to the eye can allow the immune system access to lens proteins, causing an autoimmune inflammatory reaction (see sidetrack 'The Privilege of Being and Seeing' in chapter 12). Currently, the term sequestered antigen is also used to describe antigens (or parts thereof) that are retained on FDCs for a long time. Such sequestered antigens have a role in affinity maturation (chapter 10).

❑ **Superantigens.** Characterized by their ability to bind antigen receptors outside the antigen-binding site, superantigens can stimulate >5% of the naïve lymphocyte pool. In comparison, conventional antigens normally stimulate less than 0.01% of naïve lymphocytes. Until recently, superantigens were thought to bind only TcRs. It is now established that both T and B cells can be activated by superantigens.

   • **T cell superantigens.** Certain bacterial toxins are powerful T cell mitogens[6] that can stimulate the proliferation of 2–20% of T lymphocytes. These include

---

[6] Mitogens are substances that cause cells to divide.

bacterial superantigens such as staphylococcal enterotoxins (A through I except F), toxins produced by *Streptococcus pyogenes* (A-C and F), and mycoplasmal and viral antigens (mammary tumour virus, Epstein-Barr virus, etc). Microbial superantigens are medium sized proteins (22–29 KD) that are resistant to proteases and temperatures of 60°C and higher, and survive in a pH range of 2.5 to 11. They can induce biological effects at femtomolar concentrations[7]. They probably evolved as mechanisms of exploiting MHC:TcR interaction to the selective advantage of the pathogens. Main characteristics of T cell superantigens are:

[7] 1 femtomole = 10^{-15} M

- Superantigens do not undergo processing by APCs prior to MHC-binding, unlike T cell epitopes.
- They bind to T cells having a particular variable region in the β chain of the TcR (called Vβ chain; chapter 6).
- Superantigens act like glue and bind MHC and TcR antigen non-specifically. Thus, TcR, MHC and superantigens form a trimolecular complex, although both the MHC peptide-binding groove and the TcR antigen-binding groove are not involved (fig. 4.6).
- Superantigens activate the immune system. Since superantigens bind both MHC and TcR, they end up stimulating both APCs (expressing MHC class II molecules) and T cells irrespective of antigen-specificity. As a result of this antigen non-specific stimulation, the immune system goes into a state of high alert where monocytes, B cells, T cells, and NK cells are in activated mode. Superantigen stimulation leads to massive production and release of cytokines by T cells (IL-2, TNF-α/β, IFN-γ), monocytes and NK cells (IL-1, IL-6, TNF-α). This massive release of cytokines is responsible for clinical manifestations such as hypotension (rapid fall in blood pressure), shock, nausea, vomitting, etc. The released cytokines in turn recruit other

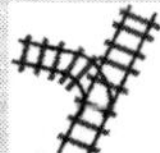

The Super Shocker:
Toxic Shock Syndrome and Superantigens

First described in 1978, Toxic Shock Syndrome is a spectrum of symptoms (high fever, hypotension, generalized skin rash, dysfunction of multiple organs associated with chills, headache, vomitting, diarrhoea, muscle pain, hallucinations, etc) found in menstruating women using super-absorbent tampons. Investigations revealed that the causative agent was an exotoxin produced by *Staphylococcus aureus* named TSST-1 (**T**oxic **S**hock **S**yndrome **T**oxin-**1**). The super-absorbent tampons afforded this opportunist pathogen an ideal environment to grow and secrete the toxin. Introduction of guidelines for tampon usage (a change every 4–6 hours) and their composition led to a dramatic decline of the disease in menstruating women. The notion of TSS being a female disorder was soon dispelled when it was found to be prevalent in the general populace as well. Anyone suffering from an infection by *S. aureus*, such as burns victims or patients with post-operative infections, is potentially likely to suffer TSS.

The list of diseases caused by superantigens has been growing steadily since the staphylococcal toxin was first identified. Superantigens are implicated in food poisoning, Necrotizing Fasciitis (rapidly spreading soft tissue infection), scarlet fever, rheumatoid fever, Kawasaki's disease (a leading acquired heart disease in children), diabetes mellitus, psoriasis, SLE, Multiple Sclerosis, Sudden Unexpected Nocturnal Death Syndrome, etc.

The potential of the superantigens is now being harnessed for novel approaches to disease treatment. For example:

- The T cell proliferating abilities of superantigens can be used in cancer immunotherapy. Fusion proteins consisting of superantigens fused with Fab fragments of antibodies against a particular peptide:MHC complex expressed by tumours allow the targeting of T cells to tumours.
- The ability of superantigens to cause anergy or deletion of a particular subset of T cells or to induce active immunosuppression could be exploited to eliminate/silence populations of T cells involved in autoimmune responses.

effector cells, resulting in a runaway immune response that is injurious and potentially fatal.

♦ They can induce anergy[8], apoptosis, and even active suppression of T cells. In addition, superantigens can mediate the killing of APCs. They can thus suppress adaptive immune response.

• **B cell superantigens.** Naturally occurring proteins that bind to antibodies via their antigen-binding site, irrespective of their antigen-specificity have been recently discovered. Staphylococcal protein A was one of the first B cell superantigens reported. Many others have been described since. These include gp120 from certain HIV isolates and protein L from *Peptostreptococcus magus*. Intriguingly, a human gut-associated sialoprotein termed **protein Fv** (pFv) also has B cell superantigen activity and may influence B cell selection in gut-associated lymphoid tissue. These superantigens bind to all Ig molecules having a particular V_H region (antigen-binding region). They have been implicated in certain autoimmune disorders. The unique features of B cell superantigens are:

♦ B cell superantigens bind Ig at a site close to but other than the antigen-binding site. Hence, binding of the superantigen to an Ig molecule does not interfere with its antigen-specific binding.

♦ They are functionally multivalent; they can bind two or more Fab regions allowing them to cross-link BcRs and activate complement.

♦ B cell superantigens cannot stimulate B cells by themselves. B cells generally require two signals for stimulation — the first being the cross-linking of BcR by the antigen and the second being the signal delivered by either T cells or accessory cells. B cell stimulation by superantigens follows this inherent B cell physiology, and a second signal is generally required for complete activation and proliferation.

♦ Superantigen activation causes the proliferation and eventual apoptosis of B cells.

♦ B cell superantigens can bind soluble Ig, since soluble Ig and BcR have the same structure. Igs can therefore compete with BcR for sites on the superantigen.

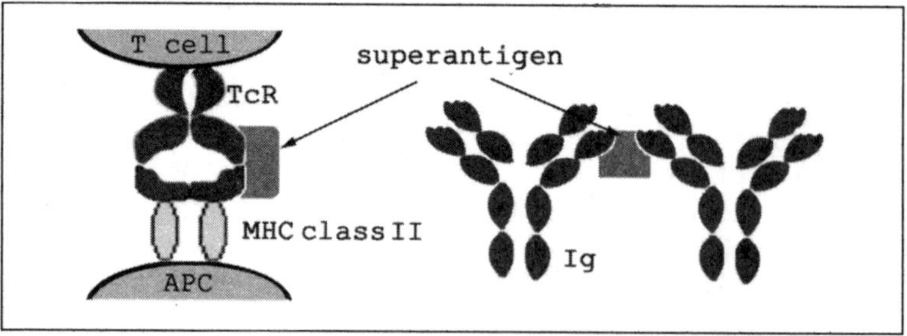

Figure 4.6 Superantigens bind antigen receptors outside the antigen-binding pocket and activate lymphocytes independent of their antigen-specificity. T cell superantigens such as staphylococcal enterotoxins bind to T cells having a particular variable region in the β chain of the TcR. They do not undergo processing by APCs and can stimulate the proliferation of 2–20% of peripheral T lymphocytes (left panel). The B cell superantigens bind to all Ig molecules having a particular V_H antigen-binding region (right panel). Since the B cell superantigens bind Ig at a site other than the antigen-binding site, binding of the superantigen to an Ig molecule does not interfere with its antigen-specific binding.

♦ Igs formed later in the immune response bind superantigens with lowered affinity. Normally, antibodies formed later in the immune response show an increased affinity for the challenging antigen due to a change in the antigen-binding region of Ig. Called 'affinity maturation' the phenomenon results

[8] Anergy literally means a lack of energy. Anergic cells do not respond to signalling via their antigen receptor.

from mutations in the DNA region encoding the antigen-combining site of the Ig molecule (chapter 10). Thanks to this change in the antigen-binding site, antibodies produced later in the immune response fit the antigen better than those produced in the initial stages. In the case of superantigens, such mutations result in a decreased rather than increased fit to the superantigen.

❑ **T-dependent and T-independent antigens.** As explained, antigens can be divided into two subtypes, depending upon their B cell activation pattern.

- **T-Dependent (TD) antigens** are unable to stimulate B cell proliferation on their own. Cell to cell contact (called cognate help) between the T and B cells is needed for B cell responses to TD antigens. Thus, two signals are required for B cell stimulation by TD antigens — the first delivered by the antigen via the BcR and the second by cognate interaction between T and B cells.

  Most proteinic antigens are TD antigens. Conventional B cells (CD5$^-$ B cells, the so-called B2 cells) respond to TD antigens. T cell associated phenomena such as germinal centre formation, isotype switching[9], and affinity maturation are only observed for TD antigens. Mice lacking T cells (eg, SCID mice, nude mice, or neonatally thymectomized mice; chapter 5) are incapable of producing antibodies to TD antigens. Thus, immune responsiveness to TD antigens is determined by the T cell repertoire of an animal, and if there is a hole in this repertoire (ie, if T cells capable of responding to a particular MHC:peptide complex are missing), the animal becomes unresponsive to that antigen.

- **T-Independent (TI) antigens.** Physical contact between B cells and T cells is not required by the B cells to respond to TI antigens. The B cell response occurs in the absence of the second signal, although soluble cytokines secreted by APCs and/or T cells can enhance this response. TI antigens are normally polysaccharide antigens with repetitive subunits and multiple antigenic determinants. Examples of naturally occurring TI antigens include the envelope of the Epstein-Barr virus, LPS, and flagellin. Synthetic TI antigens are dextran-sulphate, Ficoll and polyvinyl pyrrolidone. The B1 subset of B cells (CD5$^+$) usually responds to TI antigens. Secondary responses to TI antigens do not essentially differ from primary responses. The main features of B cell responses to TI antigens are listed below.

  ♦ TI antigens do not lead to germinal centre formation.
  ♦ Affinity maturation does not occur; the overall affinity of antibodies to TI antigens remains low.

  TI antigens are further divided into type 1 and type 2.

  ♦ **TI type 1** antigens are truly T-independent, since the response to these antigens does not decrease in nude mice. They are large polysaccharide antigens that are mitogenic to B cells and can stimulate neonatal as well as mature B cells by antigen-non-specific mechanisms, eg, via TLRs. Therefore, at high concentrations they behave as polyclonal B cell activators. Some B cells are bound to express a BcR that can specifically recognize these antigens. In such instances, they activate the B cell in an antigen-specific manner (fig. 4.7). LPS is the prototypical type 1 antigen.

  ♦ **TI type 2** antigens are highly repetitious molecules; the multiple, identical epitopes bring about extensive cross-linking of BcR, thereby stimulating B cells. They are not B cell mitogens and do not polyclonally activate B cells (ie, by antigen-non-specific mechanisms). Although type 2 antigens do not need the direct involvement of T$_H$ cells, some cytokine production by T cells (eg, IL-2, IL-5) is required for efficient B cell stimulation. Type 2 antigens are incapable of eliciting an immune response in neonatal mice or T cell deficient mice. They can activate complement and stimulate only mature B cells. Bacterial flagellin and the synthetic polysaccharide TNP-Ficoll are examples of TI type 2 antigens. The exact mechanism by which

[9] Isotype switching is the phenomenon wherein a clone of B cells can change the class of Ig produced from IgM to IgG/IgA/IgE without any change in the antigenic specificity of the molecule.

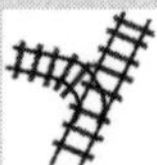

Defending the Defenceless: New Approaches to Fighting Childhood Infections

Children under the age of four are subject to a number of invasive bacterial infections. Many of these infectious agents such as *H. influenzae* type b, *N. meningitides* and *S. pneumoniae* cause severe infection because infants and young children are unable to mount an effective immune response to the capsules of these organisms. These capsules allow the organisms to escape phagocytosis and therefore T cell involvement in the ensuing response. The carbohydrate nature of the capsules makes them poor immunogens. Although purified capsular polysaccharides can be used in vaccines in immunocompetent individuals, their TI nature precludes them from being used in infants and children. Thus, they fail to protect the people most at risk of contracting these infections (infants, the elderly, and immunocompromized individuals). Different strategies are therefore used to convert the TI response to a TD type.

❑ Conjugating purified capsular polysaccharides or oligosaccharides to a protein carrier renders the carbohydrate immunogenic even in the very young. Four such vaccines have been approved for clinical use in the USA. They consist of a conjugate of the capsular antigen of *H. influenzae* type b attached to a protein carrier. A greater than 97% reduction in disease has been shown to result from the vaccination in the USA, UK, and Finland. Efforts are now underway to develop conjugate vaccines against *Salmonella typhi*, *Shigella* spp., type B streptococcus, etc.

❑ The use of peptides that mimic the carbohydrate's antigen structure can result in a TD immune response. Such antigens have the advantage of being stable, easy to produce, and of a defined chemical nature. Unlike conjugated vaccines, this approach has not reached the clinical trial stage.

  • Anti-idiotypic antibodies can be used to define specific peptides that mimic carbohydrate antigens. Such peptide mimics have been used successfully in some animal models of bacterial, viral, and parasitic infections

  • Peptide mimics of carbohydrate antigens can also be identified by screening a phage-display library with anti-polysaccharide monoclonal antibodies.

  • Nucleic acid vaccine technology and peptide mimicry can be combined in a novel approach which involves the cloning of an oligonucleotide encoding a peptide mimic into a eukaryotic expression plasmid. Such peptide mimic-DNA vaccines have been developed against the capsular polysaccharide *S. pneumoniae* serotype 4 and have been shown to confer protection in laboratory animals.

type 2 antigens activate B cells is not clearly understood. Immuno-compromised individuals (such as HIV seropositives), people older than 65, and children under two seem unable to respond to these antigens.

The TI antigen pathway seems to provide a quick protective response against common bacterial, viral, and fungal pathogens. Many pathogens have extracellular

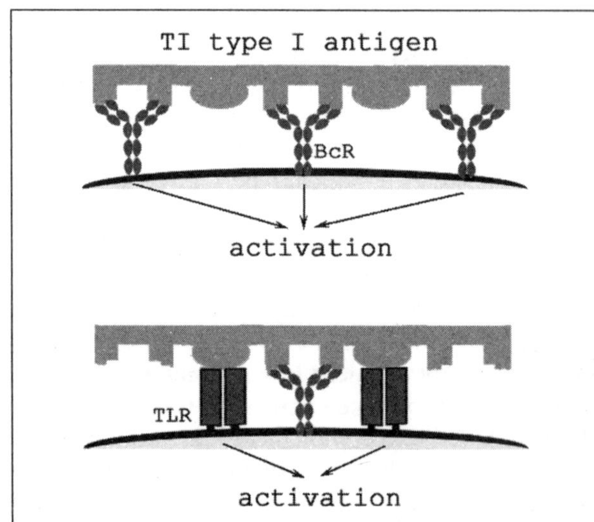

Figure 4.7 Engagement of the multiple repetitive epitopes on T-Independent antigens by BcRs generates a signal large enough to activate the B cells in the absence of T cell help. TI type I antigens such as LPS can stimulate B cells by antigen-specific (top panel) and antigen non-specific mechanisms (bottom panel). Type I antigen can therefore behave like B cell mitogens and cause their polyclonal activation. In this respect, type I antigens differ from type II antigens. Type II antigens can stimulate B cells only by antigen-specific mechanisms.

TYPES OF ANTIGENS

❑ Heterophile antigens are antigens shared by unrelated species.

❑ Isophile antigens are antigens present in some but not all individuals of a species. They are caused by allotypic variation in genes encoding the proteins. Examples include blood group antigens and MHC antigens.

❑ Sequestered antigens are self-antigens that are normally isolated from the developing immune system and elicit an immune response if cells of the immune system gain access to them. Examples include lens antigens of the eye and sperm protein.

❑ T cell superantigens form tri-molecular complexes with TcR and MHC; they bind both MHC molecules and TcR outside the peptide- and antigen-binding groove respectively.
- They do not undergo processing by APCs.
- T cell superantigens only bind certain Vβ region containing TcRs.
- Naïve T cells proliferate in response to superantigen stimulation but later get anergized; antigen-primed T cells, on the other hand, proliferate but do not get anergized.
- T cell superantigens activate the immune system antigen non-specifically; the resultant massive cytokine release causes disease.
- T cell superantigens lead to suppression of the adaptive immune response due to their effect on T cells and APCs.
- Examples of T cell superantigens include staphylococcal and streptococcal enterotoxins.

❑ B cell superantigens bind BcR outside the antigen-binding site and cause activation of B cells because of BcR ligation.
- They cause antigen non-specific activation of B cells; the activated cells eventually undergo apoptosis.
- Examples of B cell superantigens include HIV gp120, staphylococcal protein A, and protein Fv.

❑ TD antigens are generally proteinic antigens that cannot activate B cells in the absence of helper T cells.
- Cell to cell contact between homologous B cells and antigen-specific T cells is required for stimulation by TD antigens.
- CD5⁻ B cells respond to TD antigens.
- They give rise to germinal centre formation, affinity maturation, and isotype switching.

❑ TI antigens are generally polysaccharide antigens with repetitive, multiple epitopes that can activate B cells independent of T cells.
- CD5⁺ B cells respond to TI antigens.
- Affinity maturation and germinal centre formation is generally not observed for TI antigens.
- LPS is the protoypical TI type 1 antigen. It can stimulate B cells to proliferate antigen non-specifically at higher concentrations and activate them via their BcR (ie, antigen-specifically) at lower concentrations.
- TI type 2 antigens such as flagellin cannot induce antigen non-specific B cell proliferation. T cell cytokines such as IL-2 or IL-5 are required for efficient B cell stimulation by these antigens.

---

polysaccharides that allow them to resist ingestion by phagocytes and escape destruction. Escaping phagocytic digestion also helps them avoid T cell activation which can only occur when APCs display peptides of pathogenic origin in context of MHC molecules. By allowing antibody production to polysaccharide antigens, the TI pathway allows for humoral immune responses to many bacterial pathogens that would otherwise have escaped immune destruction.

4.4 Factors Influencing Immunogenicity

Immunogenicity is not an intrinsic property of a molecule. It is determined partly by the nature of the molecule, and partly by how an animal responds to it. Substances that are immunogenic in one animal need not be so in another. **Properties of the immunogen** that influence its immunogenicity include:

❑ **Foreignness.** According to the self-non-self theory of immune recognition, an immunogen must be recognized as non-self (ie, foreign) to elicit an immune response. Molecules present in the tissues or tissue fluids of an animal fail to elicit an immune response in that animal[10]. Thus, bovine serum albumin can elicit an immune response in mice while mouse serum albumin cannot. This failure to mount an immune response to self-antigens is due to the elimination of

[10] It needs no stretch of imagination to realize that the mounting of an immune response against self-antigens will prove disastrous for an animal. Diseases that result from such an immune response to self-antigens are called autoimmune diseases.

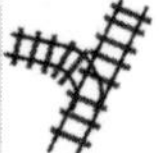

The Art of Being Provocative: Immunogenicity of Natural Molecules

Proteins. Many naturally occurring globular proteins are highly immunogenic. A globular protein is a chain of amino acids folded and refolded to yield a tight tertiary structure, or when associated with other chains, a quaternary structure. Determinants on the surface of the proteins, especially the more exposed areas, such as loops and cones of the folded chains are important in determining antigenic specificity of the protein. The whole protein may be visualized as a carrier-hapten complex — the larger globular part (comprising the internal as well as surface non-distinctive peptides) being the carrier and the antigenic determinants being the haptens. The presence of lipids or polysaccharide molecules on the proteins enhances their immunogenicity. As a rule of thumb, the density of determinants is in the range of one determinant per 5 KD MW. A single amino acid in a highly exposed position may, however, contribute largely to the specificity of the entire molecule. In the absence of the characterization of different determinants, the immunogens are referred to by the whole proteins themselves, eg, bovine serum albumin and casein. Since a large globular protein will have many determinants, different antisera raised against the same proteins may react with different determinants of that protein. These different antisera may differ in their specificities, since they may consist of antibodies directed against different epitopes on that protein. Unlike B cell responses, T cell responses to proteinic antigens are determined by the primary amino acid sequence of that protein. T cell clones raised against a particular protein will be specific for particular peptides of that protein. Both the protein and the MHC (its class and haplotype) in whose context the protein is being recognized need to be stated. Thus, a T cell clone raised against human serum albumin in mice may be referred to as anti-HSA 64-72 (sequence of amino acids in the protein that constitutes the peptide recognized) IA^k (MHC class II haplotype in whose context the peptide is recognized).

Polysaccharides. These are serologically important components of cells. Many polysaccharides are weakly- or non-immunogenic by themselves, but dominate serologic specificity of the proteins they are attached to. Ubiquitous polysaccharides such as starches, dextrans, and glycogens are by themselves largely non-immunogenic. The monosaccharides that are most frequently encountered in serologically important polysaccharides in one or more positions are pentoses and hexoses — either unsubstituted or substituted. Cell surface polysaccharide antigens are often conserved in a group of bacteria. Their presence can hence be used as an important taxonomic character. Antibodies against such conserved antigens are used for grouping bacteria and even for distinguishing between various subspecies and strains. This grouping of microbes on the basis of their antigens is called serotyping. Serotyping is an important distinguishing character in streptococci, pneumococci, salmonella, etc. The highly heat stable, micro-capsular Vi antigen found in many pathogens is also a polysaccharide. It consists primarily of polymers of O-acetyl and N-acetyl aminohexuranic acid. It is thought to help bacteria resist phagocytosis. Type specific substances by which human blood groups are recognized are also polysaccharides. The so-called blood group antigens can also be found in bacteria and in the various tissues and secretions of humans and other animals (chapter 13).

Lipids are tri-esters of organic acids with various alcohols, nitrogenous bases, and radicals such as PO_4^{-3}, SO_4^{-2}, etc. Lipids are largely non-immunogenic. When conjugated with proteins or polysaccharides, they can be immunogenic. Recent research shows the presence of CD1, an MHC-like molecule, on the cells of the immune system. These molecules can load and present lipid antigens to NKT cells, a subset of NK cells that express both NK and T cell surface markers. NKT cells are discussed in chapter 8.

Nucleic acids are, for understandable reasons, poor immunogens, and they have to be complexed with a larger molecule, or altered in some way, to be immunogenic. In SLE, an autoimmune disease, the body produces antibodies against nuclear proteins.

self-reacting clones during the process of T cell maturation in the thymus. The presence of regulatory T cell clones that suppress immune responses in an antigen-specific manner further strengthens this ban on the response to self-antigens (regulatory T cells or T$_R$ cells; chapter 8). For the same reason, ubiquitous proteins that have a highly conserved structure across a variety of species (cytochrome c and dextran) are not immunogenic. Cytochrome c of bovine origin is too similar to the cytochrome *c* of mouse origin to be recognized as foreign. T cells that can react with self-antigens not expressed in the thymus during this process of maturation escape elimination (eg, proteins from eye lens, testes, etc). Consequently, these antigens can elicit an immune response. The self-non-self theory of immune recognition is thought to be too simplistic and is now being challenged (chapter 1).

❑ **Degradability.** Processing and presentation of the antigen in the context of MHC molecules is indispensable to the development of a humoral and/or cell-mediated immune response. Macromolecules like polystyrene that cannot be degraded for presentation are therefore poor immunogens. Polymers of D-amino acids are also poor immunogens. These stereoisomers of naturally occurring L-amino acids cannot be processed by APCs since their enzymes are incapable of degrading the D-isomer. Conversely, substances that are rapidly broken down by plasma enzymes are weakly- or non-immunogenic. This is because they do not survive the highly proteolytic environment in the lysosomes of the APCs — the resulting fragments are too small to load on MHC molecules.

❑ **Molecular size and complexity.** Molecular shape is not important in determining a substance's immunogenicity. Proteins and polypeptides with rod-like, globular, or random coil configuration can all be potent immunogens. Molecular size, on the other hand, does influence immunogenicity. Generally, substances with a **Molecular Weight** (MW) of 6 KD and above tend to be better immunogens than those having a low MW. Even the polymerization of a low MW substance can increase its immunogenicity. Thus, bovine insulin (MW 6 KD) is a poor immunogen, but if polymerized by chemical methods or aggregated by heat, it is immunogenic. Similarly, intact flagellum is more immunogenic than polymerized flagellin which is in turn more immunogenic than flagellin itself. Some molecules may bind tissue proteins and thereby become immunogenic. For example, picryl chloride, formaldehyde, or drugs like penicillin and sulphonamides (all with MW <1 KD) can elicit an immune response. These molecules behave like haptens; they bind to tissue proteins and act as antigenic determinants of the tissue protein-drug complex.

Increasing complexity generally increases immunogenicity. Obviously, a complex molecule has a larger variety of potential determinants. The larger the variety of determinants, the greater the chance that one or more of these will preferentially stimulate cells of the immune system. This could partly be the reason for an increase in immunogenicity with an increase in MW or size. Cross-linking of antigen receptors on the surface of B cells is necessary to stimulate B cells (section 6.2.3). A complex molecule with multiple epitopes is therefore more likely to stimulate B cells. Structural stability or rigidity seems to be another factor that can influence immunogenicity. Molecules like gelatin that lack structural stability are poor immunogens. A linear homopolymer (a linear polypeptide of an amino acid) is usually non-immunogenic, but a branched poly amino acid structure tends to be immunogenic. Presence of aromatic amino acids in a molecule enhances its immunogenicity, probably because these amino acids lend rigidity to the molecule. The physical form of the antigen is also important. In general, particulate antigens are more immunogenic than soluble ones, and denatured antigens are more immunogenic than the native forms. Particulate antigens, probably being more irritable, are better immunogens. Moreover, the physical state of an antigen influences immunogenicity — aggregated bovine γ-globulin is immunogenic, whereas its monomers are tolerogenic.

Since it takes two for this immune response tango, the induction of an immune response depends not only on the immunogenicity of the molecule, but also on the **nature of the animal and the method of administration.**

❑ **Genetic makeup.** An immunogen may elicit a prolonged response in an individual of one species but fail to do so in another. Many studies have clearly established that some aspects of the immune response are genetically determined. This immune responsiveness is partially under the control of the MHC genes located on chromosome 6 in humans and chromosome 17 in mice. These genes and their impact on immune responsiveness is discussed in chapter 7. For obvious reasons, genes that encode BcR, TcR, and other proteins involved in immune regulation also influence the animal's ability to respond to different macromolecules.

❑ **Age.** As a rule, it is difficult to induce an immune response in very young animals. If an animal encounters an immunogen before it is immunologically mature (ie, neonatally), T cells capable of reacting to that antigen are eliminated. The animal then becomes tolerant to that antigen. Conversely, the capacity to respond to immune stimuli is also impaired with increasing age. A variety of changes occur with aging, including the appearance of new differentiation antigens, modification of cell membranes, and quantitative differences in surface Ig expression on B lymphocytes. It is thought that age also leads to an impaired B lymphocyte, T lymphocyte, and macrophage function. Consequently, appearance of autoantibodies, production of paraproteins, and immune deficiencies can occur with increasing age. It is therefore essential to consider the age of an animal when interpreting the results of immunological experiments.

❑ **Method of antigen administration.** The dose of the immunogen, its route of administration, and the presence of adjuvants all influence the outcome of antigen administration.

    • **Dose of the immunogen.** Every immunogen has an optimal immunogenic dose. Amounts much larger than the optimal dose generally lead to a tolerance (ie, failure to elicit an immune response) called the high zone tolerance, while much smaller doses may lead to low zone tolerance. This is especially true of TI antigens. Generally, a single dose of an immunogen is less effective than repeated administrations in eliciting an immune response. The dose of the antigen can also influence the type of immune response; small repeated antigen doses have been found to induce IgE antibody responses; larger doses result in an IgG antibody response in experimental animals.

    • **Route of administration.** For deliberate immunization of experimental animals, an immunogen is usually injected in the body by specific routes. The most common routes of administration are intradermal or subcutaneous (sc), intramuscular (im), intravenous (iv), and intraperitoneal (ip). Regardless of the route, most antigens eventually reach the nearest draining lymph node, and once there, activate antigen-specific T and/or B lymphocytes. When given iv, the antigen reaches the spleen, which acts as a filter for blood and traps all antigens entering the blood. As a rule, an immunogen will elicit a better response if introduced parenterally[11] into the body. This is because the immunogen is more likely to be digested before it reaches an APC if introduced by the digestive route or through epithelial tissue. The route of administration also influences the type of immune response elicited. Minute doses repeatedly inhaled via respiratory mucosa or given sc tend to result in an IgE response, but mucosal administration of large doses of the antigen elicits an IgA response. Also, soluble antigens tend to be immunogenic when injected in tissues but tolerogenic when given ip.

    • **Use of adjuvants.** Adjuvants (from Latin *adjuvare* — to aid or help) are agents that are administered along with the antigen and can enhance the humoral or cellular immune response by non-specific mechanisms. Thus, a substance that can accelerate, prolong, and/or enhance the quality of specific immune responses to an immunogen can be labelled an adjuvant. A highly heterogeneous group of molecules or compounds has such immunostimulatory properties. The mode by which these molecules stimulate the immune system varies widely. Since

---

[11] Parenterally: *para* — around, *enterally* – gut, ie, by routes other than the digestive tract.

adjuvants have diverse mechanisms of action, they must be chosen for use with a particular immunogen depending upon the route of administration and the desired immune response. The exact mechanism of action of the adjuvants is unclear, although six broad modes of action can be delineated.

♦ **Enhanced translocation of the immunogen from site of administration to the local draining lymph node**. Immune responses are not initiated at the site of immunogen injection. An immunogen can trigger an immune response only when it reaches the local lymph node. Adjuvants may promote such translocation by protecting the immunogen from rapid non-specific elimination at the site of injection; immunogenicity of peptide antigens that would normally be cleared rapidly from the site of injection can be improved with the use of particulate adjuvants that associate with or otherwise hold the antigen.

♦ **Improved antigen delivery to or antigen processing and presentation by the APCs.** By promoting phagocytosis, adjuvants can assist in the translocation of an immunogen besides increasing its presentation to T cells.
  – Adjuvants like purified saponins, ISCOMs (**I**mmune **S**timulatory **Com**plexes; see sidetrack 'Spicing the Cocktail'), and liposomes have been shown to improve induction of MHC class I restricted cytotoxic T lymphocyte responses by delivering the antigen directly to the cytosol for presentation by class I molecules.
  – Particulate antigens such as liposomes, ISCOMs, polymer microspheres, and MF 59 can be used to target antigen to phagocytic cells; macrophages and DCs that have internalized the antigen move rapidly to the draining lymph node, where the phagocytosed antigen is processed and presented.

♦ **Increased biological or immunological half-life of the antigen.** Many adjuvants are good adsorbing agents. They can cause a slow and prolonged release of the immunogen, ie, they have a depot effect; adjuvants like aluminium salts, Freund's adjuvant, and oil based adjuvants are thought to owe their adjuvant action to this depot effect.

♦ **Engagement of PRRs.** Many cells of the innate immune system express receptors that specifically recognize patterns or motifs on pathogenic organisms. Engagement of these PRRs is known to enhance immune responses.
  – Adjuvants based on microbial components such as pertussis toxin, LPS (or its active derivative monophosphoryl lipid A), mycobacterial cell wall derived muramyl dipeptide, and CpG rich motifs are all known to increase immune responses by the engagement of TLRs on the cell surface and thereby stimulate the innate immune system (chapter 2).
  – Fusing of an antigen to the complement component C3d can result in antigen-specific antibody responses by acting as a molecular adjuvant of innate immunity.
  – The cage-like structures of ISCOMs may also mimic PAMPs and stimulate immune responses.

♦ **Induction of local reaction at the site of injection.** Signals from damaged or stressed cells are known to induce immune responses. The ability to cause a local reaction is seen in many commonly recognized adjuvants such as aluminium salts, $Ca_3(PO_4)_2$, and mineral oils. Still, the efficacy of the adjuvant must be weighed against the severity of the local reaction. It is for this reason that Freund's adjuvant (complete or incomplete) is unacceptable for use in humans.

♦ **Induction of costimulatory molecules or immunomodulatory cytokines.**
  – Some adjuvants, like the Freund's adjuvant, cause a strong local inflammatory reaction, inducing the expression of costimulatory molecules and the production of pro-inflammatory cytokines (chapter 8 describes

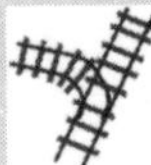

Spicing the Cocktail: Adjuvants 101

Complete Freund's Adjuvant (CFA) is one of the most effective adjuvants ever discovered. It has a stimulating effect on almost all immune responses. It is a water-in-oil emulsion containing suspended live or dead mycobacteria. An intense inflammatory response develops around the site of injection. The adjuvant activity of mycobacteria is largely due to a complex glycolipid — **M**uramyl-**d**i-**P**eptide (MDP). The complete adjuvant causes a reaction that is too strong to be of use to humans. **Freund's incomplete adjuvant,** consisting of the water-in-oil emulsion but not the mycobacterial suspension, is less inflammatory but even then too strong for human use. Its use is restricted to animals. Derivatives of MDP when administered in saline induce a mainly humoral immunity. Water-in-oil emulsions of MDP can modulate both humoral and cell-mediated immunity and may be used in humans.

Mineral salts. One of the first adjuvants to be licensed for use in humans, compounds containing aluminium are popular adjuvants [$Al(OH)_3$, $Al_2(SO_4)_3$, alum, etc], especially when humoral responses against proteinic antigens are desired. Calcium phosphate nanoparticles have been used in a variety of vaccines (diphtheria, pertussis, tetanus, polio, etc). It has been found to induce a predominantly T$_{H}$1 response.

Immunostimulatory adjuvants. Adjuvants that exert their effect primarily at the cytokine level are called immunostimulatory adjuvants.

- **LPS,** although a powerful immunostimulant, is not suitable for clinical applications. **Monophosphoryl lipid A** is a less toxic derivative of LPS that retains adjuvant activity. It has been shown to promote the release of IFN-γ in clinical trials. If used alone, it does not promote a potent antibody response.

- **Saponins.** Triterpenoid glycosides derived from *Quillaia saponaria* have long been used in veterinary medicine. Saponins have been shown to intercalate in cell membranes through their interaction with cholesterol and result in pore formation. The antigen can then penetrate the cell easily and thereby get carried to the regional lymph node. The immunostimulatory fraction of saponin — Quil-A — was useless for clinical applications because of its toxicity. QS21, a pure fraction of Quil-A, has low toxicity and was found to induce T$_{H}$1 type responses (induction of IFN-γ, IL-2, cytototoxic T lymphocytes, and IgG2a antibodies). It has been used in clinical trials for multiple immunogens (cancer, HIV-1, influenza, malaria, and hepatitis B).

- **CpG DNA.** The investigation of the tumour reducing effects of the BCG vaccine led to the discovery of the immunostimulatory capability of bacterial DNA. This effect was later linked to the presence of unmethylated CpG dinucleotides. This CpG motif is common in bacterial DNA but rare in vertebrate DNA. Unmethylated CpGs in the context of selective flanking sequences can be recognized by TLRs. CpGs are found to release pro-inflammatory cytokines (TNF-α, IL-1, IL-6, and IL-12). Hence, they are potent inducers of T$_{H}$1 responses. A number of pre-clinical and clinical trials are underway to test the possible use of CpG DNA, especially in cancer immunotherapy.

- **Cytokines** are being evaluated as adjuvants (IL-1, IL-2, IL-12, IFN-γ, and GM-CSF). Toxicity, however, remains an issue, since they all show dose-related toxicity. A high manufacture cost, stability problems, and a short *in vivo* shelf life make cytokine use in routine vaccination unlikely. Neverthelss, they do hold immense promise in the field of cancer immunotherapy.

Particulate adjuvants. These adjuvants have dimensions comparable to those of pathogens (10–100 nm in diameter) and are easily taken up by DCs and macrophages.

- **MF59** is an oil-in-water emulsion of biodegradable oil (squalene) that has been shown to increase the immunogenicity of the influenza vaccine. It targets the antigen to macrophages and DCs and induces a potent antibody response. It has been licensed for human use in a variety of vaccines (HIV, influenza, hepatitis B, herpes simplex, etc).

- **Liposomes** are particles made of concentric lipid membranes containing phospholipids and other lipids in a bilayer configuration separated by aqueous compartments. These are often used in combination with other immunostimulators, such as monophosphoryl and Lipid A. A liposomal hepatitis A vaccine is now in the final stages of commercial development. The development of polymerized liposomes is also being investigated. Similarly, modified liposomal structures called chochleates are being evaluated for mucosal delivery of vaccines. Virosomes, consisting of a liposome and inactivated viruses, are now being allowed for human administration.

> ❑ **ISCOMs.** The incorporation of Quil A into lipid particles comprising cholesterol, phospholipids, and cell membrane antigens are called **I**mmuno**S**timulating **COM**plexes, or ISCOMs. ISCOMs, like QS21, are found to induce T$_{H1}$ type responses, and an influenza ISCOM vaccine is nearing the end of a successful clinical trial. ISCOMs have relatively low toxicity and target the antigen directly to APCs.
>
> ❑ **Polymeric microparticles** made of poly(lactide-co-glycolides) are also being investigated for targeting antigens to APCs. Poly(lactide-co-glycolides) are biodegradable polyesters that have been used in humans as suture material for many years, so their safety is well established. They are used to encapsulate the antigen. By allowing the controlled release of antigen, they can induce prolonged immunity to the antigen. They have been shown to induce potent mucosal and systemic immunity on administration by the oral route.
>
> **Mucosal adjuvants.** Apart from polymeric microparticles, several other adjuvants are being investigated for mucosal antigen delivery.
>
> ❑ **Bacterial toxins,** including the cholera toxin and the enterotoxin of *E. coli* are the most potent mucosal adjuvants available. Sadly, their toxicity limits usage. Recombinant mutated toxins are now being studied as possible adjuvants. The mutated cholera toxin is reportedly being investigated as an adjuvant to be used in topical skin applications.
>
> ❑ **Transgenic plants** expressing antigens and adjuvants are the most recent development in the field of mucosal adjuvants. Their acceptance and applicability remains questionable.

the importance of costimulatory molecules in immune responses). These events in turn lead to the recruitment of macrophages and DCs to the site of antigen injection.

– Costimulatory molecules by themselves can also be used as adjuvants. Two signals are required for naïve T cell activation. Engagement of TcR by MHC:peptide complexes delivers the first signal. Binding of costimulatory molecules (such as CD80/CD86) on APCs to their ligands on T cells delivers the second and results in T cell activation (section 8.3.3). Thus, DNA encoding antigen-CD86 fusion proteins deliver both the signals required for T cell activation. Administration of these along with the antigen was found to result in enhanced T cell responses.

– Adjuvants can selectively modulate cytokine responses, thereby inducing the desired T$_{H1}$ or T$_{H2}$[12] type response. Bacterial toxins like the cholera toxin and pertussis toxin preferentially drive T$_{H2}$-responses and enhance IgA and IgE antibody production. Monophosphoryl Lipid A, on the other hand, has been shown to induce IFN-γ and hence a T$_{H1}$ response. Cytokines themselves may also be used as adjuvants. IL-12 for instance, when administered with an antigen, has been shown to selectively induce a T$_{H1}$ response. IFN-γ and GM-CSF are two other cytokines being evaluated for their adjuvant activity.

Choosing the appropriate adjuvant is crucial for both the end result (high antibody/cytotoxic T lymphocyte response) and the welfare of the immunized animal. Adjuvant selection is based upon antigen characteristics (size, net charge, and the presence or absence of polar groups). Adjuvant choice is also dependent upon the species to be immunized. Admittedly, in spite of all the advances in knowledge, adjuvant selection remains largely empirical. Perhaps the most desirable feature of an adjuvant is its ability to specifically enhance an immune response to the antigen it is administered with. An adjuvant with broad, non-specific effects is more likely to induce adverse immunological effects. The benefits of incorporating adjuvants into vaccine formulations must be weighed against the risks of adverse reactions. Adjuvant induced local adverse reactions include inflammation at the site of injection, induction of granulomas, or abscess formation. Systemic reactions may include malaise, fever, adjuvant arthritis, and anaphylactic shock. This risk of adverse reactions and concerns about the safety of adjuvants has restricted their

[12] T helper cells fall in two broad groups — type 1 (T$_{H1}$) and type 2 (T$_{H2}$). They differ in the cytokines they produce, the Ig isotypes they promote, and the type of immune response they drive. They are described in chapter 8.

development after the introduction of alum in the first half of the 20th century. Many experimental adjuvants currently undergoing clinical trials have been shown to be highly immunostimulatory. The acceptability of side effects often depends upon intended use. For standard prophylactic use in healthy individuals, only adjuvants with minimum side effects are acceptable (hence the popularity of the rather weak alum salts!). For adjuvants that are designed to be used in life-threatening situations (eg, cancer), the acceptable side-reaction levels are likely to be higher. Other issues important to adjuvant design and usage include biodegradability, stability, ease and cost of manufacture, and applicability to multiple immunogens. Future adjuvants will probably exploit more site-specific delivery systems and target antigens better for optimal immune response induction with minimal side effects.

Entities of the Adaptive Immune Response: The Lymphoid System

5

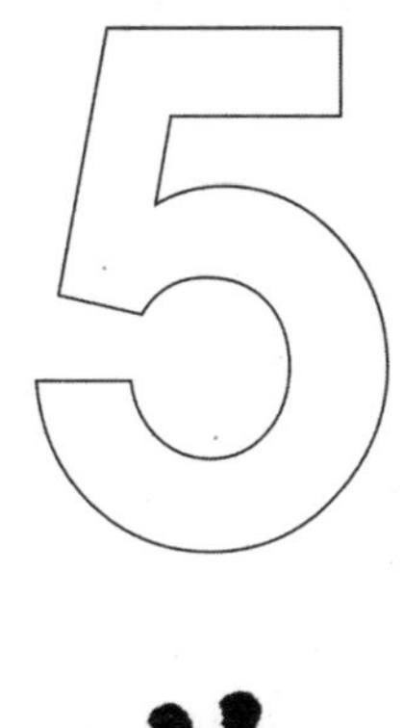

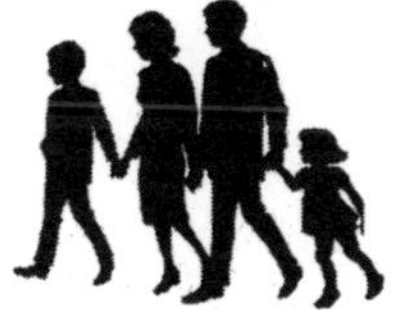

Win or lose, sink or swim
One thing is certain we'll never give in
Side by side, hand in hand
We all stand together
Play the game, fight the fight
But what's the point on a beautiful night?
Arm in arm, hand in hand
We all stand together

— Paul McCartney, *We All Stand Together*

BALT: Bronchus-associated lymphoid tissue
CALT: Cutaneous-associated lymphoid tissue
CTLs: Cytotoxic T cells
GALT: Gut-associated lymphoid tissue
HEV: High endothelial venule
IELs: Intraepithelial lymphocytes
MALT: Mucosa-associated lymphoid tissue
NALT: Nasopharynx l-associated lymphoid tissue
PALS: Periarterialor lymphoid sheath
SALT: Skin-associated lymphoid tissue
SCID: Severe combined immunodeficiency
sIgA: Secretory IgA
VIP: Vasoactive intestinal peptide

5.1 Introduction

Cells of the immune system are organized into tissues and organs which are collectively referred to as the lymphoid system (fig. 5.1). This system comprises cellular components responsible for antigen-specific host defence and consists of lymphocytes, epithelial cells, and stromal cells[1] arranged either in discretely encapsulated organs (thymus, spleen, etc) or accumulations of diffuse lymphoid tissue (eg, Peyer's patches). **Organs and tissues of the lymphoid system are connected to each other by the lymphatic system.** Plasma tends to seep into surrounding tissues through thin capillary walls because of the high pressure under which blood circulates. A major portion of this plasma re-enters the blood through capillary membranes. The remainder, called lymph, flows into a separate system of tiny, open capillaries — the lymphatic capillaries — and from there, into progressively larger lymphatic vessels. Eventually, the lymph enters blood circulation so that the

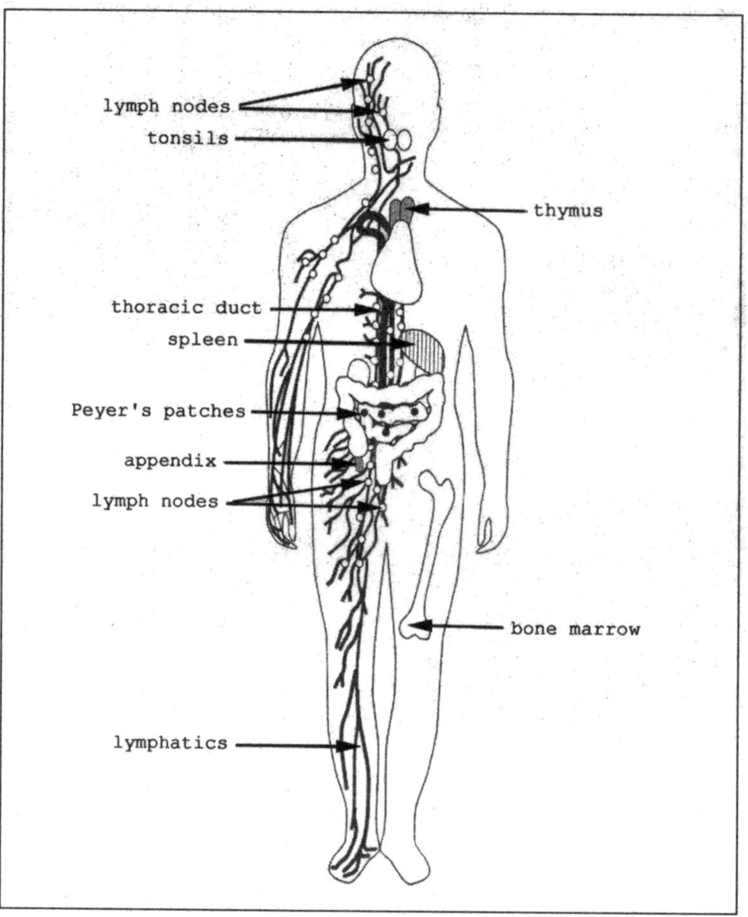

Figure 5.1 The lymphoid system consists of lymphocytes, epithelial cells, and stromal cells arranged either in discreetly encapsulated organs or accumulations. The thymus and the bone marrow are primary lymphoid organs of humans. These are the site of lymphopoiesis and lymphocyte maturation. The lymphocytes that have matured in the primary organs get lodged in the secondary lymphoid organs (lymph nodes, spleen, and MALT), where they undergo further differentiation on antigenic challenge. The lymph nodes are found at the junction of lymphatic vessels traversing the body. They drain and filter lymph from the tissue spaces and internal organs. The lymph eventually collects in the thoracic duct from where it drains in the left subclavian vein and then enters the blood stream. Epithelium-associated lymphoid tissue is found in a variety of organs such as tonsils, intestinal epithelium, Peyer's patches, appendix, urinogenital epithelium, skin, and bronchial lining (Courtesy of the Department of Immunology, Erasmus MC, The Netherlands).

[1] The connective tissue, nerves, and vessels that form the frame-like support of an organ or a part thereof are called the stroma. Stromal cells are the cells that form this supporting framework.

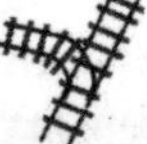

They Have Feelings Too: Lymphoid Organs as Neuroendocrine Organs

Although we think of the thymus as a purely immunological organ, it is also rich in nerve fibres. Noradrenergic and peptidergic fibres enter the thymus with nerve bundles and plexuses around blood vessels, penetrate the cortex from subcapsular plexuses, and branch out among lymphocytes in the thymic cortex. The vasculature and lymphatic tissue of the outer and deep cortex are enervated by these fibres. Neuropeptides are present in thymic neurons. *In vitro* studies indicate that T cell responses can be affected by neurosecretory products, and anatomical studies clearly show the association of nerve fibres with aggregates of lymphoid cells *in vivo*. Other organs of the immune system, including the bone marrow, lymph nodes, spleen, and lymphoid tissue in the MALT such as Peyer's patches and tonsils show extensive enervation and penetration by noradrenergic nerve fibres. Little is known about the function of this enervation outside its assumed role in controlling blood flow. Many cells of the lymphoid system, including T cells and DCs, express receptors for hormones and neuromediators such as **V**asoactive **I**ntestinal **P**eptide (VIP)[2], somatostatin, calcitonin generated peptide, substance P, etc. These neuropeptides are released from unmyelinated nerve endings in the lymphoid organs. Reciprocally, neural cells express receptors for cytokines, and lymphoid cells can secrete neuropeptides. Thus, both neural cells and immune cells can influence each other in a paracrine and autocrine manner. The central nervous system and the immune system have been suggested to have bi-directional circuits. Thymosins, interleukins, complement components, enkephalins, adrenocorticotropic hormones, and thyroid-stimulating hormones present in thymic cells produce neuroendocrine effects on both systems. The precise relation of the anatomy and physiology of neuroimmune functions in T cell development and differentiation, however, remains unresolved. Recent research further stresses the relation between the immune system and the neuroendocrine system — thymectomy in mice not only reduces the immune response but also deteriorates learning performance. Increasingly, we face evidence that we cannot think of the body in terms of isolated systems; it must be viewed holistically.

levels of fluid in the circulatory system remain constant. Mature lymphocytes continuously circulate between various lymphoid organs and other tissues via the lymph and the blood stream, increasing their chances of encountering an immunogen. Approximately 1–2% of the available lymphocyte pool circulates every hour. Most lymphocytes leave blood circulation through a specialized section of the post-capillary venule (ie, a very tiny vein) known as the **High Endothelial Venule (HEV[3])**. Here, lymphocytes react with the high endothelial cells. Some lymphocytes can leave blood circulation through non-specialized venules. All lymphocytes eventually re-enter the blood stream through the lymphatics. Adaptive immune responses do not occur at the site of the entry of immunogens or agents perceived as a threat to the well-being of the individual. Instead, immunogens or pathogens are transported by the lymph to the tissues of the lymphoid system. Immunogens deposited in peripheral tissues are carried via the lymphatic channels and trapped in the lymph nodes directly downstream of the site of infection. Pathogens entering the blood are trapped in the spleen; those infecting the mucosal surfaces accumulate in the tonsils or Peyer's patches. Thus, the whole lymphatic system and the architecture of the lymphoid organs is designed to maximize chances of trapping any immunogen entering the system. The juxtaposition of the cells further increases response efficiency; cells that have to interact with each other for the generation of an immune response are found in the proximity of each other.

5.2 The Primary Lymphoid Organs

The primary or central lymphoid organs are the major sites of lymphopoiesis, ie, generation of lymphocytes. In the primary lymphoid organs, lymphoid stem cells divide and differentiate into lymphocytes. The rate of cell division and differentiation

[2] Recent studies indicate that in lymphoid organs, lymphocytes themselves are the major source of VIP. It has potent anti-inflammatory effects and promotes T cell differentiation to T$_{H2}$ type while inhibiting T$_{H1}$ pathways (section 8.3.5.1). Thus, this neuropeptide seems to behave suspiciously like a cytokine.

[3] The name HEV alludes to the fact that the endothelial lining of these venules consists of cells having a plump cuboid morphology and not the flat morphology observed in other blood vessels. The 'high' in the name, thus, refers to the thickness of these cells.

is stupendous. Around 10^8 lymphocytes are formed daily in the bone marrow through cell division. **Newly formed lymphocytes undergo a process of proliferation and maturation in the primary lymphoid organs before migrating to secondary lymphoid organs**. Two primary lymphoid organs have been recognized in mammals — the thymus and the bone marrow. Recent evidence suggests that in humans, the intestinal epithelium is also a primary lymphoid organ[4]. Both primary and secondary lymphoid organs are often called 'lymphoepithelial', since they consist of a mass of lymphocytes and a smaller number of epithelial cells.

5.2.1 The Thymus

In mammals, the thymus is located in the thorax, which overlies the heart and the major blood vessels. Immature lymphocytes produced by the yolk sac or liver in the early stages of development or by bone marrow stem cells later in life migrate to the thymus for maturation. These lymphocytes that mature in the thymus are called the T lymphocytes, or simply, the T cells. Unlike other lymphoid organs, the thymus is not involved in lymphocyte circulation and does not receive lymph from other tissues.

The thymus is a bi-lobed, encapsulated organ. Each lobe is organized into lobules or follicles. Strands of connective tissue, called trabeculae, separate the lobules. These lobules are organized structures consisting of an outer cortex and inner medulla. A three-dimensional network of stromal cells, consisting of epithelial cells, interdigitating DCs, and macrophages, criss-cross the cortex and the medulla. The cortex is densely packed with immature lymphocytes (also called thymocytes) with a few scattered macrophages. The medulla, however, appears epithelial because of a relative scarcity of lymphocytes. The lymphocytes found in the medulla are mature thymocytes. The bulk of the macrophages are found at the cortico-medullary junction and the medulla. Most of these thymic macrophages originate in the bone marrow and migrate to the developing thymus. The medulla also shows the presence of DCs, which like the macrophages, originate in the bone marrow (fig. 5.2).

A single layer of epithelial cells — called subcapsular thymic epithelial cells — lines the internal surface of the thymus. Both the cortex and medulla also have their own layers of epithelial cells. They show heterogeneity in their ultrastructural morphology as well as in their origin. The cortical epithelial cells are stellate cells with long cytoplasmic extensions, and medullary epithelial cells are spindle-shaped. Some epithelial cells in the outer cortex are referred to as 'thymic nurse cells', since each 'nurse cell' seems to almost completely surround many thymocytes, thus appearing to nurse them. These nurse cells are postulated to play a role in T cell maturation.

The thymic epithelium, like the skin, undergoes progressive keratinization and maturation. The subcapsular thymic epithelium contains less mature keratin than the specific agglomerations of epithelial cells found in the medulla — called Hassal's corpuscles — where the most mature keratin is found. The Hassal's corpuscles are filled with whorls of keratinized epithelium, leukocytes, and cell-debris. It is postulated that the epithelium of the thymus may not be static but may in fact undergo continuous turnover like the epithelium of the skin. Hassal's corpuscles are thought to be the internal site for the endocytosis, degradation, and carrying away of exfoliated epithelium by leukocytes.

Chemotactic peptides elaborated by thymic epithelial cells and/or mononuclear cells are believed to initiate the migration of circulating lymphocytes to the developing thymus. The thymus is populated with lymphoid cells in three discrete 24–36 hour waves which are separated by refractory periods. Temporally expressed receptors or periodic releases of chemotactic factors by thymic epithelial cells are believed to regulate this population of the thymus. Epithelial cells also have an important role in T lymphocyte maturation. It is now recognized that thymic epithelial cells have immunomodulator and neuroendocrine functions which affect the functioning of

---

[4] It represents a major site of T cell lymphopoiesis and has a substantial fraction of T cells in the body.

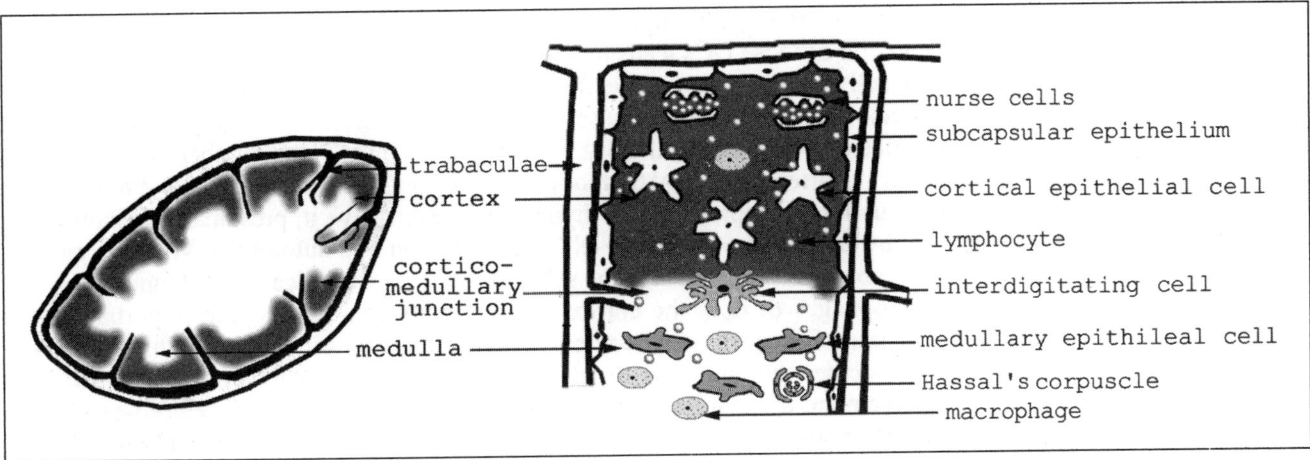

Figure 5.2 The thymus is a bi-lobed primary lymphoid organ where T lymphocytes mature. *Each lobe of the thymus is organized into lobules that are separated by strands of connective tissue called trabaculae. The lobules consist of an outer cortex and an inner medulla and are lined by subcapsular thymic epithelial cells. Both the cortex and medulla have their own layer of epithelial cells called cortical epithelial cells and medullary epithelial cells. Some cortical epithelial cells seem to completely surround many thymocytes and are called nurse cells. The cortex is densely packed with immature lymphocytes. It also contains a scattering of macrophages. Interdigitating cells found at the cortico-medullary junction are thought to be important in the process of thymic maturation. The medulla shows the presence of Hassal's corpuscles, stellate medullary epithelial cells, macrophages, and relatively few thymocytes that have survived the process of maturation.*

T cells inside and outside the thymus. They produce soluble thymic hormones such as thymulin, thymosins, thymopoietin, the thymic humoral factor, and cytokines like IL-3 and IL-7 that regulate the proliferation, differentiation, and maturation of T cells. Granular deposits of IL-1 are found to be present in thymic cortical epithelial and/or mononuclear cells. Thymosin-α1 and the thymic humoral factor are detected in both cortical and medullary epithelial cells, whereas thymosin β3 has been found only in the cortical population. These hormones are involved in thymocyte maturation. Thymic epithelial cells express MHC molecules in three basic patterns. The subcapsular epithelial layer is MHC class II negative. The remaining cortex, including thymic nurse cells, is strongly MHC class II positive. The inner membrane of thymic nurse cells also expresses MHC class I molecules strongly. The medulla is strongly MHC class I and II positive. All cells in the thymus express MHC class I molecules, but the highest expression is on non-epithelial cells.

In the thymus, T cells 'learn' to distinguish between self and non-self antigens; the process is referred to as 'thymic education'. T cells undergo both positive and negative selection — positive selection for those T cells capable of recognizing antigens bound to self-MHC molecules and negative selection to ensure the deletion of self-reacting clones. Both these processes are discussed in chapter 8. The earliest cells to enter the thymus lodge in the subcapsular region of the cortex and form a distinctive population. They undergo a phase of intense proliferation to give rise to large, self-renewing lymphoblasts. The stream of newly produced thymic lymphocytes goes from the cortex to the medulla. As the thymic lymphocytes go deeper in the cortex, they are subjected to selection processes. In the medullary region, interdigitating cells derived from the bone marrow lie superimposed on the epithelial cells. Both these cells are rich in MHC class I and II molecules. They are thought to be important in the twin processes of self/non-self education and acquisition of MHC restriction (ie, the capacity to recognize antigen only in the context of self-MHC molecules). The relative contribution of the epithelial cells *vis á vis* other stromal cells in these processes is not known. Although MHC class II expressing epithelial cells are thought to be important in thymic education, it is the non-epithelial DCs in the thymus that are thought to control the development of CD4[+] T$_H$ cells, since depletion of these DCs leads to a loss of T$_H$ cells in the periphery.

T cell precursors that arrive from the bone marrow to the thymus reside there for a week before entering a phase of intense proliferation. 5×10^7 thymocytes are estimated to be generated daily in young adult mice. This number corresponds to about a quarter of the total thymocytes in the young thymus. About 95–98% of these cells undergo apoptosis in the thymus and never leave it, presumably because they fail the twin tests of self/non-self discrimination and autologous MHC restriction. Only about 10^6 cells survive the selection processes and leave the thymus each day. Macrophages in both the cortex and the medullary regions are important in the digestion of those T lymphocytes that are dead or destined to die. Thus, immature lymphocytes that enter the thymus at the cortex journey towards the medulla and receive maturation and survival signals *en route*. Only mature T cells co-expressing TcR for non-self proteins and the appropriate MHC co-receptor (CD4 for class II, CD8 for class I) finally survive to reach the medulla, from where they may eventually leave the thymus. Mature T cells that leave the thymus:

❑ are capable of recognizing antigen only in context of self-MHC molecules,
❑ take part in cellular interactions,
❑ possess homing receptors, and
❑ are equipped with all properties necessary to perform the immune functions of T lymphocytes.

The thymus is relatively large at birth. Once peripheral tissues are populated with diversified T cells, its major function is over. The thymus was believed to atrophy as an animal reached maturity (attained puberty). It is now established that this is not entirely correct, and reduction in true thymic tissue starts as early as at one year of age and continues at the rate of 3% per year until middle age. The adult thymus is nonetheless functional and continues to produce precursors of T lymphocytes at a slow rate.

5.2.2 The Bone Marrow

It was discovered that in birds, some lymphocytes mature in the Bursa of Fabricus (an organ found only in birds and reptiles), and these cells were called the B lymphocytes or the B cells. In mammals, the foetal liver and the adult bone marrow[5] are sites of B cell maturation[6]. Apart from giving rise to B cells, the bone marrow is also an important site of antibody production, ie, unlike the thymus, the bone marrow also acts as an important secondary lymphoid organ.

The bone marrow is physiologically the most important site of haematopoiesis. In adults, pleuripotent stem cells in the bone marrow give rise to platelets, erythrocytes, lymphocytic cells — T cells, B cells, and NK cells. Bone marrow stem cells also give rise to the myeloid lineage cells (neutrophils, basophils, eosinophils). They are also the source of DCs (fig. 5.3). The aggregate volume and weight of the bone marrow surpasses that of the liver. It is a highly organized anatomical structure comprising vascular and non-vascular components. It is divided into wedge-shaped haematopoietic compartments filled with proliferating and differentiating blood cells in connective tissue matrices bordered by venous sinuses. It has a closed circulation in which arterioles flow out into venous sinuses, finally emptying into a large central sinus that is connected with the efferent (*efferent* — conducting outwards) venous system. Several observations suggest that the haematopoietic cells move centripetally as they differentiate and mature from the bone marrow periphery (ie, near the surrounding bone) inward towards extravascular tissue spaces. Thus, cells near the bone are immature, whereas those near the central sinus are mature. As with the thymus, stromal cells of the bone marrow are essential for the regulation of haematopoietic cell development. The microenvironment of the bone marrow consists

---

[5] A fortuitous occurrence ☺. Otherwise, we would have to come up with yet another name for these lymphocytes!

[6] The bone marrow does not perform the function of a primary lymphoid organ in all mammals. In ungulates such as cattle and sheep, B cell maturation occurs in the Peyer's patches.

THE THYMUS

❑ It is a bi-lobed lymphoepithelial organ which is the site of T lymphocyte proliferation and maturation.
❑ T cells undergo positive and negative selection in the thymus.
  • Positive selection ensures recognition of antigen bound to self-MHC molecules.
  • Negative selection ensures deletion of self-reacting clones.
❑ The cells also acquire appropriate homing and antigen receptors in the thymus.
❑ The thymus consists of two regions — the cortex and medulla, each having its own epithelial layer of cells.
❑ The epithelial cells have several functions.
  • Chemotaxins secreted by thymic epithelial cells are responsible for migration of lymphocytes to the developing thymus.
  • The epithelial cells have immunomodulatory and neuroendocrine functions.
  • Hormones and cytokines produced by the epithelial cells are responsible for T cell development and maturation.

BONE MARROW

❑ It is the most important site of haematopoiesis.
❑ It is also a site of B cell maturation and selection.
❑ It is the major site of antibody production.

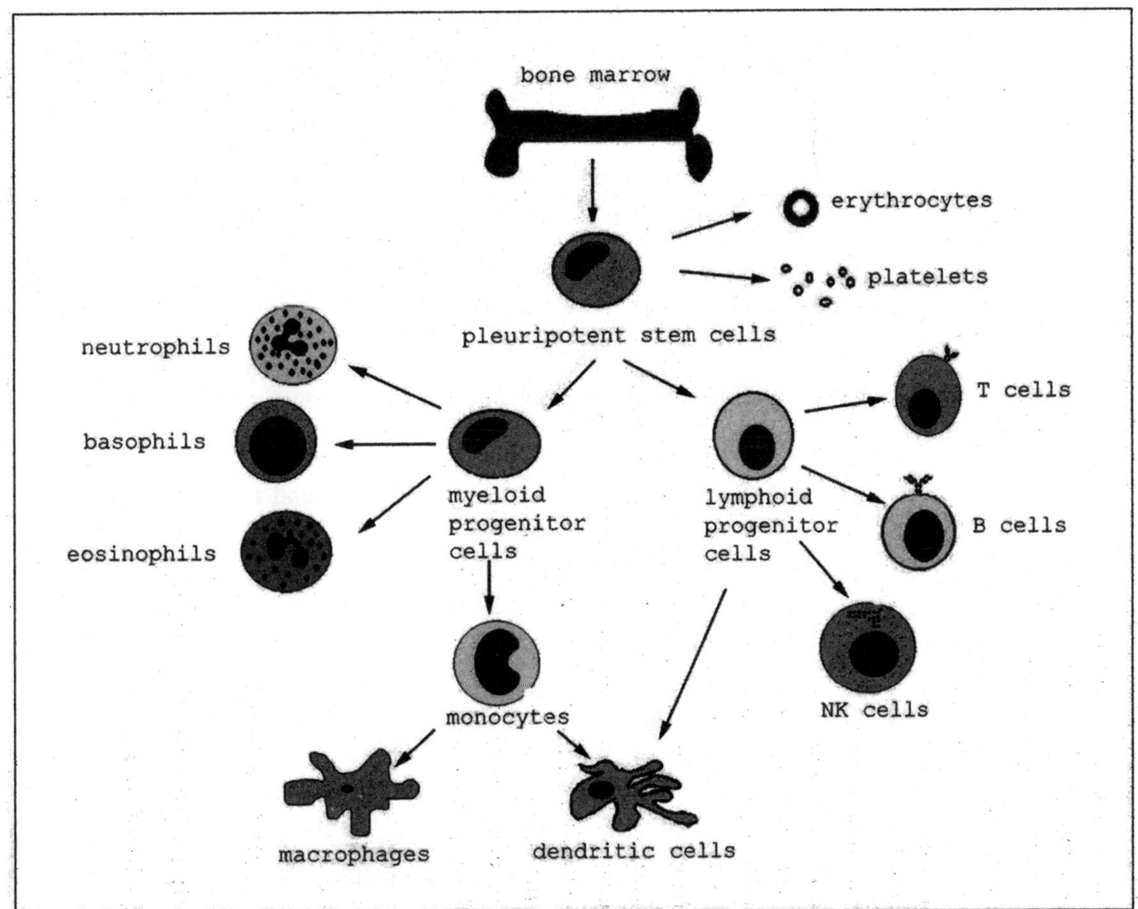

Figure 5.3 The bone marrow is the most important site of haematopoiesis. *Pleuripotent stem cells in the bone marrow give rise to platelets, erythrocytes, lymphoid progenitor cells, and myeloid progenitor cells. The lymphoid progenitor cells further differentiate to T lymphocytes, B lymphocytes, and NK cells. The lymphoid progenitor cells also give rise to a type of DC called plasmacytoid DC. The myeloid progenitor cells give rise to the myeloid lineage cells (neutrophils, eosinophils, and basophils). They also give rise to monocytes that can further differentiate to macrophages or DCs, depending upon the cytokine environment they are exposed to.*

of a unique endothelium and connective tissue stroma combined with locally deposited cytokines that regulate haematopoietic stem cell compartmentalization, proliferation, and differentiation. The signals and factors involved in this development are not as yet fully characterized. It is known that the stroma assists in haematopoiesis through the glycosaminoglycan-rich extracellular matrix that binds and distributes growth factors such as GM-CSF. Stromal cells also secrete IL-7, a growth factor for lymphocyte development.

The emerging lymphocytes are subjected to various influences in the microenvironment of the bone marrow to become mature B cells capable of Ig production. Like T cells, B cells are also subjected to a selection process that eliminates self-reactive clones. Those pre-B cells that do not form functional Ig molecules or that possess Ig molecules which recognize and bind self-antigens undergo apoptosis in the bone marrow. B cells that survive this selection process leave the bone marrow through efferent blood vessels.

5.3 The Secondary Lymphoid Organs

Lymphocytes that have matured in the primary organs are lodged in the secondary or peripheral lymphoepithelial organs. These organs create an environment in which lymphocytes can interact with each other and the antigen. **They also act as the centre through which the immune response, once generated, is disseminated in the body.** Secondary lymphoid organs are the site of further maturation and differentiation of lymphocytes. The secondary lymphoid organs consist of the following.

❑ **The lymph nodes** are distributed throughout the body. These are encapsulated organs found at the junction of lymphatic vessels. They act as filters for the lymph and trap antigens and cells containing antigens that flow into them via afferent (*afferent* — to bring, conducting inwards) lymphatics. They also provide a site for activation of naïve lymphocytes and clonal expansion of activated lymphoid cells.

❑ **The spleen** acts as a filter that traps blood-borne organisms or antigens.

❑ **Epithelium-associated lymphoid tissue** comprises non-encapsulated lymphoid tissue found in a variety of organs. It can be broadly divided into two categories.
  • MALT (**M**ucosa-**A**ssociated **L**ymphoid **T**issue) is found in the submucosal areas of the gastrointestinal, respiratory, and urinogenital tract, eg, tonsils, adenoids, and lining of the bronchi.
  • CALT (**C**utaneous-**A**ssociated **L**ymphoid **T**issue) or SALT (**S**kin-**A**ssociated **L**ymphoid **T**issue) that helps in defending the outermost surface of the body.

5.3.1 The Lymph Nodes

Human lymph nodes are encapsulated, kidney-shaped structures between 1–25 mm in diameter, found at the junction of lymphatic vessels (fig. 5.1). These lymphatics drain and filter lymph from tissue spaces. The lymph eventually collects in the thoracic duct, from where it drains in the left subclavian vein and then enters the blood stream. The capsule covering the lymph node is a collagenous structure that penetrates it. The radial trabeculae formed by the capsule, along with reticulin fibres, form the supporting structure for various cellular components within the lymph node. Just beneath the capsule is the subcapsular sinus, lined with phagocytic cells. Lymph passes from the surrounding capsule in this sinus via the afferent lymphatic vessels. The lymph leaves the node via the efferent lymphatic vessels (fig. 5.4). Blood vessels enter and leave the node through the hilus. Lymphocytes travel to the lymph nodes through the blood stream and enter it across the HEV. Thus, lymph nodes are fed by two vascular systems:

> The way the immune system responds to an antigenic challenge is a good lesson in business management. Don't believe us? Read this description of how 'the BEANS factory', a provider of e-commerce solutions, deals with customer requirements.
>
> 'Our dynamic, highly responsive and flexible organizational structure is centred on a customer-oriented, market and innovation-driven focus. Our strategic business units are structured such that different teams of specialists with the necessary knowledge and skills are assembled to address specific market, project or client needs. These project teams are created, managed and then dissolved over the project cycle.'
>
> Q.E.D. We rest our case.

❑ the lymphatic system that delivers antigens and antigen-transporting cells from peripheral tissues to the nodes and returns fluid and cells to circulation, and
❑ the blood vasculature which brings circulating lymphocytes into the system.

Histologically, the lymph node can be divided into two zones — the cortex and the medulla (fig. 5.4). The cortex consists of an outer cortex and inner paracortex. The outer cortex lies just under the subcapsular sinus and consists of a macrophage rich zone and B cell follicles. It is often referred to as the 'B cell area'. The cells of the cortex are localized to discrete follicles. Around each follicle is a condensation of reticular cells. These are termed the primary follicles. The primary follicles are present in lymph nodes as early as the second trimester of human foetal life. They consist of a network of FDCs and recirculating small B lymphocytes. Primary follicles are found in the spleens of germ-free as well as normal animals. This implies that they are formed independent of pathogenic challenge. They seem to provide the microenvironment essential for B cell survival, although the nature of the signals from the primary follicles that allow this survival is not known. Naïve B cells emerging from the bone marrow have to lodge here briefly before entering circulation. Failure to enter the primary follicles results in B cell death within a matter of days. Primary follicles develop into secondary follicles upon antigenic stimulation. These secondary follicles contain many FDCs and macrophages as well as a fine network of interdigitating cells that are rich in MHC class II molecules. B cells that have encountered antigen in the lymph node migrate from the primary to the secondary follicles and differentiate to plasmablasts that give rise to antibody-secreting plasma cells[7]. These plasma cells then migrate to the medullary cords, from where a majority leave for the bone marrow. Unstimulated B cells migrate through the primary follicle and leave the lymph node via the efferent lymphatic.

The paracortex lies interior to the outer cortex and consists mostly of T cells. It is a high traffic zone where migrant or recirculating T and B lymphocytes enter from the blood. Lymphocytes in the paracortex are directed towards specific B or T cell microenvironments by fibroblastic reticular cell corridors where the lymphocytes encounter APCs. The paracortex is populated with T cells and many APCs — the interdigitating cells — rich in MHC class II molecules. If the lymphocytes are not activated by twin signals of antigen (displayed in the context of MHC class II molecules) and costimulatory molecules, they crawl out of the lymph node through the lymphatic channels. For a naïve lymphocyte that does not encounter its cognate antigen, such a circuit through the node is thought to take fewer than 24 hours.

The medulla lies to the inner side of the paracortex and consists of medullary strands separated by the medullary sinuses and interconnected medullary cords. Scavenger phagocytic cells are arranged along the medullary strands. During passage of the lymph across the lymph node, the phagocytic cells trap any particulate antigens present. Antigens that escape phagocytosis within one lymph node face phagocytes in other lymph nodes through which the lymph must pass before entering major efferent collecting ducts. Antigens that succeed in eluding lymph node entrapment will ultimately be captured by blood monocytes or macrophages in the spleen, liver, or bone marrow.

---

[7] Antigenic stimulation also increases extravasation of the lymphocytes into the lymph nodes near the site of stimulation. Together with the proliferation of the lymphocytes, this gives rise to what is popularly called 'swollen glands'.

When an animal is challenged by a TD antigen, germinal centres consisting of rapidly multiplying lymphoblasts appear in the secondary follicles. Germinal centres are discrete lymphoid compartments where B cells (that are stimulated by the twin stimuli of antigen and T cell help) divide, switch the isotype of Ig expressed, and differentiate. B cell follicles are found in all peripheral lymphatic tissues, including the foci of chronic inflammation. A germinal centre develops in a follicle as proliferating B cells displace cortical reticular fibres into a bask-like enclosure that separates central lymphoblasts from the peripheral mantle of small B cells. Lymphoblasts, FDCs, and macrophages reside in this enclosure. Proliferating B cells in the germinal centres have a clearly defined nuclear shape (something that is handy for identification). The size and number of germinal centres is related to the intensity of antigenic stimulation. Germinal centres show a well-defined architecture consisting of a dark zone, light zone, and mantle (fig. 10.5). They last for about three weeks after antigen administration and are the sites of antigen-dependent B cell proliferation, selection and differentiation, and affinity maturation (see below).

FDCs in the germinal centres bind and retain antigen unchanged for long periods of time. During the process of antigen-dependent proliferation, B cells undergo extensive mutation in the genetic region that codes for the antigen-combining site of the Ig molecule. As a result, they give rise to clones of cells that express Ig with an altered — and better fitting — antigen-combining site. Antibodies produced by such cells react much more strongly with the antigen, ie, they have a higher affinity for the antigen. FDCs help in selection of the clones with increased affinity for the antigen. Macrophages in the follicles are thought to phagocytose those newly emerging B cells that have a reduced complementarity of fit (and hence, lowered affinity) for the antigen (chapter 10). Antibodies produced later in the immune response therefore have an increased affinity for the antigen. This phenomenon is called affinity maturation.

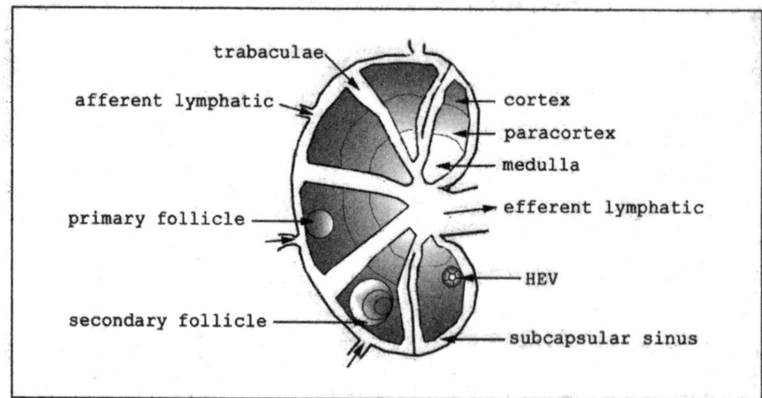

Figure 5.4 Lymph nodes are encapsulated structures that provide a site for the activation and clonal expansion of lymphocytes. The capsule covering the lymph node forms radial trabaculae that penetrate into the lymph node. Lymph passes from the surrounding capsule into the subcapsular sinus via the afferent lymphatic vessels; it leaves the node via the efferent lymphatic vessels. Lymphocytes travel to the lymph nodes through the blood stream and enter it across the high endothelial venule (HEV). The lymph node can be divided into three regions — cortex, paracortex, and medulla. The cortex lies beneath the subcapsular sinus and is called the B cell area, since it is rich in B lymphocytes. The cells of the cortex are localized to discrete follicles termed the primary follicles. They provide the microenvironment essential for B cell survival. The cortex also shows the presence of secondary follicles. These are formed on antigenic stimulus and are the site of antigen-stimulated B cell proliferation and differentiation. The paracortex lies interior to the outer cortex and is the T cell area; the medulla lies to the inner side of the paracortex and is rich in scavenger macrophages.

THE LYMPH NODES

❑ These are encapsulated bean-shaped organs found at the junction of lymphatic vessels.
❑ Afferent and efferent lymphatics maintain a continuous, active flow of lymphocytes to these organs.
❑ Lymph nodes filter and trap antigens or antigen-containing cells in lymph.
❑ They are the site of activation and clonal expansion of antigen-specific B and T lymphocytes that get lodged there.
❑ They consist of a cortex (B cell area), paracortex, and medulla (together, T cell area).
- Cells of cortex arranged in discrete areas are called primary follicles.
- Antigen stimulation with TD antigen gives rise to secondary follicles — the site of memory B development, isotype switching, and affinity maturation.

THE SPLEEN

❑ It is an encapsulated organ lying just behind the stomach; it consists of red pulp, white pulp, and the marginal zone separating the two.
- The red pulp is the site of erythrocyte disposal.
- The white pulp represents the organized lymphoid compartment. It contains PALS, which has primary and secondary germinal centres.
- The marginal zone is involved in antigen trapping; MZ B cells respond to TI antigens.

5.3.2 The Spleen

A fist-sized organ that lies at the upper left of the abdomen, behind the stomach, and close to the diaphragm, the spleen contains up to 25% of the body's mature lymphocytes. It is surrounded by a dense fibrous collagenous capsule with muscular trabeculae that penetrate the organ and subdivide the spleen into lobules. As with other encapsulated lymphoid organs, these intrusions along with the reticular framework, support the variety of cells found in the spleen. The spleen consists of three types of tissue.

❑ **The red pulp** (medulla) encloses the cortical area and makes up the bulk of the spleen. It contains erythrocyte-rich blood in the cords of the reticulum and contains erythrocytes, lymphocytes, macrophages, granulocytes, and plasma cells. Aged or damaged erythrocytes are removed from circulation in the red pulp.
❑ **The white pulp** is formed of cylindrical collections of lymphocytes around the arteries. It represents the organized lymphoid compartment in which regulated activation and maturation of antigen-dependent B and T cells can occur.
❑ **A border region called the marginal zone** separates the red and the white pulp. A principal function of the marginal zone is antigen trapping, and it seems to be important in generating rapid humoral responses to blood-borne antigens. The marginal zone of the spleen contains a heterogeneous assortment of mononuclear cells with specialized functions. It is home to a subset of B cells called MZ B cells (section 8.2.3) that respond to predominantly TI type 2 antigens. Macrophages and DCs present in the marginal zone appear to be important in MZ B cell generation, maintenance, and functioning.

Unlike the lymph nodes, the spleen has a single vascular supply. Immune cells and antigens enter the tissue via blood flowing in from the splenic artery, which is the only point of entry to the spleen. The splenic artery branches several times before entering the splenic hilus. After branching into trabecular arteries, it further branches into central arterioles that penetrate the white pulp nodules. Ultimately, these vessels terminate in small arterioles which empty into the reticulum of the red pulp cords or white pulp sinuses. The bulk of the lymphoid tissue of the white pulp is arranged around the central arterioles and consists of a coaxial layer rich in T cells, called the **Periarterialor Lymphoid Sheath (PALS)**. The PALS also contains abundant interdigitating DCs that are thought to act as APCs early in the immune response. In the white pulp, B cells are organized into two compartments. The first consists of predominantly naïve cells and includes cells from the marginal zone that lie adjacent to the marginal sinus. The second compartment is composed of cells associated with follicles, which in the resting state, are primary follicles (fig. 5.5). Secondary follicles develop on antigenic stimulation. Both primary and secondary follicles are similar in composition and structure to those found in the lymph nodes (section 5.3.1).

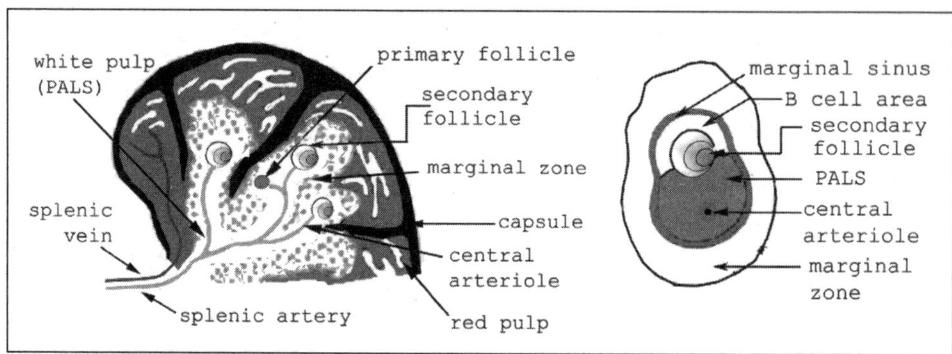

Figure 5.5 The white pulp of the spleen is the centre through which immune response to blood-borne antigens is initiated and disseminated. The spleen is an encapsulated organ that is divided into lobules by its capsule. A schematic cross-section of the spleen is shown in the left panel. The right panel is an enlargement of a small section of the white pulp. The bulk of the spleen consists of the red pulp that is the site of erythrocyte disposal. Blood carrying lymphocytes enters the spleen at the hilus via the splenic artery. After branching into trabecular arteries, the splenic artery further branches into central arterioles. Cells (and antigen) then pass into a marginal sinus and empty into the trabecular vein. Cylindrical collections of lymphocytes are present around the trabeuclar arterioles and constitute the white pulp. A border region called the marginal zone separates the red and the white pulp. The bulk of the lymphoid tissue of the white pulp is arranged around the central arterioles and consists of a coaxial layer rich in T cells called the Periarterialor Lymphoid Sheath (PALS) flanked by the B cell area containing B2 cells. Primary and secondary follicles are found in this area. The marginal zone that separates the white pulp and red pulp contains a special subset of B cells that have characteristics similar to B1 cells.

Lymphocyte traffic in the spleen moves across a blood:tissue interface into sites of antigen presentation in the marginal zone and PALS. **The spleen is the primary site for the initiation of immune responses to blood-borne antigens and pathogens in addition to being a partner in every immune response in the body.** 48–100 hours after antigen priming, antigen-laden mononuclear cells and lymphoblasts are released into efferent lymph from other lymphatic tissues. These cells lodge in the spleen and set up satellite zones of T and B cell proliferation. During active immune responses, lymphoblastic B cells committed to plasma cell differentiation lodge in the red pulp cords and sinuses where they mature and begin secreting antibodies.

5.3.3 Epithelium-associated Lymphoid Tissue

Non-encapsulated lymphoid tissue is found at two major sites in the body — tissue associated with the mucosa or that associated with the skin.

5.3.3.1 MALT

Mucous membranes that cover the digestive, respiratory, and urogenital tracts are spread over an area of approximately 400 m^2. They are the major portals of immunogen entry into the body. Being the primary sites for immunogen encounter, mucosal epithelia need to be well-defended. The number of plasma cells in MALT exceeds that found in the lymph nodes, spleen, and bone marrow combined. **MALT can either be well organized, eg, the appendix and Peyer's patches, or barely organized, as in the lamina propria of the intestinal epithelium.** Organized lymphoid tissues of the respiratory and gastrointestinal tracts contain the largest numbers of lymphocytes and are most fully characterized. Afferent lymphatics carry the immunogens that have gained entry at the mucosal surface to draining lymph nodes where specialized APCs present them to the immune system. Some of the important MALTs include:

- ❑ **NALT (N**asopharynx-**A**ssociated **L**ymphoid **T**issue). It includes the tonsils found in Waldeyer's ring — lingual tonsils at the base of the tongue, palatine tonsils at the sides of the back of the mouth, tubal tonsils at the pharyngeal openings of the Eustachian tubes, and nasopharyngeal tonsils (adenoids) in the roof of the nasopharynx.
- ❑ **BALT (B**ronchus-**A**ssociated **L**ymphoid **T**issue). In humans, BALT is normally found only in the lungs of children and adolescents. It may be found in adult lungs in certain pathological states.
- ❑ **GALT (G**ut-**A**ssociated **L**ymphoid **T**issue) includes the lymphoid tissue of the epithelium of the gastrointestinal tract. The outer mucosal epithelium contains dispersed **I**ntra**e**pithelial **L**ymphocytes (IELs) with unknown functions. The lamina propria under the epithelium has large numbers of B cells, T cells, plasma cells, and macrophages in follicles. The submucosal layer contains the Peyer's patches, which are nodules of 30–40 lymphoid follicles.

The mucosal immune system is the most dispersed diverse, and complicated lymphocytic system in the body. It is now clear that the microenvironment in these mucosal barriers has a marked influence on the immune response. Like the thymus, it plays a role in generating antigen-reactive lymphoid cells that can further mature into effector cells. The mucosal lymphatic tissues are also responsible for inducing tolerance to antigens that are commonly experienced in the enteric canal. Mucosal tolerance is manifested by antigen-specific suppression of delayed cutaneous hypersensitivity (chapter 15) and reduced IgG expression. Thus, MALT has to achieve a fine balance between two opposing immune functions — amplifying the

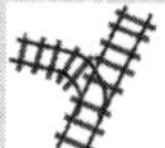

Better Throat of: Tonsils

The tonsils are lymphoepithelial structures found at the openings of the respiratory and digestive tract. The Swiss scientist Waldeyer first noted the importance of this ring of lymphoid tissue in the pharynx (hence the name Waldeyer's ring). The ring is comprised of the tonsils and the sub-epithelial lymphoid tissue in the mucosa of the pharynx. Tonsils are secondary lymphoid organs containing aggregations of lymphoid cells located in the lamina propria of the pharyngeal wall. The subepithileal lymphoid compartment of the tonsils consists of secondary follicles (B cell areas) surrounded by interfollicular T cell areas. Cells ultrastructurally similar to M cells have been found in the epithelium and are thought to act as a portal to antigens. The mucosa of the pharynx has a complex secretory immune system. B cells stimulated by the antigen in the mucosa of the pharynx migrate to nearest lymph nodes for differentiation to Ig-producing plasma cells. Most of the Igs are IgA polymers that are exported by the serous salivary cells by a special protein complex that is formed between the J chain of the Ig and a receptor protein (section 9.8). Thus, the key to successful protection lies in the ability of IgA polymers to prevent the adherence of bacteria and viruses to the pharyngeal epithelium.

In the past, the tonsils had been accused of causing or exacerbating a number of diseases (rheumatoid arthritis, myocarditis, glomerulonephritis, and gout, to name just a few), and the Greeks were reported to have performed tonsillectomies as early as 3000 BC. Tonsillectomies have now declined, thanks to an appreciation of the immune function of the tonsils. Nonetheless, tonsils can act as routes of entry for viral infections (Epstein-Barr and measles virus) as well as post-viral bacterial infections. Recent evidence suggests that the tonsils could also serve as sites of HIV entry and replication.

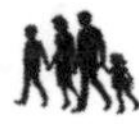
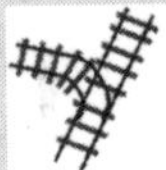

'M'ing for the Gut

M cells are found in the epithelium overlaying Peyer's patches. They originate from epithelial cell precursors that are induced to differentiate into actively pinocytosing cells containing few lysosomes and low levels of phosphatases. M cells serve as a channel for the entry of molecules and particles into the underlying mucosal follicular region. Following bacterial binding, M cells may engulf the organism in a kind of phagosome. Bacterial binding to M cells may be favoured over binding to other epithelial cells. The mechanism for the selectivity of this binding is still unclear. M cells do not seem to take up normal intestinal flora, although this is done by the absorptive cells of the intestine. The normal flora may lack the surface molecules necessary for adhesion to M cell surface. Alternatively, this exclusion could also be attributed to specific immunity resulting from previous contacts with the microflora. For example, specific **s**ecretory **IgA** (sIgA) antibodies have been shown to affect the inhibition of macromolecule absorption by absorptive cells. sIgA antibodies binding to bacteria may reduce their M cell uptake or stop the expression of adhesions by these cells. Indeed, sIgA antibodies to *Salmonella typhimurium* appear to prevent their entry into the Peyer's patches. Uptake by M cells provides an easy entrance into host tissues. Conversely, for opportunistic organisms living adjacent to the mucosa, the possibility of uptake by M cells might be a negative virulence factor. Once taken up by M cells, the bacteria will be transferred to follicular macrophages. Not having the capacity to resist lysosomal action in these macrophages, they may be killed following transfer and prime the system to elicit a non-inflammatory immune response.

development of committed B cells to IgA-secreting plasma cells in response to environmental antigens and inducing systemic tolerance to others.

A great deal remains to be learned about the mucosal immune system, but the best studied component of this important yet enigmatic system is the GALT. **GALT is the collective name given to multiple types of lymphoid tissue found at various sites in the gastrointestinal tract.** The intestinal epithelium has a dual role — it has to allow nutrient absorption while disallowing pathogen entry. The cells of the epithelium have 'tight junctions' that do not allow the passage of molecules more than 2 KD in size. The outer mucosal epithelial layer contains the IELs. IELs are a large heterogeneous population of immune cells[8] in the intestinal epithelium consisting mostly of T lymphocytes. One type expressing the $\alpha\beta$TCR and the CD4 or CD8 coreceptor seems to have originated from the thymus. The other group expresses CD8$\alpha\alpha$ homodimers and may express $\alpha\beta$ or $\gamma\delta$TcR. Some IELs are CD4$^-$, CD8$^-$, and thy-1$^+$ cells that express $\alpha\beta$TcR and show NK-like activity. These NKT lymphocytes are thought to be of extra-thymic origin, since they are found in neonatally thymectomized or nude mice. Their precise ontogeny (ie, origin and development) is still being investigated. IL-7, secreted by epithelial enterocytes, is thought to be important for their development. Recent work in the mouse model suggests that some of them may develop in the crypt of the lamina propria. They have a limited diversity, and their precise function remains unknown; they have, however, been postulated to be important in innate immune responses.

The lamina propria lies just under the epithelial layer and contains loose clusters of lymphoid cells consisting of B cells, plasma cells, T$_H$ cells, and macrophages. Progenitors of T cells are also found in the crypts of the lamina propria of both large and small intestinal villi. The submucosal layer of the lamina propria contains aggregations of lymphoid follicles called Peyer's patches (fig. 5.6). These patches are found primarily in the distal ileum of the small intestine. Peyer's patches have a unique dome-shaped epithelium that is specialized to sample environmental antigens. The dome epithelium covering is composed of cuboidal absorptive epithelial cells interrupted by delicate membranous cells that have luminal microfolds on their surface. These cells, called 'M' cells[9], endocytose and transport various materials without lysosomal degradation[10]. Peyer's patches contain lymphoid compartments

---

[8] Since the lymphocytes are dispersed within the epithelium and not in the epithelial cells, 'intraepithelial' lymphocyte is a misleading term for them.

[9] Not 'M' as in "Bond, James Bond". The M in the name is for membranous.

[10] M cells were originally thought to be the only cells involved in the transport of antigens from the intestinal lumen. Recently, DCs have been found to be involved in antigen sampling too. They extrude in and out of the epithelial tight junctions to capture and transport a sampling of the antigens present in the intestinal lumen.

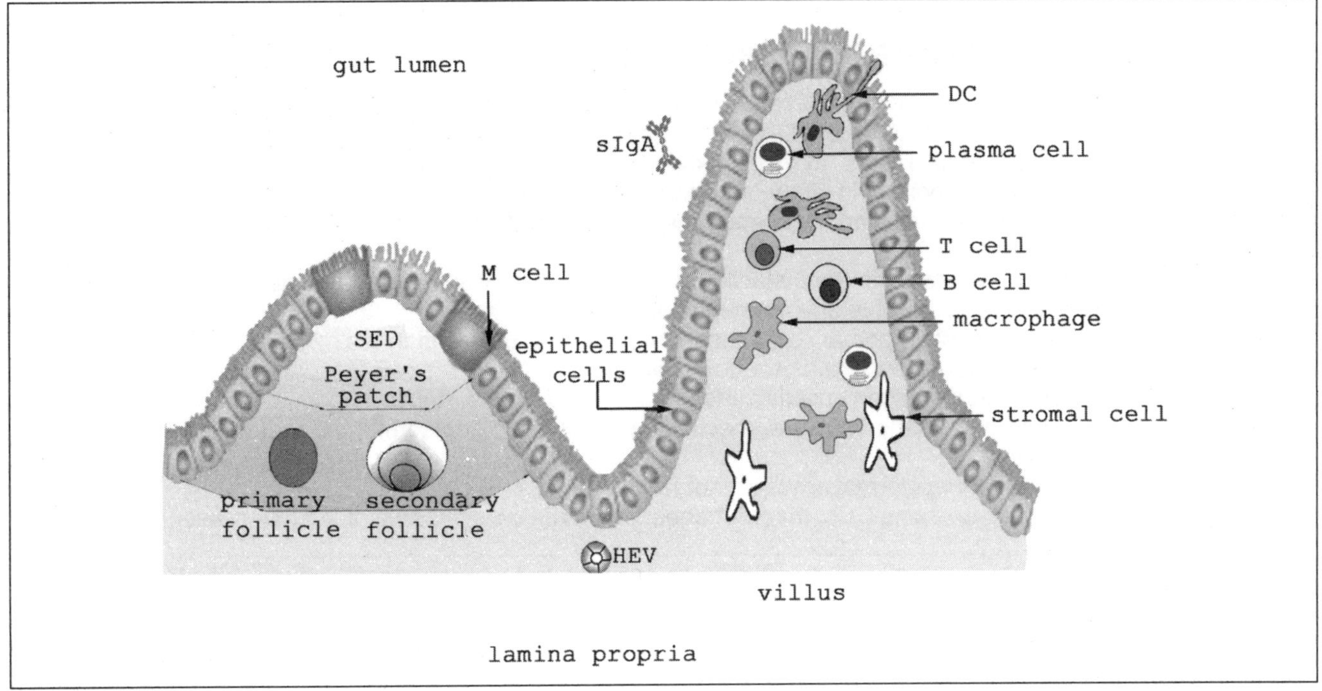

Figure 5.6 *GALT is the collective name given to multiple types of lymphoid tissue found at various sites in the gastrointestinal tract. The lamina propria lies just under the intestinal epithelium and contains loose clusters of lymphoid cells consisting of B cells, plasma cells, T cells, and macrophages interspersed with stromal cells. The diffuse tissue of the lamina propria is rich in IgA-secreting plasma cells. This secretory IgA (sIgA) is important in the defence of the mucosal tissues. The submucosal layer of the lamina propria contains aggregations of lymphoid follicles called Peyer's patches. The Peyer's patches have a unique subepithelial dome (SED) that is specialized to sample environmental antigens. Delicate membranous cells that have luminal microfolds on their surface (M cells) are found interspersed in the cuboidal absorptive epithelial cells of the dome. These M cells along with DCs are important in sampling antigens in the gut lumen. Located beneath the SED are numerous primary and secondary follicles surrounded by a mantle of B cells. The interfollicular area is rich in T cells. The B cells undergo isotype switching and affinity maturation in the secondary follicles (Adapted from Nature Reviews in Immunology (2002) 3:63).*

that are analogous to the deep cortex and follicles of lymph nodes. Each Peyer's patch contains multiple individual B cell follicles located beneath the dome epithelium and separated by interfollicular areas rich in T cells. A mantle of B cells surrounds each germinal centre in the follicle. Antigen is deposited into the small lymphocytes, small mononuclear phagocytes, or DCs immediately beneath the M cells and above the B cell mantle of germinal centres. Minute quantities of intact antigens and products of digestion are transported to the lamina propria by ordinary absorptive epithelial cells found anywhere in the small bowel. Peyer's patches facilitate the generation of an immune response within the mucosa. B cell precursors and memory cells are stimulated by antigen in Peyer's patches. These then migrate to the mesenteric lymph nodes where they undergo further proliferation and maturation. Mature lymphocytes then enter systemic circulation and migrate throughout the MALT and finally travel home to the gut via HEV, thus maximizing their chances of antigen encounter. Current research points towards the existence of two types of Peyer's patches in humans which behave like primary and secondary lymphoid organs. **Peyer's patches are important sites of IgA-secreting plasma cells.**

5.3.3.2 SALT or CALT

The skin, being exposed to the external environment, is under continuous assault by micro-organisms. The impervious epidermis is important in keeping most invaders out. It is also equipped with its own lymphoid system to help control breaching of

---

EPITHELIUM-ASSOCIATED LYMPHOID TISSUE

❑ It comprises non-encapsulated lymphoid tissue in skin and mucosa.
❑ MALT — consisting of NALT, BALT, and GALT — is the most diverse and dispersed of the lymphocytic systems.
- IELs in GALT consist of $\alpha\beta$ T cells, $\gamma\delta$ T cells, and NKT cells.
- IELs are thought to be important in innate immune responses.
- In humans, GALT also acts as a primary lymphoid organ — crypts in the lamina propria are the site of T cell lymphopoeisis.
- Peyer's patches, found mainly in the distal ileum of the small intestine, have a unique epithelium. M cells and DCs in the epithelium sample environmental antigens.
- Peyer's patches also contain primary and secondary follicles; B cells in these follicles are responsible for antigen specific mucosal defence and produce mainly IgA.
❑ SALT or CALT is involved in antigen specific defence of the external surfaces of skin.
- Keratinocytes and Langerhans cells are specialized APCs of the epidermal layer; intraepidermal layers contain B and T cells.
- Langerhans cell monitor epidermal environment for antigens.
- The dermal layer also contains DCs, macrophages, and mast cells capable of antigen presentation.

---

the outer layer. Keratinocytes, specialized cells found in the epidermis, secrete cytokines that can induce inflammatory responses. These cells also present antigens to T_H cells. The Langerhans cells, a type of DC found interspersed in this epidermal matrix, are perhaps the most important component of SALT. They are specialized APCs that reside in the epidermis and constantly monitor the epidermal microenvironment by internalizing any micro-organisms (or immunogens) that penetrate the epidermal layer. Following microbial uptake, Langerhans cells migrate to regional lymph nodes. Here, they differentiate into interdigitating DCs that are potent activators of naïve T cells and initiate an immune response. The epidermis also contains intraepidermal lymphocytes that are similar to the IELs of MALT. Additionally, the dermal layer underlying the epidermis also contains scattered DCs, T cells, macrophages, and mast cells. Thus, immune responses initiated in the SALT are effective in maintaining cutaneous immunity and are normally sufficient to prevent systemic entry of invaders.

5.4 Accessory Cells

Lymphocytes by themselves cannot initiate an adaptive immune response. Antigen capture and T cell activation are integral to triggering the adaptive immune response. Accessory cells (or APCs) intimately involved with the lymphoid system are essential in the development and expression of immune responses. **Physical interaction between APCs and T cells is required to initiate an immune response.** Since they are so intimately involved with the functioning of the immune system, they are described in this chapter, although they are not really a part of the lymphoid system. Many types of cells can process and/or present antigen to T cells (DCs, macrophages, B cells, FDCs, vascular endothelial cells, epithelial cells, eosinophils, mast cells, etc). Antigen presentation, however, is considered an important function of only the first three cell types.

5.4.1 Antigen Processing and Presentation

Presentation of antigen by specialized accessory cells is the first step in triggering an immune response. Recognition of the antigen by T cells is largely determined by how the antigen is processed by APCs. A complex series of steps generates peptides (or glycolipids) from the antigen. The type of MHC (like) molecules that bind these peptides (or glycolipids) in turn determines the subset of T cells stimulated — MHC class I molecules stimulate Cytotoxic T lymphocytes (CTLs), MHC class II molecules

---

APCs

❑ APCs capture antigen, migrate to T cell areas, present antigen to T cells, induce activation and proliferation of T cells, and modulate immune responses.

❑ They can internalize antigen by pinocytosis, phagocytosis, receptor mediated endocytosis, etc.

❑ They process internalized antigens, load fragments of digested antigens on MHC molecules, and present them to T cells.

❑ Professional APCs such as DCs, macrophages, and B cells deliver two signals to T cells and activate them.

  • The first signal is antigen-specific — delivered by the recognition of peptide-loaded MHC molecules.

  • Secondary signals are antigen non-specific signals delivered via costimulatory and/or adhesion molecules.

❑ Non-professional APCs such as fibroblasts and endothelial cells normally deliver only antigen-specific signals and anergize T cells.

---

stimulate T$_H$ cells, and glycolipid loaded CD1 molecules activate NKT cells. Of these, T$_H$ cells are indispensable for generating an immune response, since only these cells can co-opt other cells in developing the response. Thus, expression and loading of MHC class II molecules is necessary for a full-blown immune response. Once the immune system is activated, stimulatory APCs must be removed from circulation in order to avoid overstimulation of the system. Hence, the APCs themselves eventually become the target of cytotoxic cells such as NK cells, K cells, and CTLs. Such removal also helps in the destruction of any intracellular pathogens that may have survived in the phagosomes of the APCs. The major steps in antigen presentation are given below.

❑ **Internalization.** The antigen must be taken up by APCs for successful presentation.

  • Soluble antigen can be taken in by pinocytosis[11].

  • Particulate antigens can be internalized by various means. The most obvious route is phagocytosis. Digested fragments derived from phagocytosed cells are then displayed in the context of MHC (or MHC-like) molecules on the surface of scavenging cells. Engagement of these MHC complexes by TcR is the first signal required to initiate an immune response; the second is provided by engagement of costimulatory molecules (see below). Scavenger cells are involved in clearing cellular debris — whether self- or foreign. Therefore, they display a sampling of both self- and non-self antigens with other mechanisms (requirement for costimulatory molecules, presence of T$_R$ cells, elimination of self-reactive clones, etc) in place to ensure the absence of autoimmune responses.

  • Non-phagocytic or poorly phagocytic cells express a variety of receptors that can bind the antigen and aid in internalization. These include PRRs like mannose receptors, TLRs, and LBP described in chapter 2. Ligands for these receptors are expressed only on micro-organisms (ie, non-self cells). This ensures that the emanating response is not self-deleterious.

  • Many accessory cells also express FcRs. Antigen-antibody complexes bind to the surface of the accessory cell via FcR. Such binding activates the cell membrane, allowing internalization of bound complexes. This method of internalization requires the presence of specific antibodies in the system, ie, it is of particular use in secondary responses. The antigen internalized via the FcR is presented more efficiently than by other routes, aiding in quicker responses.

  • B cells can take up and internalize soluble antigen via their antigen receptor. B cells are unique in this respect, since unlike other accessory cells they behave as antigen-specific APCs. They are especially important in presenting soluble antigen, since neither macrophages nor DCs can efficiently take up soluble antigens.

---

[11] Similar to drinking, pinocytosis is the ingestion of dissolved materials by endocytosis. The cytoplasmic membrane invaginates and pinches off, placing small droplets of fluid in a pinocytic vesicle. The liquid contents of the vesicle are then slowly transferred to the cytosol.

❑ **Antigen processing.** The internalized antigen is transported across a series of endocytic compartments rich in proteases. These compartments gradually decrease in pH and consequently have increased degradative capability. Peptides of a size suitable for binding to MHC molecules (about 8–20 amino acid long) are produced by these degradative pathways and can even be secreted from the cell. The generated peptides are then loaded onto MHC molecules (chapter 7). Evidence suggests that some proteins may not undergo internalization; instead, they are degraded by surface proteases and loaded onto MHC molecules at or near the cell surface.

❑ **Antigen presentation.** 'Professional' antigen presentation consists of two separate interactions (fig. 5.7).
- Recognition of the MHC:peptide complex by TcR constitutes the first signal delivered to T cells. CD4/CD8, the coreceptors for MHC molecules, are also engaged in this primary interaction.
- The second signal is delivered by the engagement of costimulatory molecules. A number of costimulatory and adhesion molecules (CD80/CD86[12], CD54[13]) are expressed by APCs. Binding of costimulatory molecules to their ligands (CD28[14], and CD11a/CD18, respectively) expressed on T cells, along with TcR engagement, leads to T cell activation. Only 'professional' APCs such as DCs, macrophages, and B cells express these costimulatory molecules. Other cells such as endothelial cells and fibroblasts, considered 'non-professional' APCs, do not normally express these molecules[15]. There is a virtual cross-talk between the professional APCs and T cells, since the interaction of TcR with the MHC:peptide complex also upregulates the expression of existing costimulatory molecules or induces expression of new molecules. Little is known about the signalling pathways that control expression of these adhesion molecules by professional APCs. It is now believed that even with professional APCs, engagement of PRRs is required to induce the expression of costimulatory

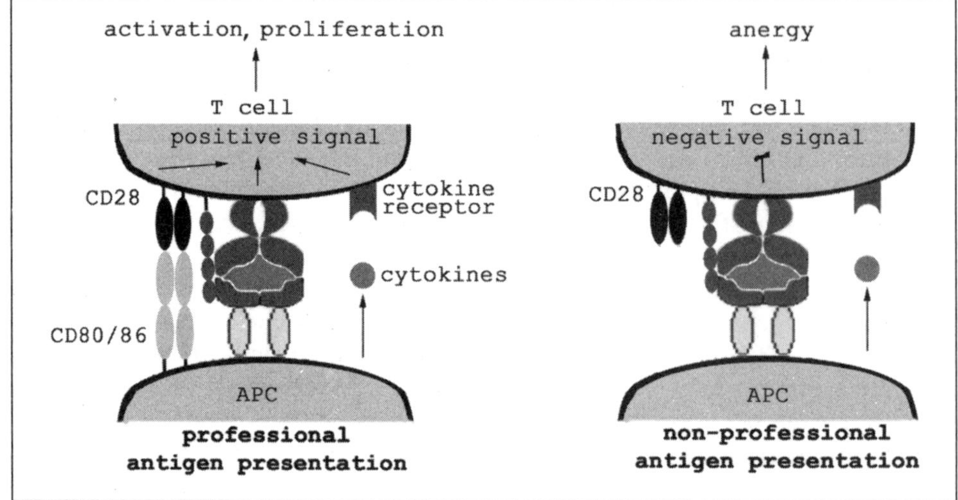

Figure 5.7 Professional APCs stimulate naïve T cells by delivering two separate signals. *The first signal is the antigen-specific signal delivered by the engagement of MHC:peptide complex on the APC by TcR and CD4 (or CD8) on T cells. The second signal is delivered by the engagement of costimulatory molecules on the APC (here represented by CD80/86) by their respective ligands (CD28) on T cells. Downstream signalling pathways activated by these signals result in IL-2 production. These events ultimately lead to proliferation and differentiation of naïve T cells to effector T cells. Non-professional APCs (right panel) can process and load antigen on MHC molecules. Since they do not express costimulatory molecules, the signal generated by only TcR and CD4 (or CD8) engagement is insufficient to stimulate T cell proliferation and results in T cell anergy instead.*

[12] Old name B7.1 and B7.2.

[13] Also called ICAM-1, CD54 binds CD11a/CD18 (old name LFA-1).

[14] CTLA-4, another molecule expressed on T cells, is also a ligand for CD80/86. Instead of stimulating T cells, however, engagement of this molecule makes them unresponsive to the MHC:peptide signal (chapter 8).

[15] Except when exposed to inflammatory stimuli like infection or exposure to IFN-γ.

molecules. Such a system allows induction of costimulatory activity by common microbial constituents, enabling the immune system to distinguish between antigens borne by infectious agents and those associated with innocuous proteins — including self-proteins. This idea is supported by the observation that often, foreign proteins cannot evoke an immune response on their own unless they are mixed with microbial constituents such as LPS that can induce costimulatory activity. Such microbial constituents are therefore co-administered with the antigen in vaccines.

Engagement of TcR in the absence of costimulatory signals (as happens in the case of non-professional APCs) leads to anergy in naïve T cells. Such T cells cannot be further stimulated by APCs. Delivering only signal 2 (ie, ligation of CD28) in the absence of antigenic stimulation, on the other hand, does not have a deleterious effect on T cells. Thus, all peptides — self- or non-self — can, in principle be presented in context of MHC molecules. Non-professional antigen presentation, absence of self-reactive clones[16], and the action of T$_R$ cells prevents a potentially deleterious immune response to self-antigens.

5.4.2 Functioning of APCs

Accessory cells have multiple functions.

- ❑ **Capturing of antigen.** APCs such as DCs and macrophages have a sentinel role. They act as sensors, continuously circulating between the lymphoid system and blood and phagocytosing dead or dying cells. Spillage of intracellular contents of either infected or apoptosing cells could prove injurious. By removing potentially infected or normal dying cells, they help contain damage to the system.
- ❑ **Migration, transport, and presentation of antigen.** APCs acquire antigens in non-lymphoid tissues and then migrate to T cell areas of the lymphoid system, thereby increasing chances of encountering the appropriate T cells. Once in the T cell areas, they present the antigen to T cells.
- ❑ **Induction of activation and proliferation of T cells.** By providing appropriate costimulation, APCs ensure induction of an immune response. Absence of such costimulatory signals induces non-responsiveness or tolerance, rather than the activation of T cells.
- ❑ **Modulation of immune response.** APCs influence the immune response in a number of ways.
  - Intracellular events in APCs determine the type of peptide generated, and hence, the epitope against which the T cell response is directed.
  - The class of MHC molecules on which the peptide is loaded in the APCs determines the type of T cell subset activated (eg, T$_H$ or CTL).
  - Cytokines secreted by APCs influence the course and extent of the immune response.

5.4.3 Types of APCs

APCs can be divided into professional and non-professional types. Antigen presentation by professional APCs is indispensable for switching on immune responses. Only these will be considered here.

- ❑ **DCs** are by far the most important of APCs. They comprise a large family of leukocytes with related morphology that possess the ability to activate naïve T cells. They are widely distributed in tissues and are found especially at environmental interfaces. These are perhaps the only cells with no known function other than activating and controlling T and B cells. Although they differ widely in terms of anatomic localization, phenotype, and function, all DCs have several common features.

[16] Strictly speaking, this is not true. Although negative selection in the thymus does weed out self-reactive clones, the process is not foolproof, and self-reactive clones do exist in the periphery. A reduced frequency (and not *absence*) of self-reactive clones would be a more accurate statement.

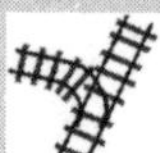

The Long Arms of the Police: Human DCs

In humans, DCs are found as CD34$^+$ precursor populations in the bone marrow and blood and as more mature forms in lymphoid and non-lymphoid tissues. The CD34$^+$ progenitor cells themselves are of two different sub-types — myeloid and lymphoid progenitors. Myeloid CD34$^+$ progenitor cells give rise to CD11c$^+$CD14$^+$ DC precursors (monocytes) that can further differentiate to interstitial DCs and CD11c$^+$CD14$^-$ precursors that give rise to Langerhans cells. The lymphoid progenitors differentiate into the CD11c$^-$ CD14$^-$ blood precursors that give rise to lymphoid DCs (or plasmocytoid DCs, as they are now called). FDCs are thought to originate from this lymphoid lineage (fig. 5.S1).

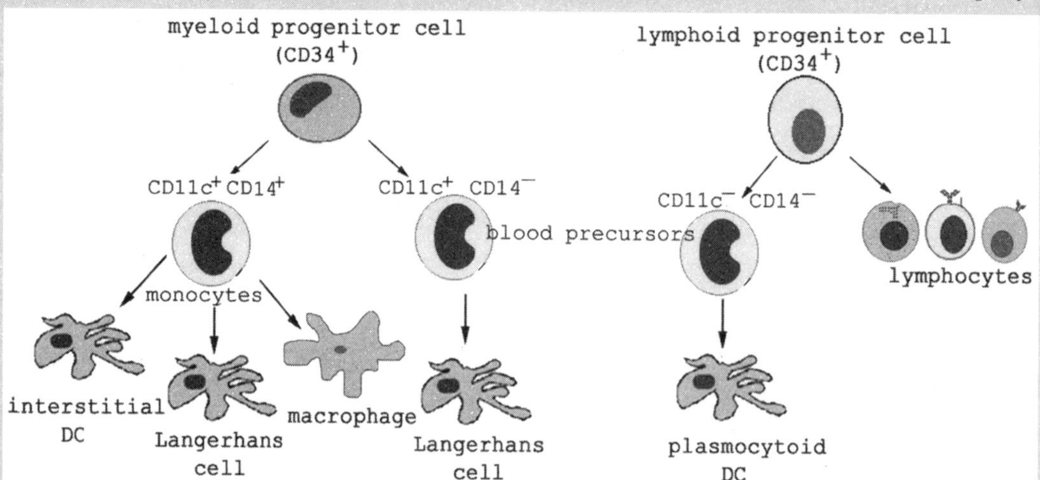

Figure 5.S1 CD34$^+$ progenitor cells can give rise to DCs, macrophages, or lymphocytes, depending upon the cytokine milieu they are exposed to (Adapted from Physiological Reviews (2001) 82:97).

Subtypes of DCs: Besides being classified according to their degree of maturation, DCs can also be classified according to their location.

☐ **Langerhans cells.** The first DCs to be discovered, Langerhans cells arise from the myeloid lineage and are found in non-lymphoid tissues, especially the epidermal layer of the skin. One distinctive feature of Langerhans cells is the occurrence of Birbeck granules. These are typical structures observed under the electron microscope and are thought to be a part of antigen processing machinery. Langerhans cells have a varied role in the capture, migration, processing, and presentation of cutaneous pathogens/parasites. They are in an intermediate stage of maturation, wherein they are highly efficient in capturing and processing antigen but not in the presentation of the antigen to T cells. As Langerhans cells start migrating to the regional lymph node, they begin to mature. The processed antigen from the endocytic pathway finds its way to the cell surface, and the ability of Langerhans cells to present antigen to T cells improves. They are extremely efficient in sensitizing hosts to low doses of antigen but appear to be damaged by high antigenic loads.

☐ **Interdigitating DCs** are found in the secondary lymphoid organs such as the lymph nodes, spleen, and tonsils. These are mature DCs that have captured antigen in the periphery and migrated to the secondary lymphoid organs to activate T and/or B cells. They are thus instrumental in presenting antigen to naïve T cells.

☐ **Interstitial DCs** are immature DCs found in almost every organ of the body — the liver, pancreas, kidney, heart, ureter, bladder, thyroid, gut, and dermis, except in parts of the brain, eyes, and testes. These DCs, along with the Langerhans cells, form a sentinel network to patrol for antigens. Derived from CD14$^+$ myeloid precursors, these DCs can prime both CD4$^+$ and CD8$^+$ T cells. They are the only DCs thought to be able to induce activated B cell differentiation to Ig-secreting plasma cells in the germinal centre.

☐ **Plasmocytoid DCs.** These cells resemble plasma cells at an ultrastructural level, and this gives them their name. They are found in the T cell zones of lymphoid organs and the thymus. Their unique ability to secrete copious amounts of IFN-α/β upon viral stimulation suggests a role in defence against viral infections.

☐ **Thymic DCs** are important in thymic education. Unlike other DCs, these DCs present self-antigens to developing T cells to induce tolerance. Thymic DCs expressing CD8α appear to be functionally different from CD8α^- cells, in that they express FasL and can induce T cell apoptosis.

- DCs originate from CD34$^+$ progenitor cells and are seeded via the bloodstream to the tissues, where they give rise to immature DCs (see sidetrack 'The Long Arms of the Police').
- Immature DCs actively internalize the antigen by both receptor mediated and non-receptor mediated mechanisms and degrade these internalized antigens in endocytic vesicles to produce fragments capable of binding MHC (or MHC-like) molecules.
- DCs mature and migrate to lymphoid organs in response to danger signals such as tissue damage, presence of pathogen-derived products, inflammatory cytokines, and chemokines.
- Mature DCs can activate antigen-specific naïve T cells. Maturation upregulates expression of peptide loaded MHC and costimulatory molecules, allowing DCs to present antigen to naïve T cells.
- Mature DCs secrete cytokines that can skew the immune response to T$_{H1}$ or T$_{H2}$ type (ie, they become DC$_1$ or DC$_2$ type) in response to microenvironmental factors. Conversely, IL-10 secreted by immature DCs can result in T$_R$ cell formation and hence, suppression of immune responses.

DCs are migratory cells that travel from one site to another, performing specific functions at each site. Derived from the bone marrow, DCs circulate via the blood before entering tissues where they become resident immature DCs that monitor their environment. Interstitial DCs and Langerhans cells are examples of such DCs. These immature DCs can migrate towards inflammatory foci where they take up and process antigens. Such immature DCs are avidly endocytic; this characteristic is downregulated upon maturation (Table 5.1). DCs then migrate to the draining lymph node and home into T cell rich areas to initiate an immune response, maturing during this migration. As they mature, they lose their ability to respond to inflammatory stimuli and upregulate surface expression of peptide loaded MHC class II molecules.

One particular subtype of DCs — FDCs — has a major role in secondary humoral responses. Although evidence strongly suggests that FDCs originate from lymphoid DCs, their ontogeny is not entirely clear. There is even some debate about them being DCs. FDCs are found in secondary follicles in B cell areas of all lymphoid tissues. These are non-phagocytic cells that can retain antigen-antibody complexes on their surfaces for prolonged periods of time. They are responsible for the increased antibody affinity for the antigen in secondary responses (chapter 10).

❑ **Macrophages and related cells.** By virtue of their antigen presentation capabilities, these mediators of innate immunity are also important in the switching

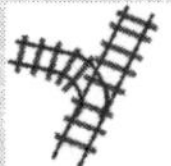 ## To Eat or not to Eat?

Recognition and ingestion of self-cells by phagocytes is crucial in protecting tissues from the toxic contents of dying cells and avoiding an inflammatory response. Exactly how phagocytes distinguish between viable and dying cells is still unclear. Dead or dying cells have been postulated to upregulate certain (as yet unidentified) receptors that are recognized by phagocytes, allowing for selective recognition of apoptotic cells. Since apoptosis involves radical changes in the cell, it is also possible that intracellular molecules normally not expressed on the cell surface gain access to the surface, enabling phagocytic recognition. These hypotheses postulate positive signals, ie, dead or dying cells express signals absent in healthy, viable cells. Recently, there is evidence for negative signalling as well, ie, active repulsion of phagocytes by viable cells. The molecule CD31 (or PECAM-1) has been shown to be involved in this process. CD31 is involved in a number of cellular interactions including lymphocyte migration. Engagement of CD31 expressed on both phagocytes and lymphocytes in viable cells was found to lead to phagocyte detachment and thus cell survival. Such detachment is disabled in dying cells. Instead, in apoptotic cells, CD31 engagement promotes tight binding and ultimately ingestion by the phagocyte.

Table 5.1 Characteristics of immature and mature DCs

Characteristic	Immature DCs	Mature DCs
Cell shape	Relatively small cells with no prominent processes	Larger cells with numerous processes (dendrites or veils)
Antigen capture	• Actively endocytic and phagocytic • Internalize antigens via receptor- and non-receptor mediated processes; active in antigen processing • Express high levels of FcRs	• Poorly phagocytic • May internalize antigens via specific receptors • FcR expression is lower; it is downregulated during maturation
Antigen presentation	• Have high levels of intracellular MHC molecules but do not express them at the surface • Costimulatory molecules either absent or expressed at very low levels • Poor in antigen presentation; may anergize rather than stimulate T cells	• Express a high density of MHC:peptide complexes on cell surface • Variety of costimulatory molecules expressed • Efficient in antigen presentation to naïve and memory T cells
Cytokine responses	• Proliferate in response to GM-CSF • Mature in response to IFN-γ, TNF-α, and non-cytokine stimuli such as LPS, CD40L, etc • Inhibited by IL-10 • Cannot secrete cytokines that skew the T$_H$ response; may secrete IL-10 that results in formation of T$_R$ cells	• Do not proliferate appreciably in response to any stimulus • Do not differentiate further; are stable end-cells • Resistant to IL-10 • Secrete IL-10 or IL-12, skewing the response to T$_{H2}$ or T$_{H1}$ type respectively

on of the adaptive response. Macrophages have already been discussed in chapter 2; only their antigen presentation will be discussed in this section.

Macrophages are potent APCs especially important in immune responses to intracellular pathogens such as *Leishmania* spp. or trypansomes. Resting macrophages have few or no MHC molecules and do not express the costimulatory molecules CD80/CD86. On engagement of PAMPs expressed by micro-organisms, expression of MHC and costimulatory molecules is upregulated. It is thought that such expression of costimulatory molecules only after the ingestion of micro-organisms might allow the immune system to discriminate between infectious agents and innocuous self-proteins and avoid tissue damage. In secondary immune responses, antibodies are already present in circulation. Macrophages can bind antigen-antibody complexes via FcRs, leading to efficient internalization and hence, better antigen presentation.

Although they are not considered professional APCs, both eosinophils and mast cells have been shown to be capable of T cell stimulation. Like macrophages, resting eosinophils do not express either MHC class II molecules or costimulatory molecules. When exposed to IL-3 and GM-CSF, however, they have been shown to express both these molecules and activate T cells. They may thus have a role in activating T cells in allergic or parasitic responses. Mast cells have also been shown to actively phagocytose Gram-negative bacteria and present immunogenic peptides to T cells, and they may have a role in the development of CTL responses to bacterial pathogens.

❑ **B cells.** Although not as important in antigen presentation *in vivo* as macrophages or DCs, B cells can present antigen to T cells. They are, in fact, the only cells capable of presenting soluble antigens. They express MHC molecules constitutively and costimulatory activity is induced only in the presence of microbial products such as LPS. This ensures tolerance to self-antigens; even if B cells present soluble self-antigens, naïve T cells cannot be activated without co-stimulation.

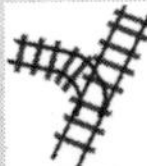

Lessons in Wanting:
Immunodeficient Mouse Models

Single-gene mouse mutants have proven useful experimental tools in immunological research. Two key single-gene naturally occurring mutations are the **nu**de *(nu)* and **S**evere **C**ombined **I**mmuno**d**efeciency *(SCID)* mutations.

❑ *nu* mutation. First reported in Scotland in 1966, mice having this mutation are called nude mice (no funny ideas please!) because the mutation results in a state of hairlessness. Later, it was realized that the thymus fails to develop to normal maturity in homozygous nude mice, ie, they are athymic. As in mice whose thymus is removed neonatally (ie, have been thymectomized), T cells areas of the lymphoid organs are heavily depleted in nude mice. Although they lack T cells, nude mice have a normal complement of bone marrow-dependent B cells. They are therefore a unique tool for the study of the role of thymus on lymphocyte differentiation, B cell functioning, etc. These nude mice can be reconstituted with populations of cells derived from normal mice, allowing for studies on selective populations of immune cells. NK cells and macrophages of these mice are found to be more potent than normal mice. The mice are used for research on NK cells as well. This is also the first animal model to be widely used in studying the factors regulating tumour growth and metastases.

❑ *SCID* mutation. These mice lack a key enzyme (DNA dependent Protein Kinase) needed for the development of a normal immune system (chapter 10). As a result, SCID mice lack both T and B cells. Dr. Bosma of the Fox Chase Cancer Centre serendipitously discovered these mice in 1980. This was the first known animal model for human SCID, a congenital syndrome that is usually fatal. Since they lack an immune system, these mice are excellent models for studying the relationship between immune defects and cancers of the lymphoid system. SCID mice have a great potential for reconstitution studies because they lack normal B and T cell compartments. The action of the *SCID* mutation in blocking lymphocyte development is not absolute, and some adult mice generate a few clones of functional B and T cells, ie, the mutation is 'leaky'. The successful implantation of functional human foetal haematolymphoid organs (including the thymus and lymph node tissues) into SCID mice has led to the development of the *SCID-hu* chimeric model that can be used in cancer research, chemotherapy, and radiation therapy.

6 Molecules of Adaptive Immune Recognition: Lymphocyte Receptors

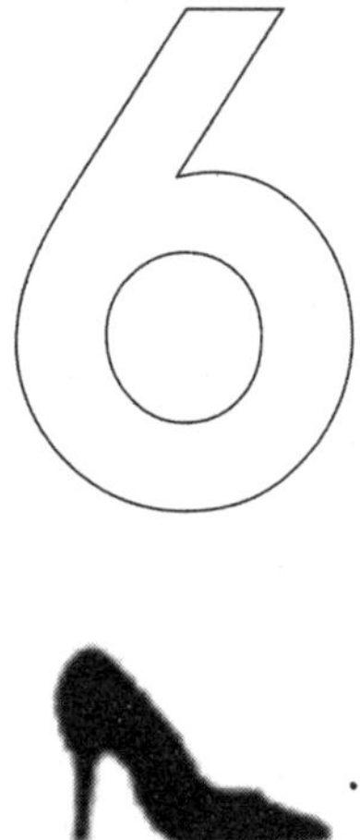

I go to sleep
Here you come again
A ghost with sweet angel eyes
I can't erase
The beauty of your face
I need you here by my side...

I'll find you
If it takes a million dreams
I'll find you
I know you're out there somewhere
I'll find you
Don't give up on me
I'll find you
I swear

— Jennifer Love Hewitt, *I'll Find You*

6.1 Introduction

A 'receptor' is a general term used for a molecule that receives signals from its ligand, ie, the molecule it binds. Receptors expressed on membranes generally have three distinct domains:

- An extracellular domain that (specifically) binds the ligand,
- A transmembrane domain that spans the plasma membrane, and
- A cytoplasmic domain that participates in signal transduction; if the receptor has a very short cytoplasmic domains (as happens with BcR and TcR), it is associated with accessory signal transducers.

Thus, the receptors themselves or the molecules associated with them link the exterior of the cell to the interior. The binding of the ligand to the receptor is usually communicated to the interior of the cell by a conformational change in the receptor. The most common result of this conformational change is either the opening of ion channels in the cell membrane or a change in the cytoplasmic domain of the receptor. The change in concentration of ions (such as Ca^{2+}) that results because of the opening of ion channels is the signal that produces an intracellular response. The change in the conformation of the cytoplasmic domain of the receptor on the other hand enables it to associate with and activate enzymes and/or signalling proteins (see box).

Antigen recognition by the lymphocyte antigen receptors causes them to cluster and ultimately results in the transcription of multiple genes. Although both BcR and TcR are involved in antigen recognition, they recognize antigens in two fundamentally different ways. Antigens are recognized in their native states by antibodies and BcR; TcR recognizes fragments of the antigen only when they are loaded on self-MHC molecules (chapter 4). This duality in antigen recognition serves in defending the body in different ways.

- **Ig molecules, the main unit of BcR, serve two purposes in the immune system.** Circulating Ig help in the defence against micro-organisms and their toxic products. They effectively neutralize toxins by eliminating them from the system or by blocking their activity after binding. Igs also trigger a host of cell-mediated clearing processes such as phagocytosis and complement activation that can kill invading pathogens. As part of the BcR complex, antibodies help activate the process that results in secretion of copies of themselves. These antibodies secreted by plasma cells remain in circulation even after the removal of the challenger, prolonging the conferred protection.
- **TcR helps in the detection of micro-organisms that can live or 'hide' inside cells.** Such organisms can optimize their ability to replicate within the cell while evading the immune system. T cells detect such intracellular parasites by probing cell surfaces for peptides derived from pathogens complexed to MHC molecules.

Both BcR and TcR are multiprotein complexes consisting of an antigen-recognition unit and associated proteins. The antigen recognizing units have similar structures and belong to the Ig superfamily (see sidetrack 'Molecular Mafias'). The two receptors differ greatly, however, both in terms of the epitopes they recognize and the cascade of events (and hence the functions) they trigger. Clustering of receptors is required to generate the initial signal. In the case of BcR, this clustering (also called cross-linking) is easily achieved by the binding of multivalent antigen to multiple BcRs on the B lymphocyte. Such clustering is more difficult to understand in the case of TcRs. It is probable that multiple TcRs on the T cell engage multiple MHC:peptide complexes on APCs or target cells. The signal generated by binding of the antigen to BcR or TcR is converted to a form recognized by the intracellular machinery, thereby initiating a series of reactions that ultimately changes gene expression in the nucleus. Both the receptors and some of the downstream signalling pathways involved in this altering of gene expression will be described in this chapter.

AP-1:	Activating protein-1
Blk:	B lymphoid tyrosine kinase
BLNK:	B cell linker protein
Btk:	Bruton's tyrosine kinase
CDRs:	Complementarity determining regions
Csk:	C-terminal Src kinase
DAG:	Diacylglycerol
ER:	Endoplasmic reticulum
GPI:	Glycosylphosphatidyl-inositol
IκB:	Inhibitors of NFκBs
IP₃:	Inositol-(1,4,5)-triphosphate
LAT:	Linker of activated T cells
CTLA-4:	Cytotoxic T lymphocyte-associated antigen-4
Lck:	Lymphocyte-specific protein tyrosine kinase
MAP kinases:	Mitogen-activated protein kinases
mIg:	membrane Immunoglobulin
NFAT:	Nuclear factor of activated T cells
NFκB:	Nuclear factor κB
PI3-kinase:	Phosphatidylinositol-3-kinase
PIP₂:	Phosphatidylinositol-(4,5)-bisphosphate
PKC:	Protein tyrosine kinases
PLC:	Phopholipase C
PTKs:	Protein tyrosine kinases
SH2 domains:	Src-homology 2 domain
SHIP:	SH2-containing protein tyrosine phosphatase-1
SHP-1:	SH2-containing Inositol polyphosphate phosphatase
ZAP-70:	70 KD ζ-Associated protein

General Concepts in Signal Transduction

Signal transduction can be defined as the process of converting a signal from one form to another. In lymphocytes, a signal is generated by the binding of a ligand to its receptor followed by receptor clustering. This original clustering signal is transduced into chemical signals in the cytoplasm by the activation of receptor-associated protein kinases. These enzymes are essentially phosphorylating enzymes, ie, they add a phosphate group to suitable amino acid residues on other proteins (or enzymes). Phosphorylation by protein kinases is a common general mechanism for the regulation of biochemical activity by the cell. Phosphorylated membrane proteins bind other signalling proteins that are normally free in the cytoplasm, transferring the signal from the membrane to the cytosol. Such binding also increases the local concentration of the signalling protein and its ability to be phosphorylated.

❑ Phosphorylation can occur on tyrosines, serine or threonines, and histidines; separate classes of kinases phosphorylate different amino acids.

❑ It may activate or inactivate enzymes; many enzymes become active when phosphorylated and inactivated when dephosphorylated, or vice versa. Some enzymes may even have two phosphorylation sites — one inhibitory and the other activatory. The enzyme is inactive when phosphorylated at the inhibitory site. Enzymes involved in dephosphorylation are called phosphatases. Phosphatases can remove an inhibitory phosphate group and allow the enzyme to be activated or alternatively deactivate the activated protein.

❑ Phosphorylation creates a binding site on the enzyme enabling it to bind other proteins in the cytosol; many receptor-associated kinases are associated with the inner surface of the cell membrane and cannot interact with their targets that are free in the cytosol. Phosphorylation of membrane-associated enzymes creates a binding site for these target proteins.

❑ It is reversed by enzymes called phosphatases that remove phosphate groups.

Phosphatases remove phosphate groups from membrane proteins and reverse the signalling event. It is important to inactivate (bring to ground level, if you will) the signal generated once the ligand is removed from the receptor. Such removal of phosphate groups adds a time factor to the signalling mechanism — the individual signal is active only for a given length of time. Thus, phosphatases limit the length of time that the signalling event occurs, preventing a runaway cellular response. CD45, associated with both BcR and TcR, is an example of a transmembrane tyrosine phosphatase. Kinase/phosphatase activities ensure that the lymphocyte is rapidly activated on encountering a homologous antigen and equally rapidly inactivated once the antigen is removed.

Adaptor proteins are small molecules that connect different receptors to common intracellular signalling components. These proteins do not have kinase activity; instead, they recruit other molecules to the activated receptor. They often contain several SH2 domains (**S**rc-**H**omology domains) flanked by SH3 domains. They bind to phosphotyrosine residue by their SH2 domain and to other proteins via the SH3 domains. Thus, adaptor proteins position the proteins bound to their SH3 domain at or near the receptor-associated tyrosine kinases.

Small G proteins are a class of GTP-binding proteins that exist in two states, depending upon whether they are binding GTP or GDP. The GTP bound form is active, and the removal of phosphate yields the inactive GDP form. Since these G proteins have phosphatase activity, they are normally inactive. Adaptor proteins bind the G proteins to membrane receptors. Receptor-activated factors then displace the GDP and allow GTP to bind and activate the G protein. Activated G proteins, in turn, stimulate a cascade of kinases — eg, MAP kinases — that phosphorylate transcription factors in the nucleus. Ras is the best-known example of a G protein.

Transcription factors bind to the promoter region of DNA and promote DNA polymerase binding and mRNA synthesis.

Coligation of activating receptors is necessary to start the signalling cascade. Signal transduction in the immune system follows the same general pathway. Thus, whether it is the antigen receptors, the costimulatory molecules, activating receptors on NK cells, or FcRs which are engaged, the general pathway remains the same. The details (the kind of enzymes and adaptor molecules, genes transcribed, etc) differ. The general pathway of antigen receptor activation is outlined below.

❑ Signal transducing units of antigen receptor complexes are associated with intracellular protein kinases localized at the inner surface of the cell membrane.

❑ Ligation of the antigen receptors (represented by a single Ig-fold in the figure) brings the protein kinases together, allowing them to act on each other and on the tyrosines on the cytoplasmic tails of the signal transducing units, thereby initiating the signalling process. Clustering of the receptors thus results in phosphorylation of tyrosines in the ITAMs of its signal transducing unit by receptor-associated kinases.

❑ Phosphorylation of the tyrosines allows cytosolic protein tyrosine kinases to dock into the activated (ie, phosphorylated) protein; adaptor proteins may help in the process by bringing the target cytosolic molecules to the cell membrane.

❑ The cytosolic kinases then get phosphorylated by other protein tyrosine kinases.

❑ This chain reaction results in the recruitment and activation of a key enzyme that can cleave the membrane-associated phospholipid **P**hosphatidy-linositol-(4,5)-bis**p**hosphate, or PIP$_2$, into two potent messenger molecules — **D**iacyl**g**lycerol (DAG) and **I**nositol-(1,4,5)-tri**p**hosphate (IP$_3$). Since one molecule of the enzyme can produce many molecules of these messengers, this represents a major amplification step in receptor-mediated signalling.

❑ The messengers further activate downstream pathways, finally resulting in activation of a number of transcription factors.

❑ Small G proteins are also activated.

❑ These proteins activate a cascade of protein kinases that result in the phosphorylation and activation of multiple transcription factors.

❑ The transcription factors translocate to the nucleus, resulting in the transcription of new genes.

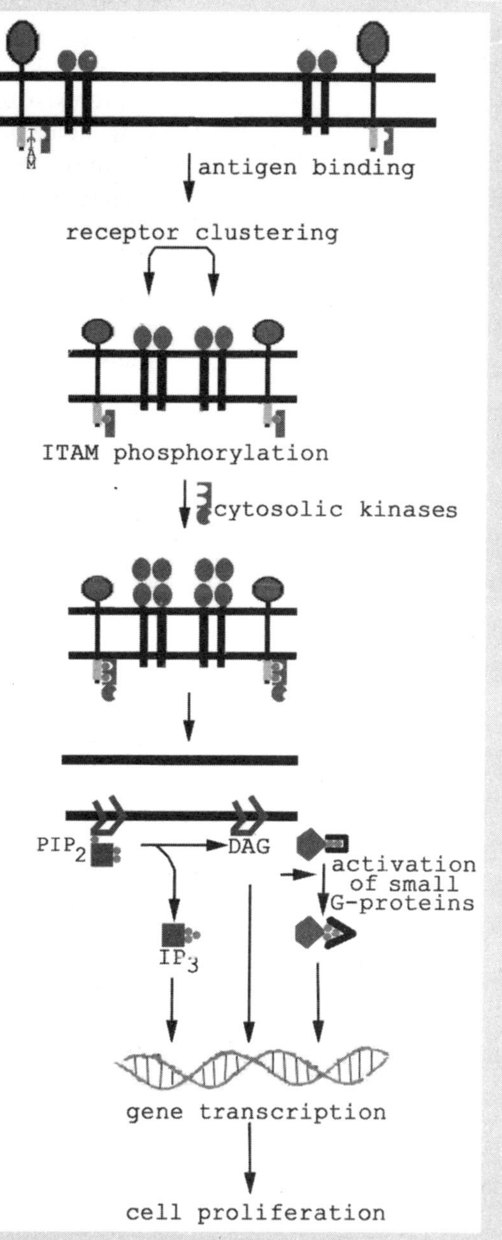

Figure 6.S1 The general pathway of signal transduction following the clustering of antigen receptors is similar in B and T cells.

A cautionary note — a plethora of new terms are being introduced here; it is important to understand the concepts instead of getting bogged down by terminology.

6.2 The B Cell Antigen Receptor

The immune system must recognize and deal with a myriad of antigens. Encoding and expressing a radically different protein for every possible antigen it may or may not encounter, however, would be a waste of energy and DNA. Faced with this dilemma, evolutionary forces came up with an ingenious solution — antigen receptors having a highly variable structure at the antigen-binding end but an invariant structure at the cytoplasmic end (distal from the antigen-binding site). This allows the same basic structure to be utilized for binding different antigens. As a further refinement, the signalling function is bifurcated from the receptor function, allowing the utilization of pre-existing cellular enzyme machinery and eliminating the need for synthesis of new molecules.

Antigen receptors and signalling molecules comprising BcRs (and TcRs) are not randomly distributed in the plasma membrane. They are found clustered in special structures called 'lipid rafts'[1]. These are specialized lipid-rich areas, or microdomains, found in the outer leaflet of the plasma membrane. Certain cellular proteins can associate with lipid rafts because of their structural features (fatty acylation, presence of a glycosylphosphatidylinositol (GPI) residue, oligomerization, specialized transmembrane domains, etc), but others are excluded from them. The fact that certain cytosolic proteins are selectively transported to lipid rafts while others are excluded from them has given rise to the idea that lipid rafts act as assembly points and platforms that facilitate the interaction of particular signalling components. The precise nature and organization of lipid rafts is unknown. Lipids rafts are found to be enriched in sphingolipids, cholesterol, GPI-linked proteins, and acylated signalling molecules. Lipid rafts are thought to facilitate immunoreceptor signalling by producing a physical environment rich in kinases, adaptor molecules, and intracellular effector molecules, while helping exclude negative regulators such as CD22 (section 6.2.2).

6.2.1 Structure of the B Cell Antigen Recognition Unit

The antigen recognition unit of the BcR is a **m**embrane-bound **Ig** (mIg) molecule associated with a plethora of signal transduction accessory molecules. The mIg provide specific epitope recognition, whereas accessory molecules allow the mIg to associate with cytosolic enzymes needed for intracellular signalling following antigen binding. A detailed description of different types of Igs is given in chapter 9. In this section, only those features that are important to antigen recognition are reviewed.

❑ The prototypical Ig molecule has a quaternary complex structure consisting of four polypeptide chains:
  - Two 50 KD H chains, each containing around 440 amino acids, and
  - Two 25 KD L chains of 220 amino acids each.
❑ The secondary structure of the Ig molecule is formed by the folding of polypeptide chains into anti-parallel β-pleated sheets. Each polypeptide of the Ig molecule is thus folded into compact globular domains which are connected to neighbouring globular domains by amino acid sequences that do not participate in the β-pleated sheet structure. This kind of polypeptide folding is a universal structural feature found in a multitude of proteins, and it is called the Ig fold or domain (see sidetrack 'Packed and Folded').
❑ Ig H chains consist of four such Ig domains and the L chains consist of two domains each.
❑ Globular domains of the adjacent L-H or H-H chains interact in the quaternary structure of the complex to form functional domains with discrete functions (fig. 6.1).
  - Globular domains at the amino-terminus of the H and L chain are non-covalently associated through an extensive hydrophobic interface. This association forms the antigen-binding pocket of the Ig molecule. Since the Ig molecule consists of two H and two L chains, it has two antigen-binding sites. The sequence of amino acids in these globular domains at the Amino– terminus, for both the H and L chains, is highly variable. These domains are therefore called **V**ariable domains (V_H and V_L respectively).
  - Globular domains at the COOH– terminus of the L chains are associated with the second globular domain of the H chain. The remaining two globular domains

---

Packed and Folded: The Ig Fold

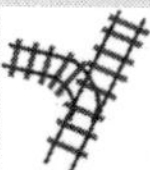

As the first protein structures were solved, it was established that proteins have structurally different lobes. Wetlauferi assigned the word 'domain' to these compactly folded structures in 1973. Such domains form an important level in hierarchical organization of the three-dimensional structure of globular proteins. Domains are important in protein folding and in biological functions and may be considered connected units which are independent in terms of their structure, function, and folding behaviour.

Each Ig domain consists of approximately 110 amino acids, and each fold consists of a sandwich of two β-pleated sheets. Each sheet consists of anti-parallel β-strands connected by loops of varying lengths. The β-strands are stabilized by hydrogen bonds that connect the amino group of one strand with the carbonyl groups of the adjacent strand. These β-strands are characterized by alternating hydrophobic and hydrophilic amino acids whose side chains are perpendicular to the plane of the β-sheet (fig. 6.S2). Side chains of the hydrophobic amino acids are oriented inwards between the two β-pleated sheets, while the side chains of the hydrophilic amino acids are pointed outward, away from the two opposing β-pleated sheets. The sandwich of the two β-pleated sheets is stabilized by hydrophobic interactions between the two β-pleated sheets and the presence of a disulphide bond which forms a loop of about 60 amino acids.

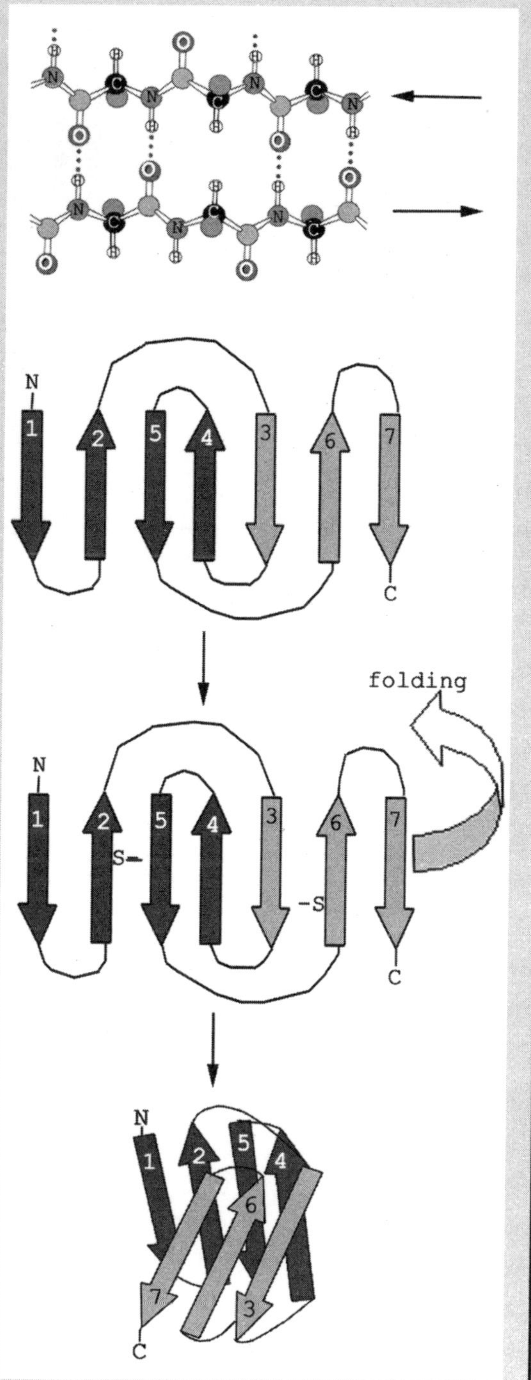

Figure 6.S2 The Ig domain consists of a sandwich of two β-pleated sheets stabilized by hydrophobic interactions and a sulphide bond.

of the two H chains are held together by non-covalent hydrophobic interactions to yield a Y-shaped molecule. Apart from in the V_H and V_L domains, the sequence of amino acids in the remaining domains of the H and L chains has little variation. These domains are therefore called the **C**onstant domains (C_H and C_L).

- C domains have seven strands — four making one sheet and the other three making the other sheet. The two sheets are packed close together and joined by disulphide linkages emanating from strand two and six, giving a stable structure with a hydrophobic core.

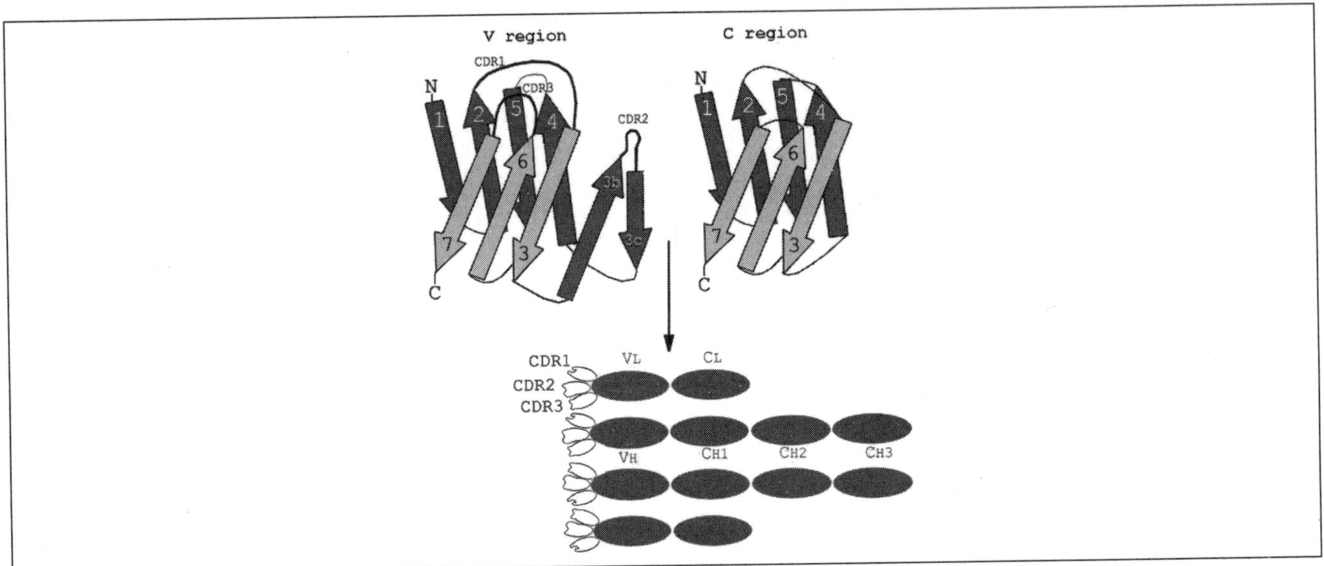

Figure 6.1 The prototypical Ig molecule consists of four polypeptide chains — two heavy (H) and two light (L) — and is bilaterally symmetrical. Each polypeptide chain consists of globular domains folded into anti-parallel β-pleated sheets that are connected to the neighbouring globular domains by amino acid sequences that do not participate in the β-sheet structure. The H chains consist of four such domains, while the L chains consist of two such domains (top panels). Globular domains of the adjacent L-H or H-H chains interact in the quaternary structure of the complex to form functional domains with discrete functions (bottom panel). The amino acid sequences in the first N– terminal domains of the H and L chains vary greatly and are called variable regions (VH and VL respectively). The remaining domains have little sequence variation and are called C (constant) regions. The L chain has one constant domain (CL); the H chain has three (CH1, CH2, CH3). The C domains consist of seven β-strands, packed in two sheets of four and three strands each. The two sheets are joined by disulphide linkages (not shown here) giving a stable hydrophobic core. The structure of the V region is similar to that of the C region except that it has two additional strands. The sequence variability is not uniformly distributed in the V region but clustered in three distinct regions called the Complementarity-Determining Regions (CDRs), and falls in the peptide loops that connect the β-strands. The less variable regions occur in the β-pleated sheets that provide the basic framework of the Ig fold. The CDRs of both the chains constitute the antigen-binding region of the antibody, and the typical Ig molecule has two antigen-binding sites.

- The V region structure is slightly different from the C region structure in that it has two additional strands.
  - In the VH and VL domains, variability is not uniformly distributed but clustered in three distinct regions called the hypervariable regions or the **C**omplementarity-**D**etermining **R**egions (**CDRs**, since they form the surface that matches the topology and physicochemical character of the antigen). The less variable regions occur in the β-pleated sheets and are called the framework regions, since they provide the basic framework of the Ig fold.
  - Each V region has three CDRs. The peptide loop that links the β-strands 2 and 3 constitutes CDR 1 (amino acids 24–34). Similarly, the loop connecting strands 3b and 3c represents CDR 2 (amino acids 50–56), and the loop linking strands 6 and 7 forms CDR 3 (amino acids 89–97).
  - CDRs are brought together to form a continuous surface that constitutes the antigen-binding site of the antibody, ie, amino acids in the CDR regions actually take part in the antigen-binding process.

Each B cell expresses about 10^4–10^5 antigen receptors per cell. Naïve cells express either mIgD or mIgM or both. Memory cells express mIg of a switched isotype (mIgG/mIgA/mIgE) alone or along with mIgM. The mIg is identical to secreted Ig except for the following.

- ❑ It has a stretch of amino acids at the COOH– terminus of the H chains that is needed for anchoring the molecule to the cell membrane.
  - Since the molecule is anchored in the cell membrane and traverses this membrane, this stretch of amino acids consists of an additional hydrophobic region that lies sandwiched between the hydrophilic portions.

- The hydrophobic portion is the transmembrane segment of the mIg, whereas hydrophilic portions are present on either side of the cell membrane.
- The hydrophobic portion forms a stretch of α-helix within the membrane. This transmembrane segment is the most evolutionarily conserved part of the mIgM H chain, and it is identical in species as far apart as mice and humans, suggesting some critical function.
- The DNA encoding this membrane part of the mIg lies beyond the last C_H domain on the C region gene. Production of the two forms of Igs is brought about by differential transcription of this gene (section 9.4).

❑ mIg exists only as a basic four-chain unit. Unlike the secreted forms of IgA or IgM, it does not form polymers of this basic unit.

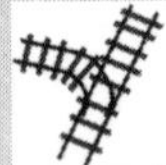

Molecular Mafias: The Ig Superfamily

Proteins having the same overall architecture can be clustered into what are called 'superfamilies'. Proteins in a given superfamily are encoded by genes derived from a common primordial gene that encoded the basic domain structure. These genes could have evolved independently and do not necessarily share genetic linkage functions.

The Ig superfamily is an ever-increasing group currently comprising about 80 members. These membrane bound proteins are found in species as diverse as insects, worms, and humans. The common factor in these molecules is the 'Ig-like' fold, consisting of an anti-parallel β-sheet sandwich formed from nine β-strands held together by a disulphide bond. This architecture is thought to make the molecule protease resistant. Human proteins belonging to this group include TcR and its accessory proteins (CD2, CD3, CD4, and CD8), MHC molecules (class I, class II, CD1, Qa1, etc), BcR and its accessory molecules (Ig-α, Ig-β, CD19, and CD22), FcRs, a number of cytokine receptors, costimulatory molecules (CD28, CTLA-4 (CD152), their ligands B7-1 (CD80) and B7-2 (CD86)), and adhesion molecules (PECAM-1 (CD31), ICAM-1 (CD54), ICAM-2 (CD102), and ICAM-3 (CD50)). Most of these proteins do not bind antigens. It is thought that the Ig fold facilitates interactions between membrane proteins, since such interactions can occur between the faces of the β-pleated sheet of both homologous and non-homologous Ig domains.

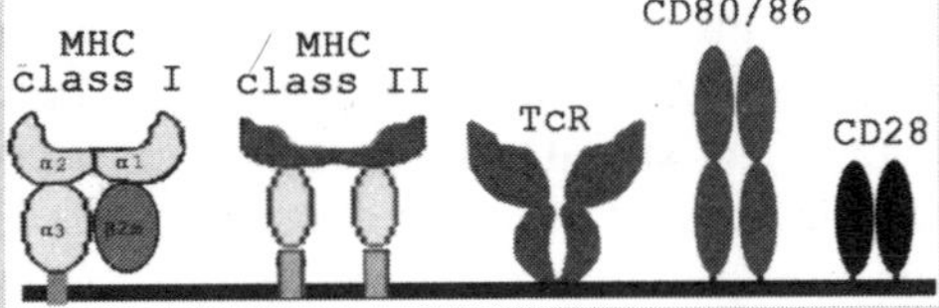

Figure 6.S3 *Many proteins involved in immune interactions belong to the Ig superfamily.*

6.2.2 The BcR Complex

The BcR is a multi-unit structure consisting of one molecule of mIg associated with an Ig-α-Ig-β heterodimer and other molecules (CD19, CD21, CD22, CD45, CD72, and CD81) involved in the signalling pathways (fig. 6.2). Of these, CD19, CD21, CD45, and CD81 are positive regulators of BcR function, while CD22 and CD72 are negative regulators.

❑ **Ig-α(CD79a) and Ig-β (CD79b)** belong to the Ig superfamily. A disulphide bond links the two molecules to form a heterodimer. Until recently, two molecules of the heterodimer were thought to be associated with one mIg molecule. However, recent work suggests that only one molecule of the heterodimer is associated with one molecule of mIg. CD79a and CD79b show a sequence homology with T cell receptor-CD3 complex components (section 6.3.1), suggesting a common origin. Ig-α is coded by the gene *mb-1* and Ig-β is coded by *B-29*. This latter gene is expressed only in B cells, and Ig-β is expressed at all stages of B cell development. *mb-1* (and therefore Ig-α) on the other hand is not expressed at the plasma cell stage.

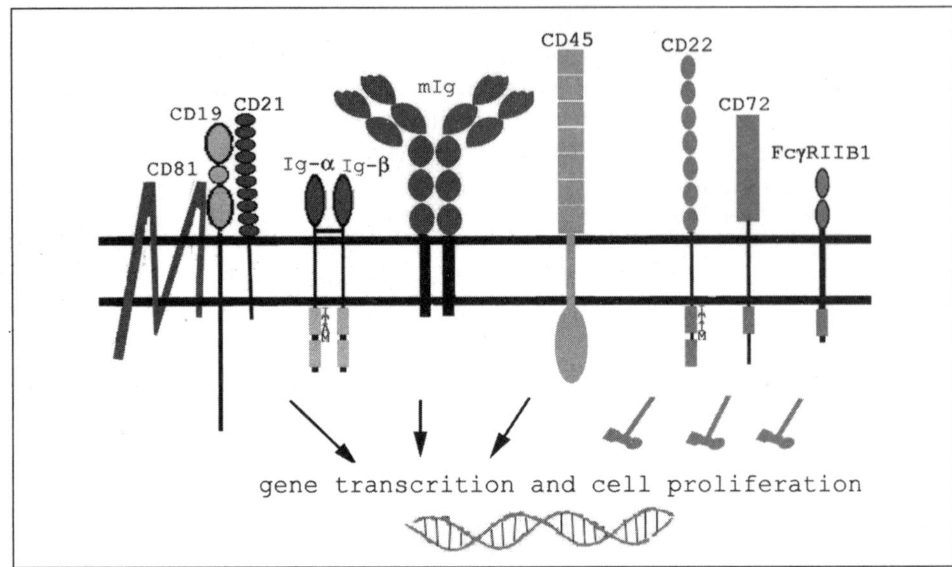

Figure 6.2   The B cell antigen receptor is a multi-protein complex consisting of one Ig molecule and a number of other associated molecules. *mIg is the antigen-recognition unit of the complex. Its short cytoplasmic tail makes it unsuitable for transduction of the signal generated by antigen binding. The Ig-α:Ig-β heterodimer associated with mIg is the signal transducing element. The BcR complex also has a molecule of CD19 covalently associated with CD81 and CD21. This CD19:CD21:CD81 complex is a positive regulator of B cell function. So is CD45, which can get recruited in the complex. Negative regulators associated with the complex include CD22, CD72, and FcγRIIB1.*

The heterodimer associates with mIg in the **E**ndoplasmic **R**eticulum (**ER**). Quality control mechanisms in the ER ensure that only mIg associated with Ig-α and Ig-β is exported to the cell surface, while unassociated mIg is retained in the endoplasmic reticulum. Both Ig-α and Ig-β have long cytoplasmic tails that can interact with intracellular signalling machinery. They undergo conformational changes when surface mIgs aggregate because of the binding of a multivalent antigen. The signal generated is then transmitted to the B cell nucleus via an intracellular signal transduction pathway. Ig-α and -β have two ITAMs each in their cytoplasmic tails. Tyrosine kinases associated with the receptors phosphorylate tyrosines in these ITAMs when mIgs are cross-linked by the antigen.

❑ **CD19**, another member of the Ig superfamily, is physically associated with BcR and is a positive regulator of BcR function. On the surface of B cells, CD19 forms a heterologous, non-covalent complex with CD21 and CD81 (TAPA-1 of the old literature).

• **CD19** is the earliest cell surface molecule related to B lineage differentiation, and all cells of this lineage express this molecule. It has a long cytoplasmic tail of 240 amino acids that is conserved across diverse species. CD19 is phosphorylated on BcR ligation. Coligation of CD19 with BcR decreases the threshold of antigenic stimulation by at least two orders of magnitude. It also regulates the phosphorylation and activation of multiple downstream adaptor proteins and enzymes (including Bruton's tyrosine kinase and MAP-kinases). Its importance in BcR signalling can be deduced from the fact that genetically engineered mice deficient in CD19 show an impaired response to TD antigens.

• **CD21** (CR2) is a receptor for complement component C3d. C3d is generated from C3 when complement is fixed (chapter 3). When BcR binds C3d coated antigen, C3d binds CD21. This coligation of the CD19-CD21complex results in an enhanced B cell response (fig. 6.3).

• **CD81** is a member of the tetraspanin family[2] of integral membrane proteins widely expressed in the body. It has recently gained notoriety after being

---

[2] The name 'tetraspanin family' alludes to the fact that the members of this family have four transmembrane domains.

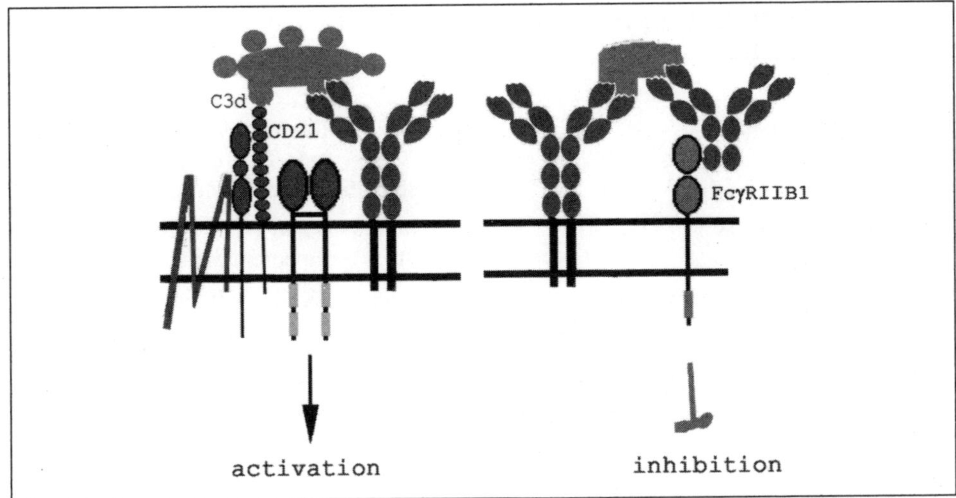

Figure 6.3 Coligation of CD21 with BcR can positively regulate its function, whereas coligation of FcγRIIB1 with it regulates its function negatively. *CD21, a receptor for cleavage products of the complement component C3, is found to be associated with CD19 and CD81 in the BcR. It is a positive regulator of BcR. Coligation of CD21 and BcR via C3d coated antigen results in an enhanced B cell response. It also reduces the concentration of antigen required for B cell activation. By contrast, coligation of the Fc receptor FcγRIIB1 with BcR by antigen-IgG complex inhibits B cell response.*

recognized as a receptor for the hepatitis C virus envelope protein. Both B and T cells express CD81. It is shown to be physically and functionally associated with CD19 along with two other members of the tetraspanin family. Although its actual role in signal transduction is unclear, there is evidence to suggest that CD81 could partially relay or amplify the signal initiated by CD19.

❑ **CD22**, a sialoadhesin that can bind to sialic acids, is constitutively associated with BcR. It carries two ITIMs in its cytoplasmic tail. It is known to limit BcR signalling by recruiting phosphatases and inhibiting the tyrosine phosphorylation of multiple cellular proteins. Its inhibitory functions are dominant over the costimulatory functions of the CD19/CD21 complex. Recent studies indicate that it may play a role in the migration of B cells to the bone marrow.

❑ **CD72** is a type II membrane protein[3] that has a C-type lectin domain in the extracellular region and an ITIM in its cytoplasmic tail. It is also a negative regulator of BcR functioning.

❑ **FcγRIIB1**, an isoform of FcγRIIB, is expressed on B cells and is shown to downmodulate BcR signalling only when it is coligated to BcR by antigens complexed with IgG. The single ITIM in its cytoplasmic tail gets phosphorylated by cross-linking with cellular Ig and suppresses phosphorylation of CD19. The lipid phosphatase SHIP is essential for this inhibitory function.

6.2.3 Simplified Outline of BcR Signalling

BcR and TcR signalling pathways are essentially similar. Ligation of receptors results in the phosphorylation of ITAMs on accessory molecules and leads to the recruitment of a key enzyme that phosphorylates **Ph**ospholipase **C** (PLC). As a consequence, potent messengers **D**iacylglycerol (DAG) and **I**nositol-(1,4,5)-triphosphate (IP$_3$) are formed, ultimately leading to the activation of multiple transcription factors. The shared nature of the enzymes and molecules involved in these downstream signalling pathways make them attractive targets for controlling unwanted immune responses (Table 6.1).

[3] Type I membrane proteins are anchored in the cell membrane at the Amino– terminus (eg, the invariant chain of MHC class II molecules and CD72); type II membrane proteins are anchored via the Carboxyl–terminus (eg, MHC class I and II molecules and Ig).

Table 6.1 Drugs targeting lymphocyte signalling pathways

Drug	Target	Effect
Cyclosporin A	Calcineurin phosphatase	Inhibits T cell activation and cytokine synthesis via TcR; cannot block T cell activation by exogenous cytokines
Tacrolimus (FK506)	Calcineurin phosphatase	Inhibits B and T cell activation; 100 times more potent than cyclosporin A
Sirolimus (rapamycin)	Affects second signals delivered to T cells via IL-2, IL-4 and IL-6; thought to affect p70^{56} kinase involved in synthesis of proteins required for cell cycle progression	Inhibits T cell proliferation by arresting the cells in the G1 phase

❑ mIg clustering, as a result of antigen binding, leads to the phosphorylation of ITAMs on CD79a and CD79b by several Src family **P**rotein **T**yrosine **K**inases (PTKs) including Lyn, Blk, Fyn and Lck.
- Phosphorylation appears mainly to occur at the membrane proximal tyrosine.
- Tyrosine phosphorylation of CD79 further facilitates the recruitment of additional molecules of these PTKs.
- Recruitment of PTKs further amplifies CD79a and CD79b phosphorylation.
- CD45 may help in the process by dephosphorylating Fyn (section 6.3.2)

❑ Only a subset of CD79a and CD79b has both their ITAM tyrosines phosphorylated. These phosphorylated molecules serve as docking sites for the SH2 domains of the cytosolic PTK Syk. This Syk recruitment by BcR is a key event that results in a plethora of downstream signalling events and results in the phosphorylation of phospholipase **C**γ (**PLC**γ).

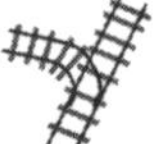

Seeing Red (or Green): ITIMs and ITAMs

ITAM (**I**mmunoreceptor **T**yrosine-based **A**ctivating **M**otif) is composed of two tyrosine residues separated by around 13 amino acids. The canonical ITAM has the general sequence of Yxx(L/I)x(6-8)Yxx(L/I), where each single letter represents an amino acid (Y = tyrosine, L = leucine, I = isoleucine, and x = any amino acid). Although these motifs were originally discovered in Ig-α and Ig-β, they are now known to be present on other molecules of the immune system. Thus, ITAMS are found on the cytoplasmic tails of numerous receptors, including FcγRIII (found on NK cells, macrophages, and neutrophils), FcεRI on mast cells, and basophils and activatory receptors on NK cells. Phosphorylation of tyrosines in the ITAMs by protein kinases allows them to recruit other enzymes/molecules involved in signal transduction. The Syk family of tyrosine kinases (Syk and ZAP-70), involved in BcR and TcR signal transduction respectively, have two SH2 domains that can bind two phosphotyrosines. These two tyrosines have therefore to be spaced precisely for proper binding. Thus, the presence of ITAMs in the cytoplasmic tail of a protein implies the involvement of the Src family and Syk family kinases in signal transduction.

    ITIM (**I**mmunoreceptor **T**yrosine-based **I**nhibitory **M**otif) has a large hydrophobic residue such as isoleucine or valine one or two residues upstream of a tyrosine that is followed by leucine two amino acids later ([I/V]xYxxL). ITIMs too are not exclusive to TcR and BcR but are found on a number of inhibitory receptors of the immune system — CD22, FcγRIIB, CTLA-4 as well as on a number of inhibitory receptors on NK cells. Tyrosine-phosphorylated ITIMs recruit **SH**2-containing **i**nhibitory **p**hosphatases (called SHP-1and SHIP) that are essential for the negative regulation of cell activity. These inhibitory phosphatases carry a SH2 domain that preferentially binds the phosphorylated tyrosines in the ITIM. SHP-1 (**SH**2-containing protein tyrosine **P**hosphatase-1) removes phosphate groups added by tyrosine kinases, while SHIP (**SH**2-containing **I**nositol polyphosphate **P**hosphatase) is thought to inhibit the activation of PLC and thus the production of DAG and IP$_3$.

Arch SAARC

The Src family of **P**rotein **T**yrosine **K**inases (PTKs), pronounced Sark (or SAARC), are a closely related group of proteins that regulate crucial cellular processes in response to the activation of transmembrane receptors. They are common components of signalling pathways involved in the control of a number of cellular processes in vertebrates — proliferation, differentiation, adhesion, migration, and survival, to name just a few. The first member was discovered as the oncogene v-src responsible for the tumour-causing ability of Rous sarcoma virus. Incidentally, v-src was established to be a modified form of c-src — a normal cellular gene that the Rous sarcoma virus had picked up. Src kinases are constitutively anchored to the inner leaflet of the plasma membrane and tend to be concentrated in lipid rafts.

Src PTKs having a key role in signal transduction in lymphocytes include Lck, Lyn, Blk, and Fyn.

- Lck (**L**ympho**c**yte-specific protein tyrosine **k**inase) is associated with the cytoplasmic domain of CD4 and α chain of CD8 in memory T cells but is distributed throughout the cytosol in naïve T cells.
- Fyn (oncogene related to SRC, FGR, YES) associates with the ζ and ε CD3 chains.
- Blk (**B l**ymphoid tyrosine **k**inase) is a B cell specific kinase. In B cells, Lck, Blk, and Fyn seem to be functionally redundant.
- Lyn (v-yes-1 Yamaguchi sarcoma viral related oncogene homologue) is the most abundant kinase in B cells.

Src PTKs are 52-62 KD proteins composed of distinct functional regions. Of special interest in lymphocyte signalling are the two small modular units known as the SH2 (**S**rc-**H**omology **2**) and SH3 (**S**rc-**H**omology **3**) domains. The SH2 domain binds short amino acid sequences containing phosphotyrosine. The ligand-binding surface of the SH2 domain has two pockets — one contacts the phosphotyrosine and the other contacts the +3 amino acid residue following the phosphotyrosine. Src kinases have a preference for leucine at this position (hence the importance of L/V in YxxL/V ITAM). The SH3 domain by contrast recognizes left-handed polyproline helices. The SH2 and SH3 domains are important in the control of Src PTKs activity. In the absence of input signals, Src proteins are kept in an inactive state. The SH2 and SH3 domains are unexposed, and they cooperate to turn off catalytic machinery. When the kinase is turned on, the SH2 and SH3 domains are exposed and target the protein kinase to appropriate sites in the cell.

Enzymatic activity of the Src family kinases is itself regulated by phosphorylation. Phosphorylation at one site activates the enzyme, and phosphorylation at another site inhibits it. The kinases are kept in an inactive state by the action of Csk (**C**-terminal **S**rc **k**inase), which phosphorylates the inhibitory tyrosine at the Carboxyl– terminus. In the resting state, constitutively expressed Csk keeps the enzymes inactive. Upon activation, CD45 dephosphorylates this site. Thus, the balance between Csk and CD45 activity regulates the action of Src kinases.

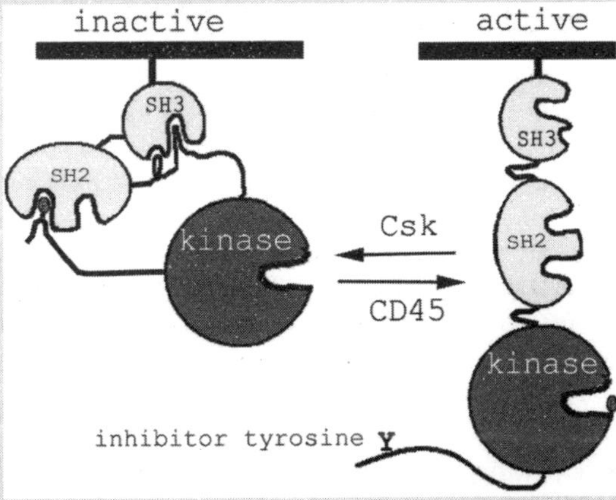

Figure 6.S4 Activity of Src kinases is regulated by phosphorylation and dephosphorylation.

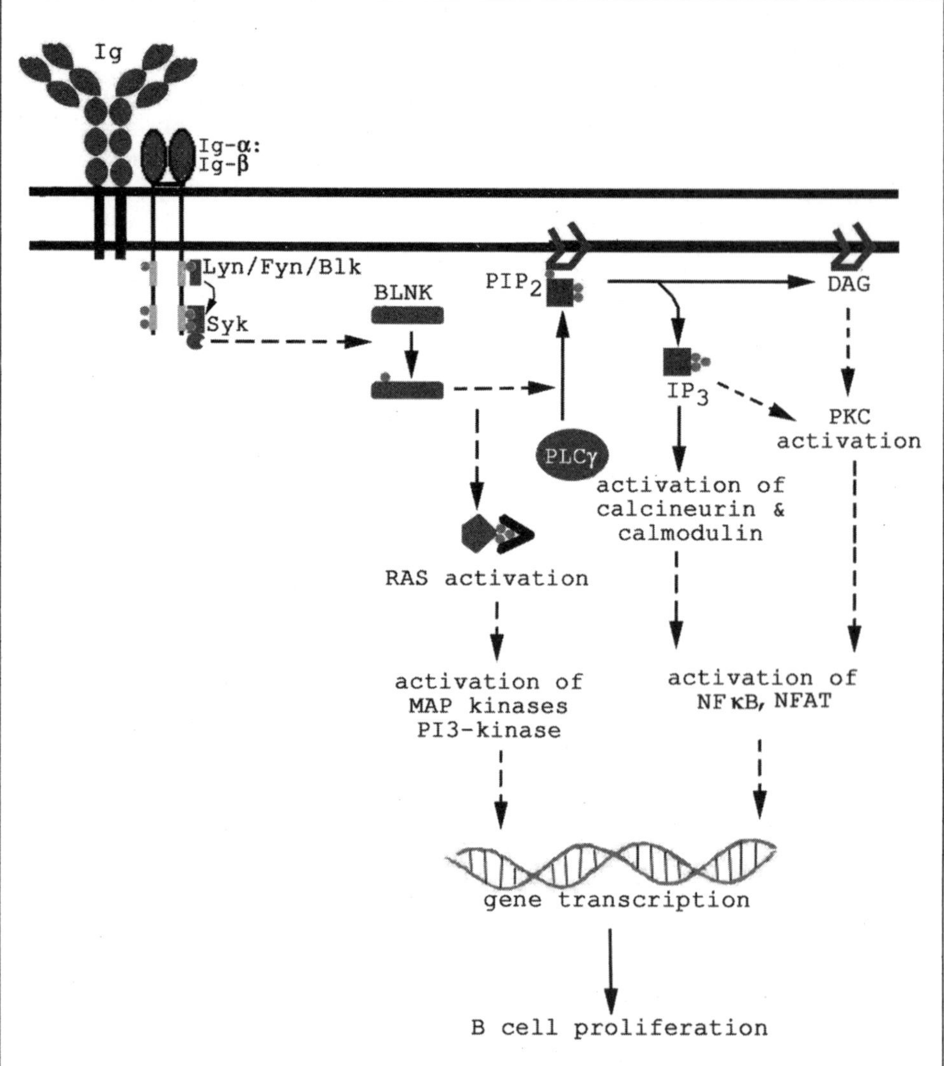

Figure 6.4 Cross-linking of antigen-recognition unit of the BcR by the antigen starts a cascade of downstream signalling events that can result in B cell proliferation. *Heterodimers of Ig-α:Ig-β are the signal transducing elements of the BcR. mIg clustering results in a change in the conformation of Ig-α:Ig-β heterodimers. Signal generated as a result of this change activates receptor-associated tyrosine kinases such as Lyn, Fyn, and Blk. They activate and phosphorylate each other and are then thought to phosphorylate ITAMs present in the cytoplasmic tails of Ig-α:Ig-β heterodimer. CD79 with both its ITAMs phophorylated serves as a docking site for Syk. Phosphorylated Syk phosphorylates the adaptor protein BLNK (B cell Linker Protein). BLNK recruits and phosphorylates the key enzyme of the cascade — PLCγ. This enzyme acts on membrane associated Phosphatidylinositol-(4,5)-bisphosphate (PIP$_2$) and splits it into two potent messengers — Diacylglycerol (DAG) and Inositol triphosphate (IP$_3$). DAG remains associated with the membrane, while IP$_3$ is released in the cytosol and interacts with ER (Endoplasmic Reticulum) receptors. IP$_3$ also activates Ca^{2+} binding calcineurin and calmodulin. Together, these molecules activate PKC and induce the transcription and nuclear localization of transcription factors Nuclear Factor of Activated T cells (NFAT) and NFκB (Nuclear Factor κB). BLNK phosphorylation also results in activation of Ras. Ras activation leads to the triggering of Phosphatidylinositol-3-kinase (PI3-kinase) and Mitogen-Activated Protein kinases (MAP kinases) and ultimately results in B cell proliferation.*

- Docking of Syk allows it to become tyrosine phosphorylated by Src family PTKs, and it is thereby activated. Lyn is important in this Syk activation, since Lyn-deficient B cells fail to induce Syk tyrosine phosphorylation.

- Phosphorylated Syk phosphorylates BLNK (**B** cell **L**in**k**er **P**rotein), an adaptor protein needed for transmitting the signal generated at the cell membrane to downstream targets.
- Multiple cell surface receptors then get rapidly tyrosine phosphorylated. These include CD19, CD22 (both of which have SH2 docking sites), and PLCγ recruited by BLNK.
  - PLCγ is phosphorylated by Syk and another PTK — Btk (**B**ruton's **t**yrosine **k**inase).
  - Phosphorylation of CD22 is a feedback loop providing for the downregulation of the escalating response. The ligation of CD22 and FcγRIIB1 is especially efficient in inhibiting signalling via BcR.
- ❏ Tyrosine phosphorylated PLCγ hydrolyses **P**hosphatidylinositol-(4,5)-bisphosphate (**PIP$_2$**) into two potent messengers — DAG and IP$_3$. These two products of PIP$_2$ cleavage activate **P**rotein **K**inase **C** (**PKC**).
  - DAG remains associated with the inner surface of the plasma membrane. It is an activator of several members of the serine/threonine protein kinase family — the most important amongst them being PKC.
  - IP$_3$, by contrast, interacts with receptors on the ER, resulting in the release of intracellular Ca^{2+} stores. IP$_3$ also leads to the opening of the Ca^{2+} channels in the plasma membrane, leading to an influx of Ca^{2+} in the cell. Together, these events result in increased intracellular Ca^{2+} levels and translocation of transcription factors.
    - The massive increase in intracellular Ca^{2+} results in the activation of the Ca^{2+} binding proteins, calmodulin, and calcineurin. Ca^{2+} released by IP$_3$ further activates PKC.
    - Calmodulin and calcineurin induce the nuclear localization of the **N**uclear **F**actor of **A**ctivated **T** cells (NFAT) and NFκB (**N**uclear **F**actor **κB**) proteins.
  - PKC activation leads to the activation of multiple transcription factors, including NFκB proteins.
- ❏ BcR stimulation also recruits adaptor proteins to the receptor site. These adaptor proteins induce activation of the small G protein, Ras.
- ❏ Ras activation ultimately leads to the triggering of **P**hosphatidylinositol-3-kinase (PI3-kinase) and **M**itogen-**A**ctivated **P**rotein kinases (MAP kinases). Several transcription factors, including AP-1 (**A**ctivating **P**rotein-**1**), which regulate the

---

B CELL ANTIGEN RECEPTOR

❏ BcR is a multimolecular complex consisting of an antigen recognition unit with associated molecules.

❏ It recognizes antigen in its native form.

❏ mIg is the antigen recognition unit of BcR; it is similar in structure to secreted Ig except that mIg contains a stretch of hydrophobic amino acids that anchors it in the cytoplasmic membrane.
- mIg consists of 2H and 2L chains; each H chain associates with one L chain, yielding a molecule that is homodimer of a heterodimer (H-L)$_2$.
- Each chain consists of a 110 amino acid V region and 110 (L chain) or 330 (H chain) amino acid C region.
- Globular domains present at the amino-terminus of the H and L chains are held together by hydrophobic interactions and form the antigen-binding pocket.

❏ Other molecules associated with BcR include:
- a heterodimer of Ig-α and Ig-β; both these molecules have ITAMs in their cytoplasmic tails and are responsible for transduction of the signal generated by mIg ligation.
- the CD19-CD21-CD81 complex; C19-BcR coligation decreases the threshold of antigenic stimulation, while CD19-CD21 coligation results in enhanced B cell response. CD19 also regulates the phosphorylation and activation of multiple downstream adaptor proteins and enzymes.
- CD22 recruits phosphatases to the signalling complex, thereby limiting BcR signalling.
- CD72 negatively regulates B cell signalling.
- FcγRIIB1; cross-linking of BcR with this molecule downmodulates BcR signalling.

expression of several genes involved in cell growth, are activated as a consequence of PI3-kinase and MAP kinases activation.

❑ The end result is B cell proliferation and differentiation (fig. 6.4).

6.3 The T Cell Antigen Receptor

TcR, like BcR, is a macromolecular complex (sometimes called a signalosome) consisting of immune-recognition receptors and associated signal transduction molecules (fig. 6.5). The antigen receptor of circulating mature T lymphocytes comprises two highly variable, clonally distributed glycoprotein heterodimers (either αβ or γδ pair) non-covalently associated with other invariant chains collectively called the CD3 complex. Also found to be associated are CD4/CD8 and CD45 molecules. The αβ and γδ heterodimers are responsible for antigen recognition and thus confer specificity. CD4 and CD8 are the coreceptors that interact with MHC molecules, while the CD3 complex and CD45 are involved in signal transduction.

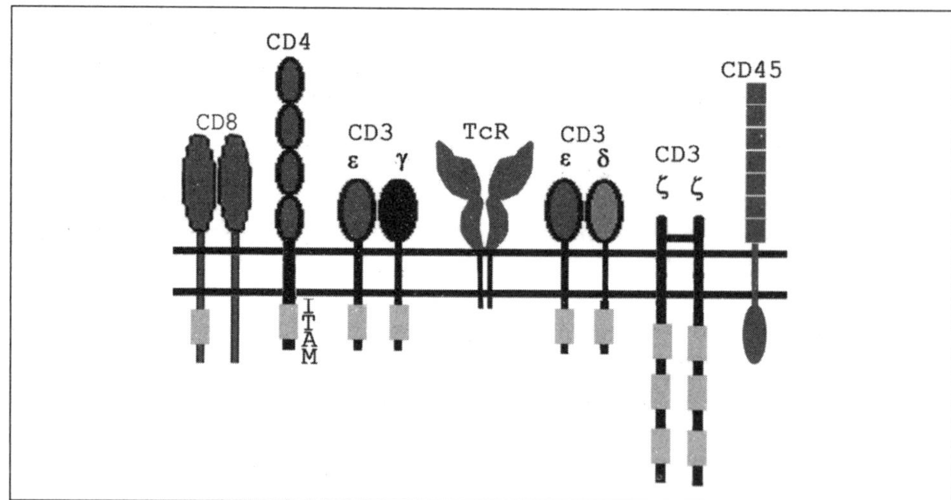

Figure 6.5 The TcR receptor complex consists of an antigen recognition unit and associated molecules such as CD3, CD45, and the coreceptors CD4/CD8. CD3 complex associated with the TcR is involved in signal transduction. It is composed of five chains (γ, δ, ε, η, and ζ) organized to form three dimers — γε, δε, ζζ. Of these γ, δ, and ε chains contain an extracellular Ig fold and a long cytoplasmic tail with one ITAM each. The ζ chain has a short extracellular fold and three ITAMs in its cytoplasmic chain. The TcR complex also contains the phosphatase CD45 and CD4 or CD8 molecules. CD4, the coreceptor for MHC class II molecules, and CD8, the coreceptor for MHC class I molecules, are found on different subset of T cells and are never present together on the same T cell. Both these molecules have one ITAM each in their cytoplasmic tail. The coreceptors must bind to the same MHC molecules as the TcR for optimal signal transduction.

T CELL ANTIGEN RECEPTOR

❑ T cell antigen receptor complex consists of an antigen recognition unit and associated molecules.

❑ The antigen recognition unit is a heterodimer of αβ chains or γδ chains held together by disulphide linkages.
  - Each of these chains has a membrane distal V region and a membrane proximal C region.
  - Both Vα and Vβ contribute to the antigen-binding pocket.
  - TcR recognizes antigen loaded on MHC class I, class II, or CD1 molecules.
  - Cytoplasmic segments of the α and β chains contain hydrophilic amino acid sequences that allow them to associate with CD3.

❑ CD3, associated with TcR antigen recognition unit, is a complex of five chains (γ, δ, ε, ζ, and η) that yield a set of three heterodimers (γε, δε, and ζζ or ζη) and is involved in signal transduction.

❑ TcR is also associated with coreceptors CD4 or CD8. CD4 is a monomeric glycoprotein, whereas CD8 is a dimer.

6.3.1 TcR Structure

The αβ complex is expressed by over 95% human peripheral blood T cells. The heterodimer consists of one chain each of an acidic α chain of 39–46 KD and a more basic 40–44 KD β chain held together by disulphide linkages. The γδ T cells have a more restricted distribution, but structurally the γδ receptor is essentially similar to the αβ receptor.

❑ The TcR heterodimer is structurally homologous to the Ig molecule in that it also consists of distinct domains — the V and C regions; the V region is distal to the cell membrane and is responsible for antigen binding, and the C region is proximal to the cell membrane.

❑ The V domain of TcR comprises CDR1, 2, and 3, corresponding to those found in the Ig molecule.
  • The CDR1 and CDR2 regions of the αβTcR interact with the α helices of MHC molecules.
  • The highly polymorphic region corresponding to CDR3 interacts with antigenic peptides bound in the MHC cleft.

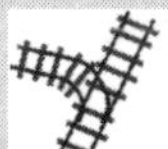

Common yet Unique: CD45

Also called leukocyte common antigen, CD45 is one of the most abundant glycoproteins expressed on immune cells. CD45 is estimated to occupy an astounding 10% of the cell surface area of B and T lymphocytes. It is a membrane-associated protein tyrosine phosphatase expressed on all nucleated haematopoietic cells. Alternative splicing generates up to eight isoforms of CD45, five of which are expressed on T cells. The cytoplasmic tail of CD45 is thought to contain the phosphatase activity and is well conserved across all mammalian species analyzed. To date, an exogenous ligand has not been found for the molecule. CD45 is associated with both BcR and TcR. Its ability to dephosphorylate Src family kinases gives it a crucial role in antigen receptor signalling. CD45 can operate both as a positive and negative regulator of Src family kinases. Two members of this family of kinases — Lck and Fyn — have been shown to be substrates of CD45. CD45 is especially important in T cell activation, as disruption of its signalling affects tyrosine phosphorylation, inositol phosphate generation, and Ca^{2+} mobilization. It also seems to regulate adhesion in T cells. B cell development is less severely affected by CD45. The B220 isoform of CD45 is a very early marker for B cell lineage, but B cell development can occur normally in its absence. CD45 is thought to promote BcR signal transduction by constitutively maintaining Src family kinases in a partially active state. Apart from its role in antigen receptor signalling, CD45 has multiple other functions. It is important in regulating survival and/or apoptosis in immune cells. Its ligation triggers apoptosis of peripheral T and B cells. Mast cell degranulation following cross-linking of FcεRI by antigen-IgE complexes has been shown to be critically dependent upon CD45 phosphatase activity. Recently, it was shown to negatively regulate the cytokine receptor-mediated activation of haematopoietic cells. Experimental data suggests that CD45 specifically inhibits Janus kinases involved in the Jak/Stat pathway of IL-4 and IFN-γ signal transduction (see sidetrack 'Cell to Cell SMS' in chapter 8). CD45 also acts as a negative regulator of cytokine receptor-mediated proliferation and differentiation of haematopoietic cells. Specifically, it is found to downregulate IL-3 and SCF-mediated activation and proliferation of haematopoietic cells. In macrophages, CD45 seems to downregulate adhesion to the extracellular matrix and to other cells.

Over- or under-expression of CD45 seems to result in a number of diseases. A loss of CD45 expression is reported in >10% of patients of Acute Lymphoblastic Leukaemia. CD45 expression is also frequently lost in patients with Hodgkin's lymphoma and multiple myelomas. By contrast, CD45 expression is upregulated on microglial cells in patients with Alzheimer's disease. In mice, disproportionate expression of certain isoforms of CD45 on T cell subsets has been implicated in autoimmune diseases such as SLE, diabetes, and experimental allergic encephalomyelitis (the mice equivalent of multiple sclerosis). Some patients of Multiple Sclerosis and SLE also show altered expression of CD45 isoforms on CD4+ T cells. Although it has been studied over the past two decades, many questions regarding this 'common antigen' remain unanswered — eg, the nature of its ligand; the importance and functions of various isoforms; its role in antiviral immunity, autoimmunity, tumour growth, and metastases.

❑ Proximal to the membrane, each TcR chain has a short connecting sequence containing a cysteine residue that is involved in the formation of a disulphide bond between the two chains.

❑ Transmembrane domains of TcR subunits have 15–20 positively charged amino acids which allow them to interact with the CD3 complex and a very short cytoplasmic chain of 5–12 amino acids.

❑ CD3 associated with TcR, like CD79 of the BcR, is involved in signal transduction. CD3 expression is necessary for αβ or γδ heterodimer expression. Antibodies to the CD3 complex can block T cell function. The CD3 complex is composed of five chains called γ, δ, ε, η, and ζ.

- The five chains are organized to form three dimers — a heterodimer of gamma and epsilon chains (γε), a heterodimer of delta and epsilon chains (δε), and a homodimer of two zeta chains (ζζ).
- Differential splicing of the zeta chain gives the eta (sometimes called nu) chain and the corresponding ζη dimer. About 90% of TcR express ζζ heterodimers and 10% express ζη heterodimers.
- γ, δ, and ε chains are members of the Ig superfamily, consisting of an extracellular Ig fold, a transmembrane domain, and a long cytoplasmic tail.
- ζ (and therefore η) chains do not have the Ig fold. They have a very short extracellular domain (only nine amino acids) and a long cytoplasmic domain (ζ has 113 amino acids, η has 155).
- Transmembrane domains of all CD3 chains are negatively charged and therefore interact with positively charged TcR transmembrane domains.
- All CD3 chains have ITAMs — one each in γ, δ, and ε chains and three each in ζ and η chains.

❑ Coreceptors CD4 and CD8 are transmembrane glycoproteins found on different subsets of T cells. CD4 is present on TH and TR cells, and CD8 is found on CTLs. These molecules are important in antigen recognition by αβ T cells. They are coreceptors for MHC molecules — CD4 for MHC class II molecules, and CD8 for MHC class I molecules. The coreceptors must bind to the same MHC molecules as the TcR for optimal signal transduction. Antibodies to CD4/CD8 inhibit T cell activation.

- Both CD4 and CD8 belong to the Ig superfamily.
- CD4 is a transmembrane monomeric glycoprotein containing four extracellular Ig domains, a transmembrane domain, and a cytoplasmic tail with serine residues that can be phosphorylated by serine/threonine kinases. It is internally associated with the Src family kinase Lck.
- CD8 is a dimer consisting of αβ or αα subunits. Each subunit consists of a single Ig fold, a transmembrane region, and a cytoplasmic tail that can be phosphorylated at several sites.

6.3.2 Simplified Outline of TcR Signalling

Like BcR, clustering of TcR leads to the nuclear localization of transcription factors and ultimately results in gene transcription that allows proliferation and differentiation of the cells (fig. 6.6).

❑ Clustering of the TcR complex and coreceptors results in the activation of PTKs associated with the cytoplasmic domains of clustered CD3 and coreceptor proteins; the signalling is initiated by CD3 and associated Fyn.

❑ Lck, a Src family kinase bound to the cytoplasmic tail of CD4 (or CD8), is brought into the proximity of the ITAMs of CD3 ζ chain and results in the phosphorylation of the Syk family kinase ZAP-70 (70 KD ζ-**A**ssociated **P**rotein).

- Both Fyn and Lck are regulated by tyrosine phosphorylation at two sites. Phosphorylation at one site induces activation, while it has an inhibitory effect

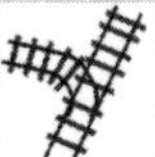

Turning it On: NFκB Proteins

The NFκB family of transcription factors has a central role in co-ordinating the expression of a number of genes involved in the control of both innate and adaptive immune responses. The family comprises five members — RelA, RelB, cREL, NFκB1, and NFκB2. The main activated form of NFκB is a heterodimer of RelA and NFκB1. The NFκB family of proteins is normally present in the cytoplasm in association with a family of inhibitory proteins IκBs (**I**nhibitors of NF**κB**s). Upon activation, IκBs get phosphorylated and subsequently degraded. The degradation of IκBs allows NFκB proteins to translocate to the nucleus and bind their cognate DNA-binding sites. NFκB proteins can thus regulate the transcription of a large number of genes, including those of antimicrobial peptides, cytokines, chemokines, stress-response proteins, and anti-apoptotic proteins.

NFκB proteins get rapidly activated in response to a variety of stimuli, including stress signals, engagement of PRRs (especially TLRs) by PAMPs on pathogens, and pro-inflammatory cytokines such as IL-1 and TNF-α produced by activated macrophages and monocytes. IL-1 and TNF-α produced by APCs can, in particular, induce NFκB phosphorylation and enhance T cell activation. Interestingly, TcR clustering alone is not enough to activate NFκB or AP-1, and this results in deficiency of IL-2 production. Engagement of the costimulatory molecule CD28 in conjunction with TcR clustering, however, results in activation of these proteins and their nuclear translocation, resulting in IL-2 production necessary for T cell proliferation. NFκB is important in a number of B cell processes such as germinal centre formation and isotype switching. It is also involved in B cell maturation, since mice lacking NFκB1 and NFκB2 show a complete absence of B cell maturation. NFκB function is thus essential for lymphocyte activation and survival and for mounting normal immune responses. The constitutive activation of NFκB pathways, on the other hand, is associated with a number of diseases, including inflammatory bowel disease, Multiple Sclerosis and asthma.

at the other site (called regulatory site). Thus, the enzymes are normally inactive because of phosphorylation at the regulatory site. CD45 helps in Lck and Fyn activation by removing the regulatory phosphate.

- Lck and Fyn phosphorylate tyrosines in the ITAMs of the CD3 complex. The tyrosine phosphorylated ITAMs in the ζ chain become specific 'docking sites' for the PTK ZAP-70. The docked ZAP-70 remains inactive until CD4 or CD8 engagement results in the activation of Lck. Lck or Fyn then proceed to phosphorylate (and therefore activate) bound ZAP-70.

❑ ZAP-70 activation is a crucial step in T cell activation. It initiates three separate cascades, each of which ultimately activates transcription factors.

- ZAP-70 phosphorylates the adaptor protein LAT (**L**inker of **A**ctivated **T** cells).
  - ◆ LAT, located in the plasma membrane, is thought to link early tyrosine phosphorylation events to distal portions of the signalling pathway. In the absence of LAT, TcR engagement does not lead to gene transcription.
  - ◆ Tyrosine phosphorylated LAT recruits PLCγ, PI3-kinase, and other molecules to the membrane.
- ZAP-70, like Syk, activates PLCγ to cleave PIP_2 into IP_3 and DAG (section 6.2.3).
  - ◆ The cleaving of PIP_2 ultimately leads to the activation of the transcription factors NFAT and NFκB.
  - ◆ Both factors enter the nucleus and activate the transcription of several genes, including the IL-2 gene.
- ZAP-70 also activates the Ras pathway.
  - ◆ Ras activation leads to the activation of PI3-kinase and MAP kinases.
  - ◆ The transcription factor AP-1 is also activated.

❑ New mRNA is synthesized as a consequence and results in the proliferation and differentiation of the T cell.

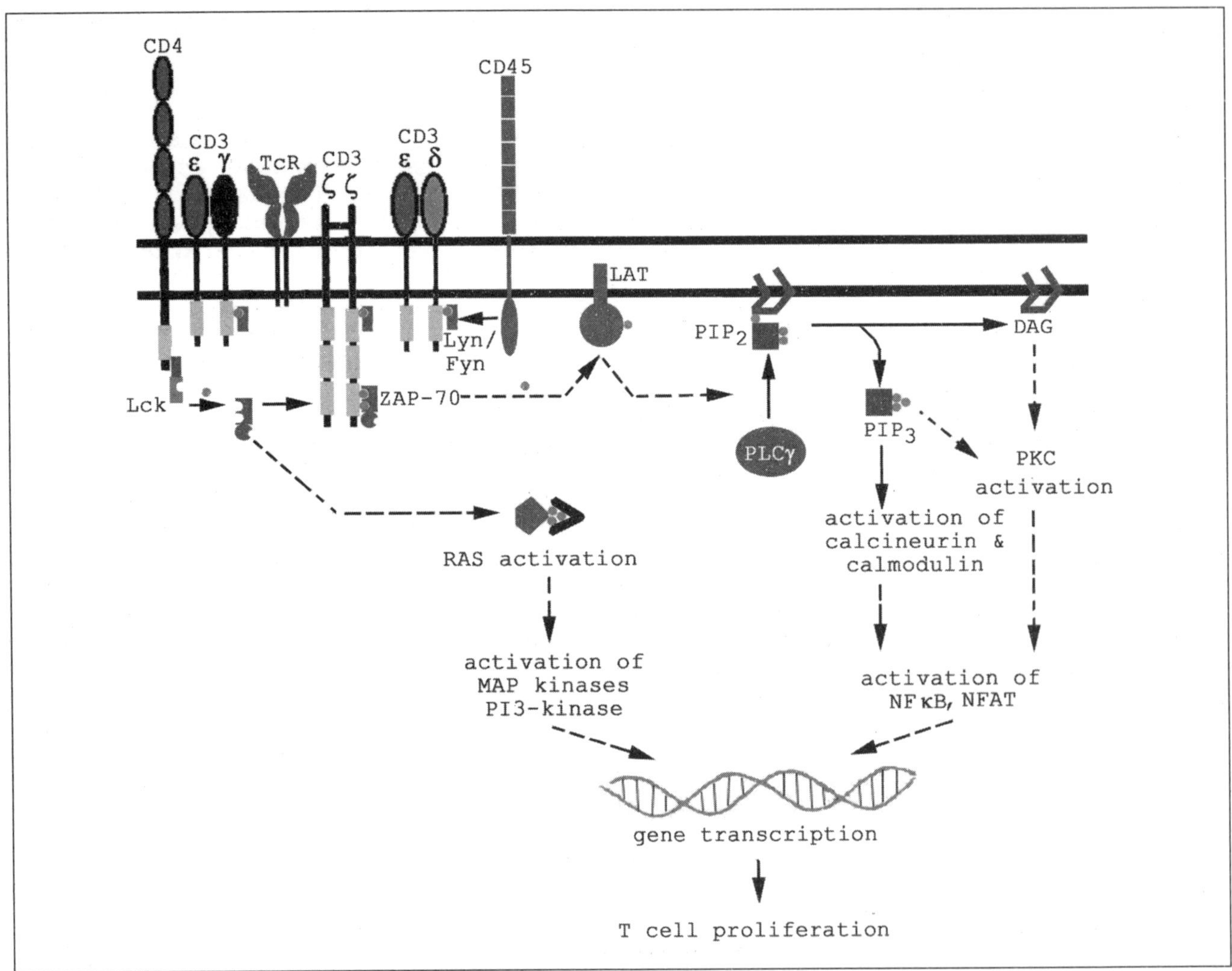

Figure 6.6 Coligation of TcRs by peptide:MHC complexes along with CD4/CD8 engagement triggers downstream events that can result in T cell proliferation. Antigen recognition by TcRs results in a change in CD3 conformation. CD3-associated protein kinases such as Lyn and Fyn are normally in an inactive state and need to be activated by CD45. CD45 removes the inhibitory phosphate and activates the enzymes. Activated Lyn and Fyn phosphorylate the ITAMS on CD3 dimers. Engagement of CD4 (or CD8) by MHC molecules activates the coreceptor-associated tyrosine kinase Lck. Activated Lck is brought into the vicinity of CD3ζ-associated ZAP-70, which it proceeds to phosphorylate. ZAP-70 activates the Ras pathway, which in turn results in the activation of MAP kinases and PI3-kinase. ZAP-70 also phosphorylates the adaptor protein LAT. LAT recruits PLCγ and other kinases to the cell membrane. Activated PLCγ cleaves PIP_2 to IP_3 and DAG. The downstream events of PIP_2 cleavage are similar in B cells and T cells and cause new gene transcription and T cell proliferation.

6.4 Effect of Costimulators on B and T Cell Signal Transduction Pathways

It is generally accepted that two signals are required for both B and T cell activation. BcR clustering by the antigen delivers the first signal required for B cell activation. However, most antigens lack the multiple epitopes required for sufficient BcR clustering (except of course, the TI antigens). A second signal delivered by cognate (physical) interaction with TH cells is therefore needed to respond to such (TD) antigens (section 8.2.4). A plethora of molecules are implicated in this cognate interaction. The most important is the engagement of CD40 on B cells by its ligand CD154 (also called CD40L) on the T cells. It has been established that CD40-CD154 interaction leads to enhanced transcription NFκB proteins. The exact molecular mechanism that leads to this increased transcription is yet to be elucidated.

MAJOR STEPS IN B CELL AND T CELL SIGNALLING PATHWAYS THAT RESULT IN THEIR PROLIFERATION

	B Cell	**T Cell**
Ligation of antigen receptor	Phosphorylation of CD79a and b by tyrosine kinases (Lyn, Blk, Fyn, and Lck)	Phosphorylation of CD3 ζ chain by Lck (associated with CD4) and Lyn/Fyn (associated with CD3)
	↓	↓
	CD79 molecules with both their sites phosphorylated serve as docking sites for Syk	Phosphorylated CD3ζ becomes a docking site for the Syk family kinase ZAP-70
PLCγ phosphorylation	Syk is phosphorylated by Src family kinases (eg, Lyn)	ZAP-70 is phosphorylated by Lck or Fyn
	↓	↓
	Syk phosphorylates BLNK; multiple receptors get rapidly phosphorylated, including CD19 and CD22	ZAP-70 phosphorylates LAT
	↓	↓
	BLNK recruits PLCγ to the membrane	LAT recruits PLCγ to the membrane
	↓	↓
	PLCγ gets phosphorylated by Syk and Btk	ZAP-70 phosphorylates PLCγ

Phosphorylated PLCγ hydrolysis PIP_2 to DAG and IP_3

Activation of PKC and translocation of transcription factors	DAG activates many kinases including PKC	Increased intracellular levels of Ca^{2+}, caused by IP3, results in the activation of calmodulin and calcineurin; it also results in further activation of PKC
		↓
		Calmodulin and calcineurin induce nuclear translocation of transcription factors (NFAT, NFκB)
Activation of PI3-Kinase, MAP Kinases, and gene transcription	BcR stimulation recruits adaptor proteins to the receptor site and results in activation of Ras	ZAP-70 activates the Ras pathway
	↓	↓

Ras activation results in activation of PI3-kinase, MAP kinases, and AP-1

Together, these lead to transcription of genes involved in proliferation and differentiation of cells

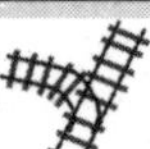

The Agonists and the Antagonists

Changing some TcR contact residues of a peptide can alter the signalling events associated with TcR clustering.

❏ Peptides that activate T cells are called agonist peptides.

❏ Structurally related peptides may not activate T cells but instead, prevent them from responding to agonist peptides; alternatively, they may deliver negative signals to the T cells. Such peptides are called antagonist peptides.

❏ Some peptides lead to only partial T cell activation and are called partial agonists or **A**ltered **P**eptide **L**igands (APL).

APLs seem to inhibit TcR signalling through the altered phosphorylation of CD3ε and ζ chains. TcR ligation in the absence of costimulation is also thought to generate such incomplete phosphorylation. It is possible that pathogens, especially viruses, may persist and survive by this mechanism which regulates T cell activation. For example, in HIV infections, mutants that circumvent CTL-killing by causing partial activation of cells are found to arise in later stages of infection. Similarly, the malarial parasite *P. falciparum* has been shown to evade the immune system by this mechanism. The reduced activation induced by APLs is now being explored for the therapeutic modulation of T cell function in diseases characterized by unwanted T cell activation (eg, autoimmune disorders or allergies) as well as for disorders of suboptimal T cell activation (eg, cancers).

With T cells, both primary and secondary signals are delivered by the same APC. TcR clustering by the MHC:peptide complex delivers the primary signal. The second signal is delivered by the engagement of costimulatory molecules. CD28 is the prototypical costimulatory molecule expressed by naïve and antigen-primed T cells. The ligand for CD28 is CD80 and CD86. Incidentally, all these molecules belong to the Ig superfamily. The molecular mechanism by which CD28 cross-linking affects T cell activation is not clearly understood. The cytoplasmic tail of CD28 lacks enzymatic activity but has several tyrosines that can be phosphorylated by Src family PTKs. Phosphorylation of the cytomplasmic tyrosines is thought to lead to the binding of PI3-kinase and result in NFκB activation. Thus, CD28 is believed to amplify TcR signal by augmented transcriptional activity and increased mRNA stability. CD28 ligation is also thought to recruit lipid rafts to the site of T cell-APC interaction, thereby causing a local increase in lipid-associated enzymes and adaptor proteins. It also promotes T cell survival by inducing the upregulation of Bcl-xL (section 16.1). LFA-1, another costimulatory molecule, is an integrin family molecule that interacts with its ligand ICAM-1 on the APC. This interaction helps in cytoskeletal reorganization during T cell activation and amplifies TcR signal by recruiting Src family kinases and PI3-kinase to the site of interaction and promoting the activation of transcription factors.

CTLA-4 (**C**ytotoxic **T** Lymphocyte-associated **A**ntigen-**4**) shows a 30% homology with CD28. It binds to the same ligands as CD28 (CD80/86). However, it is a negative regulator of T cell activation. CTLA-4 ligation is found to reduce TcR dependent activation of MAP kinases and the transcription factors NFAT, NFκB, and AP-1. Ligation of CTLA-4 during TcR stimulation results in reduced cytokine production and cell cycle arrest. The molecular mechanisms behind these effects are still being investigated (see sidetrack 'The Need for Stimulating Company', chapter 8).

Molecules of Adaptive Immune Recognition: Antigen Presenting Molecules

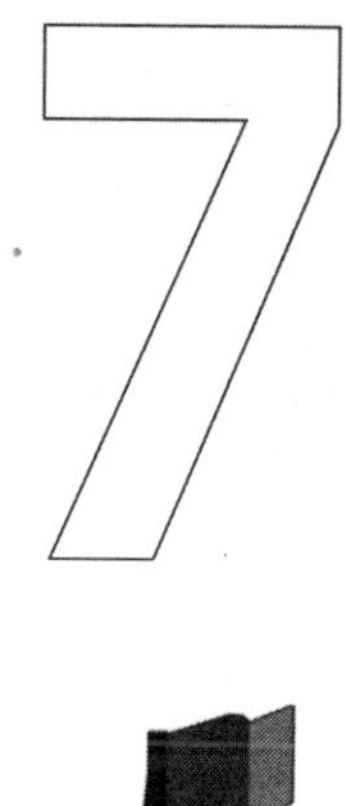

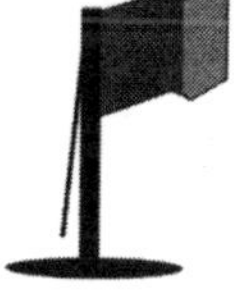

I know I left too much mess and destruction
to come back again
And I caused nothing but trouble
I understand if you can't talk to me again
And if you live by the rules of "it's over"
Then I'm sure that that makes sense

Well, I will go down with this ship
And I won't put my hands up and surrender
There will be no white flag above my door

— Dido, *White Flag*

CLIP:	Class II-associated invariant chain peptide
HSP:	Heat shock proteins
Ii:	Invariant chain
Ir genes:	Immune response genes
LMP:	Low molecular weight peptide
MECL-1:	Multcatalytic endopeptidase complex like-1
TAP:	Transporter associated with antigen processing
β_2-m:	β_2-microglobulin

7.1 Introduction

The adaptive immune system is activated through the specific recognition and binding of B or T cell antigen receptors to their respective ligands. The preceding chapters have shown that B cell recognition is rather simple, since BcRs recognizes native ligands. The story gets more complicated with T cells. The TcR ligand has to be processed and loaded onto specific molecules that are expressed on the surfaces of APCs. These molecules on which the antigen fragments are loaded are the MHC or MHC-like molecules[1]. One can think of MHC molecules as flagpoles; the kind of the flag displayed will depend upon the availability of flags and the wherewithal of the cell. MHC molecules are unique, in that they bind a variety of peptides, ie, different flags can be flown from the same MHC poles. TcRs are the flag-recognition systems of the T cells. MHC molecules can be loaded with fragments of any proteins that the cells have internalized or synthesized and expressed on the cell surface. Molecules loaded with self-peptides act as white flags and spare the cell from the ferocity of the adaptive immune system. The presence of fragments derived from an infecting agent or from proteins synthesized because of infection or transformation serve the exact opposite purpose. They behave like the proverbial red flags, signalling potential danger and target the cell for destruction.

7.2 MHC Class I Molecules

Located on chromosome 6 in humans and chromosome 17 in mice, the MHC region codes for polypeptides of three different classes. Two of these are highly polymorphic[2] peptide receptors involved in T cell antigen recognition; the third class of molecules includes some complement components, cytokines, enzymes that are important in innate immunity, and proteins involved in growth and development.

Except for a few cell types such as neurons, almost all nucleated cells of the body express MHC class I molecules[3]. The degree of expression differs for different cell types. Lymphocytes show the highest level of expression, while the expression is very low in fibroblasts, neural cells, muscle cells, etc. **Pro-inflammatory stimuli such as IFNs (including α, β, and γ), TNF-α, and LPS upregulate the expression of these molecules on most cell types.** Murine class I molecules are called H2-K, -L, or -D, with the haplotype indicated by a letter in superscript (eg, H2-K^d); human equivalents are HLA-A, -B, or -C, with the haplotype indicated by a number (eg, HLA-A1).

7.2.1 Structure

Although class I, II, MHC and MHC-like molecules differ in the structure of their subunits, they are closely related in their overall three-dimensional structure. These are transmembrane glycoproteins that have an Ig fold in their membrane-proximal domain; the membrane distal domains form a cleft or groove for peptide binding (or glycolipid) binding. Class I molecules are composed of a glycosylated 45 KD polypeptide chain called the α (or heavy) chain that is non-covalently associated with a non-glycosylated peptide — β_2-microglobulin (β_2-m). β_2-m is a 12 KD peptide sometimes referred to as the light chain of class I proteins. Both heavy and light chains belong to the Ig superfamily. Calling β_2-m 'light chain' is actually misleading since it is *not* encoded by the MHC genes but by genes located on chromosome 15 in humans and chromosome 2 in mice. It is a soluble protein that can be found by itself in serum or urine. Although β_2-m can be synthesized independent of the class I molecule, the reverse does not hold true. β_2-m is necessary for the processing and expression of class I molecules. Individuals with a congenital defect in β_2-m production fail to express class I molecules.

---

[1] 'Major histocompatibility complex' seems a strange name to give to molecules involved in antigen presentation to T cells. The name had been coined long before the function of these molecules was established. The 'major' and 'histocompatibility' in the name came from the observation that this genetic region appeared to play an important role in transplant (allograft) rejection. The term 'complex' referred to the fact that the region consisted of numerous loci closely linked to each other and sub-serving different functions. Since these molecules could give rise to antibodies, they were called 'MHC antigens'. The MHC complex is called the H-2 complex (Histocompatibility antigen-**2**) in mice, because it represents the second antigen originally defined by Gorer, a British scientist who studied mouse MHC. Human MHC is called the HLA (**H**uman **L**eukocyte **A**ntigen).

[2] In genetics, *poly* which is Greek for many, and *morph,* Greek for shape, is taken to mean variation at a single genetic locus and its variation within a species. The individual variant genes are called alleles. Each set of alleles is called a haplotype or allotype.

[3] Human erythrocytes, being non-nucleated, do not express class I molecules.

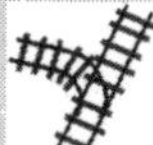

Class Interference:
Viral Interference in MHC Class I Antigen Presentation

MHC class I molecules on the surface of infected cells present virus-derived peptides to naïve CD8[+] T cells. Activation of naïve CD8[+] T cells results in the generation of an anti-viral CTL response and the recruitment of other components of the immune system to this response. Hence, downregulation of MHC class I expression can help a virus escape recognition and targeting by the immune system. Nevertheless, a complete shut down of class I expression is not advantageous to the virus, since it can leave the infected cell susceptible to NK cells. As you can imagine, it requires some juggling on the part of the virus to successfully evade immune detection. Ideally, the virus should downregulate but not completely shut down MHC class I expression. Viruses have evolved ingeneous ways of reducing MHC class I expression and antigen presentation.

❑ Kaposi's Sarcoma virus (a gamma herpes virus) encodes two proteins, K3 and K5, that increase endocytosis of class I molecules from the cell surface, effectively decreasing surface expression of these molecules and preventing recognition by CTLs.

❑ The Nef protein encoded by HIV relocates cell surface MHC class I molecules to the *trans*-golgi network, thereby downregulating their surface expression.

❑ Vpu, expressed by HIV-1, induces the degradation of newly synthesized class I molecules.

❑ Human cytomegalovirus encodes a virtual catalogue of proteins that can interfere with MHC class I molecule surface expression and peptide loading.

- Two proteins, US2 and US11 encoded by the cytomegalovirus, induce the translocation of newly synthesized MHC class I molecules to the cytosol for degradation. At the same time, NK cell activation is avoided, since US2 and US11 downregulate only some MHC class I alleles. The alleles that are allowed to be expressed at the cell surface deliver inhibitory signals to NK cells.

- UL18, a virus encoded MHC class I homologue, is thought to help in preventing NK cell-mediated lysis.

- US6 inhibits TAP-mediated peptide loading of MHC class I molecules. The exact mode of this inhibition is not yet elucidated.

- The glycoprotein US3 retains MHC class I molecules in the ER.

- The encoding of UL40 brilliantly illustrates how a chance mutation bestows a survival advantage. A peptide generated by the processing of UL40 is similar to the HLA-E ligand (a nonamer derived from HLA-C signal sequence) and helps stabilize and express HLA-E at the surface of the infected cell. The HLA-E:UL40-derived peptide complex delivers an inhibitory signal to NK cells and hence protects the virus from NK cell-mediated lysis.

❑ Adenovirus types 2 and 5 express a protein that binds to MHC class I molecules, causing their retention in the ER/*cis*-golgi.

❑ Adenovirus type 12 represses the transcription of LMP, TAP, and MHC class I molecules.

❑ Herpes simplex virus blocks the transport of MHC class I molecules from the ER to the cell surface. The immediate early protein ICP47 encoded by the virus binds TAP, thereby inhibiting the binding and translocation of peptides from the cytosol to the ER lumen — interference with peptide loading causes the molecules to be retained in the ER.

❑ The **E**pstein-**B**arr virus encoded **n**uclear **a**ntigen-**1** (EBNA-1) is resistant to proteasomal degradation and escapes antigen processing.

The α chain of the class I molecule is a type II membrane protein anchored in the cell membrane at the COOH– terminus by a hydrophobic structure that traverses the cell membrane and a short hydrophilic cytoplasmic tail about 30 amino acids in length. The majority of the polypeptide is external to the transmembrane region. The extracellular NH_2– terminus of the class I molecule has three globular domains termed α1, α2, and α3, each about 90–92 amino acids in length. The α3 domain is closely associated with $β_2$-m and also has a site for the binding of the CD8 coreceptor. $β_2$-m is not anchored in the cell membrane but is held in position solely because of its interaction with the α chain. The α1 and α2 domains, consisting of two α-helices resting on a sheet of eight β-strands, form the peptide-binding groove. The α1 domain is highly polymorphic, and along with α2, is responsible for the great variations observed in peptide binding by class I molecules (fig. 7.1).

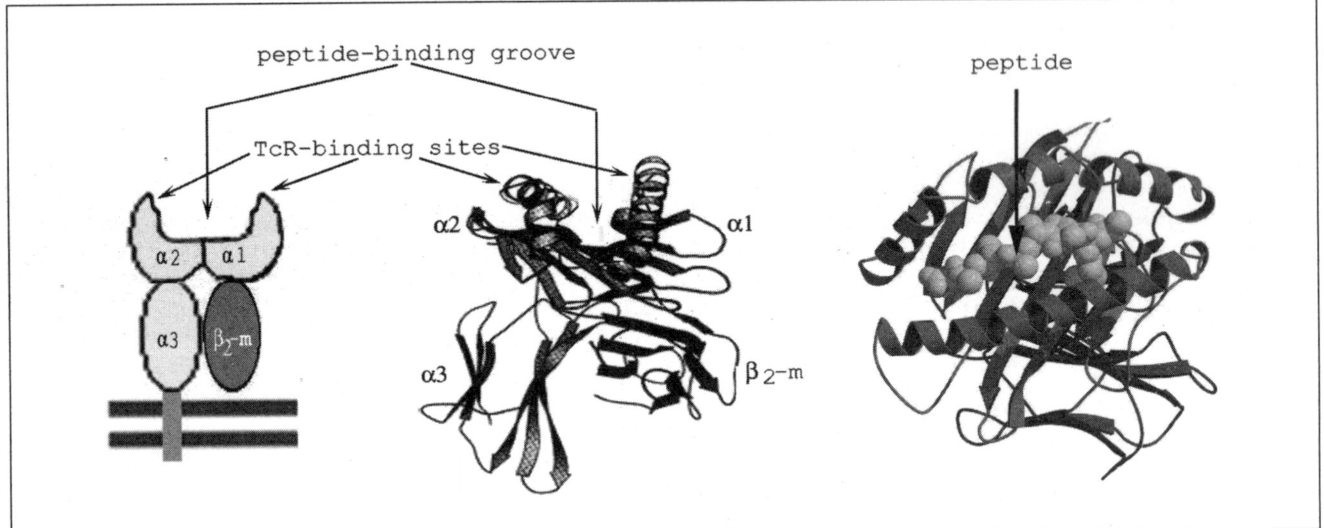

Figure 7.1 The peptide-binding groove of the MHC class I molecules is present at the membrane distal region of the α chain that is non-covalently associated with β2-m. β2-m is not anchored in the cell membrane but is held in position solely because of its interaction with the α chain. The extracellular region of the class I molecule has three globular domains termed α1, α2, and α3. The α3 domain is closely associated with β2-m and also has a site for the binding of the CD8 coreceptor. The left panel is a schematic depiction of the molecule, whereas the centre panel is a ribbon diagram of the molecule. The top view of the peptide-binding groove (ie, looking down into the groove) is depicted in the right panel. The floor of the groove is formed by β-pleated sheets, and the walls are formed by α-helices. The α1 and α2 domains contribute to the formation of the peptide-binding groove. These domains also have sites that contact TcR. The peptide lies in an elongated conformation along the peptide-binding groove with both Amino– and Carboxyl– termini tightly fixed in this groove.

Both MHC class I and class II molecules differ from other peptide-binding proteins in two major respects.

- Each MHC molecule can bind multiple peptides (but not at the same time). An individual can be infected by a wide variety of pathogens whose proteins differ widely in amino acid sequences. In order to activate T cells, MHC molecules, whether class I or II, must be able to bind stably to different peptides.
- The binding of the peptide is essential for the correct folding and stabilization of MHC molecules. The MHC-peptide complex is extremely stable, and the peptide co-purifies with the MHC molecule in experiments designed to isolate MHC molecules from cell lysates.

The peptide lies in an elongated conformation along the peptide-binding groove with both Amino– and Carboxyl– termini tightly fixed in this groove. The peptide-binding groove contains pockets that accommodate particular peptide side chains — termed anchor residues — that help anchor the peptide in the groove. These pockets vary in depth and chemical nature between allelic variants and thus determine the set of peptides that can be bound by a particular class I allele. Six pockets have been identified in the class I groove (P1 through P6). P1 and P6 react with the N– and C– termini of the peptide respectively and P2–P4 react with the peptide side chains. For human class I molecules, the C– terminal anchor residue of the peptide needs to be either hydrophobic or basic[4]. **The terminal anchor residues of the peptide form multiple hydrogen bonds and salt bridges with conserved amino acid residues in the two pockets located at the ends of the peptide-binding groove.** These interactions are essential for stable association between the peptide and the class I molecule, and they constrain the length of bound peptides to about 8–10 residues.

[4] Murine class I molecules are generally more hydrophobic than human class I molecules and can bind only peptides having a hydrophobic residue at the C– terminus.

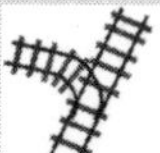

When Harry Meets Sally: MHC and Mate Selection

MHC genes are known to play a central role in immune recognition. What is not so well known is that MHC genes are a source of individual odours that influence individual recognition, mating preferences, nesting behaviour, and the selective blocking of pregnancy in animals. Experiments in rodents clearly establish that mice prefer mates that are genetically as far removed from their MHC haplotyes as possible. Soluble MHC found in the urine and sweat of animals seems to influence the choice of mates in rodents. In animals, the chances of bringing a pregnancy to full term are maximized when the foetus and mother have different MHC alleles. Since the MHC is directly linked to host defence, it is hypothesized that this is probably a way of ensuring that MHC diversity is maintained in a population, maximizing the chances of survival of the species.

The role of MHC in human mate selection is difficult to study, since the MHC loci are the most polymorphic loci in the human genome. Recent experiments in humans seem to indicate that the same compulsions observed in other animals are operative in *Homo sapiens sapiens*. Individuals describe body odours as pleasant (*parfum au naturel!*) when the odours are from people who have few HLA alleles that match their own. Research suggests that at least in women, mate preference seems to be dictated by paternal MHC and women prefer mates with MHC haplotypes different from their own. There is some evidence to suggest that oral contraception may reverse this choice. Further research is needed to establish if this is indeed true, and what, if any, are its repercussions.

7.2.2 Synthesis and Assembly

Both the light and heavy chains of class I molecules are synthesized in the ER. A newly synthesized heavy chain binds to a number of ER resident chaperone proteins, beginning with calnexin, during the assembly process. The interaction with calnexin is thought to facilitate folding of the nascent heavy chain and promote assembly with β_2-m. The Ig-binding protein BiP can substitute for calnexin. Erp57 (a thiol reductase) also associates with this complex. Once the heavy chain:β_2-m heterodimer is formed, it dissociates from calnexin and associates with calreticulin. The whole complex then interacts with TAP (**T**ransporter associated with **A**ntigen **P**rocessing; see below). This interaction promotes loading of peptides on the class I molecule. A TAP-associated transmembrane glycoprotein called tapasin[5] is involved in stabilizing this process. Tapasin is thought to promote the stability and peptide transport activity of TAP and hold the class I molecule in its peptide-receptive conformation. Once loading is accomplished, class I molecules are released from TAP. The peptide:MHC class I complex is then transported through the *trans*-golgi network to the cell surface, where it undergoes periodic recycling between the endosomes and the cell surface (fig. 7.2). Eventually, the molecules are internalized and degraded. Under physiological conditions, binding of a peptide is essential for the stability and transport of class I molecules. Heavy chains that do not get associated with β_2-m are not loaded with the peptide (ie, are empty), and are retained in the ER by these chaperones. Eventually, these incompletely assembled units are translocated to the cytosol and degraded by the proteasome.

7.2.3 Antigen Processing and Presentation

MHC class I molecules predominantly present peptides derived from proteins in the cytosol and endogenous biosynthetic pathways. Two distinct proteolytic processes are important in the generation of these peptides.

❑ **Proteasomal degradation.** The first step in antigen processing is the degradation of proteins by the 26S proteasome.
  - The proteasome is the main proteolytic system in the nucleus and cytosol of all eukaryotic cells. To ensure that the proteasome degrades the correct protein, it

[5] Except for tapasin, all other chaperones (calnexin, clareticulin, and BiP) involved in class I assembly are 'housekeeping proteins' that participate in the folding of a variety of multimeric proteins in the ER. The only known function of tapasin is in class I peptide loading. It is encoded by the MHC, and its expression is induced by IFNs.

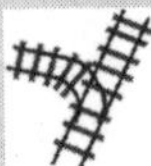

Cutting Across Class Lines: Cross-presentation

Naïve CD4[+] T cells have a limited circulation; they circulate between the lymph nodes, blood, and spleen. They rely on macrophages and DCs to capture pathogens or their products from the site of infection, transport them to the draining lymph node, and present them in the context of MHC class II molecules. Naïve CD4[+]T cells need to scan only the surfaces of DCs and macrophages in order to obtain a sampling of antigens in the body. The story is more complicated with naïve CD8[+] T cells. These cells recognize antigen loaded on MHC class I molecules. Since MHC class I molecules present endogenous antigens, only infected DCs or macrophages would be able to activate naïve CD8[+] T cells. A mechanism of presenting exogenous antigen by the MHC class I pathway is therefore needed to trigger CTL activation in the absence of APC infection. This is achieved by cross-presentation. Antigen processing of exogenous antigens in the MHC class I pathway is called cross-presentation; cross-priming is the priming of CTLs by exogenous antigens. Although both the DCs and macrophages are efficient scavengers, macrophages are poor at stimulating naïve T cells. DCs, on the other hand, are the most efficient APCs of the body and hence, a logical choice for cross-priming. Current experimental data are in agreement with this idea, and recent research suggests that different subsets of DCs are capable of cross-presentation under different conditions.

DCs have been shown to internalize apoptotic and necrotic cells and cross-present the antigens derived from such cells. Since apoptosis is a part of normal cell turnover, it is hypothesized that a tolerogenic response is initiated when macrophages or immature DCs internalize apoptotic cells and cross-present the antigen to naïve T cells. Conversely, if the immature DCs are exposed to inflammatory stimuli such as LPS, cytokines, dsRNA, or CpG DNA, peptides from the apoptosed cells will be loaded on MHC class I molecules because of cross-priming. The end result will be an immunogenic CTL response that causes the lysis of the cross-priming DCs. Cells undergoing necrotic cell death as a result of infection or trauma provide both the antigen and the stimulus necessary for immunogenic cross-priming. Cross-priming is thought to be especially important in immunity to viral infections that are localized to peripheral, non-lymphoid compartments (eg, human papilloma virus infection, in which the infection is confined to epithelial cells of the skin). Cross-priming may also be vital in generating immunity to viruses that infect professional APCs and inhibit or interfere with MHC class I antigen processing and presentation. Under these conditions, uninfected DCs can internalize infected DCs and induce immunity by priming naïve CD8[+] T cells via cross-presentation.

is 'tagged' by ubiquitination. In this process, multiple molecules of ubiquitin are covalently attached to the ε-amino group of lysine residues in the protein.

- It consists of two regulators (one 19S, and the other, 11S) that can attach like caps to a core 20S proteolytic unit (fig. 7.3). The polyubiquitin chain is recognized by the 19S subunit of the proteasome. The association of the 20S proteasome with two 19S regulators at either end yields the 26S proteasome involved in ATP-dependent degradation of ubiquitin-conjugated proteins. The core 20S structure is a barrel-shaped multi-catalytic complex. It is composed of two heptameric outer rings of structural α subunits and two heptameric inner rings of catalytic β subunits which together, form a hollow cylinder. The β subunits are encoded as inactive precursors which get activated by autocatalysis. The 20S proteasome is involved in the degradation of unfolded proteins and polypeptides and can function independently of or in association with regulatory subunits.

- IFN stimulation[6] leads to induction of the 11S regulator and three additional subunits of the proteasome. Two of these, LMP-2 (**Low M**olecular weight **Peptide-2**) and LMP-7, are encoded by the MHC genes whereas MECL-1 (**M**ultcatalytic **E**ndopeptidase **C**omplex **L**ike-**1**) is non-MHC encoded. These subunits seem to be important for the generation of MHC class I peptides. Together, they alter the catalytic activity of the proteasome to generate peptides having the basic or hydrophobic C– terminal residues required for efficient binding to class I molecules. LMP-2 and LMP-7 containing proteasomes are

---

[6] This is a good example of the links between innate and adaptive immunity. As a result of the innate immune response, cells at the site of viral invasion secrete IFNs (type I and type II); IFN stimulation leads to upregulation of MHC class I and/or MHC class II expression. Induction of the immunoproteasome further ensures that viral proteins are efficiently loaded on class I molecules and thus trigger an adaptive immune response.

labelled 'immunoproteasomes', since they generate a different spectrum of peptides than the constitutive proteasome.

- Majority of the peptides that result from proteasomal degradation are too short to be loaded onto class I molecules and are rapidly destroyed by endopeptidases and exopeptidases; the amino acids are recycled for protein synthesis.

❑ **Peptide trimming**. Oligopeptides generated by the proteasome are often longer than those required for loading onto class I molecules. Aminopeptidases in the cytosol or ER trim these oligopeptides to antigenic peptides of the length (8-10 amino acids long) needed to bind to MHC class I molecules with high affinity. Thus, the C– terminus of the antigenic peptide is determined by the proteasome, while the N– terminus is often the result of peptide trimming.

Peptides produced in the cytosol have to be translocated to the ER in order to enable their association with class I molecules. A heterodimer called TAP, consisting of two transporter proteins (TAP-1 and TAP-2), is involved in this translocation.

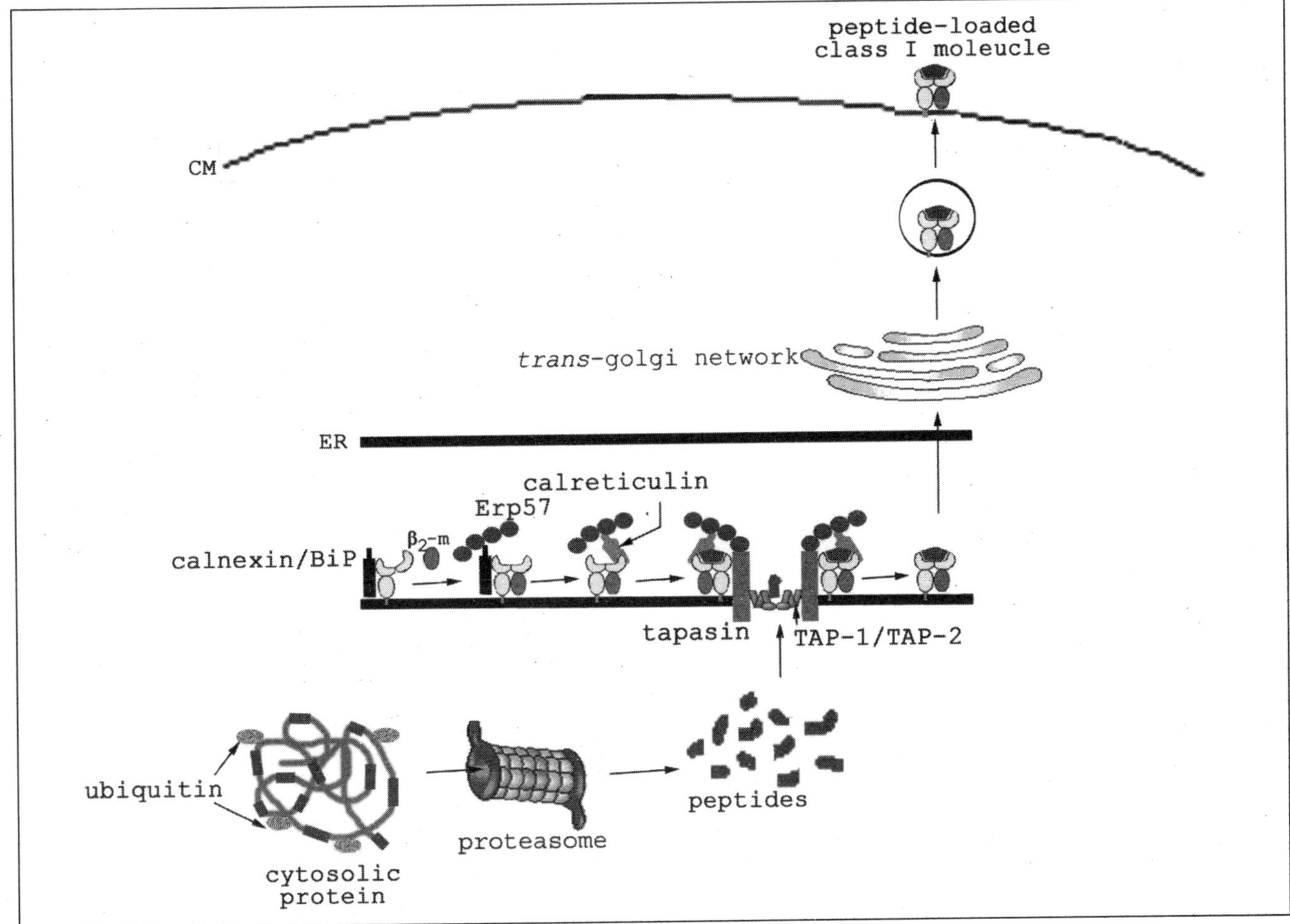

Figure 7.2 MHC class I molecules are synthesized and loaded with peptides in the ER. *A number of chaperones are involved in MHC class I synthesis. Calnexin or BiP associate with the newly synthesized α chain of the class I molecule. Another chaperone — Erp57 — also associates with this complex. The chaperones help in the folding of the α chain and also promote its association with β₂-m. The α:β₂-m heterodimer dissociates from calnexin and associates with calreticulin. Class I molecules present peptides derived from cytosolic proteins. In the cytosol, poly ubiquinated proteins are degraded by the proteasome to yield oligopeptides that may be further trimmed by cytosolic endopeptidases. The peptides are translocated across the ER membrane and into the ER lumen by the heterodimeric protein TAP (**Transporter associated with Antigen Processing**) consisting of two subunits — TAP-1 and TAP-2. TAP proteins are thought to form a pore into the ER membrane that allows peptide translocation. Another protein, tapasin, is involved in the translocation process. It is thought to stabilize the TAP complex and hold the class I molecule in its peptide-receptive conformation. Once loaded, class I molecules are transported across the trans-golgi network to the cell surface.*

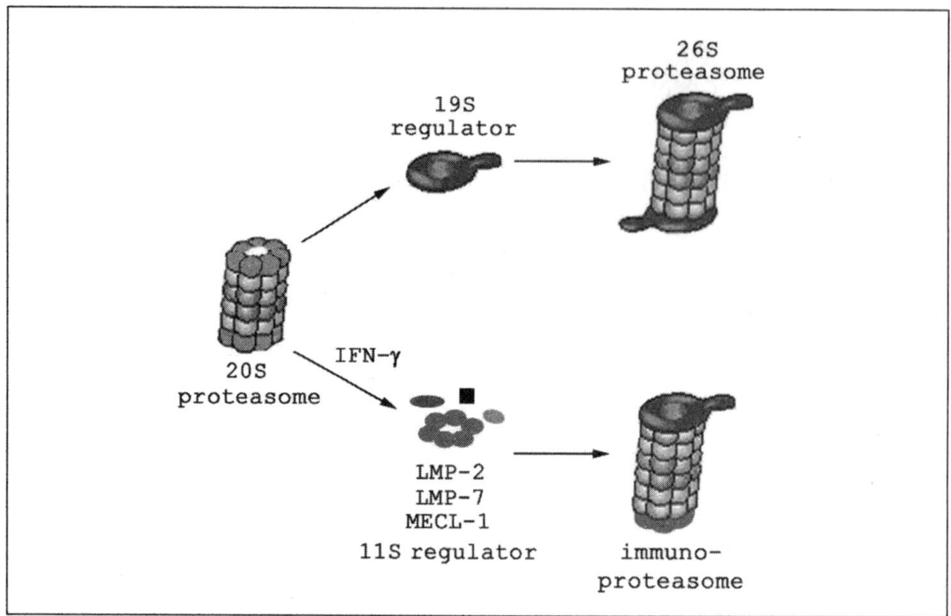

Figure 7.3 The majority of the peptides loaded on MHC class I molecules are generated by proteasomes. The proteasome is the main proteolytic system of eucaryotes and is responsible for the degradation of most of cytosolic and nuclear proteins. It consists of a barrel-shaped core 20S subunit of about 700 KD. This core subunit is composed of two heptameric outer rings of α subunits and two heptameric inner rings of β subunits, which together, form a hollow cylinder. Association of this core subunit with two 19S regulators at either end yields the 26S proteasome involved ATP-dependent protein degradation. The immune system has evolved mechanisms to modify this pathway to enhance the efficiency of peptide generation. IFN-γ produced by NK cells, T cells, macrophages, etc in response to infection, induces the formation of additional proteins that can associate with the proteasome. These include LMP-2 (Low Molecular weight Peptide-2), LMP-7, MECL-1 (Multcatalytic Endopeptidase Complex Like-1), and an 11S regulator. It is thought that the 20S subunit can associate with either the 11S regulator alone or simultaneously with one 11S and one 19S subunit. These novel forms of proteasomes are called immunoproteasomes. Incorporation of LMP-2, LMP-7, and MECL-1 in the immunoproteasome results in the formation of the kind of peptides suitable for MHC class I loading.

Genes encoding both TAP-1 and TAP-2 also lie within the MHC, near the genes encoding proteasome subunits. TAP is a member of the ATP-binding cassette family of transport proteins. The generated peptide is first bound to TAP and then translocated to the ER. Both TAP-1 and -2 co-operate in this translocation. They are thought to jointly form a pore in the ER membrane through which the peptide is translocated from the cytosol to the ER lumen. Peptides having a hydrophobic or basic C–terminus are preferentially translocated by TAP. Initial binding of the peptide is ATP-independent, but the pumping of peptides across the ER membrane is an ATP consuming process. Peptides that are not bound to class I molecules are exported from the ER to the cytosol by a translocon and eventually degraded by resident peptidases.

Since almost all proteins that are resident in the cytosol and ER are synthesized by the APC, MHC class I molecules display a 'sampling' of the genes expressed by that cell in peptide form to the immune system. In most cases, these peptides are derived from autologous proteins and ignored by the immune system because of self-tolerance. However, if the MHC class I:peptide complexes are recognized as foreign, the immune system is triggered, and this results in activated CTLs killing the offending cell. **MHC class I molecules are thus important in presenting intracellular parasite-derived or tumour-derived peptides.** Since many infected/ transformed cells are deficient in MHC class I expression, absence of MHC class I molecules results in NK cell-mediated lysis of these cells. This is because the engagement of inhibitory receptors on NK cell by certain peptide:MHC class I complexes on the target cell delivers a negative signal to the NK cell (section 2.2.2.2). Surface expression of class I molecules is thus needed to spare the cell from NK cell-mediated lysis. Through these checks and balances, the immune system maximizes the chances of eliminating potentially infected or transformed cells. MHC class I molecules are, in this respect, double-edged swords. On the one hand, recognition of a particular MHC:peptide complex by TcRs on activated CTLs results in the lysis of APCs bearing that MHC:peptide complex. A complete lack of class I molecules, on the other hand, makes the cell susceptible to NK cell-mediated lysis.

Recent experiments have established that some DCs are capable of MHC class I presentation of exogenous antigens. Called cross-presentation, this pathway of antigen presentation may play an important role in the initiation of CTL responses to a variety of pathogens and intracellular bacteria. Although the exact mechanism is unclear, three general pathways have been described.

❑ Direct translocation of pathogen-derived antigenic material in the cytosol of host APCs by the pathogen itself or by specialized mechanisms of transport allows processing of the protein by normal cytosolic machinery of the MHC class I pathway. This mode of gaining access to the cytosol is observed for certain viruses and bacteria like *Listeria monocytogenes*.

❑ Direct endosomal loading of preformed (recycling) MHC class I molecules with peptide determinants that are generated in the endosomal compartments is the second mode of cross-priming. Alternatively, the peptide antigen may be exocytosed (regurgitated) from the endosomal compartment onto the cell surface for association with preformed MHC class I molecules.

❑ Diversion of exogenous proteins from the endosomal compartments, or from extracellular fluid, into the cytosol for processing by the conventional MHC class I pathway.

MHC CLASS I MOLECULES

❑ Class I molecules are expressed on all nucleated cells of the body.

❑ They are transmembrane glycproteins consisting of an α chain that is non-covalently associated with one molecule of β_2-m.

- The α chain is anchored in the cell membrane by its COOH– terminus; the extracellular NH_2– terminus consists of three globular domains (α1, α2, α3).
- The peptide-binding groove is formed by the α1 and α2 domains and is closed at both ends.
- The terminal anchor residues of the peptide form multiple hydrogen bonds and salt bridges with amino acid residues in the two pockets located at the ends of the peptide-binding groove.
- The α3 domain associates with β_2-m and also has a site for CD8 binding.

❑ MHC class I molecules predominantly present peptides derived from endogenous antigens and are important in presenting parasite-derived or tumour-derived peptides.

- Under certain conditions, class I molecules can be loaded with peptides derived from exogenous antigens; the phenomenon is called cross-presentation.
- Both the carboxy- and amino- termini of the peptide are tightly fixed in the peptide-binding groove.
- Due to the closed peptide-binding groove, class I molecules bind only peptides 8–10 amino acids in length.
- The proteasome in the cytosol generates the peptides for loading.
- TAP, a heterodimer of two transporter proteins, translocates the peptides from the cytosol across the ER membrane and into the ER lumen.
- The peptide-loaded class I molecule is eventually transported to the cell surface.

7.3 MHC Class II Molecules

MHC class II molecules are vital to the functioning of the immune system. T$_H$ cells must recognize peptide:MHC class II complexes on APCs to initiate or co-operate in an immune response. MHC class II molecules have a limited tissue distribution, being essentially restricted to cells of the immune system. They are found on professional APCs (DCs, B cells, macrophages and related cells) as well as on thymic epithelial cells. The degree of expression varies not only amongst the cell types but also according to the maturational and activation status of the cell. Immature DCs do not express class II molecules on their cell surface, but mature DCs express these molecules at very high levels. Similarly, only mature B cells constitutively express MHC class II molecules. Human but not murine activated T cells also express MHC class II molecules. Expression of class II molecules is also upregulated in cells of the monocyte/macrophage lineage upon activation. IFN-γ can induce the expression of these molecules in many cell types that do not normally express them. Murine class II molecules are referred to as IA or IE, with the haplotype written as a superscript (Balb/c mice are IA^d read as IA of d). Human class II molecules are HLA-DR or DP or DQ, followed by a number that defines the haplotype.

7.3.1 Structure

The class II molecules are heterodimers composed of two glycosylated subunits, a 33–35 KD α chain, and a 25–29 KD β chain held together by non-covalent bonds. Both chains are anchored in the cytoplasm at the COOH– termini. They have a short cytoplasmic domain of 10–15 amino acids and an extracellular domain of 90–100 amino acids. The hydrophobic transmembrane region is about 30 amino acids in length. Both the α and β chains consist of two domains each (α1, α2 and β1, β2). The β2 domain contains the binding site for CD4. The membrane distal domains of both chains, ie, α1 and β1 domains, form the peptide-binding groove. The floor of this groove consists of β-pleated sheets, α-helical regions form the walls. The peptide-binding groove is open at both ends. An MHC class II ligand can therefore vary in length from 12–25 residues. **The peptide lies in an extended conformation along the class II peptide-binding groove. Both peptide ends hang out of the groove**; this is in contrast to the MHC class I molecule where peptide ends are deeply buried

---

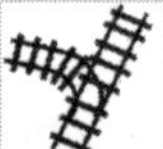

The Determinants of Survival: Immune Responsiveness and MHC

McDevitt and Chinitz were the first to observe that the capacity to respond to several antigens is controlled by a cluster of genes termed the **Immune response (Ir) genes**. Later, Ir genes were found to encode MHC class II molecules. All immune response genes, however, are not MHC-linked. MHC class II genes can control immunological responsiveness essentially through their effect on the functioning of T cells. The failure to respond to a particular antigen may be due to a number of reasons.

❑ **Failure of association.** An immune response is triggered when naïve T cells recognize a peptide in the context of MHC class II molecules. Failure of a particular MHC class II allotype to interact/associate with a given peptide will result in the failure to activate anti-peptide T cells and the individual will be termed a 'non-responder' for the antigen that gave rise to that peptide.

❑ **A hole in the T cell repertoire** is caused when T cells recognizing a particular peptide:MHC complex are either absent or unable to respond to it. Mechanisms that could lead to a hole in the T cell repertoire include:

- an absence of genes that code for a particular TcR or set of TcRs,
- deletion, anergization, or strict regulatory control of T cells reacting to a particular MHC:peptide configuration — autoreactive T cells are deleted or anergized during thymic selection; if association/interaction of a given epitope with MHC class II molecule results in a conformation similar to a self-antigen, T cells responding to such complexes will either be absent or unable to respond because of the action of T$_R$ cells, and
- failure to positively select particular T cell clones during thymic education which can result in unresponsiveness to certain antigens.

within the molecule (fig. 7.4). Similar to the class I molecule, the peptide-binding groove of the class II molecule also contains pockets to accommodate particular peptide side chains (anchor residues). The side chains of the amino acids in the centre of the group protrude out of the groove and make contact with TcR residues, whereas those of the remaining amino acids point into the groove and are accommodated in the pockets. The anchor residues determine the set of peptides that can be loaded onto the molecule. The highly polymorphic β1 domain is the major determinant of the binding specificity of different MHC class II haplotypes. Of the nine pockets identified, P1, P3, and P7 seem to be particularly important for binding. **The peptide is held in the groove by multiple hydrogen bonds formed between the backbone of the peptide and the amino acids lining the binding groove.** This is in contrast to class I molecules where the hydrogen bonds are clustered at terminal residues.

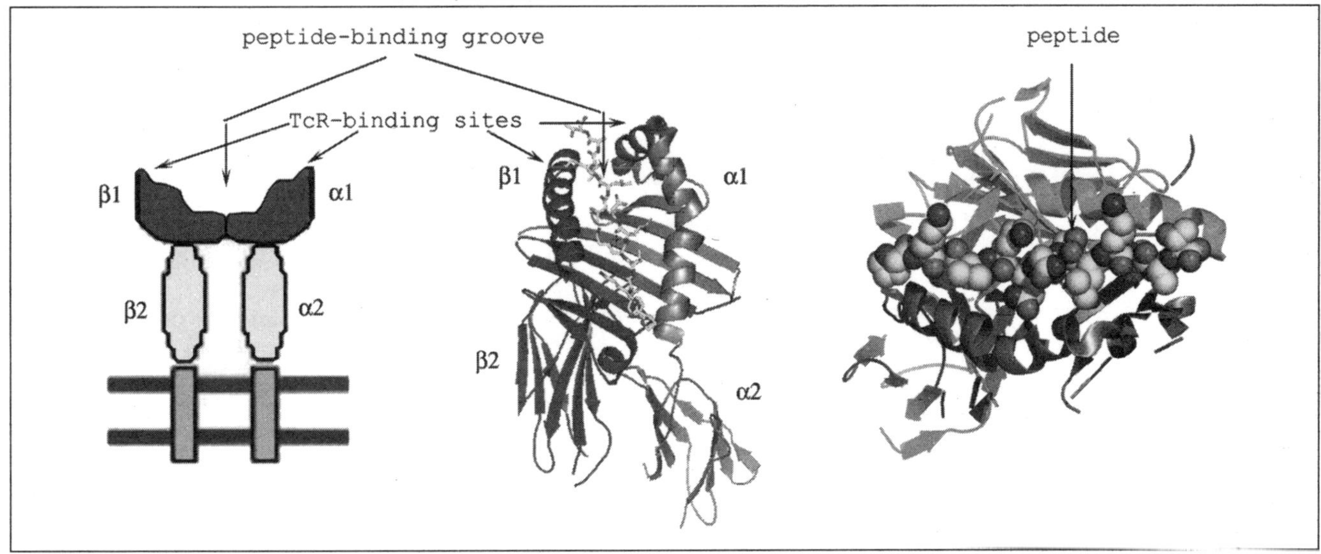

Figure 7.4 MHC class II molecules are heterodimeric proteins consisting of an α and a β chain held together by non-covalent interactions. They are anchored in the membrane by a small cytoplasmic region. Both chains contribute to the peptide-binding groove which lies at the membrane distal region. Each chain consists of two domains (α1, α2, β1, and β2). The β2 domain has the CD4 binding site. The left panel is a schematic depiction of the molecule, whereas the centre panel is a ribbon diagram of the molecule. The top view of the peptide-binding groove is depicted in the right panel. Both α1 and β1 domains contribute equally to the peptide-binding groove. It is essentially similar to the class I groove in that the floor of the groove is formed by β-pleated sheets and the walls are formed by α-helices. The peptide-binding groove is open at both ends and the peptide lies in an extended conformation along it with both the peptide ends hanging out of the groove. The peptide is held in the groove by multiple hydrogen bonds formed between the backbone of the peptide and the amino acids lining the binding groove (Courtesy of I. Strug, U. Mass. Med, Woecester MA).

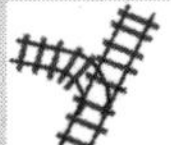

The Day After:
Fates of Interacting TcR and MHC Molecules

Receptor internalization is often accompanied by receptor-mediated ligand internalization. Upon physiological stimulation, receptors of the tyrosine kinase family, eg, BcRs, complement receptors, and FcRs are rapidly internalized. TcR also belongs to this family of receptors. It is rapidly down-modulated following stimulation by a variety of ligands (peptide:MHC complexes, superantigens, anti-TcR antibodies, etc). The internalized TcR is then degraded along with some of the molecules involved in signal transduction. In most cases, the ligands are soluble molecules that bind to their receptor with high affinity, and they are co-internalized along with the receptor. It is more difficult to establish the fates of membrane-bound ligands such as MHC:peptide complexes. Membrane-bound MHC:peptide complexes are now known to be extracted from APCs by T cells. In addition, other membrane-bound ligands such as costimulatory molecules (CD80/86) and adhesion molecules that take part in T cell-APC interaction are also acquired by T cells. The exact method of extraction and the fates of the acquired molecules remain to be determined.

The interactions of MHC class I and class II molecules with their peptides is governed by similar principles. The product of a particular allele of MHC class I or class II molecules is capable of binding any one of a large number (thousands) of peptides. These peptides differ in their sequences but share two or three amino acid residues (called motifs) that fit into anchoring pockets on MHC molecules. Thus, peptides binding to different alleles can be distinguished by their motifs. Figure 7.5 depicts the manner in which the TcR interacts with MHC: peptide complex.

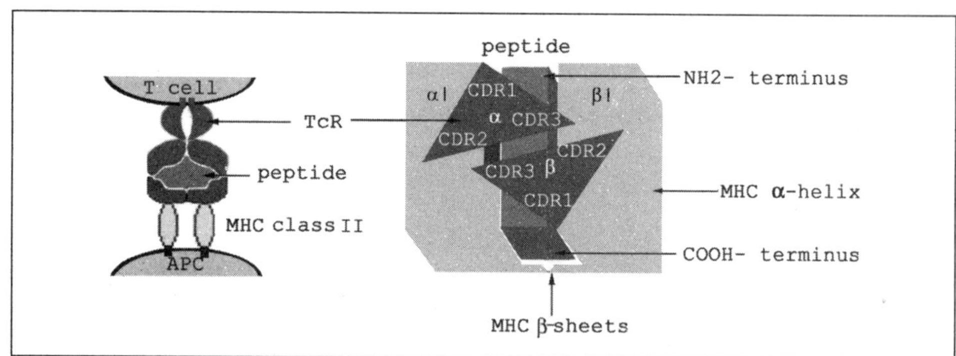

Figure 7.5 The antigen receptor of the T cell physically interacts with MHC:peptide complexes on the APC. *The left panel is a schematic side view of the trimolecular complex formed between the TcR, MHC class II molecules, and the peptide present in the peptide-binding groove. Viewed from the top, the β-sheets of the MHC class II molecules (right panel) form the floor of the peptide-binding groove. The peptide in the groove forms a rather flat surface in the middle and is bordered by the α-helices of the MHC molecule. The TcR sits diagonally across this surface with the CDR1 and CDR2 loops of the TcR α chain positioned above the Amino– terminus of the peptide, while the CDR1 and CDR2 loops of the β chain loom over the Carboxyl– terminus of the peptide. The less variable CDR1 and CDR2 loops of the TcR make contact with the relatively less variable α-helices of the MHC molecules, while the most variable CDR3 region of the TcR makes contact with the most variable parts of the peptide. TcR:MHC class I:peptide contact occurs on similar lines (Adapted from New England Journal of Medicine (2000) 343:702).*

7.3.2 Synthesis and Assembly

Like all proteins, MHC class II molecules are synthesized in the ER along with a chaperone molecule, called the **I**nvariant chain[7] or **Ii**. A trimer of Ii forms a scaffold on which newly synthesized αβ chains are added. Absence of Ii leads to misfolding and the aggregation of class II molecules. A nonamer, consisting of three subunits each of Ii, α, and β subunits, is formed at the end of this process. The insertion of the CLIP (**C**lass II-associated **I**nvariant chain **P**eptide) region of Ii into the peptide-binding groove of the class II molecule stabilizes Ii-class II interaction. CLIP protects the peptide-binding groove and prevents premature loading by peptides present in the ER.

The newly synthesized $(\alpha\beta Ii)_3$ nonamer is exported across the *trans*-golgi network to endosomal peptide loading compartments. Cytoplasmic motifs present in the tails of the Ii and β chain of class II molecules are thought to be responsible for this targeting of class II molecules to endosomal compartments. Once the nonamer reaches the endosomes, the Ii trimer scaffold is cleaved to yield three αβIi units. Ii then undergoes sequential proteolysis from the N- and C- terminus, leaving CLIP in the peptide-binding groove until it is displaced by the peptide ligand. Removal of CLIP and loading of the peptide onto the MHC class II molecule is facilitated by two other molecules — HLA-DM and HLA-DO (H2-M and H2-O in mice). The peptide loaded class II molecules are then exported to the cell surface (fig. 7.6). The cell surface peptide:class II complexes are fairly stable (average half-life of around 48 hours), allowing ample opportunity for a T cell encounter.

[7]Unlike MHC class II molecules, the sequence of amino acids in this chaperone does not vary in different haplotypes and is therefore termed 'invariant'. It is non-MHC protein encoded by genes on chromosome 5 in humans and 18 in mice. Originally thought to be involved only in MHC class II synthesis, the Ii is now known to have multiple functions, including roles in B cell maturation and chaperoning the protease Cathepsin L and the MHC-like CD1 molecule.

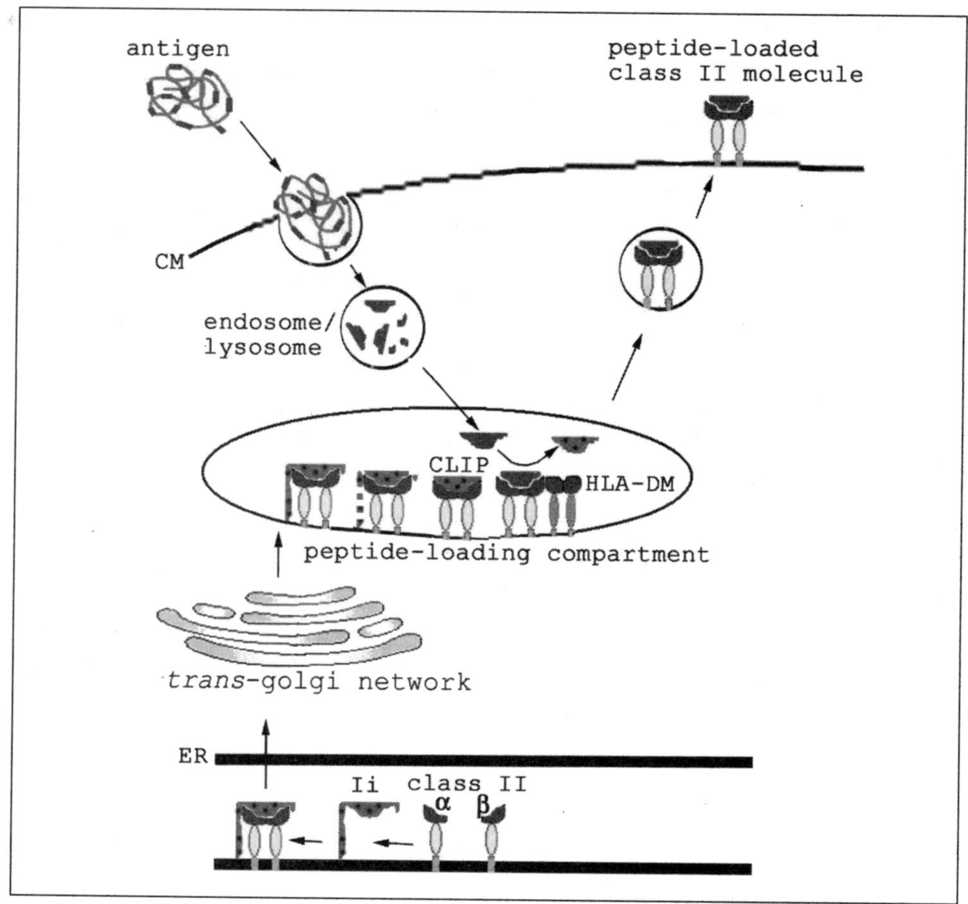

Figure 7.6 MHC class II molecules are synthesized in the ER and loaded with peptides in the lysosomal peptide-loading compartments. *The α and β chains of the molecule are synthesized with a chaperone molecule called invariant chain or Ii. A part of Ii is inserted in the peptide-binding groove of the αβ heterodimer. This interaction stabilizes the complex and prevents premature loading of class II molecules. Nonamers consisting of three molecules of α:β:Ii are formed in the ER and transported across the* trans-golgi network *to the peptide-loading compartments. Ii undergoes sequential proteolysis in these compartments. The class II-associated invariant chain peptide or CLIP remains in the groove until it is displaced by peptides generated in the endosomal/lysosomal compartments. This peptide-loading is facilitated by HLA-DM and -DO. Any proteins (whether self- or foreign) that are internalized by the cell enter the endosomal/lysosomal pathway. Due to the increasing proteolytic environment in these compartments, the proteins undergo degradation. Peptides of appropriate length and motifs are loaded on MHC class II molecules. The loaded MHC:peptide complexes are then exported to the cell surface. Recognition of these complexes by $CD4^+T$ cells results in the triggering of an immune response.*

7.3.3 Generation of the Peptide Ligand and its Loading

The peptides presented by MHC class II molecules are generated mostly by the degradation of proteins that access the endocytic pathway. Lysosomal proteases and other hydrolases process (via degradation) these proteins and generate peptides that can be loaded on MHC class II molecules. Thus, they present exogenous antigens that have been endocytosed by the APCs. Since endosomes/lysosomes are also sites of endogenous protein degradation, class II molecules also display a fair sampling of a cells' own proteins.

Exogenous antigens enter the endocytic pathway by a variety of mechanisms — pinocytosis (DCs), phagocytosis (macrophages, DCs), receptor-mediated endocytosis (B cells, DCs, and macrophages), etc. The importance of the different routes of

---

MHC CLASS II MOLECULES

❑ The class II molecules are expressed mainly by cells of the immune system.
❑ They are heterodimers of an α chain and a β chain held together by non-covalent bonds.
- Both chains consist of two domains each (α1, α2 and β1, β2), and are anchored in the cell membrane by their –COOH terminus.
- Binding site for CD4 lies in the β2 domain.
- The peptide binding groove is formed by the α1 and β1 domain.
- The binding groove is open at both ends; both ends of the peptide hang outside the groove.
- The peptide is held in the groove by multiple hydrogen bonds.

❑ MHC class II molecules are synthesized in the rough ER along with Ii.
- Ii promotes proper folding of the molecule.
- It protects the peptide-binding groove from premature loading.
- In the peptide-loading compartments of the endocytic pathway, Ii undergoes sequential proteolysis to leave behind CLIP.

❑ Class II molecules can be loaded by endogenous or exogenous peptides.
- Exogenous antigens are degraded in the endocytic lysosomal compartments.
- Peptides generated by these degradative processes are then loaded on the class II molecules.
- Peptide-loading occurs by displacement of CLIP.
- HLA-DM (H2-M) and HLA-DO (H2-O) facilitate the loading process and also influence the spectrum of loaded peptides.
- Peptide loaded class II molecules are then exported to the cell surface.

---

internalization differs in various APCs. As a result of this internalization, antigens are enclosed in endocytic vesicles and transported along the endosomal-lysosomal pathway. These vesicles have an increasingly acidic pH and are rich in proteases/hydrolases. Thus, antigens are exposed to increasingly denaturing and proteolytic conditions during transport and the antigen is reduced to peptides of varying lengths by the time it reaches the lysosomal peptide-loading compartments. **The formation of MHC class II:peptide complexes therefore occurs as a result of the intersection of two endocytic pathways — one transporting the exogenous antigen along the endocytic route and the other exporting class II molecules from the ER to the endocytic route.**

In the peptide-loading compartments, peptides encounter CLIP-loaded MHC class II molecules. Loading of the peptide on class II molecules entails exchange of CLIP for the peptide ligand. The MHC encoded, non-polymorphic HLA-DM facilitates the loading process. HLA-DM has a structure similar to MHC class II molecules (ie, it is a αβ heterodimer), but its peptide-binding groove is closed. HLA-DM is thought to facilitate peptide loading by physically associating with the MHC class II molecule and holding it in an 'open' conformation conducive to the dissociation of CLIP and subsequent re-association with the peptide ligand. HLA-DM is said to act like a peptide editor, since the spectrum of peptides presented by an APC is influenced by the presence or absence of HLA-DM. HLA-DO, another class II-like molecule, has been shown to modulate HLA-DM functioning.

7.4 Organization of MHC Genes

The MHC gene complex contains a large number of individual genes. Although the complex performs similar functions in different species, detailed arrangement of the genes differs amongst different species. Originally, different genetic loci of the MHC were identified by functional and serological analysis. The result has been a rather complicated mess as far as the names of the various genes and gene products is concerned (no, it was really not done to test your patience ☺). Identification by serology has also led to the gene products being referred to as *antigens*. Recent establishing of genetic maps of human and mouse MHC has helped in identifying the different genes that encode particular polypeptides. Only genes with known functions will be described here, using the simplest and most accepted nomenclature to minimize confusion (so we hope!). Many other genes with possible functions in

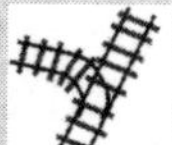

A Class Apart: MHC Class III Molecules

The MHC represents about 0.1% of the human genome and is traditionally divided into class I, II, and III regions. It is one of the most gene-dense regions of the genome. MHC class I and II regions encode proteins involved in antigen presentation. Although the entire class III region has now been sequenced, the functions of all the proteins encoded by this region are far from understood. Products of the MHC class III region are not involved in antigen presentation. Some proteins encoded by the telomeric end of the class III region appear to be involved in inflammatory responses and are often dubbed MHC class IV molecules. These include members of the TNF family and HSP70 (**H**eat **S**hock **P**rotein 70). Complement components and other molecules involved in growth and differentiation remain in class III. Products of class III and IV genes seem to be associated with a number of immune and non-immune diseases. The more important proteins with known functions include:

❑ Components of the complement cascade — C2, C4a, and C4b of the classical pathway and Factor B of the alternative pathway are encoded by the MHC class III region.

❑ Several products critical to growth, development, and differentiation:
- NOTCH4, a transmembrane receptor that determines cell fate and differentiation through cell-to-cell interaction, is encoded by this region. Murine NOTCH4 is a proto-oncogene. There is some evidence to suggest that this molecule may regulate morphogenesis of epithelial cells during development of the mammary gland.
- TNXB (**Ten**ascin-**XB**), an extracellular matrix protein involved in connective tissue cell migration and muscle morphogenesis during embryonic development, is clustered close to the NOTCH4 gene.
- PBX2, a transcription factor probably involved in regulating expansion of haematopoietic precursors, is also encoded by the class III region.

❑ Enzymes related to metabolism of lipids or steroids:
- LPAAT-α (**Lipo**phosphatidic **a**cyl **t**ransferase-α) is required for the acylation of glycerols for lipid biosynthesis.
- PPT2 is a **p**almitoyl **p**rotein **t**hioesterase required for the hydrolysis of lipid thioester from lipoproteins.
- CYP21B (21-hydroxylase) is an enzyme required for the hydroxylation of steroids important in the biosynthesis of glucocorticoids and mineral-corticoids.

❑ The **R**eceptor for **A**dvanced **G**lycation **E**nd-products (RAGE), a member of the Ig superfamily, binds AGE (**A**dvanced **G**lycation **E**nd-products) that accumulate with aging and is thought to play an important role in the chronic inflammation that contributes to complications in diabetes, inflammatory bowel disease, Alzheimer's disease, etc.

❑ Two proteins distantly related to class I molecules — MIC-A and MIC-B. They seem to activate NK cells, $\gamma\delta$ T cells, and CD8$^+$ T cells which carry the NKG2D receptor.

❑ Three related cytokines, TNF-α, lymphotoxin-α (also called TNF-β), and LT-β (TNF-χ) (encoded by the so-called class IV region).
- TNF-α is a pro-inflammatory cytokine important in innate immune responses. Lack of TNF-α leads to an absence of splenic primary B cell follicles.
- TNF-β has a similar mode of action as TNF-α but with a limited tissue distribution. Deletion of the TNF-β gene leads to a specific absence of lymph nodes, Peyer's patches, and splenic germinal centres in mice, leading to the suggestion that TNF-α and -β are involved in the development of secondary lymphoid organs.
- LT-β is a membrane bound protein that forms a heterodimer with TNF-β and can induce activation of the transcription factor NFκB.

❑ HSP70, a member of the heat shock protein family is also placed in MHC class IV under the alternative scheme. HSPs are a family of chaperone molecules induced by environmental stress such as oxidative injury. HSP70 is thought to be involved in the processing and presentation of bacterial and tumour antigens.

immunity also map to this DNA region but will not be discussed. This is because with some genes, the proteins they code have been identified, but the exact functions of these proteins are not known; in the case of others, the proteins encoded have not been fully characterized.

Figure 7.7 shows the genetic organization of the human and mouse MHC. The entire complex extends over 4×10^6 base pairs. The organization of murine and human MHC is essentially similar. Separate regions of the complex code for MHC class I and class II molecules; several genes within these regions encode each chain.

❑ **In humans, the MHC class I region is located on the same stretch of the chromosome. Three genes — *HLA-A, -B, -C* — are found to encode MHC class I heavy chains;** the HLA class I loci are highly polymorphic and more than 80 alleles for HLA-A, 180 for HLA-B, and 40 for HLA-C have been identified so far. Both alleles of each locus are expressed, so an individual can express up to six different MHC class I molecules. **Murine MHC class I genes are called *H2-K, -D*.** The murine class I region seems to be translocated compared to human

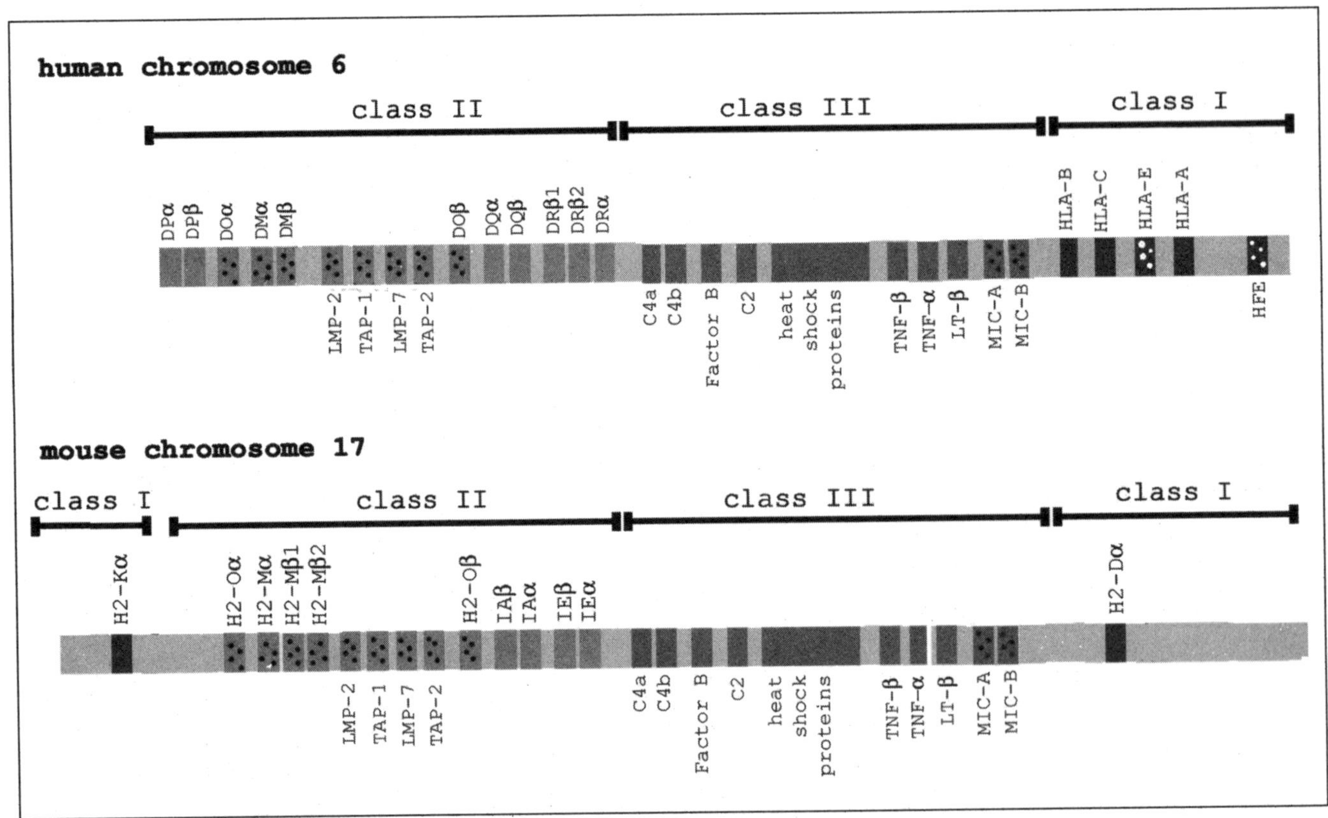

Figure 7.7 The genes encoding MHC molecules are located on chromosome 6 in humans and chromosome 17 in mice. *Conventionally, the complex is divided into class I, II, and III regions. A schematic representation of the organization of human (top panel) and mice (bottom panel) MHC genome is depicted here and does not reflect the actual distances between the genes. In humans, the class II region codes for the α and β chains of MHC class II molecules. This region also codes for molecules involved in loading of class II molecules (HLA-DM and HLA-DO) as well as molecules involved in the processing and loading of class I molecules (LMP-2, LMP-7, TAP-1, and TAP-2). Adjacent to this region is the region encoding MHC class III molecules. These molecules are not involved in antigen processing and presentation and include components of the complement pathway (C4a, C4b, Factor B, and C2), a number of heat shock proteins (here depicted by a single large box), cytokines (TNF-α, -β, LT-β), and the MHC-like molecules MIC-A and MIC-B. The α chain of the MHC class I molecules is encoded by the class I region. It also encodes for hematochromasis protein (HFE) involved in iron metabolism. The organization of the mouse MHC genome is essentially similar to the human genome with the class II region encoding for α and β chains of murine class II molecules (IA and IE) and molecules involved in loading of class I and class II molecules. The murine class I region, unlike its human counterpart, is split into two coding for H2-K and H2-D. In some haplotypes, a third MHC class I molecule (H2-L; not shown here) is encoded by genes lying adjacent to H2-D.*

MHC class I; it is split in two in the mouse, with the class II and class III regions located in between the two class I regions.

❑ **Three pairs of MHC class II α and β chains are found in humans — HLA-DR, -DP, and -DQ.** Some individuals contain upto three β chain genes in their HLA-DR cluster (represented by a single β gene in the figure). These DRβ gene products can also associate with the DRα chain, yielding four sets of DR molecules. **Two sets of genes encode murine class II molecules — H2-A (also called IA) and H2-E (also called IE).**

❑ HLA-DM and -DO (and their murine equivalents H2-M and H2-O), involved in peptide loading onto MHC class II molecules, are also located in the class II region.

❑ LMP genes in the MHC class II region code for two subunits of proteasome involved in the cytosolic breakdown of proteins. Genes encoding TAP molecules involved in class I loading also lie in this region, in close association with the LMP genes.

❑ MHC class III region encodes a variety of proteins (see sidetrack 'Conforming Non-confirmists').

7.5 Polygenism and Polymorphism in MHC Molecules

The ability of the immune system to respond to a multitude of foreign immunogens can be attributed to the ability of MHC molecules to bind a vast range of peptides. This ability is the result of two characteristics of the MHC: polygenism and polymorphism. MHC genes are polygenic, ie, several sets of MHC class I and class II genes encoding proteins with different ranges of peptide binding specificities are found in the same individual. An individual inherits one set of genes from each parent; hence, one set of MHC haplotype will be inherited from both the parents by the offspring. Since the genes are polymorphic (see below), most individuals are likely to be heterozygous at these loci. MHC alleles are codominant, ie, products of both alleles are expressed, and both function in presenting antigens to T cells. This means that the potential number of distinct MHC molecules expressed by each cell of an individual is doubled. With three sets of MHC class I genes and three sets of class II genes on each allele, an individual human can typically express six class I and class II molecules each on his or her cells. Since MHC class II molecules consist of two chains (α and β), and since α and β chains from different chromosomes may combine to give functional molecules — two α and two β chains giving rise to four different products — the number of class II molecules expressed by an individual may be even greater.

MHC genes are the most polymorphic genes known. Human MHC genes are highly polymorphic at each locus, ie, there is a great variation in individual genes and their products within a single species. Maximal polymorphism is observed for residues that line the peptide-binding groove of the molecules, and thus, the binding specificity. **MHC polymorphism directly affects antigen recognition by T cells.** Generally speaking, T cells can only be activated by APCs that have the same MHC allele. If APCs of one mouse haplotype (say H2-K^b) infected with a particular virus are mixed with CTLs of another strain (H2-K^k) induced by the same virus, the H2-K^b APCs will not be killed. This is because CTLs of H2-K^k haplotype will not recognize peptide:MHC complexes presented by APCs of H2-K^b haplotype. This is called the histocompatibility (or MHC) restriction of cellular interaction. The restriction implies that T cells are programmed (or restricted) to respond to cells bearing only a particular histotope[8] (MHC molecule). Histocompatibility restriction along with antigen-specificity develops during the thymic maturation of T cells (chapter 8). Thus, **TcR specificity is defined both by the peptide and the MHC molecule on which the peptide is loaded.** Direct contact of TcR with polymorphic

[8] Although it is well established that T cells are MHC restricted, between 1–7% T cells can recognize particular non-self MHC (allogeneic) molecules, ie, between 1–7% T cells are alloreactive. The exact mechanism of this alloreactivity is not clear. TcRs recognize peptides loaded on self-MHC molecules. However, if the configuration of a peptide:non-self MHC complex is similar to that recognized by the TcR, alloreactivity is the result. Some TcRs also respond to distinctive features of the non-self MHC, independent of the peptide bound by it. Alloreactivity is of special significance in transplantations and graft rejections.

residues on the MHC molecule has been shown to affect antigen recognition. MHC restriction in antigen recognition reflects the combined effect of differences in peptide binding and of direct contact between the MHC molecule and TcR.

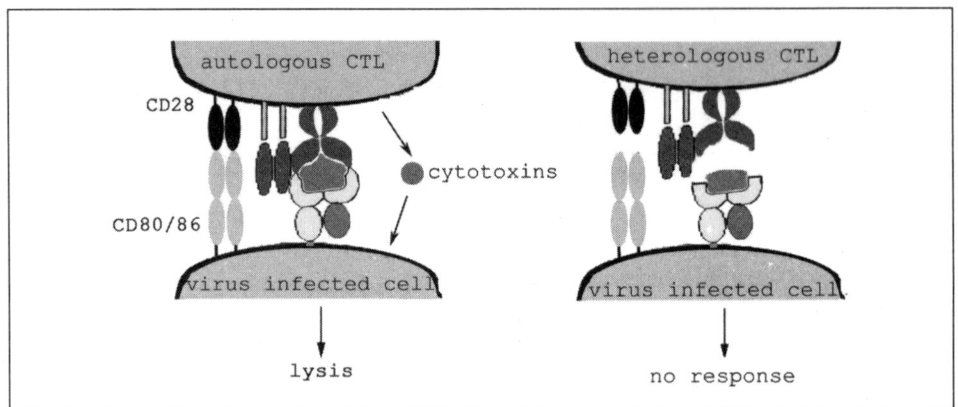

Figure 7.8 T cells are self-MHC restricted. *In the thymus, T cells get programmed to recognize and respond to self-MHC molecules. Only T cells expressing TcRs recognizing self-MHC molecules are allowed to survive so that the TcR specificity is defined both by the peptide and the MHC molecule on which the peptide is loaded. Due to this MHC restriction, CTLs induced by a virus will kill only autologous APCs (ie, derived from the same host) infected with that virus (left panel). They will fail to recognize and kill heterologous APCs (ie, derived from a genetically non-identical host) infected with the same virus.*

It is important to understand the need for MHC diversity and the advantages that this diversity bestows on the species. Although MHC genes do not directly encode TcR, by virtue of their association with the antigens, they are part of the T cell antigen recognition process. Polygenism and polymorphism in MHC proteins extend the range of antigens to which the immune system can respond. Polymorphism along with codominance doubles the number of different MHC molecules expressed by an individual. It increases diversity in MHC molecules, and consequently, the peptides presented to the T cell. The population as a whole will benefit from such diversity, since a pathogen that may be able to evade the immune system of one individual will not be able to evade that of another. In the large evolutionary scheme of things, individuals are expendable but the species must survive[9]. The discovery of superantigens and the emergence of the AIDS pandemic help us appreciate the dynamic nature of the host-parasite relationship. Whenever man comes up with a better mouse trap, nature corresponds with a better mouse — every strategic evolutionary change in the host results in a corresponding, survival-bestowing mutation in the parasite.

If indeed MHC diversity bestows an evolutionary advantage, the question, 'why limit the MHC loci?', also needs to be considered. Each addition of a distinct MHC molecule to the MHC repertoire would increase the number of peptide:MHC conformations that would be recognized as self, and this in turn would necessitate the silencing of a greater number of T cell clones in order to maintain self-tolerance. Already, less than 5% lymphocytes entering the thymus survive the selection process. If the number of MHC loci were increased, even less T cell clones would be selected. Since between 100–200 identical MHC:peptide complexes (representing about 1% of a particular MHC haplotype) are required to activate a T cell, an increase in MHC molecules will mean an effective decrease in the concentration of a single type of MHC molecule expressed on a cell surface (provided the total number of MHC molecules expressed by the cell remains constant). Given that only a portion of the MHC molecules are loaded with peptides, this would mean that the number of particular peptide:MHC complexes on the APCs would be insufficient to activate

[9] Communism, anyone?

T cells. By having multiple MHC loci but limiting their numbers, the system achieves a balance between the advantages of diversity and the disadvantage of an increased presentation of self-peptides.

7.6   CD1

Until recently, T cells were thought to recognize exclusively protein-derived antigens that were presented in the context of MHC class I and class II molecules. In the last few years, a growing body of research has established that antigen presentation is not restricted to proteins and that the immune system has evolved the capability of presenting lipid antigens to T cells. CD1 molecules are involved in this presentation.

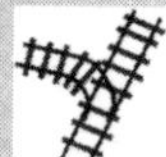

Conforming Non-conformists: Non-classical MHC Molecules

The MHC superfamily consists of class I and class II molecules that are highly polymorphic and are called the classical MHC molecules. In contrast, non-classical MHC molecules show little polymorphic variation, and only some are capable of binding peptides or peptide surrogates (eg, lipids) for presentation to T cells. Figure 7.S1 is a schematic representation of some non-classical human MHC molecules. Numerous such molecules are now under investigation.

❑ HLA-DM and HLA-DO, similar in structure to MHC class II molecules, are incapable of peptide-binding but influence peptide loading on classical class II molecules.

❑ HLA-E, also called a non-classical (or MHC class Ib) molecule, is a cognate receptor for members of the CD94/NKG2 family of NK receptors. It presents TAP-derived peptides from the signal sequences of other HLA-molecules in the cell and is a readout of cellular MHC class I synthesis. Incorrect processing of class I alleles within a cell suppresses the display of HLA-E-peptide complexes at the cell surface, thus reporting to NK cells the impairment of intracellular processing essential for antigen presentation and making the cell susceptible to NK cell-mediated lysis.

❑ HFE protein is called the haemochromatosis protein, since mutations in this protein cause the hereditary iron-overload disease, haemochromatosis. It has a class-I like structure ($\alpha\beta_2$-m), but the peptide-binding groove is very narrow because of the altered positioning of the $\alpha 1$ helix. It cannot bind peptides, but the molecule plays a major role in iron metabolism.

❑ ZAG (**Z**n-α2 **G**lycoprotein) has an MHC class I-like α chain but does not associate with β_2-m. It is thought to be involved in lipid metabolism.

❑ CD1, the first human differentiation antigen to be identified by monoclonal antibodies, is important in antigen presentation to T cells (section 7.6). It is not encoded by the MHC genes.

❑ MIC-A and MIC-B are MHC encoded proteins (MHC Class IV). They do not associate with β_2-m. MIC-A is a ligand for NKG2D.

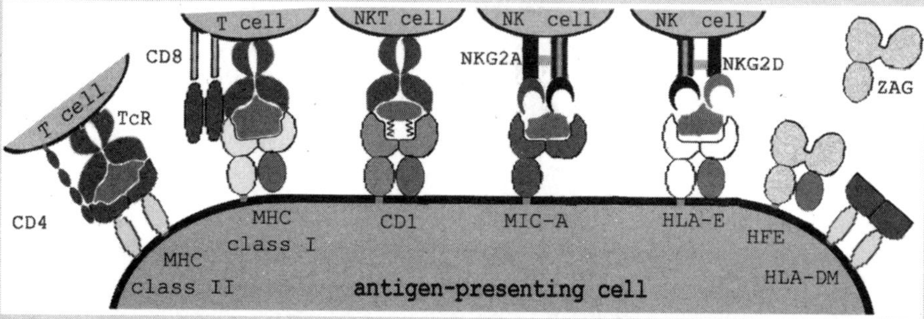

Figure 7.S1   A number of molecules expressed by APCs belong to the MHC superfamily. *These include the antigen-presenting molecules (MHC class I, II, and CD1), HLA-DM and HLA-DO (not shown here) that facilitate class II loading, non-classical MHC molecules such as MIC-A and HLA-E involved in NK cell activation, HFE involved in iron metabolism, and ZAG involved in lipid metabolism.*

CD1 MOLECULES

- ❑ CD1 molecules are expressed by thymocytes and professional APCs such as monocytes, DCs, and B cells.
- ❑ They are similar to MHC class I molecules in structure; they consist of an α chain non-covalently associated with one molecule of β_2-m.
- ❑ CD1 synthesis seems to follow the general pathway of MHC class II molecules.
- ❑ Five isoforms of the molecule are identified in humans; only one is found in mice.
- ❑ CD1 molecules present lipid antigens to NKT cells.
  - The CD1antigen-binding groove contains two large, deep pockets.
  - The inner surface of the groove is lined almost exclusively with non-polar amino acids.
  - Lipids such as diacylglycerols, sphingolipids, polyisoprenoids, and mycolates can be loaded in this hydrophobic groove.

CD1 molecules are β_2-m associated glycoproteins that are structurally related to MHC class I molecules (fig. 7.9). **Their primary function is the presentation of lipid antigens.** The CD1 groove contains two large, deep pockets, and the inner surface of the groove is lined almost exclusively with non-polar amino acids. This lining provides a hydrophobic surface for interaction with the aliphatic hydrocarbon chains of the amphipathic glycolipids presented. The insertion of aliphatic hydrocarbon chains of antigen into the hydrophobic CD1 groove is postulated to position the rigid and hydrophilic elements of the antigen on the α-helical surface of the groove, so they are available to interact with TcR. This implies that the hydrophilic cap of the antigen, including the carbohydrate, phosphate, or polar substituted groups of the lipid, is likely to determine the specificity of the interactions of the antigen with TcR. Supporting this model is the fact that CD1-restricted T cells have been found to be highly discriminating. They can distinguish between monosaccharides that differ in the orientation of even a single hydroxyl group on the lipids. Most lipids presented by CD1 such as diacylglycerols, sphingolipids, polyisoprenoids, or mycolates have two hydrophobic tails and a relatively small, polar head group (fig. 7.10).

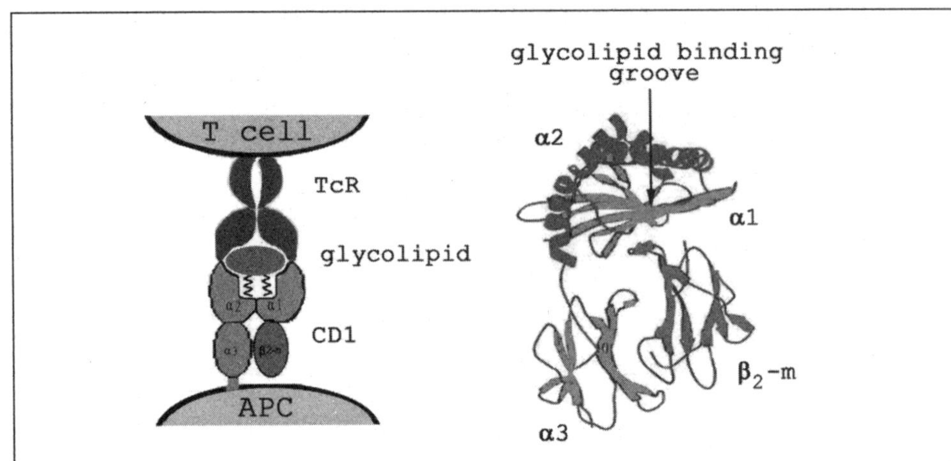

Figure 7.9 CD1 molecules are structurally similar to MHC class I molecules and present lipid antigens to NKT cells. CD1 molecules consist of an α chain that is non-covalently associated with β_2-m. The left panel is a schematic depiction of the molecule, while the right panel is a ribbon diagram of the molecule. The $\alpha1$ and $\alpha2$ domains form the antigen-binding groove, and the $\alpha3$ region anchors the molecule in the cell membrane. The antigen-binding groove is lined with non-polar amino acids allowing interaction with the aliphatic chains of the antigen. This allows the polar region of the molecule to make contact with TcR residues (Adapted from Immunology (2001) 104:243).

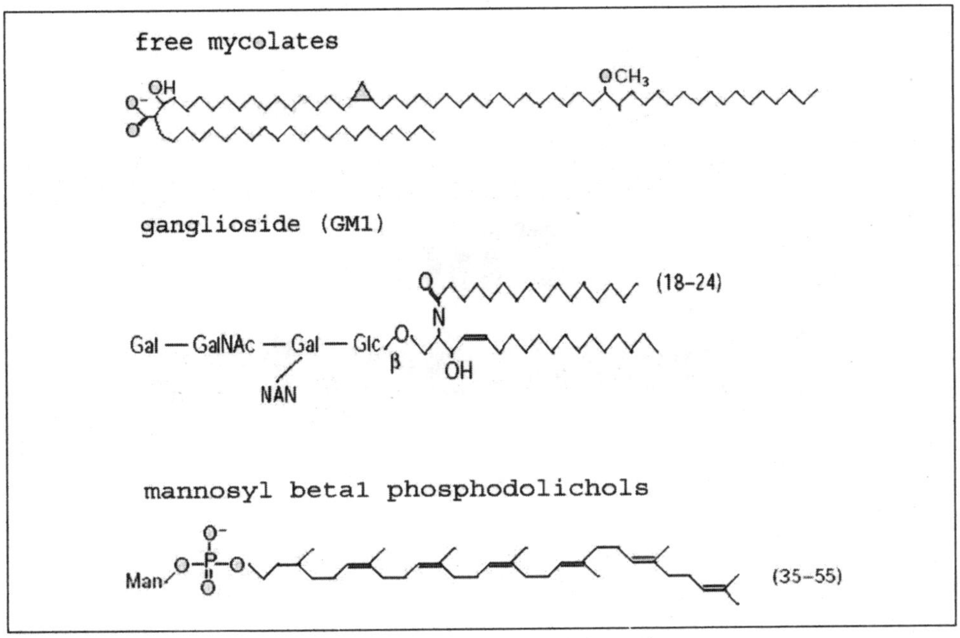

Figure 7.10   A variety of lipids, phospholipids and glycolipids can be loaded on CD1 molecules. *The antigens presented include those derived from microbial origins as well as self-molecules (Adapted from Immunology (2001) 104:243).*

CD1 molecules are mostly expressed by thymocytes and APCs such as monocytes, DCs, and B cells. Being non-polymorphic, these proteins are called non-classical MHC molecules. Five CD1 isoforms (CD1a to CD1e) encoded by genes located on chromosome 1 have been identified in humans; only one isoform (CD1d) is found in mice. These isoforms have been placed in different homology groups — CD1a, 1b, and 1c are called group 1 isoforms, CD1d belongs to group 2. The elusive CD1e isoform was recently isolated and seems to be sufficiently different to justify a third group. Only the first three isoforms are known to function in T cell responses to naturally occurring self- and foreign antigens. Group 1 CD1 proteins have been shown to mediate T cell recognition of glycolipid components from the mycobacterial cell wall. CD1d presents antigen to NKT cells, and recent evidence suggests that these molecules may be involved in immunity to intracellular parasites such as *Leishmania* spp. and *Plasmodium* spp. as well as autoimmune diseases. Thus, CD1 proteins, like classical MHC molecules, are thought to have a dual role in immune responses.

- ❑ **They present exogenous antigens to T cells** to activate host defence against infections; such presentation may be especially important for immune responses to pathogens like mycobacteria that have glycolipid-rich cell walls. *M. tuberculosis* downregulates CD1 expression as part of its immune evasion strategy.
- ❑ **CD1 molecules present self-sphingolipids**, such as gangliosides and ceramides, and have a role in tumour surveillance, autoimmunity, and immunoregulatory interactions with other cells.

The exact mechanism of synthesis and assembly of these molecules is still being elucidated, but it seems to follow the general pattern of MHC class II molecules. Ii has been shown to act as a molecular chaperone for at least the CD1d molecules during its synthesis in the ER. Cellular lipids may be loaded on CD1 molecules in the ER or lysosomes, and these could be exchanged for exogenous lipids at the cell surface. Lipid antigens are likely to be processed for presentation, analogous to proteinic antigens presented by MHC class I and class II molecules. The exact mechanisms involved in antigen processing are yet to be established.

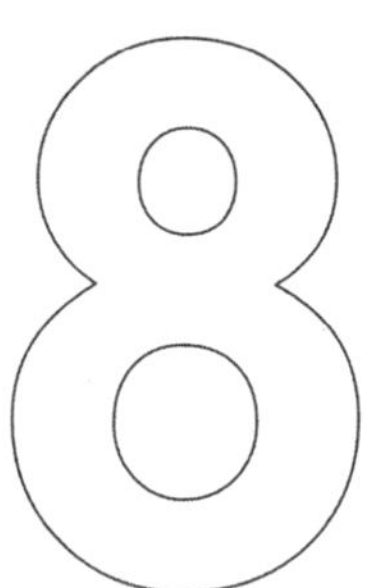
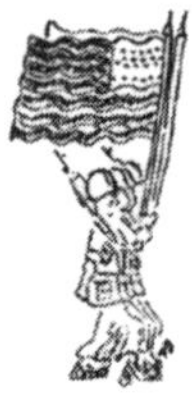

8

The Lymphocytes

In valley green, on towering crag,
Our fathers fought before us,
And conquered 'neath the same old flag
That's proudly floating o'er us.
We're children of a fighting race,
That never yet has known disgrace,
And as we march, the foe to face,
We'll chant a soldier's song

— Irish National Anthem

8.1 Introduction

Lymphocytes develop from self-renewing pleuripotential haematopoietic stem cells that can give rise to multiple cell lineages. Some progenitors give rise to erythroid cells that eventually differentiate into erythrocytes. Others give rise to myeloid lineages from which the phagocytes and the granulocytes develop. Yet others develop into lymphocytes in the specialized environment of the primary lymphoid organs (fig. 5.3). Different markers expressed on their cell surfaces help distinguish the different lineages. Lymphocytes have a central characteristic differentiating them from other cell types — they are committed to react to a group of structurally related chemical entities. This intrinsic reactivity is due to specific receptors that enable them to recognize and bind antigens. The commitment is predetermined, ie, it exists in the lymphocytes even before contact with the antigen, and it develops in the primary lymphoid organs. Once committed, the lymphocytes retain this commitment for the rest of their lives. Their progeny also have the same antigenic specificity, ie, they possess a population of receptors having identical combining sites. A given clone or set of lymphocytes, therefore, differs from every other clone or set of lymphocytes in

❑ The structure of its antigen receptor's combining site, and
❑ The range of antigenic substances that can stimulate the lymphocyte and, therefore, the range of antigenic substances to which it can respond. This response can be varied, ranging from activation and proliferation, to production of effector molecules (antibodies, cytotoxins, cytokines, or other soluble factors), to anergy.

Lymphoid stem cells give rise to lymphocytes in the microenvironment of the primary lymphoid organs (chapter 5). The newly formed lymphocytes undergo maturation in these organs to give rise to lymphocytes that differ in their functional properties. B lymphocytes mature in the bone marrow (in mammals) or Bursa of Fabricus (in birds) and are responsible for humoral immunity. Lymphocytes that mature in the thymus are called T lymphocytes. These are multifunctional cells involved in multiple aspects of adaptive immunity. Lymphocytes produced in the primary lymphoid organs are called naïve (or virgin) cells, because they have not yet encountered the molecules recognized by their antigen receptors. These naïve lymphocytes are exported to the periphery and localize preferentially in organized secondary lymphoid organs. Following antigenic stimulation, mature lymphocytes complete their differentiation to effector cells in the secondary lymphoid organs. B cells give rise to antibody-secreting plasma cells and T lymphocytes give rise to T$_H$ cells, CTLs, or T$_R$ cells. A subset of T lymphocytes expressing markers for both NK cells and T cells has been recently identified and is called the NKT cells. The maturation and differentiation of NKT cells is still under investigation.

The immune system is capable of reacting to a virtually limitless number of antigens. This ability to react to a variety of antigens is due to the existence of a very large number of sets (or clones) of lymphocytes, each bearing receptors specific to a particular antigen. In this sense, lymphocytes may be thought of as a heterogeneous collection of cells differing from each other in their ability to combine with and respond to different antigens. Analyses of genetic and molecular factors leading to antigen receptor diversity have led researchers to believe that the human genome has the potential to encode for about 10^{18} different antigen receptors. This implies that our body has the potential to produce at least 10^{18} differing clones of lymphocytes, each capable of reacting to a different antigen. How these diverse clones arise from the lymphoid stem cells is dealt with in chapter 10.

As discussed in chapter 6, T and B lymphocytes differ in the natures of their antigen receptors. The Ig molecule itself behaves as the antigen receptor of a B cell, but for T cells the antigen receptor is a non-Ig glycoprotein belonging to the Ig superfamily. Different lymphocytes subsets can be distinguished by the presence of

AICD:	Activation-induced cell death
AIRE:	Autoimmune regulator
ANAE:	α-naphthyl acid esterase
BAFF:	B cell activating factor of the TNF family
BCA-1:	B cell attracting chemokine-1
BLC:	B lymphocyte chemoattractant
Blimp-1:	B lymphocyte induced maturation protein-1
BLS:	Bare lymphocyte syndrome
CAMs:	Cell adhesion molecules
CD:	Cluster of differentiation
CTLA-4:	Cytotoxic T lymphocyte antigen-4
CVID:	Common variable immunodeficiency
DD:	Death domain
DISC:	Death-inducing signalling complex
DN:	Double negative T cells
DP:	Double positive T cells
DTH:	Delayed-type of hypersensitivity
ELC:	Epstein-Barr virus induced molecule 1-ligand chemokine
FADD:	Fas-associated death domain
gld:	Generalized lymphadenopathy
HSA:	Heat-stable antigen
IAPs:	Inhibitors of apoptosis proteins
ICOS:	Inducible T cell costimulator
IL-1Ra:	IL-1 receptor antagonist
lpr:	Lymphoproliferation generalized lymphadenopathy
MCF:	Macrophage chemotactic factor
MCP-1:	Monocyte chemoattractant protein-1
MIF:	Macrophage inhibitory factor
MIP:	Macrophage inflammatory protein
MZ:	marginal zone of the spleen
PD-1:	Programmed death gene-1
RAG:	Recombination activating genes
RANK:	Receptor activator of NFκB
RANK-L:	Receptor activator of NFκB ligand
RIP:	Receptor interacting proteins
SCF:	Stem cell factor
SCID:	Severe combined immunodeficieny
SDF-1:	Stromal cell derived factor-1
SLC:	Secondary lymphoid tissue chemokine
SP:	Single positive T cells
STAT:	Signal transducer of activation and transcription
TdT:	Terminal deoxynucleotidyl transferase
TECK:	Thymus expressed chemokine
TIM:	T cell immunoglobulin- and mucin-domain-containing molecule
TNFR:	TNF receptor

TRADD:	TNFR-1-associated death domain
TRAF:	TNFR adaptor factors
TRAIL:	TNF-related apoptosis inducing ligand
VCP:	Vaccinia complement protein
VIP:	Vasoactive intestinal peptide

particular cell surface markers on their cell membranes. These markers used to have peculiar names (lyt, lyb, thy, leu, etc), usually given by the different (groups of) scientists who identified them. Now, an internationally accepted nomenclature identifies these markers by using a single prefix CD (**C**luster of **D**ifferentiation)[1]. This book includes the older names in parentheses wherever possible to facilitate reference to older papers/books. Appendix I summarizes the major CD antigens.

8.2 The B Lymphocytes

B cells are the only cells capable of producing Igs. They represent between 5–15% of the circulating lymphoid pool. They are found in the bone marrow, blood, lymphoid organs, and lymph. B cells form and mature in the bone marrow and from there, they migrate to the lymph nodes via the blood stream. In the absence of antigenic stimulus, they pass through the primary follicles and return to circulation via the lymphatic system to eventually die a few days later. If, however, they encounter an antigen, they form a primary focus of proliferating cells and leave the primary follicle to form the germinal centre of the secondary follicle. Here, the B cells undergo proliferation and differentiation to give rise to antibody-secreting plasma cells and memory cells. The plasma cells subsequently migrate to either the medullary cords of the lymph node or the bone marrow, whereas memory cells re-enter circulation.

8.2.1 Markers

Mature cells of a specific lineage express a number of molecules and receptors (called markers or antigens) on their cell surfaces. Such markers help identify cell type. They also aid the understanding of the function and biology of that cell. Mature human B cells express many markers.

- ❑ **B cell receptor complex** is the most distinctive marker of B cells. It consists of mIgM or mIgD along with a host of other molecules — Ig-α, Ig-β, CD19, CD21, CD22, CD72, CD81, etc (section 6.2).
- ❑ **CD45,** also associated with BcR, is a leukocyte common antigen found on all haematopoietic cells. Different isoforms of this marker are expressed on different lymphocytes or even at different stages of development of the same lymphocyte — memory cells have a different isoform from naïve cells. B220, a heavier isoform of this marker, is one of the earliest markers for B cell lineage.
- ❑ **Receptors for complement components,** CR1 (CD35) and CR2 (CD21), are expressed by B cells (chapter 3).
- ❑ **CD5** is expressed by a subpopulation of B cells. It is normally expressed by T cells. CD5$^+$ B cells, called B1 cells, are involved in innate immune responses (chapter 2).
- ❑ **CD32 (FcγRII),** a low affinity receptor for the IgG, is also expressed by B cells.
- ❑ **MHC class II molecule** expression allows B cells to present antigen to T cells.
- ❑ **Costimulatory molecules** such as CD80/CD86 (together referred to as B7 or B7.1/B7.2) as well as molecules like CD40 and CD134 that are important to T cell-B cell interaction are expressed by activated B cells.

8.2.2 Ontogeny

B cells are formed by the multiplication and differentiation of pleuripotent stem cells derived from mesenchymal cells that migrate to the foetal yolk sac. B cell formation begins in the yolk sac, shifts to the foetal liver, and finally shifts to the bone marrow. Lymphocyte formation continues in the bone marrow throughout adult life. About 2×10^7 to 5×10^7 B cells are estimated to be produced daily in the bone marrow, but a large number of them die by apoptosis before reaching the peripheral

---

[1] Whew!

The Wars Within: The B Cells — **Neill Harris**

"I want to tell you about myself. I want you to understand where I come from and what I stand for. And I want you to see, finally, why you can never win.

In the beginning, it was dark and confusing. There were so many of us then, all crammed into such a tiny space. We clung to our surroundings as best we could, listening to the babel of voices speaking to us and we learnt. We learnt about ourselves — where we came from, what we are and what we are capable of.

It was a hard, dark time. As we moved through our home, staying for the most part close to the boundaries, we saw generation after generation of our kind struck down by some mysterious malaise. All around us lay the detritus of dead and dying cells. Soon — horribly soon — we too became affected. Over half of us fell then and there was not a one of us that did not feel the changes occurring deep within our bodies, not a one of us that did not shudder at the thought of the gruesome fate that could so easily have claimed each of us. We took what solace we could from our continued existence, although it seemed meaningless then and resolved to increase our numbers once more. Then, the second change came. By some small mercy, it was less severe than the first and most of us survived. When finally it was all over, we found ourselves different; bigger, stronger. There was nothing for us there anymore and so we left the comforting walls of our home behind and ventured out into the cavernous interior.

As we travelled, I looked around at my brothers and marvelled at the variation I saw. Each of us now wore a different uniform; the same colours applied in magnificent, unique designs.

We reached our destination, the core of the marrow and saw that others like us had come from all corners of our home. We rejoiced, for our numbers were great and together we were strong. If we had known that our trials were not yet over, we would not have been so unwary. Before we knew it, once again our numbers were being culled — and this time the enemy was without, rather than within. Cell after cell withered and died at the touch of the deadly molecules floating amongst us. It was then that we learnt our purpose: to protect our home against invaders. Those who died were traitors to the cause, cut down because they would sabotage our home at the first opportunity. A few repented, taking on new coats. Those who would not were destroyed. We were better off without them.

And so, we left our birthplace behind and moved out into the world. We looked in awe upon the highways of this place, always busy, night or day. We marvelled at the elegantly organized structures we found. Everywhere we looked, we saw life and activity, thousands upon thousands of cells going about their business, all playing their roles in the great machine. This is what you would destroy with barely a thought.

The greatest marvel of all, though, was the Node. It was vast and it seemed a home away from home for us and our kinds. A centre for gossip, a haven for wanderers and sanctuary for refugees.

The illusion was soon stripped away, though. The Node was not big enough for all who wished to use it and cells squabbled bitterly over what little resources there were. I was one of the lucky ones; I found a pass, no doubt dropped in a brawl, which gained me admittance to the follicle, where there was food and shelter. I watched cells I had lived alongside for days wander lost and confused, unsure of where to go or what to do.

I watched them waste away and die.

And so life fell into a routine, for a time; I would leave the Node and travel the world for a while, seeing the sites, ever vigilant for incursions of your kind. Every so often I would return to my new home, checking in, as it were and resting before my next trip. Gaining entry to the follicle was still a struggle, but it became easier with time.

Then I came here and I sensed you. As if you could have hidden! You may have outwitted my macrophage comrades once, but they just needed to be shown where to go. And so, I returned to the Node to start the Call. I hadn't felt so alive in days! This time, I didn't go to the follicle; a T cell took me to one side and told me what I must do. He showed me the way to the germinal centre, where I increased my numbers. Some were inferior and were culled. Most were stronger. All recognized your presence and were outraged.

I can sense you, you know. You're still there, aren't you? The last few cells, trying in vain to cling to life whilst wave upon wave of phagocytes sweep through your ranks. You might as well give up; you haven't a prayer. 'Maybe next time', you think. I wouldn't count on it; I know your face, now. And I never forget a face."

(Reproduced with permission of the author.)

B LYMPHOCYTES

❑ These are the only cells capable of producing Ig.

❑ They mature in the bone marrow in mammals or Bursa of Fabricus in birds.

❑ B cells express mIg on their surface; mIg is the B cell antigen receptor and is associated with a host of other molecules.

❑ They also express MHC class I and II molecules; expression of MHC class II molecules allows them to present antigen to T cells.

❑ Three major subsets of B cells are recognized on the basis of phenotypic, topographic, and functional characteristics.

- B1 cells are CD5 expressing, non-recirculating, self-renewing cells found in pleural and peritoneal cavities. They respond predominantly to TI antigens and have a role in innate immune responses.
- B2 cells are CD5$^-$ mature, recirculating B cells found in the periphery.
  - ♦ These are the 'conventional' B cells responsible for long-lasting humoral immunity.
  - ♦ B2 cells respond to TD antigens and undergo affinity maturation and class-switch recombination.
  - ♦ Two signals are required to activate B2 cells. Cross-linking of BcRs delivers the first signal; engagement of costimulatory molecules on the surface of B cells by their ligands on T cells delivers the second.
  - ♦ Cytokines released by the T$_H$ cells further helps in the activation, proliferation, and differentiation of these cells.
  - ♦ BcR ligation in the absence of T$_H$ help anergizes these cells.
- MZ B cells are non-recirculating cells located in the marginal zone of the spleen. They respond predominantly to TI antigens.

❑ Cross-linking of the surface Ig (with/without T$_H$ cell help) leads to activation, proliferation, and differentiation of B cells. In the case of B2 cells, it results in the formation of memory cells and plasma cells.

- Memory cells are small B cells capable of reacting to smaller amounts of antigen than naïve cells, are less dependent on T cell help, and produce Ig of higher affinity for the antigen; the Ig produced is of an isotype different from (that produced by) naïve B cells.
- Plasma cells are end cells responsible for the antibody production.

---

lymphoid organs. A whopping 95% of the B cell populations that develop in the bone marrow and primary/secondary germinal centres perish there for a variety of reasons — faulty gene rearrangement, anti-self receptor expression, lack of stimulation, etc. The total repertoire of B cell specificities approaches 10^9, whereas the total number of B cells in adults is about 10^{11}.

All lymphoid cells arise from a common lymphoid progenitor cell. These CD34$^+$ common lymphoid progenitors go through a series of steps before emerging as naïve B cells. **B cell development can be divided into four broad stages — pro-B[2] cell, pre-B cell, immature B cell, and mature B cell.** These stages can be distinguished by stage-specific differentiation markers expressed by the developing B cell and successive steps in the rearrangement and expression of Ig genes. The initial stages of B cell development are often referred to as the antigen-independent[3] phase. In the next phase, called the antigen-dependent phase, naïve B cells undergo a process of differentiation to become plasma cells or memory cells. None of these steps or changes are spontaneous. Rather, each step requires the interaction of extracellular signalling molecules with specific receptors on the B cell surface. This interaction may be between proteins expressed on the surface of other cells (such as the stroma of the bone marrow) and the surface of B cells, between cytokines and their receptors on the surface of B cells, or between the antigen and mIg.

As they mature, B cells migrate from the subendosteum, adjacent to the inner bone surface, to the central axis of the marrow cavity. The non-lymphoid stromal cells found in the bone marrow microenvironment are essential for early B cell development. The CAMs (**C**ell **A**dhesion **M**olecules) on stromal cells form specific adhesion contacts with corresponding ligands on B cells and thereby deliver signals required for their development. For example, interaction between SCF (**Stem Cell Factor**) on stromal cells and its receptor called c-kit (CD117) on the lymphocyte

[2] The pro- in the pro-B stands for progenitor and the pre- for precursor.

[3] Not to split hairs, but calling the development from lymphoid progenitor to naïve B cells 'antigen-independent' is not strictly correct, since self-antigens are involved in B cell selection and survival!

Unwelcome, Unwanted B: B cell lymphomas

B cell precursors go through a number of developmental stages before becoming mature B lymphocytes. Upon antigenic stimulation, mature B cells proliferate and differentiate to antibody-secreting plasma cells or memory cells. B cells thus undergo extensive gene rearrangements throughout their life cycle and are under strict regulatory controls. Pro-apoptotic signals ensure homeostasis of the exploding B cell population. If something goes amiss, malignant transformation of B cells can occur at any step of their development — from early B cell progenitors to mature B cells and further differentiation to plasma cells. B cell lymphoma is a cell population arising from a single B lymphocyte that gets arrested at a particular developmental stage. Lymphomas are the pathological outcomes of genetic accidents that have occurred during lymphocyte development and have greatly helped in furthering the understanding of B cell development and biology. Amino acid sequencing and elucidation of Ig domains was only made possible because of the discovery of Bence-Jones proteins secreted by patients suffering from multiple myeloma (a type of plasmacytoma). Plasmacytoma patients have large quantities of a single type of Ig in their serum (so-called myeloma proteins) secreted by a clone of immortalized plasma cell. Additionally, they excrete excess Ig L chains produced in their urine (called paraproteins). Since myeloma proteins and paraproteins from a single patient are of monoclonal origin, they are identical in their amino acid sequences. Analysis of these proteins therefore allowed the determination of the amino acid sequences of a complete Ig molecule and the comparison of paraproteins from different patients allowed the study of variability in these sequences. Modern monoclonal antibody technology is based on the same principle of immortalizing plasma cells.

Lymphomas are divided into two major groups. Hodgkin's lymphomas are composed of unique malignant cells thought to be of B cell origin. Non-Hodgkin's B cell lymphomas arise during lineage differentiation signalled by productive rearrangements of Ig genes. Mature B cell lymphomas often arise because of occasional errors in the rearrangement process that results in reciprocal chromosomal translocations which juxtapose Ig genes with novel genes. Many translocations place a proto-oncogene such as *Bcl-2* or *myc* next to the Ig locus. The juxtaposed gene is placed under the control of the Ig enhancer and becomes activated, leading to the dysregulation of normal differentiation and initiation of proliferation instead.

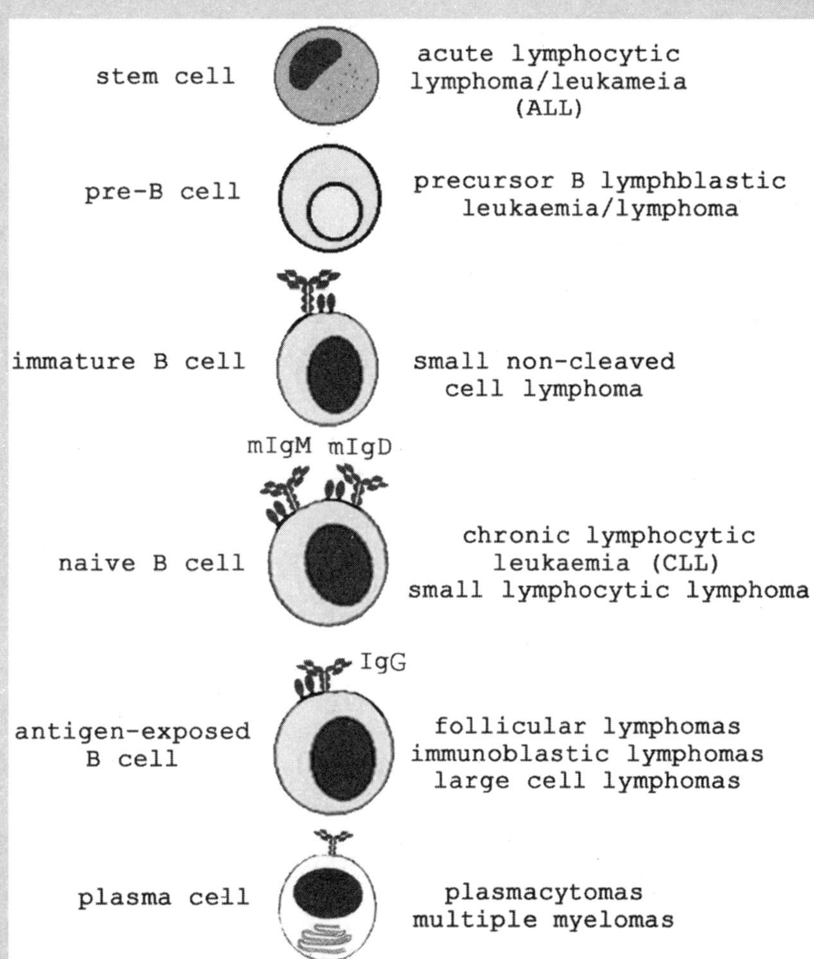

Figure 8.S1 B cell lymphomas can arise at various stages of B cell development (Adapted from lymphoma information network; www.lymphomainfo.net).

membrane is essential for the development of both B and T cells in the bone marrow. Additionally, stromal cells also secrete growth factors. For example, IL-7 secreted by stromal cells is indispensable to B and T lymphocyte development. The later B cell developmental stages are much less dependent on such stromal contacts. The ligand-receptor binding initiates the signalling cascades that result in the altered expression of the proteins required for development. The transcription factor Pax-5 has been identified as a key regulator of B cell development. It is essential for commitment to B cell lineage and for repression of alternative lineage differentiation. The major steps in the ontogeny of B cells are outlined below (Table 8.1).

❑ The **earliest committed B cell precursors are the pre-pro-B cells.** These cells have their Ig loci in the germline[4] configuration. **They do not express components of BcR** and have low expression of **R**ecombination **A**ctivating **G**enes (*RAG-1* and *RAG-2*). Cytokines induce the synthesis of RAG-1 and RAG-2 proteins and the nuclear enzyme **T**erminal **d**eoxynucleotidyl **T**ransferase (TdT) in pre-pro-B cells, resulting in their becoming early pro-B cells[5].

❑ **Early pro-B cells express a precursor BcR** composed of Ig-α, Ig-β, and the chaperone, calnexin. Ig gene recombination is initiated with D-J segment rearrangement on the H chain chromosome. The cells also begin expressing CD45 (B220) and class II MHC molecules.

❑ **In the late pro-B stage, V_H genes become accessible to V(D)J recombinase,** and the assembling of the whole H chain completes the late pro-B cell stage. This recombination event seems to require Pax-5 and IL-7.

❑ **The large pre-B cell has a functional H chain but lacks a functional L chain.** The TdT gene is switched off at this stage. Consequently, N-nucleotide additions

[4] The Ig molecule consists of H and L chains. The V_H region is encoded by *V* (Variable), *D* (Diversity), and *J* (Joining) segments; the V_L region is encoded by *V* and *J* segments. In the germline, multiple loci exist for each of these segments and a productive H or L chain is obtained through gene recombination that joins one of the multiple *V* gene segments with any one of the multiple *D* (H chain only) and *J* segments (chapter 10).

[5] Products of *RAG-1* and *RAG-2* are required in the recombination of *V*, *D*, and *J* gene segments for productive BcR and TcR gene rearrangements. TdT increases *V* gene diversity even further by adding N-nucleotides at the rearrangement joints.

Table 8.1 B cell developmental stages

	Stem cell	*Pre-pro-B cell*	*Early pro-B cell*	*Late pro-B cell*	*Large pre-B cell*	*Small pre-B cell*	*Immature B cell*	*Mature B cell*
H chain	Germline	Germline	D-J joining	VDJ joining	VDJ rearranged	VDJ rearranged	VDJ rearranged	
L chain	Germline	Germline	Germline	Germline	Germline	V-J joining	VJ rearranged	VDJ rearranged
RAG	−	±	+	+	+	+	+	−
TdT	−	±	+	+	−	+	+	−
Surrogate L chain (λL)	−	−	+	+	+	−	−	−
Surface Ig	−	−	−	−	μ chain in pre-BcR	Surface and cytoplasmic μ chain	mIgM	mIgM, mIgD
Ig-α, -β	−	−	+	+	+	+	+	+
Other surface markers	CD34	CD34	CD34 B220 Class II*	B220 Class II* CD19 CD40	B220 Class II* CD19 CD40	B220 Class II* CD19 CD40	B220 Class II* CD19 CD40	B220 Class II* CD19 CD21 CD23 CD40

to gene segment joints in L chains are not as common as in H chain sequences. The *RAG-1* and *RAG-2* genes needed for the rearrangement of L chain genes remain operational. Cells start expressing a pre-BcR consisting of Ig-α, Ig-β, μ heavy chain, and two 'surrogate' L chain molecules, called λ5 and Vpre-B, on their surfaces. The surrogate light chain λ5 resembles the constant region of the λ chain but is encoded by a different gene. λ5 associates non-covalently with Vpre-B, which resembles an Ig V domain. The pre-BcR is a key checkpoint regulator in B cell development. Lymphocytes that fail to assemble a pre-BcR fail to develop further and are deleted. Pre-BcR seems to

- trigger B cell differentiation,
- initiate clonal expansion, and
- enforce heavy chain allelic exclusion[6].

An individual B cell expresses only one species of functional H and L chains, despite having two H chain alleles and four L chain alleles. This phenomenon is known as allelic exclusion (chapter 10). Somatic recombination leads to allelic exclusion for both H and L chains in individual B cells, since each B cell productively recombines only one H chain and one L chain gene. In a heterozygote, each allele (allotype) is represented on about half the B cells and half the serum Ig molecules. Experiments have clearly shown that mIgμ expression in pre-B cells inhibits further H chain recombination, enforcing heavy chain allelic exclusion. The Src kinases are believed to play a role in activating pre-B cell development and allelic exclusion.

❑ **Clonal expansion of large pre-B cells results in small pre-B cells.** These cells are arrested in the G1 phase[7]; Igκ germline transcripts are expressed and pre-B cells undergo VJL gene recombination. Successful L chain gene rearrangement leads to BcR assembly and replacement of the 'surrogate' L chains in the pre-BcR by Igκ or Igλ. The cell is then referred to as an immature B cell.

Allelic exclusion must be operative in the L chains like in the H chains; however, the exact mechanism of this exclusion is not clear. L chains also show isotypic exclusion, since an individual cell or molecule has only κ or λ chains. κ and λ are not represented equally on B cells or serum Igs. In humans, 65% Ig have the κ light chain, while only 35% have λ. In mice, serum Ig is 95% κ, in cats it is 95% λ. The ratio of κ to λ reflects the relative numbers of V region segments in each isotype and the relative efficiency of their recombination into functional L chain genes.

❑ **Immature cells are the first B lineage cells to express surface BcR.** They display surface IgM but little or no IgD. B cells remain in this stage for about three to four days. Immature B cells are particularly susceptible to BcR-induced apoptosis. It is at this stage that B cells undergo negative selection and self-reactive B cells are deleted or anergized.

- **Cross-linking of BcR by self-antigens leads to the elimination of B cells.** Thus, B cells expressing high affinity Ig for self-antigens are sent down the road to apoptosis.

- **B cells expressing BcR with intermediate affinity for self-antigens are anergized.** Anergic B cells are short-lived and have difficulty in reaching maturity. BcR signalling seems to be downregulated in anergic cells, and chronic exposure to antigens can lead to decreased BcR expression in these cells.

- **Exposure to soluble antigens that bind to but do not cross-link BcR also induces anergy** in immature B cells.

Immature B cells retain the capacity for gene rearrangement even after the assembly of functional BcRs. Hence, although many self-specific B cells undergo clonal deletion or are anergized, some can escape elimination by further rearranging their BcR. These secondary rearrangements can occur at both H and L genes. The exact mechanism of this secondary gene rearrangement, called receptor editing, is still to be determined. A survival signal appears to be required for this 'second

[6] Allelic exclusion is the expression of genes from the maternal or paternal chromosome but not both because of chromosomal inactivation. In B lymphocytes, allelic exclusion assures that all antibodies expressed are derived from the same allele.

[7] Eukaryotic cellular activities are in cyclic phases G1 to M. G0 phase is the resting phase. In the G1 phase, enzymes for DNA replication are synthesized along with other proteins needed for cellular growth. In the S phase, DNA as well as other related proteins are synthesized. The G2 phase is recognized by the synthesis of proteins and the cellular material of the mitotic apparatus, whereas actual mitosis occurs in the M phase.

chance', and it is likely that receptor editing is influenced by interactions between small pre-B/immature B cells and bone marrow stromal cells. Whether this is due to successful receptor editing or due to the elimination of self-reactive clones, the newly formed B cells lose the ability to bind self-antigens and start expressing mIgD on their cell surfaces. These B cells lack the adhesion molecules necessary for extravasation and emigrate to the red pulp of the spleen to complete the final phase of development.

❑ **Newly formed B cells in the bone marrow or the red pulp of the spleen are called transitional cells.** After lodging in the red pulp for about a day, these B cells pass through the T cell areas of the PALS to colonize the lymphoid follicles of the spleen and become IgD^{hi}IgM^{lo}CD23^{+}(CD23 is FcεRII). They start expressing homing receptors that confer the ability to recirculate and become naïve follicular B cells. Survival signals received in the follicles enable them to enter the mature peripheral B cell compartment; B cells that fail to lodge in the follicles die within a matter of days. The need for survival signals continues throughout the life of these B cells so that they must circulate through the follicles periodically. The signals promoting this survival and differentiation are not well understood. It is now established that some survival signals are received via the BcR and Bruton's tyrosine kinase[8] and CD45 seem to be critical in this signalling. KO mice lacking either of these molecules involved in BcR signalling fail to develop mature B cells, although transitional B cells are formed. Another factor important to B cell survival is BAFF (**B** cell **A**ctivating **F**actor of the TNF **F**amily). This pro-survival factor secreted by macrophages and DCs is thought to promote survival of both transitional and mature B cells. Thus, only a fraction of transitional cells succeed in entering the long-lived, recirculating, follicular B cell pool.

There is method to this madness of producing a large number of cells and then killing most of them. The immune system tries to achieve a balance between two opposing forces — the need to have a ready pool of naïve B cells at any given point of time and the need to avoid an unnecessary build-up of mature B cells. Since the naïve B cell pool needs to be continually replenished, the system continues to produce these cells in copious numbers. If all these cells are allowed to mature, the body will find itself unable to support this humungous population of B cells. To maintain homeostasis, a large fraction of newly formed B cells have to be sent down the road to apoptosis. Competition for survival signals between newly created B cells and older B cells probably maintains this B cell homeostasis and prevents build-up. B cells that survive and enter the peripheral pool may yet be sent down the road to death or anergy, this time to ensure absence of self-reactivity. Since not all self-antigens are present in the bone marrow, such mechanisms ensure the silencing of autoreactive clones.

- Mature B cells that are exposed to multivalent self-antigens in the periphery are deleted or rendered anergic.
- Exposure of a mature B cell to a high concentration of soluble self-antigen can also render the cell anergic.
- Antigen recognition in the absence of T cell help blocks B cell activation.

8.2.3 Heterogeneity

On the basis of phenotypic, topographic and functional characteristics, three major subsets of B cells are recognized (Table 8.2). The exact lineage relationship between these subsets is not very clear. However, the size of the B1 compartment *vis à vis* the B2 compartment appears to depend upon the expression and composition of the BcR.

❑ **B1 cells express CD5.** They have the IgM^{hi}IgD$^{-/lo}$CD23$^{-/lo}$ CD21^{lo}CD5^{+} phenotype[9]. These are self-renewing cells, ie, they can give rise to mature naïve cells like themselves. By contrast, the pool of naïve conventional B cells is

[8] This enzyme involved in downstream signalling via BcR plays a pivotal role in activating a network of intracellular signalling. Its deficiency causes agammaglobulinaemia (complete absence of Ig).

[9] hi: high levels of expression; int: intermediate levels of expression; –/lo: either absent or present in very low concentrations.

Table 8.2 B cell subsets

Characteristic	B1	B2	MZ
Phenotype	IgM hi IgD lo CD21 lo CD23 lo CD9 lo CD5 lo CD1 +/–	IgM lo IgD hi CD21 int CD23 hi CD9– CD5 – CD1 int	IgM hi IgD lo CD21 int CD23 lo CD9 lo CD5 – CD1 int
Recirculation in lymph	Do not recirculate	Recirculate to and from blood and lymph	Essentially confined to the spleen; MZ B cells migrate to and from PALS; plasma cells arising from these cells may exit the spleen
Renewal	Self-renewing	Replenished from bone marrow	Replenished from bone marrow
Response to antigen	TI hi TD +/–	TI – TD hi	TI hi; especially type 2 TD lo
Binding of multiple ligands	int	—	int
Proliferation	LPS hi anti-IgM +/– CD40 +/–	LPS lo anti-IgM int CD40 lo	LPS hi anti-IgM +/– CD40 –
Type of Ig	IgM, IgG3, IgA	IgG1	IgM, IgG3
Resistance to Fas mediated apoptosis	int	—	—
Apoptosis after anti-IgM treatment	—	lo	hi

Legend: hi – high, int – intermediate, lo – low, +/– uncertain response, – negative or no response

constantly replenished by the bone marrow. The majority of B1 cells develop from the foetal liver and are found predominantly in the peritoneal and pleural cavity. B1 BcR is produced preferentially from only some Ig gene segments, does not have additional N-nucleotides at the joints between segments, and is specific for mostly common bacterial carbohydrate antigens. Thought to be responsible for 'natural' IgM antibodies, B1 cells mainly respond to TI antigens and do not undergo affinity maturation. They also seem to be incapable of differentiating to memory cells. The BcR of the B1 cells seems to recognize antigens on multiple pathogens with low affinity. Hence, these cells and their secreted antibodies are called 'polyreactive'. The role of B1 cells in immunity is discussed in chapter 2.

❑ **B2 cells or follicular B cells.** Mature, recirculating CD5⁻ B cells found in the periphery and located in the follicles of the lymph nodes and spleen are called the B2 cells (ie, are 'conventional' B cells). They express the $IgM^{lo}IgD^{hi}CD23^{hi}$ $CD21^{int}$ phenotype. B2 cells are capable of isotype switching and affinity maturation and they are responsible for long-lasting humoral immunity. Unless otherwise specified, the term 'B cell' is used in reference to these cells throughout this book.

❑ **MZ (Marginal Zone) cells.** Marginal zone is the spleen compartment located at the outer limit of the white pulp. It is bordered by the MZ sinus on the inner side and by the red pulp on the outer side. The marginal sinus surrounds B cell follicles and the PALS of the white pulp. Several concentric layers of macrophages are found in the MZ. DCs and macrophages in this area filter particulate antigens from the blood and present them to T cells. Long-lived, apparently naïve B cells that localize in close proximity to the concentric rings of macrophages are called the MZ B cells[10]. Colonization of the MZ by these B cells seems to occur after 1–2 yrs of age in human infants. They are non-circulating B cells that have a partially activated phenotype ($IgM^{hi}IgD^{lo}CD23^{–/lo}CD21^{hi}$). Both B1 and MZ B

[10] Long-lived memory B cells responding to TD antigens have also been shown to reside in this compartment for prolonged periods. As the central arteriole that carries blood to the spleen empties into the marginal sinus, newly formed B cells and different types of T cells can also be found transiting through this zone.

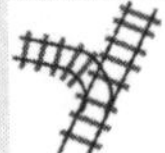

A BAFFling, RANK-Ling TRAIL: TNF Family

Proteins of the TNF and TNF Receptor (TNFR) superfamily are important in the control of such disparate processes as death, proliferation and differentiation of immune cells, modulation of innate and adaptive responses, and organogenesis of lymphoid organs. New research indicates that these proteins may also be involved in bone remodelling and lactation. Noteworthy members include TNF-α, TNF-β, CD95-CD95L, CD134-CD134L, CD40-CD154, BAFF, TRAIL, RANK, and RANK-L.

TNF receptors lack tyrosine kinase domains. They also do not interact with cytosolic proteins capable of phosphorylation. Members of this ever-growing superfamily are trimeric proteins defined on the basis of the homology of their extracellular domains that has repeats of cysteine-rich domains. Presence of cysteines allows the formation of an extended rod-like structure (called a jelly role) that is responsible for ligand binding. Trimerization of the receptor allows cytosolic proteins called TRAFs (**TNFR A**daptor **F**actors) to bind to the cytoplasmic domains of the receptors and initiate different signalling cascades, depending upon the composition of the TRAFs. Members of the family that induce apoptosis are called death receptors. They have a **D**eath **D**omain (DD) in their cytoplasmic tail that is essential for transduction of the apoptotic signal. Upon activation, the DD serves as a docking site for DD-containing adaptor proteins. A **D**eath-**I**nducing **S**ignalling **C**omplex (DISC) is formed within seconds of receptor engagement, leading to recruitment of caspase-8 or -10. Initiation of the caspase cascade results in cell death. Other members of the family that lack DDs can cause proliferation and may even confer resistance to apoptosis if appropriate TRAFs are recruited (fig. 8.S2).

❑ CD95 (Fas), involved in transducing the death signal, has a significant role in the immune system. It is expressed primarily on haematopoietic cells, but can also be found on epithelial cells. CD95 expression can be boosted by cytokines such as IFN-γ and TNF-α. Additionally, lymphocyte activation also upregulates expression of this molecule and downregulates its inhibitor FLIP. CD95-mediated apoptosis is triggered by its natural ligand CD95L (FasL). It has a much more restricted expression than CD95. Interestingly, cleaved, soluble human CD95L can also induce apoptosis unlike murine CD95L. Activation of CD95 causes the recruitment of the adaptor protein FADD (**F**as-**A**ssociated **D**eath **D**omain) and induces apoptosis. This is one of the major pathways of inducing death in target cells by cytotoxic lymphocytes (chapter 11).

❑ Exposure of cells to TNF-α can have varied results.
   • The receptor TNFR-1 is expressed by all human tissues and is the major signalling receptor for TNF-α. Depending upon the adaptor proteins recruited, TNFR-1 can cause induction of proliferative/inflammatory responses or apoptosis. Like Fas, it has a DD in its cytoplasmic tail. If it binds the adaptor molecule TRADD (**TNF**R-1-**A**ssociated **DD**), TNF-R1 causes apoptosis. Alternatively, TNFR-1 activation can lead to the recruitment of RIP (**R**eceptor **I**nteracting **P**roteins), which causes activation of the transcription factor NFκB. If TRAFs are recruited, however, MAP kinases get activated.
   • TNFR-2 is expressed mainly on cells of the immune system. It binds both TNF-α and TNF-β. It lacks DD. Instead, it allows the binding of TRAFs, which can result in recruitment of **I**nhibitors of **A**poptosis **P**roteins (IAPs) that may confer resistance to apoptosis.

❑ Activated T cells express TRAIL (**TNF**-**R**elated **A**poptosis **I**nducing **L**igand), yet another member of this family involved in the induction of apoptosis. TRAIL is involved in cytotoxic lymphocyte-mediated apoptosis. It is also important in T cell induced DC apoptosis. Thus, DCs presenting antigen to T cells are effectively eliminated, avoiding excessive activation of the immune system. New research also implicates TRAIL in the apoptosis of neutrophils.

❑ CD40 is widely distributed on the cells of the immune system. It is constitutively expressed on B cells, but its expression is lost at the plasma cell phase. CD154, the ligand for CD40, is expressed primarily on T cells. It is also found on NK cells, masts cells, basophils, monocytes, DCs, etc. CD40 ligation promotes B lymphocyte proliferation, survival, and affinity maturation. It also upregulates Fas expression, and unless the cell receives overriding signals, it can lead to apoptosis of the B lymphocyte. CD40 ligation can enhance survival and cytokine secretion by DCs and monocytes.

❑ BAFF, expressed by DCs, macrophages, monocytes, etc is a fundamental factor required for B cell survival and is found to enhance immune responses. It has been shown to control maturation of B cells in the spleen. It is thought that BAFF receptors induce NFκB transcription and promote anti-apoptotic signals in B cells.

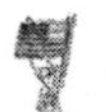

- ❑ RANK-L (**R**eceptor **A**ctivator of **NF**κB **L**igand) and its receptor RANK are the newest additions to the TNFR stable.
  - RANK-RANK-L (expressed by DCs and T cells respectively) interactions regulate DC-T cell communications, DC survival, and lymph node formation.
  - Both RANK and RANK-L are crucial to lymph node organogenesis.
  - RANK-L and RANK are expressed in mammary gland epithelial cells and control the development of lactating mammary glands during pregnancy.
  - These molecules are key regulators of bone remodelling and are essential for development and activation of osteoclasts (cells involved in bone resorption). Additionally, TNF-α and IL-1 have been shown to induce osteoclast formation and cause bone resorption independent of RANK. Recent research indicates that a balance between RANK/RANK-L controls bone remodelling and bone loss. In animal models, systemic activation of T cells was found to result in RANK-L dependent osteoclastogenesis followed by bone loss, suggesting a role for T cells in regulation of bone physiology.

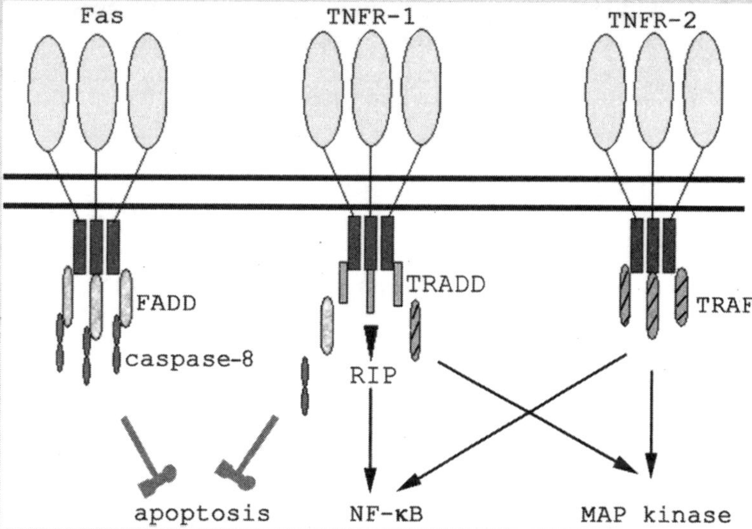

Figure 8.S2 *TNF receptors are trimeric proteins lacking tyrosine kinase domains. Trimerization of the receptors initiates different signalling pathways, depending upon the adaptor proteins recruited to the receptor (Adapted from Immunity (2000) 13:419).*

cells express CD9 — a member of the tetraspanin family (it crosses the cell membrane four times). CD9 has been shown to be important in cell adhesion and migration, signal transduction, and cancer metastases in other cell types. Its role in B cells is yet to be established. The overwhelming majority of MZ cells have germline V_H segments in their BcR. Like B1 cells, MZ cells are thought to have originated from the foetal liver, although some transitional B cells may also become MZ cells. They can present antigen efficiently and they differentiate rapidly to plasma cells when activated by antigen. They seem to primarily respond to TI antigens, although they may also respond to TD antigens in some instances (section 4.3). MZ and B1 cells respond most rapidly to antigen, giving rise to the earliest antibody response to immune challenge.

8.2.4 Activation

Mature B cells emerging from the bone marrow are in the G0 phase. Contact with antigen or polyclonal activators triggers their entry into the G1 phase. They then move through the successive phases of S and G2 before undergoing mitosis and repeating the cycle. Activated cells thus undergo clonal expansion. Activation can be achieved by antigen non-specific and specific means. Some non-specific B cell activators are listed on the next page.

- **Lectins** are plant proteins that can bind to specific cell surface glycoproteins and thereby deliver an activation signal. Lectins are 'polyclonal activators', since they activate B cells irrespective of their antigenic specificity.
- **Anti-IgM**[11] antibodies cross-link surface IgM, delivering a signal similar to antigenic stimulation. Cells expressing mIgM proliferate in response to anti-IgM antibodies. Anti-IgD antibodies may also be used to stimulate antigen-non-specific B cell proliferation. Both polyclonal activators and anti-IgM/IgD antibodies have an important application in studying B cell proliferation *in vitro*.

The mechanism of antigen-specific activation of B cells is to some degree dictated by the nature of the antigen. **TI antigens can activate B cells independent of T cell involvement.** The strength of the signal generated by the engagement of multiple BcRs by repetitive epitopes of the TI antigen is enough to activate the B cells. Cytokines secreted by T cells enhance activation by TI type 2 antigens. With TD antigens, however, activation is a two-signal process. The first signal is delivered by cross-linking of the BcR by the antigen. Activated antigen-specific T_H cells deliver the second signal. This contact-mediated signal, called cognate interaction, requires close physical contact between the two cells. Many receptor-ligand pairs contribute to cognate interaction.

❑ **MHC class II molecules.** Engagement of class II molecules on B cells by TcR stimulates early biochemical signalling events in B cells. This results in enhanced B cell response to the activation signals emanating from T_H cells. MHC:TcR binding enhances the physical proximity of the two cells, assisting in the delivery of contact-mediated signals and soluble molecules. It also seems to stimulate the proliferation and differentiation of B cells. This interaction is reciprocal, as it also affects T_H cells. TcR recognition of peptide:MHC complexes on B cells induces transient expression of new molecules on these cells, allowing them to enter into a prolonged relationship with antigen-specific B cells.

❑ **CD40**, since it is constitutively expressed, is perhaps the most important molecule in cognate interaction. Engagement of this member of the TNF family by its ligand CD154 (CD40L in older literature), upregulated on activated T_H lymphocytes promotes proliferation, cytokine production, antibody secretion and isotype switching in B cells. It is also critical in upregulating molecules involved in antigen presentation by B cells. Interaction between CD40 and CD154 is also essential in the development of germinal centres, survival of B cells in the germinal centres, and affinity maturation.

❑ **CD134L (OX40L).** This is another member of the TNF family that is important in cognate interaction. Engagement of CD134 (OX40) on T_H cells with the ligand (CD134L) on B cells is thought to be important in isotype switching and secondary antibody responses.

❑ **Adhesion molecules.** Both B and T cells express a myriad of transmembrane adhesion molecules such as CD54 (ICAM-1) and CD11a/CD18 (LFA-1) which bind to each other and are capable of mediating homotypic and heterotypic adhesion[12]. Apart from enhancing physical association of the two cells, both LFA-1 and ICAM-1 have been shown to transmit activation signals to both B and T cells. Such signals increase antigen presentation by B cells and work together with CD40-mediated signalling.

❑ **CD72.** Engagement of the CD72 molecule on B cells by CD100 on T cells enhances B cell activation mediated by CD40. This interaction seems to be particularly important in developing high affinity IgG responses to TD antigens.

❑ **CD95/Fas.** Interestingly, CD40 signals upregulate CD95 on B cells so that they become increasingly susceptible to the CD95L expressed on activated T cells; CD95 engagement leads to apoptosis unless the B cell receives overriding survival signals.

[11] When murine IgM antibodies are injected in a rabbit, the rabbit's immune system recognizes the mouse IgM as foreign and mounts an immune response. Repeated immunizations result in a rabbit serum rich in antibodies against murine IgM. The rabbit serum so generated is used as a ready source of high affinity anti-IgM antibodies.

[12] Homotypic adhesion occurs when similar molecules are involved in adhesion (eg, LFA-1 to LFA-1); heterotypic adhesion occurs when two different molecules participate in the adhesion (eg, LFA-1 and ICAM-1)

This feature of the humoral response, wherein both T_H cells and B cells must recognize antigenic determinants on the same molecule for B cell activation, is called associative or linked recognition. This requirement for cognate interaction may be advantageous in regulating the immune response. Elimination of self-reactive clones appears to be more efficient in T cells than in B cells. Thus, if a cognate antigen-specific T cell clone is not available, autoreactive B cell clones cannot get activated, decreasing the potential for an autoimmune reaction. This also limits a bystander response, since the B and T cells need to be activated and in physical contact for delivery of the second signal. The requirement for antigen-specific T cell help also explains the carrier effect noted in chapter 9. However, how an antigen-specific B cell encounters a T cell has been a puzzling feature of cognate interaction, since the two cell types occupy separate zones of peripheral lymphoid tissue. Normally, when B cells enter the lymphoid tissue through HEV, they rapidly move through the T cell zone and enter the primary follicles in the B cell zone. Upon antigen activation, B cells start expressing adhesion molecules and chemokine receptors. Consequently, they get trapped in the T cell zone, maximizing their chances of encountering the appropriate T cells. The sequence of events in B cell activation and eventual differentiation is summarized below.

1. B cells internalize the antigen either by pinocytosis or (BcR or other) receptor-mediated endocytosis.
2. The antigen is processed and loaded on MHC class II molecules; MHC:peptide complexes appear on the surface of the B cell within 30–60 minutes of encountering the antigen.
3. The B cells start expressing adhesion molecules and are trapped in the T cell zone of lymphoid organs.
4. Costimulatory molecules, such as CD80/86 required for antigen presentation, are also upregulated.
5. Recognition and binding of the MHC:peptide complex by TcR on T_H cells leads to close physical contact between the two cells.
6. A T cell-B cell conjugate is formed; the T cell shows a reorganization of its golgi apparatus.
7. The T_H cell is activated; expression of CD154, CD134 and CD100 is upregulated.
8. Ligation of various ligands on B cells (CD40, CD134L and CD72 respectively) results in the activation of tyrosine kinases and ultimately results in the activation of the transcription factor NFκB; these signals also override the apoptotic signal generated by CD95 on the B cell.
9. There is a unidirectional release of cytokines from the T_H cell to the B cell. The cytokines released include IL-4, IL-5, IL-6, TGF-β, and IFN-γ and are dictated by a number of factors such as the type of T_H cell, nature of the antigen, and site of interaction.
10. Signals transmitted through the cytokine receptors support B cell activation and also result in B cell proliferation. Thus, B cells establish a primary focus of clonal expansion.
11. T cells are also stimulated to proliferate so that both B and T cells proliferate at the border between the B and T cell zones.
12. After several days, the rate of B proliferation decreases, and the primary focus of proliferation begins to involute.
13. Some of the proliferating B cells differentiate to antibody-forming plasma cells and migrate to the red pulp of the spleen or the medullary cords of the lymph node. They are responsible for the Ig with relatively low affinity for the antigen that is found in the initial stages of the immune response.
14. Other B cells migrate into a primary lymphoid follicle, where they continue to proliferate and give rise to germinal centres.

15. B cells undergo somatic hypermutation in the germinal centres, and selection and survival of cells with increased affinity to the antigen results in affinity maturation (explained in chapter 10).
16. The cells also undergo class switch recombination giving rise to B cells secreting antibodies with the same antigenic specificity but different isotype (section 10.4.3).
17. Some germinal centre B cells also undergo differentiation to plasmablasts that continue to divide rapidly but are already committed to become non-dividing, Ig-secreting plasma cells.
18. Other germinal centre B cells differentiate to memory cells.

8.2.5 B Cell Differentiation

B cells encountering antigen and receiving appropriate T cell help in the T cell areas undergo blast transformation. In the lymphoid organs this is seen as the emergence of blast cells and formation of germinal centres. The cells enlarge; their nucleolus swells; polysomes, rough ER, etc develop and the rate of nucleic acid and protein synthesis increases rapidly. Germinal centre B cells are inherently on the road to apoptosis and require specific signals in order to survive (see sidetrack 'Not Immune to Death'). Continued ligation of BcR by the antigen along with physical interaction between B and T cells has been shown to be necessary for B cell survival. B cell survival is also enhanced by the engagement of CD40 by CD40L on T cells. The nature of the other survival signals delivered by T cells is unclear. Those B cells that receive survival signals in the germinal centres undergo somatic hypermutation and selection for cells expressing receptors with higher affinity for the antigen (chapter 10). They also undergo differentiation (fig. 8.1). The germinal centre reaction peaks in about 10–12 days after antigenic challenge and gives rise to

❑ small, relatively non-descript, non-secreting memory cells, and
❑ large, rapidly dividing plasmablasts that give rise to Ig-secreting plasma cells.

Factors that determine the fate of the proliferating B cell (differentiation to memory cell or plasma cell) are not well understood. Some studies suggest that expression of high affinity antibody may favour plasma cell rather than memory cell development. Experiments also indicate that signals received via CD40 favour a memory phenotype, but the absence of such signals promotes plasma cell differentiation, especially in the presence of IL-2 and IL-10. Signalling via OX40L (CD134L) also seems to promote differentiation to plasma cell. IL-4 has been found to favour memory cell formation. IL-6, on the other hand, is required for differentiation to plasmablasts and antibody secretion. Blimp-1 (**B l**ymphocyte **i**nduced **m**aturation **p**rotein-**1**), also called the master regulator for terminal B cell differentiation, is a key protein driving activated B cells to become antibody-secreting plasma cells. It is present in all plasma cells, whether formed from naïve cells during a primary response or from memory cells in a secondary response. How the proteins drive the plasma cell differentiation programme is unclear.

Both memory cells and plasmablasts migrate from the germinal centre. Memory cells are found predominantly in the marginal zone of the spleen, the subcapsular sinus of the lymph nodes, and under the intestinal epithelium in the Peyer's patches and crypt epithelium of the tonsils; a few are also found in the blood. The plasmablasts leave the germinal centre and develop into terminally differentiated plasma cells that secrete high affinity antibodies. Some of these cells home to the bone marrow, where they receive survival signals from stromal cells via cell adhesion molecules. These bone marrow plasma cells continue to secrete antibodies for many months. Others may be found in the medullary cords of the lymph nodes, the red pulp of the spleen, and mucosal lamina propria. Plasma cells found at mucosal sites are predominantly IgA-secreting plasma cells.

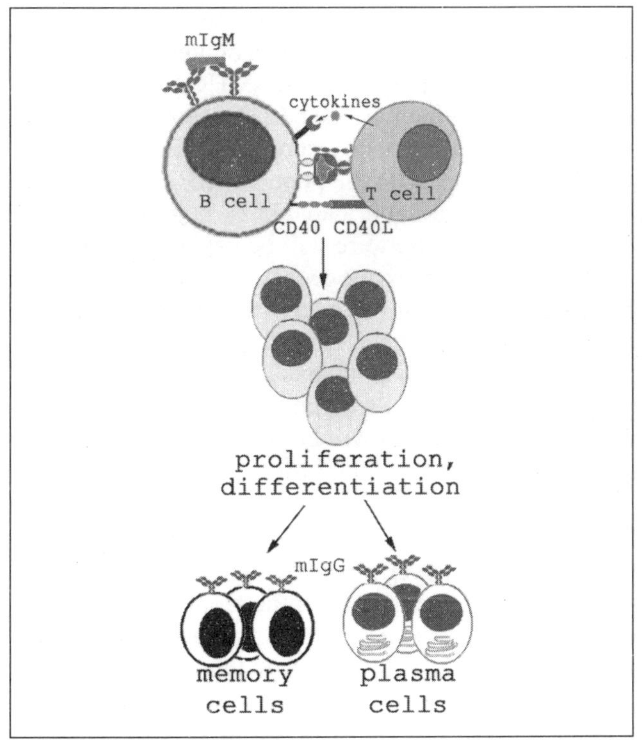

Figure 8.1 When antigen-activated B cells receive the appropriate T cell help, they undergo clonal expansion and differentiation to plasma cells and memory cells. Antigen-driven coligation of BcRs triggers downstream signalling pathways and activates the B cell. It also results in upregulation of adhesion molecules and costimulatory molecules. The internalized antigen is processed and presented to T_H cells. Recognition and binding of the MHC:peptide complex by TcR on T_H cells leads to close physical contact between the two cells. Engagement of ligands such as CD40 on B cells by their receptors on T cells delivers survival signals to B cells. Cytokines released by T_H cells support B cell proliferation and differentiation. This differentiation results in the formation of plasma cells and memory cells. The proliferating B cells also undergo class-switch recombination and somatic hypermutation in their Ig V region genes. The plasma cells have a prominent, distended rough ER and are cellular factories of Ig production.

8.2.5.1 Memory B Cells

Memory B cells develop in the germinal centre, although the exact developmental pathway that leads to their formation is not entirely clear. A degree of uncertainty also surrounds the phenotype of memory cells. It is a small, relatively undifferentiated cell. The vast majority of memory B cells express Igs other than IgM/IgD on their cell surfaces, although some may express either one or both of these isotypes. Memory B cells also express low levels of a **H**eat-**S**table **A**ntigen (HSA) and the adhesion molecule L-selectin (CD62L), whereas most naïve cells express high levels of both these molecules. The best hallmark of a memory B cell is a somatically mutated Ig gene that codes for Igs with greater affinity for the antigen. Memory B cells are long-lived cells that can survive for prolonged periods even in the absence of antigens and do not secrete antibodies. Upon leaving the germinal centre, memory B cells recirculate or home to draining areas of the lymph node and spleen. Following antigen encounter, memory cells are biased to become plasma cells. Although CD40 is important for memory B cell development, it does not appear to be required for the development of plasma cells in the secondary response.

Memory cells are more easily triggered by the immunogen than the virgin B lymphocyte. This is because they have a different isoform of the CD45 molecule that is more efficient in signal transduction. They proliferate in response to lower amounts of antigen and can differentiate to plasma cells even in the absence of T cell help. Once memory cells are formed (whether B or T), these are the cells that respond to subsequent antigenic challenges. The presence of memory cells inhibits activation of naïve cells by the same antigen. This makes good sense, since the memory cells are better equipped to deal with the antigenic challenge, and it would be a waste of energy (and time) if naïve cells were to respond to the secondary challenge. Many pathogens exploit this inhibition by undergoing antigenic variation (see sidetrack 'Trying to Fit In' in chapter 9).

Memory cell formation is responsible for the prompt and heightened antibody responses observed on secondary exposure to the immunogen. It is a simple yet elegant device to create a large pool of cells capable of responding to an immunogen that the body has encountered before (fig. 8.1). Upon first encounter, the antigen must reach the local lymph node, be taken up and loaded on MHC molecules by APCs, and be scanned by thousands of naïve lymphocytes, before a specific reaction between an APC and lymphocyte can be achieved. The response will be slow, since the T cells must be activated following contact with the peptide:MHC complex on the APC, proliferate, and differentiate before being capable of helping B cells. Moreover, only a small fraction of the B cell repertoire will be capable of binding (either weakly or strongly) to epitopes on the immunogen. It is only after B cells differentiate following T cell help that Ig production can commence. Following the first encounter, however, the animal will have a much larger repertoire of memory T and B cells capable of reacting to an antigen. Also, thanks to affinity maturation, the antigen receptor of memory B cells will bind the antigen more strongly than that of the naïve B cell. Hence, fewer antigen molecules will be sufficient to trigger the immune response, and the speed of the response will be faster.

8.2.5.2 Plasma Cells

Plasmablasts originating in the follicles of the Peyer's patches and mesenteric lymph nodes migrate via lymph to the blood and eventually the lamina propria of the gut or other epithelial surfaces. Those originating in the peripheral lymph nodes or splenic follicles migrate to the bone marrow. There, they differentiate to Ig-secreting plasma cells. **Plasma cells are terminally differentiated cells that are essentially cellular factories for the manufacture and export of Igs.** They can secrete several thousand Ig molecules per second. Two types of plasma cells can be distinguished based on their longevity and somatically mutated mIg.

❑ Short-lived plasma cells seem to represent an early response to antigen exposure that is T_H cell-dependent but germinal centre independent (eg, those formed at the primary focus of B cell proliferation). Consequently, these cells do not have a somatically mutated receptor.
❑ Long-lived plasma cells are a product of the germinal centre reaction and hence show evidence of affinity maturation and isotype switching. These cells are thought to home preferentially to the bone marrow, where they secrete the high affinity antibodies observed typically in the second week of a primary response. They are credited with maintaining significant levels of serum Ig, often for the lifespan of the animal. It is possible (though not clearly established) that this pool of plasma cells is replenished by the occasional differentiation of memory cells. Although the germinal centres last for only 3–4 weeks after initial antigen exposure, a small number of B cells continue to proliferate in them for months and may be the precursors for plasma cells in subsequent months or years.

Differentiation to plasma cells leads to the downregulation of numerous B cell-specific surface proteins. These include MHC class II molecules, CD45, CD19, and CD21. Similarly, chemokine receptors that allow homing to the B and T cell areas of the lymph nodes and spleen are reduced. However, plasma cells continue to express CXCR4, which allows their movement out of the follicles. Histologically, the plasma cell is distinct from a small lymphocyte. The nucleus is eccentric, containing coarse, radially arranged chromatin. The cytoplasm has a conspicuous and abundant rough and smooth ER as well as a prominent golgi apparatus. The ER is usually packed into thin lamellae and is sometimes even distended with Igs. The mechanism of Ig synthesis and secretion by plasma cells has been dealt with separately in section 9.4.

8.3 The T Lymphocytes

Lymphocytes that originate in the foetal liver and adult bone marrow migrate to the thymus for maturation and are called T lymphocytes. The majority of T lymphocytes in human circulation are ultrastructurally similar to small lymphocytes, possessing a large nucleus with very few intracytoplasmic organelles. T cells have a central role in immune responses and are functionally and phenotypically heterogeneous. They can be divided into two categories (CD4$^+$ or CD8$^+$), depending upon the type of coreceptor expressed[13]. Functionally, they fall into four broad groups.

❑ **CTLs** involved in the lysis of altered self-cells, eg, virus-infected cells, cells harbouring intracellular parasites, and tumour cells
❑ **Tн cells** which perform the dual function of
  • co-operating with B cells in humoral responses and
  • facilitating CMI responses by activating macrophages
❑ **Tʀ cells** which control immune responses and help in the prevention of auto-immune diseases
❑ **NKT cells** which recognize lipid antigens and are important in defence against intracellular parasites and tumours[14]

8.3.1 Markers

Mature T cells show the presence of several distinctive markers on their cell surface.

❑ **TcR.** The most important and distinguishing marker of a T cell is its antigen receptor complex.
  • T cells involved in an adaptive immune response express the αβTcR; those expressing γδTcR are a part of innate immune responses and are discussed in chapter 2.
  • CD3 and CD45 molecules are a part of the TcR complex and are found on all T cells.
  • Coreceptors CD4 and CD8 are expressed by distinctive subsets of T cells — Tн and Tʀ subsets express the coreceptor CD4 that binds to MHC class II molecules, whereas CTLs express the CD8 coreceptor that binds to MHC class I molecules.
  • NKT cells express αβTcR that recognizes antigen in context of CD1; most NKT cells express either CD4 or CD8 molecules, although some NKT cells are both CD4 and CD8 negative.
❑ **CD7.** This is probably the first molecule to appear during T cell ontogeny. It is a pan T cell marker that is expressed by prethymic, intrathymic, and post-thymic T cells. However, it is also expressed by most NK cells.
❑ **ANAE.** Both human and mouse T lymphocytes contain a number of lysosomal acid hydrolases. The **α-N**aphthyl **A**cid **E**sterase (ANAE) is localized in one or a few regions of the cytoplasm that appear as 'dots' on cytochemical staining. This pattern of cytochemical staining is distinctive of T cells. Most B cells stain negative for ANAE. Monocytes show a diffused staining pattern.
❑ **CD2.** Human T cells express CD2 (LFA-2/T11), an adhesion molecule that can fortuitously[15] also bind to sheep red blood cells.
❑ **Activation markers.** Some molecules are only expressed by activated T cells.
  • MHC class II molecules are not expressed by resting human T cells, but expression is induced upon activation. In contrast, murine T cells do not express MHC class II molecules.
  • Activation also induces the expression of α chain of the IL-2 receptor (CD25) and CD69.
  • Some costimulatory molecules like CD28 are expressed by resting as well as activated T cells; others, like CD154 (CD40L) are found only on activated CD4$^+$ T cells and NKT cells.
  • CTLA-4 (CD152) expressed only on activated T cells is, like CD28, a ligand for CD80/86. However, it is a negative receptor that arrests proliferation of

---

[13] Some NKT cells, however, express neither CD4 nor CD8.

[14] Unless otherwise mentioned, the description in section 8.3 applies to conventional T cells and not NKT cells.

[15] Fortuitously, because this property can be used for the relatively easy and selective physical separation of human T cells from B cells or, indeed, any non-T cells!

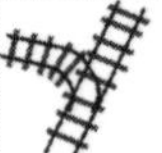

The Need for Stimulating Company: Costimulatory Molecules and T Cells

The primary event required for T cell activation is the engagement of TcR by a peptide:MHC complex. Lysis by CD8$^+$ T cells has been shown to be triggered by as few as 1–50 MHC class I molecules. Experiments show that MHC molecules need not engage all TcRs simultaneously but may serially engage several TcRs, thereby progressively amplifying intracellular signals emanating from the engagement. The ligation of costimulatory molecules, in addition to TcR engagement, is required for a productive immune response. Members of the B7–CD28 superfamily are crucial to this costimulation.

❑ **CD28**, a 44KD glycoprotein that binds CD80 and CD86, is the most effective costimulatory molecule expressed by naïve and primed T cells. TcR engagement in the absence of CD28 ligation results in apoptosis or anergy. Anergic T cells do not produce IL-2 and cannot proliferate on subsequent stimulations. Apart from increasing cytokine production, CD28 engagement also promotes T cell survival by inducing the upregulation of the anti-apoptotic Bcl-xL. CD28 ligation has also been suggested to promote TH2 pathways. Signals delivered via CD28 are also important for isotype switching in B cells. The cytoplasmic domain of CD28 is associated with Src kinases. Upon stimulation, phosphorylation of CD28 is thought to recruit PI3-kinase which ultimately leads to NFκB activation (chapter 6), IL-2 production, and T cell proliferation.

❑ **ICOS** (**I**nducible T cell **Cos**timulator) is another stimulatory molecule expressed on activated T cells. Its ligand, ICOSL, is expressed on B cells, DCs, macrophages, etc. Signals through ICOS are thought to be more important in cytokine production by recently activated and effector T cells. The ICOS pathway seems to enhance production of both TH1 and TH2 cytokines, though some recent reports suggest that engagement of ICOS preferentially induces IL-10 production.

❑ **CTLA-4** (**C**ytotoxic **T** **L**ymphocyte **A**ntigen-4; CD152) is an inhibitory receptor expressed on activated T cells and showing ~30% homology to CD28. It binds the same ligands as CD28 (ie, CD80 and CD86) but with a higher affinity. CTLA-4-KO mice develop fatal lymphoproliferative disease. Taken together, these facts suggest that CTLA-4 helps in the termination of immune responses. CTLA-4 inhibits T cell activation by reducing IL-2 production and IL-2R expression and by arresting T cells in the G1 phase of the cell cycle. Experimental data suggests that specific TcR and CD28 signals are essential in triggering the initial activation of CD4$^+$ T cells and secondarily of CD8$^+$ T cells and that the normal function of CTLA-4 is to stop this proliferation. CD4$^+$CD25$^+$ TR cells have been found to constitutively express CTLA-4, suggesting a possible suppressive role for this molecule. CTLA-4 cross-linking has been shown to inhibit activation of MAP kinases as well as several transcription factors, including NFκB, AP-1 and NFAT.

❑ **PD-1** (**P**rogrammed **D**eath gene-1) is an inhibitory molecule expressed by activated (but not resting) CD4$^+$ and CD8$^+$ T cells, B cells and myeloid cells. PD-1 has an ITIM in its cytoplasmic tail. Its ligands (PD-1L1 and PD-1L2) are expressed by not only haematopoietic cells but also cells in non-lymphoid tissues. Expression of the ligand in non-lymphoid tissue has led to the suggestion that it may be involved in the regulation of self-reactive responses in the periphery and/or regulation of inflammatory responses at these sites. Engagement of PD-1 by its ligands is thought to control the proliferation and cytokine expression of these cells.

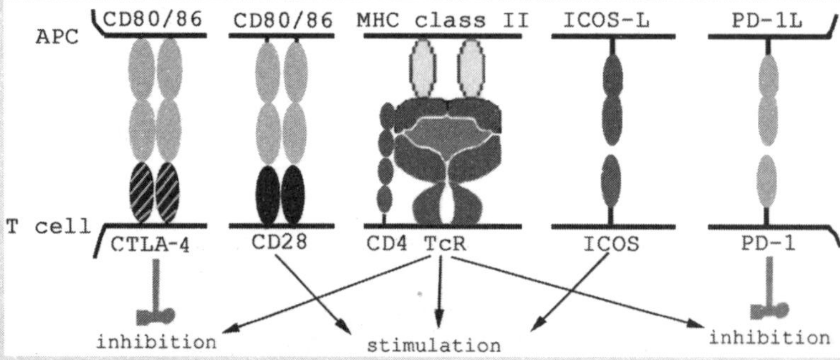

Figure 8.S3 *The eventual outcome of antigen recognition by T cells is dictated by the engagement of costimulatory molecules on T cells by their ligands on APCs.*

activated T cells and renders them tolerant instead; it is constitutively expressed on T_R cells.

8.3.2 Development

T cells, like other cells of the blood-forming system, are derived from pleuripotent haematopoietic stem cells present in the foetal liver or adult bone marrow. These haematopoietic stem cells are confronted with successive cell fate specification events and the choices made determine the type of lymphocyte as well as the functions it performs.

1. The cells take the path of the common lymphoid progenitor cells — these cells have lost the potential to become erythroid or myeloid cells but they retain the capability to give rise to lymphoid cells (B, T, NK) and possibly, DCs.
2. The cells become committed to the T cell lineage.
3. The cells must choose the path of development into $\alpha\beta$ or $\gamma\delta$ T cells.
4. The $\alpha\beta$ T cells must silence either the CD4 or the CD8 genes to become CD8$^+$ or CD4$^+$ T cells.
5. The last phase occurs only after antigenic challenge, and it is commitment to memory cell or effector cell fate.

The development of T cells is thus a very complicated process. Factors and cells involved in this development are still being identified. The development of NKT cells is even less understood. A simplified version of T cell development is described below. Students new to the subject are strongly encouraged to read these sections only after becoming knowledgeable about thymic architecture, TcR structure, and gene rearrangement and T cell functions. T cell development can be divided into two broad stages.

❑ In **phase I** (also called the early phase) lymphoid progenitor cells give rise to
  - $\gamma\delta$ T cells and
  - $\alpha\beta$ T cells expressing CD4 and CD8 (called DP or **D**ouble **P**ositive cells).
❑ In **phase II** (late phase), DP cells give rise to mature SP (**S**ingle **P**ositive; expressing either CD4 or CD8) $\alpha\beta$ T cells that leave the thymus and migrate to the periphery.

8.3.2.1 $\alpha\beta$ T Cell Development Phase I

The initial stages of thymocyte differentiation are outlined below (fig. 8.2).

❑ CD34$^+$ committed lymphoid progenitor cells arise in the bone marrow and migrate to the thymus via the blood. These cells can develop into T cells, B cells, NK cells, or DCs, depending upon the signals they receive. As a first step towards becoming T cells, the progenitors lose the potential to develop as NK cells, B cells, or DCs, giving rise to DN (**D**ouble **N**egative, ie, neither CD4 nor CD8) precursors. They do not express RAG-1 and RAG-2 proteins.
❑ DN cells express surface molecules that are characteristic of the early phase of T cell development. The first membrane molecule to be expressed is c-kit, a receptor for SCF. They also express the receptor for IL-7. Both IL-7 and c-kit ligand are essential factors for early T progenitor maintenance. IL-7 and IL-15 seem to be the only cytokines indispensable for development from the DN cells to SP cells. Signalling via IL-7 is thought to rescue thymocytes from apoptosis by inducing the expression of anti-apoptotic Bcl-2. It seems to have a role in the development of $\gamma\delta$ T cells as well. Experiments show that IL-15 is needed for the generation and maintenance of $\gamma\delta$ intraepithelial T cells and CD8$^+$ memory T cells.

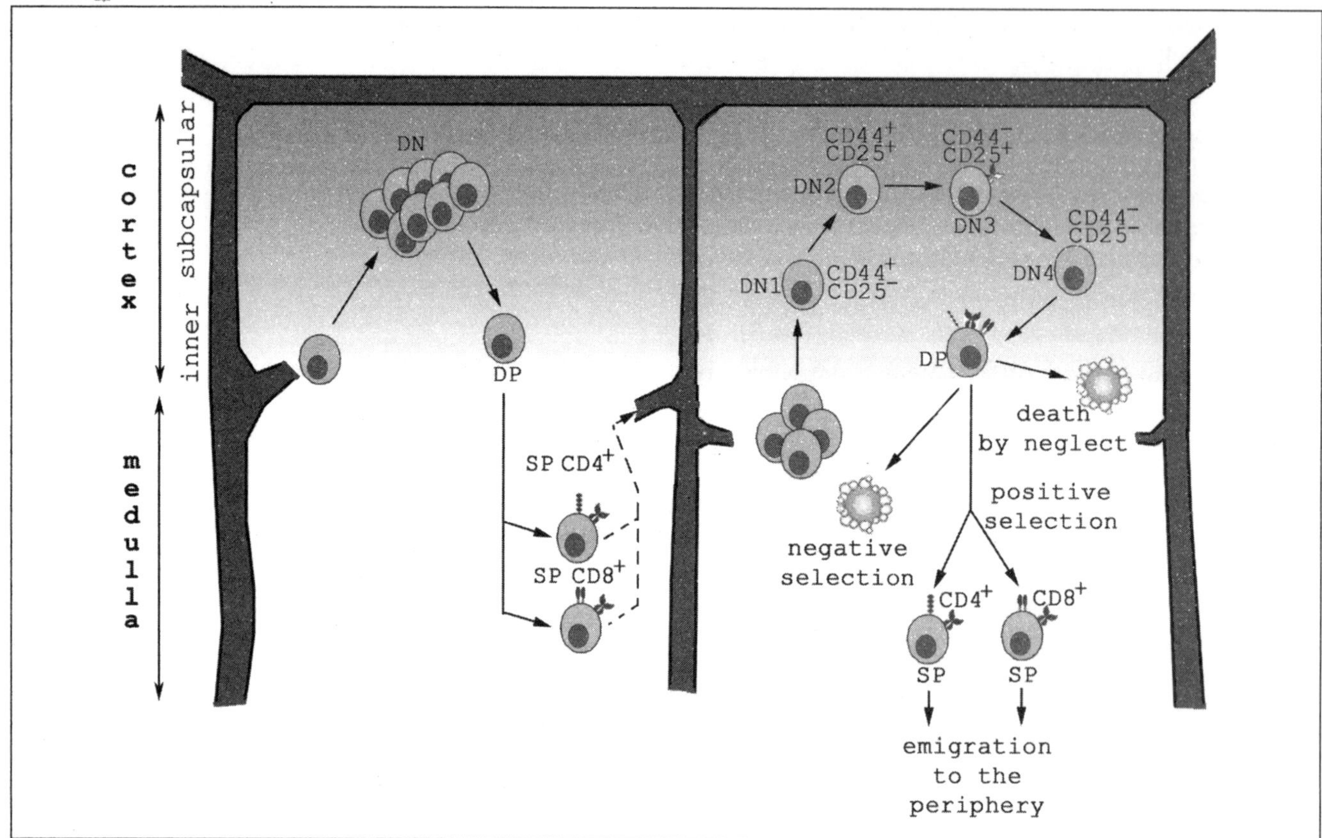

Figure 8.2 T lymphocytes undergo a complicated process of development in the thymus. *CD34⁺ lymphoid progenitors committed to the T cell lineage enter the thymus at the cortico-medullary junction. These are DN (Double Negative) cells that do not express either CD4 or CD8 coreceptors. The left panel in the figure depicts the migratory path of the thymocytes; the right panel depicts the different stages of development. After entering the thymus, thymocytes begin moving inwards to the cortex where they start dividing while migrating towards the subcapsular cortex. Thymic stromal cells differentially influence the developing thymocytes on their developmental pathway. The thymocytes undergo four phases of differentiation distinguished by their CD44 and CD25 expression. DN1 cells express the adhesion molecule CD44. They enter the DN2 phase when they start expressing CD25 as well. Cells in the DN3 phase downregulate CD44 expression but express pre-TcR consisting of a pre-TcRα chain (white subunit) and a rearranged TcRβ chain (grey subunit). TcR expression is downregulated in the DN4 (CD44⁻CD25⁻) stage when the α chain is undergoing rearrangement. The cells start expressing rearranged TcR and both CD4 and CD8 molecules as they enter the DP (Double Positive) phase. In the inner cortex, DP cells undergo further maturation and positive and negative selection. Their development into mature, SP (Single Positive) cells is absolutely dependent on the ability of the TcR to interact with MHC class I and class II molecules on stromal cells. Those cells that fail to obtain survival signals undergo death by neglect. DP cells that bind self-ligands with too high an affinity or the MHC molecules with too low an affinity are weeded out by negative selection. Cells recognizing self-MHC molecules with moderate affinity are allowed to survive. Cells that survive the selection processes enter the medulla for the final stage of development before leaving the thymus. These cells eventually lose expression of either CD4 or CD8 to become SP cells and exit the thymus to migrate to the periphery (Adapted from Trends in Immunology (2002) 23:305).*

- ❑ When the thymocytes start expressing CD44 (a cell adhesion molecule), they enter the first of four stages (DN1 to DN4) of differentiation of DN cells, distinguished by CD44 and CD25 expression.
- ❑ Cells in the DN1 phase of maturation are CD44⁺CD25⁻; these cells start expressing CD25 and enter the DN2 stage.
- ❑ CD44⁺CD25⁺ DN2 cells also express CD127 — those that are CD127^{lo} enter the αβ lineage, whereas CD127^{hi} cells seem to be predisposed to the γδ lineage.
- ❑ Cells proceeding along the αβTcR pathway downregulate their CD44 and c-kit expression as they enter the DN3 stage. These cells have the CD44⁻CD25⁺ phenotype and start expressing a surrogate α chain — pre-TcRα. This is analogous to surrogate L chain expression by B cells. pre-TcRα chain is encoded by a

non-rearranging locus. The cells also express RAG-1 and RAG-2, the enzymes needed for TcR gene rearrangement.

❏ The TcRβ chain is the first to be rearranged. The pre-TcRα pairs with a rearranged TcRβ to give pre-TcR that is expressed on the cell surface. This pre-TcR is also associated with the CD3 complex.

❏ Cells in the late DN3/early DN4 stage (CD44$^-$CD25$^+$pre-TcRαβ$^+$) must receive signals through the CD3 complex to allow further development. Interaction of the pre-TcR with an unknown ligand leads to activation of the Src family kinases (Lck, Syk) and ZAP-70. As in the B cells, signalling through pre-TcR suppresses further gene rearrangement of the β chain, ensuring the allelic exclusion of this chain.

❏ Eventually, CD25 expression is downregulated, and the cells enter DN4 stage (CD44$^-$CD25$^-$).

❏ They undergo a short burst of proliferation (six to eight cell divisions) before the TcRα chain undergoes gene rearrangement. TcR expression is low at this stage, since the pre-TcRα disappears from the cell surface and the rearranged TcRα chain is yet to be expressed. Thymocytes also begin to express coreceptors at this stage — first CD8 and then CD4.

❏ The DN4 stage thus ends with the cells becoming DP (expressing both CD4 and CD8) and having a rearranged TcR associated with the CD3 complex.

❏ These DP immature cells expressing αβTcR constitute 90% of the lymphoid compartment of the young thymus. Their development into mature cells is absolutely dependent on the ability of the TcR to interact with MHC class I and class II molecules on stromal cells — especially thymic cortical epithelial cells (nurse cells). *En route* to maturation, thymocytes are subjected to four different selective processes:

- **Death by neglect.** Unlike in the other selective processes, death by neglect (as the name suggests) is caused by the failure to obtain survival signals. In order to survive and progress further than the DP stage, T cells must obtain survival signals via TcR. However, a large fraction of DP cells fail to bind MHC molecules expressed on thymic stromal cells. Such cells that do not encounter their restricting MHC molecule on the thymic epithelium undergo death by neglect within 3–4 days.

- **Negative selection.** DP cells that bind self-ligands with too high an affinity are weeded out by negative selection. A transcription factor called AIRE (**A**utoimmune **R**egulator), expressed in the epithelial cells of the medulla, promotes expression of tissue-specific proteins that are not normally expressed in the thymus. AIRE enables the epithelial cells of the cortex and medulla to display a sampling of peptides derived from tissue-specific proteins normally expressed in various tissues of the body. In addition, cortex and medullary epithelial cells also display peptides derived from proteins brought to the thymus by the blood stream as well as those derived from thymic cells. High affinity binding of the TcR to these MHC:peptide complexes generates an apoptotic signal in developing thymocytes.

- **Positive selection.** If binding of the TcR to the self-ligands is too weak, the signal generated by the TcR is not enough to sustain survival and the cell dies. Positive selection thus allows the survival of cells recognizing self-MHC molecules. Thymic epithelial cells have a major role in this positive selection[16].

- **Lineage-specific development.** In the late phase of development, DP cells lose one of their coreceptors and finally mature to CD4$^+$ or CD8$^+$ T cells. If the coreceptor expressed mismatches the MHC molecule engaged (eg, if the TcR binds best to MHC class I molecule but the cell expresses CD4 coreceptor or vice versa), the signal generated by TcR engagement is not sufficient to sustain survival, and the cell undergoes apoptosis. Only a small fraction (5%) of cells survive these selective forces and are allowed to mature and migrate to the periphery (fig. 8.2).

[16] This is sometimes referred to as the 'tickling rule'. Cells that are tickled too much or too little die; only those cells that are tickled moderately survive to tell the tale ☺.

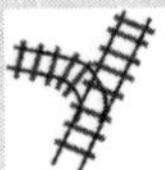

Not Immune to Death?

The immune system must achieve a balance between the need to be able to react to a multitude of antigens and the danger of autoimmunity. It must also maintain homeostasis so that the total number of lymphocytes after an antigen-specific clonal expansion reverts to baseline level. It achieves this by fine-tuning a balance between expansion and death. As a general rule, the immune system produces more cells than needed and eliminates them by apoptosis. Apoptosis is thus a central regulatory feature of the immune system. A group of enzymes called caspases are central to causing death. These enzymes are normally present as proenzymes that have to be cleaved to yield the active form of the enzyme[17]. Death is achieved by two different downstream pathways (section 11.2).

B cell death. Three cell surface molecules are key elements in the regulation of B cell survival and death — BcR, CD95, and CD40. As a general rule, BcR activation induces apoptosis by the mitochondrial pathway. The stage of maturation, the quality and quantity of signals provided, cytokines, and other factors in the microenvironment are vital in dictating whether or not the death signal is overridden. Costimulation by way of CD40 (via CD40L on T cells or macrophages) can rescue B cells from apoptosis. B cells in the germinal centre can be rescued from death by the combined effects of BcR and CD40 engagement, since signalling through these molecules upregulates the anti-apoptotic protein Bcl-xL. However, other signals that promote B cell survival and differentiation are yet to be determined. Factors that can cause plasma cell death and the anti-apoptotic signals that can rescue them are also unclear.

T cell death. Only 3–5% of immature thymocytes leave the thymus as mature T cells. The rest undergo apoptosis due to death by neglect or during positive and negative selection. Understanding of the molecular basis of this apoptosis, however, remains fragmentary. Mature peripheral T cells undergo apoptosis. Death by neglect occurs in those T cells that are insufficiently stimulated by growth signals. It also occurs at the peak or down phase of the immune response, allowing the downregulation of the number of reactive cells and termination of the immune response. Activation of T cells induces CD95L expression. However, in the initial clonal expansion phase of the response, T cells are relatively resistant to CD95-induced cell death. Similarly, memory cells are also resistant to apoptosis. Effector T cells, on the other hand, are susceptible to apoptosis via the DISC pathway and the expression of Bcl-xL can rescue them. Like B cells, T cells can also be rescued from apoptotic death by costimulatory signals via CD28.

Apoptosis and disease. Since apoptosis is fundamental to the regulation of the immune system, its derailment can lead to severe diseases. Dysfunction of CD95 causes the autoimmune lymphoproliferative syndrome in humans. Children with this disease show massive non-malignant lymphadenopathy and severe autoimmunity. In many cases, the disease has been traced to mutations in the death domain of CD95. In mice, the *lpr* (**lymphopro**liferation) and *gld* (**g**eneralized **lympha**denopathy) mutations are found to cause a disease similar to SLE. In lpr mice, a point mutation in the death domain of CD95 abolishes apoptotic signal transmission; the gld mice carry a point mutation in the Carboxy– terminal of CD95L. Failure of apoptosis also leads to tumour survival. Translocation of *Bcl-2* into the Ig H chain locus causes the deregulation of *Bcl-2* expression and results in follicular lymphomas. HIV uses this same apoptotic signal to its own advantage. Regulatory viral gene products (like Tat-1 of HIV-1) penetrate non-infected T cells and render them hypersensitive to TcR-induced CD95-mediated apoptosis. Further sensitization of CD4$^+$ T cells results from the binding of HIV gp120 to CD4 and cross-linking of the bound gp120 by anti-gp120 antibodies produced in response to the infection. The massive death of CD4$^+$ T cells leaves the patient defenceless against opportunistic pathogens and neoplasms, and ultimately, it results in the death of the patient.

This process of overproducing cells and then sending them down the road of apoptosis may appear to be insanely wasteful. To appreciate the logic behind this phenomenon, the constraints under which the T cells operate have to be understood. T cells have to function for the well-being of the individual in the cellular environment of that individual. They must bind the antigen in the context of self-MHC molecules, ie, they must respond to self-MHC molecules. At the same time, this recognition

[17] This is a common feature of all potentially harmful proteins (eg, complement components, caspases, etc.), since it gives greater regulatory control on their activity.

should not be of a high affinity, since that increases the danger of autoimmune responses. Similarly, T cells recognizing self-peptides in the context of self-MHC molecules also cannot be allowed to survive. Although the unselected repertoire of TcR is biased towards MHC recognition, the gene rearrangement and protein pairing processes that generate TcR are random. Thus, the likelihood that the TcRs produced will recognize MHC:peptide complexes present in the individual is slim. Hence, a large fraction of T cells will fail to bind MHC molecules and will undergo death by neglect. Conversely, a percentage of the T cells that do recognize MHC:self-peptide complexes in the individual will bind too well to self-ligands. These cells will be removed by negative selection. Only cells that express TcRs that recognize self-ligands but generate signals that have an intensity that is between these two extremes (no binding or high affinity binding) can initiate the multi-step positive selection process that results in lineage-specific differentiation to mature CD4$^+$ or CD8$^+$ T cells. The function of the T cell will be dictated by this choice — CD4$^+$ T cells are destined for a predominantly helper/regulator role, CD8$^+$ T cells are destined to be cytolytic cells. Optimal T cell function depends upon matching the MHC class specificity of the coreceptor and TcR. Nevertheless, it is important to point out that the selection procedures are imperfect and autoreactive clones are found in the periphery. Peripheral regulatory mechanisms are therefore needed to ensure absence of self-reactivity.

8.3.2.2 αβ T Cell Development Phase II

αβ thymocyte differentiation involves a change from the DP to the SP state by the silencing of the transcription of one coreceptor locus and the accompanying genetic events that determine the effector potential of the mature T cell. Progression from DP to SP state (ie, either CD4$^+$CD8$^-$ or CD4$^-$CD8$^+$) seems to comprise a series of intermediate states.

1. The DP cells initially downregulate both CD4 and CD8 to become CD4^{lo}CD8^{lo}TcR^{int} and are uncommitted cells.
2a. Commitment to CD4 lineage leads to upregulation of CD4 expression and the cells become CD4$^+$CD8^{lo}. TcR expression may also be upregulated at this stage. Eventually, these cells loose CD8 expression and emerge as CD4$^+$ SP with a high level of TcR expression.
2b. Cells committed to become CD8$^+$ T cells show the CD4^{lo}CD8^{hi}TcR^{hi} phenotype on the road to becoming CD8$^+$ T cells. Eventually, CD4 expression is silenced altogether and the cells become CD8$^+$TcR^{hi} SP cells.

The development of SP cells from DP cells has been a matter of intense research, much debate, and some degree of confusion. The 'strength of signal model' outlined below has gained general consensus now (fig. 8.3). This model proposes that commitment to CD4 or CD8 lineage depends upon the intensity or duration of signalling from the TcR. Short duration signals lead to the CD8 pathway; more prolonged signalling leads to the CD4 pathway. The CD4 in CD4$^+$CD8$^+$ thymocytes is more extensively associated with the lymphocyte specific protein tyrosine kinase (Lck). Thus, the binding of MHC class II molecules on the thymic epithelial cells by the TcR and CD4 tends to produce a prolonged signal, whereas TcR-CD8 engagement by MHC class I molecules produces a weak signal. Depending upon the receptors engaged, four different outcomes are possible.

❑ TcR-CD4-MHC class II engagement results in a prolonged signal and allows immature thymocytes to develop along the right pathway (ie, expressing MHC class II binding TcR and CD4).
❑ If the TcR binds MHC class II molecules on the thymic stromal cells weakly, the cells will dissociate rapidly, and the signal generated will be of a short duration. As a result, CD4 expression will be downregulated and CD8 expression

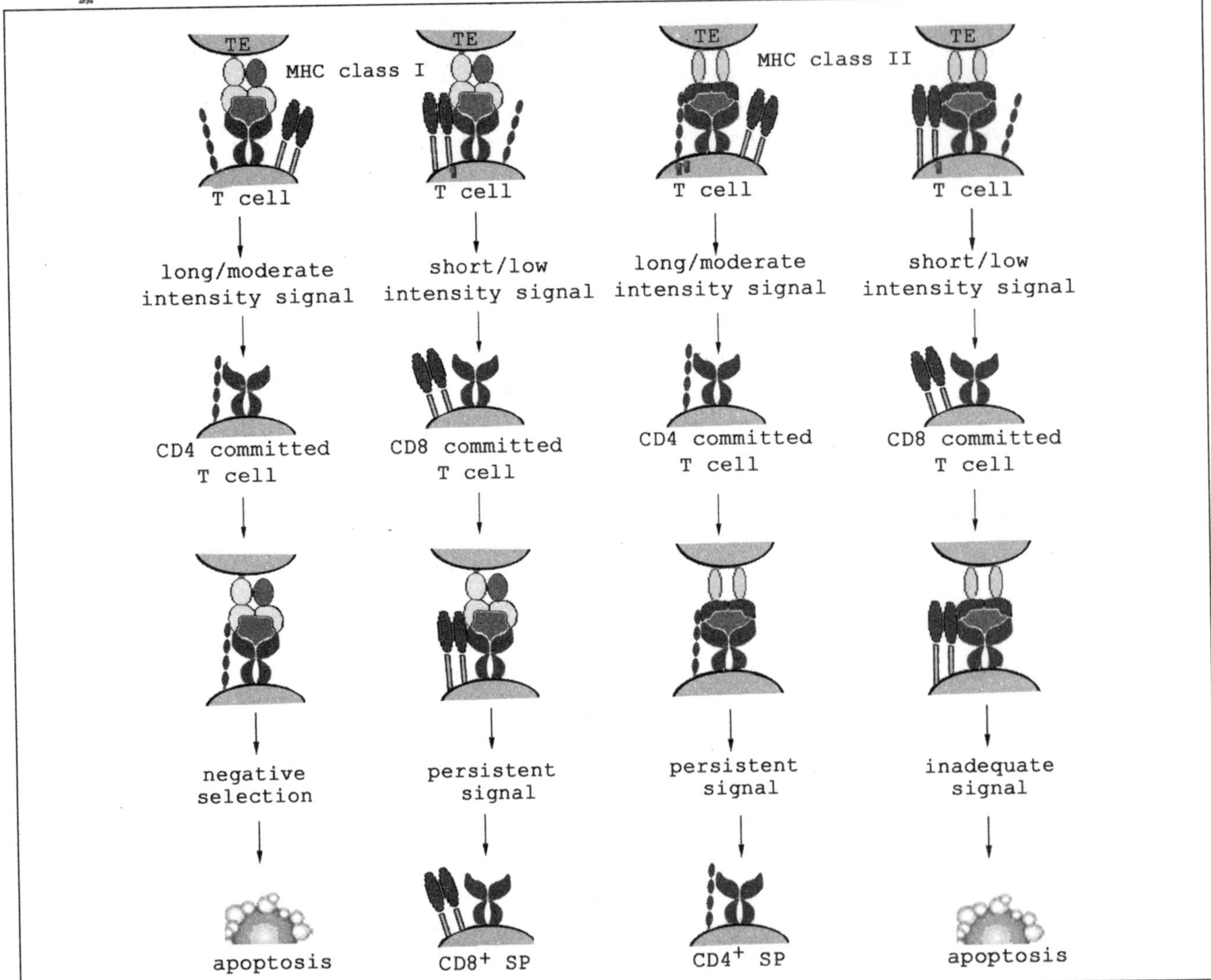

Figure 8.3 The strength of signal model for development of SP (single positive) cells from DP (double positive) cells proposes that commitment to CD4 or CD8 lineage depends upon the intensity or duration of signalling from the TcR complex. Signals generated by the engagement of MHC:peptide complexes on thymic epithelial cells (TE) by TcR dictate the further development of T cells. Short duration/low intensity signals send the cell on the CD8 path, whereas long duration/moderate intensity signals send them on the path of CD4 development. CD4 is more extensively associated with the kinase Lck than CD8. MHC class II:CD4 binding of TcR will therefore produce a more prolonged signal than MHC class I:CD8 binding, and most immature thymocytes will end up making the 'correct' choice (two central panels). If, however, the TcR expressed by the T cell binds peptide:MHC class II complex with low affinity, the signal generated by the MHC:TcR engagement will be of low intensity, and the cell will end up in the incorrect path of CD8 development. It will express CD8 and yet have a TcR that binds MHC class II molecules (extreme right panel). The signal generated will be insufficient to support further development of such mismatched cells, and they will eventually die. Conversely, if the TcR binds the MHC class I:peptide ligand with high affinity, a long signal will be produced, resulting in a cell being committed to the inappropriate CD4 lineage (extreme left panel). These cells that bind self-peptides with high affinity will be eliminated by negative selection (Adapted from Nature Reviews in Immunology (2002) 2:309).

upregulated. Such cells will fail to complete the maturation process, since the signalling capacity of TcR in the absence of CD4 will prove inadequate to support subsequent development.

❑ If, on the other hand, the immature thymocytes bind MHC class I molecules with too high an affinity, they will generate too strong a signal and enter the CD4 pathway. These 'mismatched' cells (having MHC class I binding TcR but CD4 coreceptor) will be eliminated by negative selection.

❑ Engagement of MHC class I molecules by TcR-CD8 generates a weak signal. As a result, CD4 expression will be downregulated, and CD8 expression will be upregulated. The cells will enter the CD8 pathway and develop into CD8+ T cells.

Information on how the signalling strength dictates lineage choice is scarce — partly because many of these molecules also have roles in earlier stages of thymocyte differentiation, making the KO mice approach non-usable. MAP kinase 1, NOTCH[18], and its ligands are known to be involved in this differentiation, but their exact role is unclear.

8.3.2.3 γδ T Cell Development

The exact steps involved in the maturation of γδ T cells are still being defined. Following definitive commitment to the T cell lineage, thymocytes start expressing CD25, RAG-1, and RAG-2 and enter the DN2 phase (CD44+CD25−) of development. These cells start rearranging their β, γ, and δ chains. Those that successfully rearrange the β chain enter the αβ lineage; those that rearrange γδ chains enter that lineage. The exact signals or events responsible for these choices or promoting these choices are unclear. γδTcR seems to promote αβ lineage development, but the extent to which γδTcR or pre-TcR play a role in the lineage commitment is also controversial.

Despite similarities in the overall structure of their genes and polypeptide chains, γδ T cells are quite different from αβ T cells with respect to development, repertoire, and extra-thymic tissue distribution. γδ T cells are found in the adult peripheral blood and lymphoid tissues as well as in epithelial tissues such as skin. This homing of the γδ subset to the peripheral organs is probably determined by distinct homing receptors. These cells are often CD4−CD8− and can recognize both proteinic and non-proteinic antigens independent of the MHC (Table 8.3).

Table 8.3 Major distinguishing features of B cells, αβ T cells and γδ T cells

Characteristic	B cells	αβ T cells	γδ T cells
Antigen receptor	Ig	αβTcR	γδTcR
Antigen recognized	Proteinic and non-proteinic	MHC:peptide complexes	Proteinic and non-proteinic
MHC restriction	−	+	Rare
Coreceptors	CD19/21 complex	CD4 or CD8	CD4 and CD8 absent, IELs — CD8αα
Frequency in blood	5–10%	65–75%	5–10% 25–60% in gut
Effector mechanism	Ig production	CTLs — cytotoxic granules and death receptor pathways TH1, TH2, or TR — cytokine release	CTLs — cytotoxic granules and death receptor pathways TH1>TH2; cytokine release
Function	Humoral immunity	Immune protection, pathogen eradication, immune regulation.	Immunosurveillance, immune regulation.

8.3.2.4 NKT Cell Development

NKT cells represent a subset of mature T lymphocytes expressing αβTcR as well as markers characteristic of NK cells such as CD56, CD57 (in humans; mice NKT cells express NK1.1), and CD122 (IL-2Rβ). In mice, mature NKT cells constitute a small percentage of T cells found in the thymus, spleen, and bone marrow, but a significant proportion (20–30%) of those are found in the liver. In humans only 4% of hepatic T cells are NKT cells. NKT cells express a restricted T cell repertoire. The best characterized subset of human NKT cells expresses the NK cell marker CD161. The TcR of these cells has an α chain consisting of a particular VJ segment

[18] *NOTCH* genes encode highly conserved cell surface receptors that regulate the development of a wide spectrum of cell types. NOTCH signalling functions in multiple cell fate decisions during lymphocyte development, including commitment to T cell lineage and differentiation to DN and SP stage.

(Vα24JαQ) with no junctional additions or deletions (hence referred to as 'invariant α chain'). It is associated with variant β chain (predominantly Vβ11).

Many aspects of the development of NKT cells are still controversial. Most NKT cells seem to develop intrathymically, although there is some evidence to suggest that a small fraction of NKT cells could originate and develop extra-thymically. The jury is still out on whether NKT cells develop from conventional DP thymocytes or from pre-committed precursor cells of a distinct lineage. Recent experimental evidence favours the former. Conventional DP thymocytes seem to get diverted to the NKT lineage as a result of CD1d engagement by randomly generated semi-invariant TcRs. The molecular requirements and main events in the development and selection of NKT cells also remain poorly understood.

8.3.2.5 Migration in the Thymus

Lymphocytes or thymocytes from the foetal liver and yolk sac migrate to the rudimentary thymus on about the tenth to twelfth day of embryogenesis. They colonize the thymus and ultimately give rise to T cells. In adults, T cell precursors, like B cell precursors, are formed in the bone marrow. These precursors enter the thymus at the cortico-medullary junction and are recruited from the blood stream by chemo-attractants that are produced by thymic epithelial cells. β_2-m has an important role in this recruitment. To enter the thymus, precursor T cells must attach to the endothelium of thymic blood vessels. CD44 expressed by the thymocytes is thought to play a role in this entry. Other adhesion molecules such as LFA-1, ICAM-1, CD2, LFA-3, and CDw90 (thy-1) are found to be important in subsequent interactions with thymic epithelial cells. Thymic stromal cells (subcapsular epithelial cells, thymic cortical epithelial cells, medullary epithelial cells, fibroblasts, macrophages, and thymic DCs) differentially influence the developing thymocytes on their developmental pathway. These stromal cells constitute the microenvironment where developing T cells receive signals to proliferate and mature, or undergo apoptosis through cell-cell interactions and contact with locally secreted hormones and cytokines. Additionally, extracellular matrix proteins such as fibronectin, laminin, and collagen expressed by stromal cells are also important in the adhesion and migration of thymocytes.

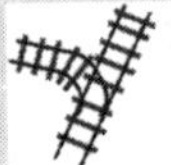

Instant Chemistry: Chemokines

Chemokines (**chemo**attractant cyto**kines**) were originally discovered because of their chemotactic properties — they were found to regulate leukocyte transport by mediating leukocyte adhesion to endothelial walls, initiation of transendothelial migration, and tissue invasion. It is now clear that chemokines are pleuripotent molecules with diverse functions in the development of the immune system and the progress of the immune response. They also regulate varied processes such as angiogenesis, haematopoiesis, and organogenesis of primary and secondary lymphoid organs. Chemokines are a family of structurally related single polypeptides (~70–100 amino acids in length). These heparin-binding proteins contain conserved cysteines at the NH_2– terminus. The number and spacing of the first two cysteines is used to characterize chemokines into subfamilies (C, CC, CXC, CX_3C), where X stands for single amino acids. CXC (α) and CC (β) are the largest of these groups.

Chemokines act through chemokine receptors. These structurally homologous receptors have seven transmembrane domains and are coupled to small G proteins. The receptors are named by the chemokine subfamily followed by a number (CCR1-9, CXCR5, etc). As is common with most newly discovered proteins, chemokines were referred to by multiple names. Additionally, single chemokines can bind to multiple receptors, compounding the confusion. According to the standardized nomenclature now adopted, chemokines are named by the subfamily they belong to followed by L (for ligand) and a number.

The role of chemokines in leukocyte adhesion and migration is well documented. Chemokines upregulate expression of adhesion molecules on leukocytes, inducing their arrest and firm adhesion. Chief amongst the secreted chemokines is IL-8 which acts on neutrophils, MCP-1 (**M**onocyte

Chemoattractant **P**rotein-**1**; CCL2) that induces adhesion of monocytes, and eotaxin (CCL11) that induces adhesion of eosinophils. Important amongst the transmembrane proteins are fractalkine (CX_3CL) and CXCL16 that mediate adhesion of NK cells and $CD8^+$ T cells.

Chemokines and their receptors are indispensable in T and B cell maturation. Both these cell types are produced in the bone marrow and must travel to other organs (thymus and spleen respectively) during their development and maturation. This migration is achieved by regulating expression of various chemokine receptors during maturation. Intrathymic migration of T lymphocytes is accomplished by the expression of different chemokines by distinct thymic areas. Chemokines also contribute to the sorting of positively and negatively selected thymocytes. They are also known to influence T cell differentiation to $T_{H}1$ or $T_{H}2$ subsets.

❑ SDF-1 (**S**tromal cell **D**erived **F**actor-1; CXCL12) prevalent at the cortico-medullary junction of the thymus is an important chemotactic factor for $CD34^+$ progenitor cells.

❑ TECK (**T**hymus **E**xpressed **C**hemokine; CCL25) seems to stimulate the migration of DN cells from the outer cortex to inner cortical regions as they differentiate to DP thymocytes. TECK may act as a chemoattractant for newly selected SP cells as they pass from the cortex to the medulla following selection.

❑ ELC (**E**pstein-Barr virus **I**nduced molecule 1-**L**igand **C**hemokine; CCL19) and SLC (**S**econdary **L**ymphoid tissue **C**hemokine; CCL21), expressed by medullary epithelial cells, have a role in intrathymic migration of SP cells. They also have a role in recirculation of lymphocytes in the secondary lymphoid organs (spleen, lymph nodes, and Peyer's patches). Naïve B and T cells express CCR7, the ligand for ELC and SLC and as a result, home to secondary lymphoid tissues expressing these chemokines. SLC expressed by HEV cells is responsible for T cell trafficking through the lymph nodes.

❑ BLC (**B** **L**ymphocyte **C**hemoattractant), expressed by stromal cells in B cell areas, helps localize B cells to this compartment of the lymphoid follicles of all secondary lymphoid organs.

❑ Chemokines regulate the movement of B cells and T cells from their respective areas to B cell– T cell border.
  - BcR stimulation promotes expression of CCR7, allowing the B cell to migrate towards T cell zones (rich in ELC and SLC) of the follicle.
  - Activated B cells also start expressing other chemokines that attract activated T cells.
  - Activated T cells express receptors for chemokines and start moving to the edge of the T cell zone.
  - These T cells also express CCR5, the receptor for BLC, further enhancing their propensity to move to the B cell area and allowing the rare antigen-specific B cell to present antigen to the rare antigen-specific T cell.

❑ MCP-1 (CCL2) is found to be a positive regulator of the $T_{H}2$ pathways; it inhibits IL-12 production by DCs and promotes differentiation to $T_{H}2$ type. Conversely, RANTES (CCL5), MIP-3α (**M**acrophage **I**nflammatory **P**rotein-**3**α, CCL3), and MIP-1β (CCL4) promote IL-12 secretion by APCs along with directly promoting differentiation to $T_{H}1$ type.

After entering the thymus, thymocytes begin moving inwards to the cortex where they start dividing while migrating towards the subcapsular cortex, which is located just under the outer border of the cortex (fig. 8.3). Thymus-expressed chemokines have been shown to play a key role — both in the initial colonization of the thymus as well as in the migration of cells within the thymus. In the inner cortex, DP cells undergo further maturation and positive and negative selection. Thymic nurse cells found in the cortex are thought to be important players in this thymic education of T cells (section 5.2.1). Since the nurse cells express neuropeptides like vasopressin and oxytocin, they may also be important in neurohormonal regulation within the thymus. Macrophages of the thymus have a major role in clearing dead or dying cells and protecting the thymic microenvironment from the potentially harmful effects of their cellular contents. Cells that have survived the selection processes enter the medulla for the final stage of development before they leave the thymus. Most mature SP cells are therefore found in the medulla. Naïve T cells leaving the thymus express homing receptors like CCR7 (see sidetrack 'Instant Chemistry') and CD62L, which allow their homing and entry into secondary lymphoid tissues.

8.3.3 Activation

Found predominantly in the T cell areas of spleen (PALS), lymph nodes and Peyer's patches (paracortex), naïve T cells (whether CD4$^+$ or CD8$^+$) circulate continuously from and to these areas via the lymph and blood. They are emptied into the marginal sinuses of the spleen along with blood. They then move into the red pulp and finally to the PALS. Upon reaching the PALS or paracortex, they tend to remain there, because they express CCR7 that binds to the chemokines CCL19 and CCL21 produced in the T cell areas. If they do not encounter their specific antigen, the cells leave the lymphoid tissue after about 24 hours and return to the blood, once again commencing their journey to a different lymphoid tissue (fig. 8.4). Naïve T cells are characterized by expression of low levels of most cell-adhesion molecules. However, they express high levels of the homing receptor, L-selectin (CD62L). It enables the cells to bind and roll across HEV, allowing their migration to and from the lymph node and permitting them to remain a part of the circulating lymphocyte pool. As they migrate through the cortical region of the lymph node, T cells bind transiently to any APCs they encounter via the adhesion molecules expressed by APCs. This gives the T cell enough time to sample the MHC molecules expressed by the APC for a specific peptide. Transient binding to APCs combined with continuous circulation allows T cells to monitor APC surfaces for peptide:MHC complexes. Only 1 in 10^4–10^6 T cells is likely to be specific for a particular antigen. The continuous circulation therefore also increases the probability that an antigen-specific T cell will come in contact with its specific peptide:MHC complex. During their normal pattern of blood to lymph recirculation, naïve T cells are metabolically quiescent and have a prolonged life span. This longevity requires at least two signals — contact with self-peptide:MHC complexes on DCs and IL-7. Recognition of these ligands probably delivers low-level signals which keep T cells sufficiently metabolically active to avoid passive death.

The migratory properties of T cells do not allow their entry into the initial site of infection. Naïve T cells are programmed to recognize antigens only in the T cell zones of lymphoid tissues, and the initiation of the immune response depends upon the transport of antigens to these areas from the site of infection. Cells involved in the transport and initiation of the immune response are given below.

❑ **DCs are the principal cells involved in antigen transport.** DCs capture antigen from the site of antigen deposition by macropinocytosis and phagocytosis and transport it to the local draining lymph node. Resting or immature DCs are incapable of stimulating T cells and need to be activated for antigen presentation. DCs express a number of PRRs on their surface. As a result, LPS or lipoproteins on the surface of most infectious micro-organisms provide the trigger needed for DC activation. Pro-inflammatory stimuli such as IFNs or cognate interaction with T cells via CD40-CD154 can also activate DCs. DCs seem to be able to present antigen from a variety of pathogens, whether viral, fungal, bacterial, or protozoan. DCs have an intrinsically high costimulatory capacity and may be particularly important in stimulating T cell responses to viruses which fail to induce costimulatory molecules in other types of APCs. DC activation

- Enhances the movement of DCs from non-lymphoid tissues to T cell areas,
- Causes DC maturation and increases the surface expression of MHC class II molecules required for maximal T cell stimulation,
- Upregulates the expression of costimulatory molecules; interaction of costimulatory molecules on T cells with their ligands on APCs (eg, CD134-CD134L, or CD28-CD80/86) can affect T cell activation by enhancing TcR signalling and may also provide additional signals that increase T cell responses, and
- Results in the synthesis and secretion of pro-inflammatory cytokines and chemokines by DCs and guides their movement to T cell areas; cytokines such

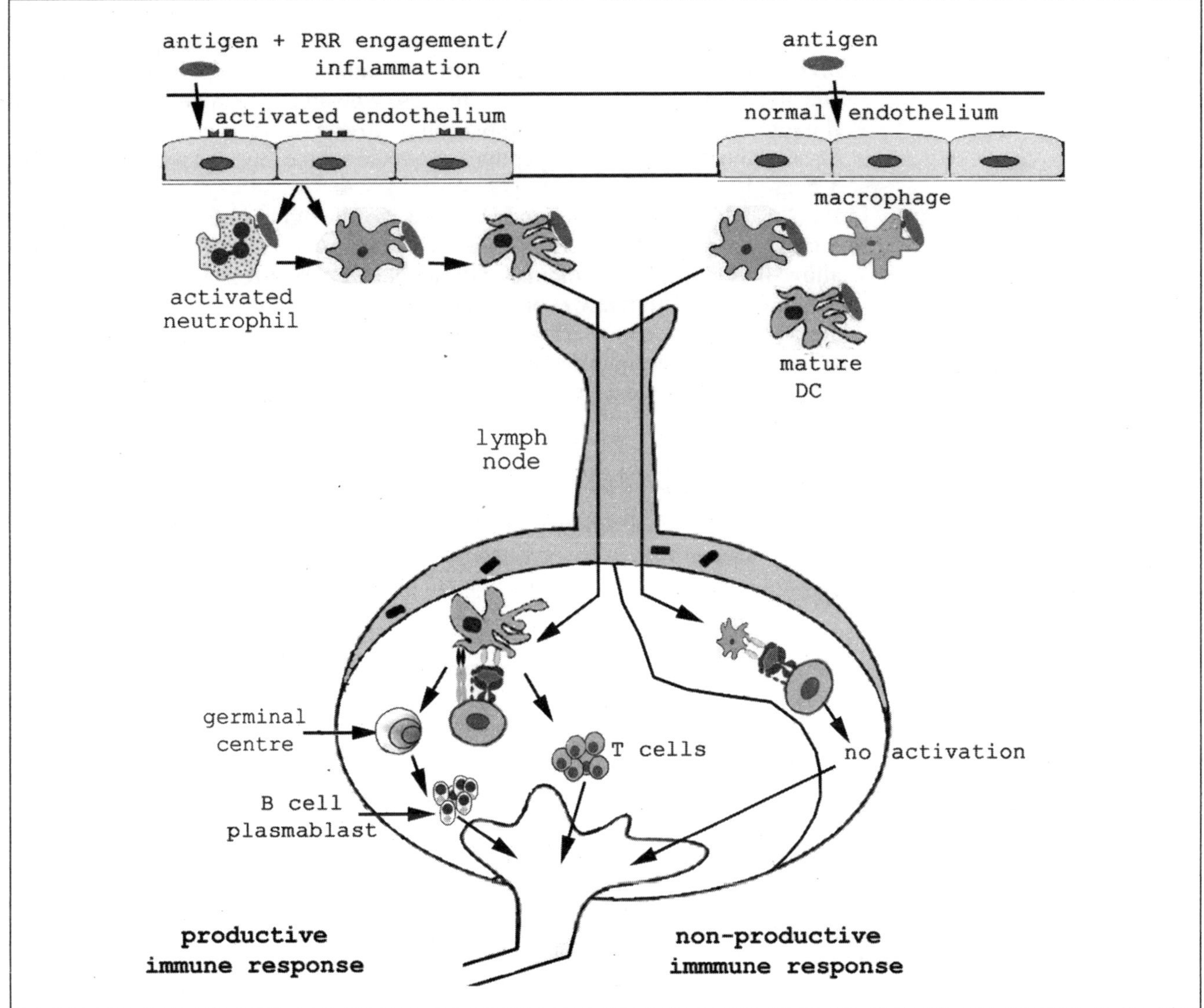

Figure 8.4 *Unstimulated APCs do not express costimulatory molecules and hence, do not trigger immune responses; exposure to pro-inflammatory stimuli induces costimulatory molecule expression and increases MHC class II expression, resulting in a productive immune response.* *Naïve T cells do not enter the site of infection. It is the job of the APCs to transport antigen to the lymphoid tissues (here represented by the lymph node) and initiate an immune response. Naïve T cells express high levels of L-selectin that enables them to bind and roll across HEVs (High Endothelial Venules) and allows their migration to and from the lymph node. T cells bind transiently to any APCs they encounter as they migrate through the cortical region of the lymph node and probe them for MHC:peptide complexes. Since unstimulated APCs express low levels of costimulatory molecules, recognition of self-peptide:MHC complexes on these cells does not activate the naïve T cells and prevents autoimmune responses (right). Recognition of pathogen-associated molecular patterns (PAMPs) or other pro-inflammatory stimuli (release of HSPs by damaged tissue cells, chemokines, or cytokines expressed by activated endothelium, etc) activates APCs and results in a productive immune response (left panel). Activation enhances their migration to the lymphoid tissues. Such activated APCs express high levels of costimulatory molecules and are efficient in antigen presentation. Antigen presentation triggers the activation, proliferation, and differentiation of naïve T cells to effector cells. Antigen recognition and signals obtained from the activated CD4$^+$ effector T cells results in activation, proliferation, and differentiation of naïve B cells in the germinal centres. Plasmablasts resulting from B cell differentiation give rise to plasma cells secreting Ig. The end result is a cell-mediated and humoral immune response.*

as IL-6 or TNF-α produced by DCs also provide secondary signals that complement CD28-CD80/86 costimulatory signals and further augment T cell activation.

❑ **Macrophages** are the body's scavengers involved in the removal of dead or dying cells. Resting macrophages express few MHC class II molecules and have no costimulatory capacity. This prevents them from activating self-reactive T cells and triggering autoimmune responses in spite of expressing self-peptide loaded MHC molecules. Macrophages express a number of receptors for microbial constituents (chapter 2). Contact with these constituents upregulates MHC class II expression. It also induces expression of costimulatory molecules like CD80/86, allowing them to present peptides derived from the ingested pathogen to naïve T cells.

❑ B cells, unlike macrophages and DCs, are capable of presenting soluble antigens internalized via BcR. B cells constitutively express MHC class II molecules that allow them to display a sampling of the antigens internalized by the cell. However, they do not constitutively express costimulatory molecules. Presentation of self-antigens by B cells therefore fails to activate naïve T cells and instead induces them to become anergic. Contact with microbial constituents, especially LPS, can induce the expression of costimulatory molecules, allowing them to become potent APCs.

The transient binding of adhesion molecules such as ICAM-1, ICAM-2, LFA-3, or DC-SIGN on APCs by LFA-1, CD2, or ICAM-3 on the T cells is of low affinity, allowing the cells to separate after brief contact. Recognition and engagement of MHC:peptide complex by the TcR results in the formation of a tight immunological synapse at the point of T cell: APC interaction within minutes.

T CELLS

❑ T lymphocytes mature in the thymus.
❑ Mature T cells
  • express either $\alpha\beta$ or $\gamma\delta$TcR that is associated with a host of other molecules,
  • mostly express either the CD4 or CD8 coreceptor, and
  • also express CD2, CD7, CD28, and MHC class I molecules.
❑ Activated T cells express CD25 and CD69 as well as costimulatory molecules; activated human T cells express MHC class II molecules.
❑ They develop from CD34$^+$ common lymphoid progenitor cells.
  • In the early phase of development, the DN cells give rise to DP cells expressing $\alpha\beta$ or $\gamma\delta$TcR.
  • The $\alpha\beta$ T cells then undergo positive and negative selection before entering the second phase of development.
  • In the late phase of development, transcription of one of the coreceptor genes is silenced to give SP $\alpha\beta$ T cells committed to CD4 or CD8 lineage.
❑ T cells are multifunctional cells.
  • TH cells are CD4$^+$ cells that co-operate with B cells in mounting a humoral response and help in activation of macrophages.
  • TR cells are also CD4$^+$ cells; they help in regulating immune responses as well as maintenance of tolerance to self-antigens.
  • CTLs are CD8$^+$ cells that kill infected, transformed, or mutated self-cells.
  • NKT cells recognize lipid antigens and are important in defence against intracellular parasites and tumours.
❑ Naïve T cells are programmed to recognize antigens only in the T cell zones of lymphoid tissues; APCs such as DCs, macrophages, and B cells transport antigen to these areas and present them to T cells.
❑ Activation of naïve T cells results in their proliferation and differentiation to effector and memory cells.
  • Antigen-specific T cells recognize MHC:peptide complexes on APC and a tight synapse is formed at the point of contact.
  • Signalling via TcR, CD3, coreceptors (CD4/CD8) and costimulatory molecules induces IL-2 synthesis in the T cells.
  • Cytokines released by APCs further aid in the process and drive T cell proliferation and differentiation.
  • Most activated T cells die within a few weeks of activation, while the rest differentiate to memory cells.
❑ Effector T cells respond to antigenic stimulation with rapid cytokine production and can participate in cell-mediated and humoral immune responses.
❑ Memory T cells produce a broader array of cytokines, proliferate, and generate effector cells more rapidly and at lower antigen concentration than naïve T cells.

1. The first direct consequence of this synapse formation is the immobilization of the T cell. Signals induced by TcR engagement result in a conformational change in LFA-1 expressed by T cells, increasing its affinity for ICAM-1 and ICAM-2. This change stabilizes the association between the two cells and allows them to enter in a prolonged association that can persist for several days. Antigen-specific trapping allows continuous recruitment of newly arriving naïve T cells in the immune response without interfering with circulation of other antigen-non-specific T cells.

2. Synapse formation is associated with the rapid clustering of TcR molecules binding to peptide:MHC complexes on APC and local accumulation of intracellular signalling molecules such as Lck and LAT.

3. Formation of lipid rafts initiates downstream signalling events that cause T cells to proliferate and eventually differentiate into effector cells.

4. TcR/CD3 signalling is aided by CD4/CD8 coreceptors and engagement of large number of costimulatory molecules/adhesion molecules on T cells. Some of these costimulatory molecules (eg, CD28) are important for inducing IL-2 synthesis by T cells, whereas others, such as CD40L, maintain or induce the activation of APCs. Yet others (eg, LFA-1-ICAM-1 interaction) act largely by enhancing TcR signalling by stabilizing synapse formation and/or recruiting signalling molecules. Some interactions, such as CD154-CD40 interaction, also stimulate B cells during B/T collaboration. Activation of T cells requires two signals. The recognition of peptide:MHC complexes provides the first signal; the second is provided by costimulatory signals generated when ligands on T cells (eg, CD28 or OX40) interact with complementary molecules on APCs (CD80/86, OX40L respectively). This two-signal model (whether for B or T cell activation) is a simple device that disallows inappropriate stimulation of the immune system. It enables the immune system to distinguish the harmful from the harmless and concentrate its efforts on the former. The requirement for costimulation ensures that a T lymphocyte must see not only the antigen, but an antigen presented only by appropriately stimulated 'professional' APCs. As explained, antigen presentation in absence of costimulatory signals results in anergizing T cells. The need for the delivery of antigen and costimulatory signals by the same cell thus ensures the absence of stimulation of self-reacting clones by other (non-APC) tissue cells. This is crucial for survival, since all self-reactive clones (especially for proteins that are expressed later in the animal's development) may not be deleted or anergized in the thymus.

5. APCs release stimulatory cytokines such as IL-1 or TNF-α that drive extensive T cell proliferation and promote their efficient differentiation into effector cells.

Thus, professional antigen presentation by the APCs triggers entry of the naïve T cells into the G1 phase. The intracellular pathways of activation involve a complex series of enzymatic steps that lead to biosynthetic events. Ligation of the costimulatory molecule CD28 by CD80/86 turns on the production of IL-2. Resting T cells express β and γ chains of IL-2R, and this heterodimer binds IL-2 with moderate affinity. Activation induces the upregulation of CD69 and CD25 (α chain of IL-2R). The expression of the α chain results in the formation of the high affinity $\alpha\beta\gamma$ heterodimer, making T cells responsive to very low concentrations of IL-2. Thus, activated T cells produce both IL-2 as well as its receptor. This cytokine is needed for the rapid proliferation and differentiation of naïve T cells into effector cells and/or memory cells. IL-2 thus acts in an autocrine fashion, inducing clonal expansion and differentiation. Activated T cells proliferate in the lymph node at a very high rate; the cells divide every eight hours for several days. The CD45 isoform changes so that the T cell becomes more sensitive to stimulation by low concentrations of peptide:MHC complexes. Late in the proliferative phase (four to five days), T cells differentiate to effector cells that are capable of acting as helper, inflammatory, or cytotoxic cells. The context in which the T cell recognizes the antigen, the concentration of this antigen, and the duration of antigen exposure can all affect the speed and nature of the immune response. Naïve T cells proliferate in response to antigen presentation. A 10–20 fold increase in the number of antigen-specific naïve T cells is observed in the lymphoid tissue three days after the subcutaneous injection of a soluble antigen like ovalbumin. However, if an adjuvant (eg, LPS or CpG DNA) is injected with the antigen, this increase could be 100-fold.

8.3.4 Differentiation

In the early phase of the immune response, rapid replication of the pathogen leads to the continuous entry of large numbers of activated APCs into the T cell zones. These APCs drive the responding T cells to proliferate rapidly (as often as every eight hours for CD8$^+$ T cells, a slower rate for CD4$^+$ T cells), synthesize a wide range of cytokines, and differentiate either into CTLs (CD8$^+$ T cells) or T$_H$ cells (CD4$^+$ T cells). Destruction of the pathogen eventually leads to a lowered inflow of APCs in T cell areas. Cytokine secretion and differentiation into effector cells is diminished. This stage of the immune response is important for memory T cell formation. Thus, upon antigenic stimulation, T cells pass through three different stages (fig. 8.5).

❑ The **expansion phase** which is initiated in the lymphoid tissue because of antigen encounter of naïve T cells. The activated cells proliferate and differentiate to effector cells.
❑ A **death phase** that occurs in the weeks that follow pathogen clearance. Greater than 90% of the effector T cells die in this 'contraction' period.
❑ **A memory phase.** Surviving antigen-specific T cells enter the memory phase. The number of memory cells stabilizes in this phase, and they are maintained for prolonged periods of time.

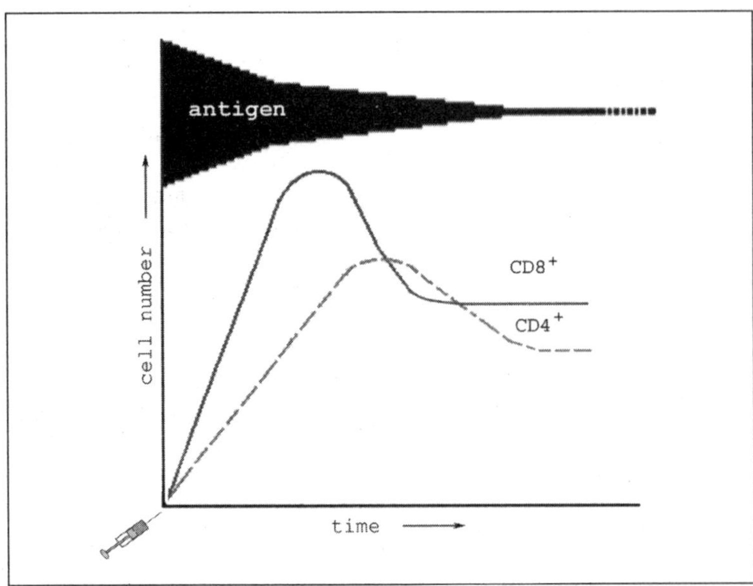

Figure 8.5 T cells pass through three different stages (expansion, contraction, and memory) upon antigenic stimulation. In the early phase of the immune response, antigen activated APCs drive responding T cells to proliferate rapidly. The proliferating cells differentiate to effector cells. As the antigen gets cleared from the system, the activated T cells enter a death phase because of Activation-Induced Cell Death (AICD). The surviving antigen-specific T cells enter the memory phase. The number of memory cells stabilizes in this phase and the cells can survive for years. Especially with viral challenges, the magnitude of CD4$^+$ T cell response is normally smaller than that of the CD8$^+$ T cell response (Adapted from Nature Reviews in Immunology (2002) 2:251).

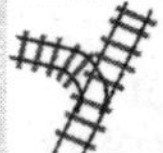

Lessons in Subversion: Virokines

Originally used to describe virally encoded cytokine homologues, the term 'virokine' is now often applied to virally encoded proteins that are secreted from infected host cells. Most virokines are powerful immunomodulatory agents created by capturing and modifying the genes responsible for regulating the host immune response. They are often homologous to but more potent than the host immune proteins. Large DNA viruses such as poxviruses and herpes viruses are a virtual cornucopia of virokines. Their structural homology and increased potency makes the virokines attractive candidates for therapy. Virokines can modulate different aspects of the host immune system.

❑ Virokines aid the virus in immune evasion by inactivating pro-inflammatory cytokines.
❑ They redirect the immune response away from the virus.
❑ They induce cell proliferation and migration, helping in the spread of the virus.
❑ Virokines control homeostasis to enhance viral replication.

Depending upon their mode of action, virokines fall into five broad groups.

❑ **Complement regulatory proteins**. One of the first virokine to be discovered was a complement regulatory protein produced by the vaccinia virus. Called VCP (**V**accinia **C**omplement **P**rotein), it is perhaps the most studied and best characterized of all virokines. It exhibits functional similarity to regulators of the complement cascade (Factor H and its structural homologues C4bp, MCP, DAF, and CR1). VCP has been shown to block antibody-mediated virus neutralization. Through its blocking of complement activation, it reduces cellular influx and inflammation at the site of infection. Additionally, VCP binds heparin-like molecules on human endothelial cells, interfering with chemotactic responses and possibly interaction with cytotoxic cells. Other complement regulatory proteins are listed in Table 3.2.

❑ **Cytokine homologues.** Several viruses encode cytokine homologues, although the advantage of producing these proteins is not always clear.
  • Human herpes virus 8, which causes Kaposi's sarcoma, has been shown to encode a homologue of human IL-6. It induces cell proliferation and is more efficient in signal transduction than IL-6.
  • Human herpes virus 8 also induces the secretion of a homologue of the chemokine MIP-2, a broad-spectrum chemokine antagonist.
  • IL-10 homologues (vIL-10) are encoded by several other herpes viruses such as the Epstein-Barr virus and cytomegalovirus. vIL-10 mimics the immunosuppressive and anti-inflammatory activity of host IL-10 but lacks its immunostimulatory properties. Like IL-10, vIL-10 can also induce proliferation, increasing the target cell pool for the virus.
  • The *Molluscum contagiosum* virus encodes a homologue of the CCβ chemokine which blocks leukocyte trafficking to the site of infection.

❑ **Cytokine binding proteins** are particularly useful to the virus as they target damaging cytokines.
  • The vaccinia virus, cowpox virus, and *Molluscum contagiosum* virus encode an IL-18 binding protein. IL-18 is a pro-inflammatory cytokine important in antiviral defence. It induces IFN-γ production, NK cell activation, and the induction of T$_{H1}$ responses. vIL-18 binding protein is shown to bind to IL-18, thereby blocking its antiviral effect.
  • The parapoxvirus Orf encodes a protein that binds GM-CSF and IL-2 — cytokines integral to development of adaptive immune responses.
  • The vaccinia virus encodes a vIFN-α binding protein that can bind IFN-α from several species.
  • Several members of the poxvirus family encode homologues of soluble cytokine receptors that often bind the cytokine with greater affinity than their host counterparts. Homologues of TNF receptors are encoded by vaccinia, cowpox, and myxoma virus. vTNFR binds to soluble TNF secreted at the site of infection, thereby blocking its antiviral and pro-inflammatory activity.
  • Variola, vaccinia, cowpox, and camelpox viruses encode a homologue of IFN-γ receptor (vIFN-γR). The importance of vIFN-γR in viral survival cannot be over-emphasized, since it binds and blocks the action of one of the most important antiviral defence mechanism of the host.
  • Vaccinia and cowpox viruses also produce vIL-1R (IL-1βR). IL-1 is expressed early in viral infections. It induces a powerful pro-inflammatory response, including induction of acute phase reaction; pyrexia; and growth and proliferation of T cells, B cells, and NK cells. vIL-1R binds to IL-1 with high affinity and blocks these antiviral pathways.

> - Cytomegalovirus encodes three different chemokine receptor homologues that bind different soluble chemokines (including RANTES and MIP-1) that are important in neutrophil chemotaxis.
> - **Serpins.** Members of the poxvirus family also encode serine protease inhibitors or serpins (chapter 3). Serpins help weaken the inflammatory response.
> - **Growth factors.** Some viruses elaborate growth factors for host cells, increasing the potential number of cells that the virus can infect. This could lead to the hyperplasia observed in some infections. For example, the vaccinia virus encodes a homologue of epidermal growth factor that causes the substantial proliferation of epidermal layers near the site of infection and has no known function in immune evasion.

8.3.4.1 Formation of Effector T Cells

Effector T cells are formed after repeated rounds of proliferation of conventional naïve T cells (fig. 8.6). These are large G1 phase cells that are nonetheless incapable of further response without some kind of stimulation. The initial interaction of the effector cell and its target is similar to that of naïve T cells, ie, dependent upon adhesion molecules (LFA-1 and CD2 on T cells and ICAMs on APCs). This initial interaction allows the more prolonged TcR-MHC:peptide engagement to occur. Effector cells are not dependent upon costimulation. When appropriately stimulated by the antigen, these effector cells can synthesize high titres of cytokines and effector molecules extremely rapidly, even in the absence of costimulatory signals. They also begin to synthesize DNA and progress through the cell cycle, either in response to the antigen itself, or cytokines such as IL-2 and IL-4. In addition, depending on their specialization, these cells participate in humoral responses ($CD4^+$ T cells) or CMI ($CD4^+$ and $CD8^+$ T cells). On the basis of their cytokine profile, effector T cells (especially $CD4^+$ T cells) are divided into type 1 or type 2 cells and are discussed later in the section on T cell subsets. Effector T cells release cytokines (or cytotoxins) at the site of cellular contact between the target and effector cells, ensuring a focussing of effector molecules on the antigen-bearing cell only.

Once the immune challenge is eliminated, the enormous number of effector cells generated become redundant and rapidly disappear. This disappearance is the combined effect of two separate mechanisms.

- **Death.** A large number of effector cells are generated in the immune response; it is important to eliminate these cells in order to avoid overburdening of the immune system (see sidetrack "Giving Up and Giving In"). The mechanisms responsible for eliminating effector cells are poorly understood. IFN-γ seems to be important in the elimination of both $CD4^+$ and $CD8^+$ T cells. $CD4^+$ T cells seem to be eliminated at a much slower rate and may involve multiple cell-death inducing mechanisms, including the Fas death pathway. Both $CD4^+$ and $CD8^+$ T cells may also undergo slow death because of a lack of contact with protective cytokines and or molecules (eg, CD40-CD40L interaction for $CD4^+$ T cells).
- **Homing to non-lymphoid tissue.** Current dogma holds that memory T cells preferentially patrol the original site of infection, ie, display tissue-specific homing. This homing is thought to be a result of a combination of adhesion molecules, chemokines, and their receptors expressed by the endothelial cells and memory cells. T cell activation results in a change in cell surface expression of a number of molecules. Expression of the homing receptor (L-selectin) is lost in a subset of activated cells; instead, these cells express higher levels of adhesion molecules such as CD2 and LFA-1. Also, activated T cells express chemokine receptors such as CCR5 and CCR2 that allows them to home to the vascular endothelium at sites of inflammation. This ensures that the effector cells recirculate and scout for infection through peripheral tissues where they may encounter sites of inflammation and their armoury can be put to use.

8.3.4.2 Formation of Memory T Cells

Resting memory cells are found after the effector response has subsided. T cell memory, like B cell memory, is long-lived and can be evoked months or years after initial antigenic encounter. Like memory B cells, once formed, memory T cells inhibit recruitment of naïve cells into the developing immune response. Thus, once they are formed, all subsequent antigenic challenges result only in the activation of memory cells. **Memory T cells are small quiescent cells that can persist for months or years and respond more efficiently to antigenic challenge than naïve cells.**

- Memory cells express the CD44^{hi} marker usually associated with activated T cells as well as a different, low MW isoform of CD45 (CD45RO).
- Upon antigenic stimulation, memory cells produce a broader set of effector cytokines than naïve cells; unlike memory cells, naïve T cells produce IL-2 and TNF-α in response to antigenic stimulation but almost no effector cytokines like IFN-γ, IL-4, or IL-5. The types of cytokines produced by memory cells depend upon the kind of cytokines present during initial stimulation.
- Memory cells proliferate and generate secondary effector cells much more rapidly than their antigen-inexperienced counterparts; they show a shorter lag time for entering the cell cycle, cytokine synthesis, and differentiation.
- They are somewhat less dependent upon costimulation than naïve cells.
- Unlike BcR genes, there is no evidence that TcR genes undergo mutation following antigenic stimulus. T cells therefore do not undergo affinity maturation in the conventional sense. However, T cells with higher affinity for the antigenic peptide:MHC complexes survive preferentially over T cells with lower affinity, and hence, secondary T cell responses do show an affinity maturation of sorts.

The source of memory T cells is unclear. Experiments have established that memory cells are generated from effector cells. Thus, some normal effector cells

---

Giving Up and Giving In: AICD

Clonal activation of antigen-specific lymphocytes is central to an effective immune response. Equally important is the removal of these expanded clones once the immunological threat has been dealt with. Apart from being a major drain on resources, the unchecked proliferation of these lymphocytes raises the dual risk of malignancy and autoimmunity. An immune response is therefore followed by large-scale death of activated lymphocytes by a process called **A**ctivation-**I**nduced **C**ell **D**eath (AICD). AICD is thought to be the default pathway of activated lymphocytes (whether B or T), avoided only by obtaining appropriate survival signals. Multiple pathways can lead to such default death.

❏ **Cytokine withdrawal.** Following TcR ligation, T cells enter a phase of IL-2 dependent proliferation. However, as infection wanes, cytokines like IL-2 that support clonal expansion can become limiting. Insufficient IL-2 can lead to cell death, unless the cells are rescued by other cytokines like IFNs or other members of IL-2 family (ie, IL-4, IL-7, and IL-15).

❏ **Fas/TNF-α pathway.** Resting T cells are relatively resistant to CD95 (Fas)-induced death. However, in the presence of IL-2, activated T cells become sensitive to CD95-induced death because of downregulation of the CD95 inhibitor, FLIP, and increased expression of CD95L. Activated T cells also express TNF-α. Engagement of the death receptors CD95L or TNF-α by their ligands (CD95 or TNFR respectively) on adjacent cells starts a signalling cascade that results in apoptosis of the cell, which is essentially suicide or homicide caused by adjacent cells.

❏ **Action of pro-apoptotic proteins.** The anti-apoptotic Bcl-2 is downregulated in activated T cells. Paradoxically, cytokines belonging to the IL-2 family inhibit this downregulation and, therefore, have a protective effect. Recent data suggests that most activated T cells die because of the activity of the Bcl-2 family protein, Bim, that may be aided by Bax and Bak in executing the apoptotic signal. This death signal can be overridden by Bcl-2.

may differentiate further to memory cells. There is some evidence to suggest that memory cells are derived not from normal effector cells but from a subset of precursors that arrive in the lymphoid tissue late in the immune response. Such 'late arrivals' or 'stragglers' are hypothesized to get insufficient contact with the antigen. This stimulation allows them to become effector cells transiently but is not strong enough to induce them into the effector cell-death pathway irreversibly. Such cells can therefore further differentiate to the memory phenotype. The factors affecting the transition of activated T cells to resting memory T cells are largely unknown. So are the factors that promote the maintenance of antigen-specific memory populations for prolonged periods of time. Formation of memory T cells necessitates the survival of some effector T cells after pathogen clearance. Administration of adjuvants is found to promote such survival, but the mechanisms underlying the escape from apoptosis are not clear. For years, there had been a controversy regarding the need for antigenic stimulation in memory T cell survival. It is now clear that long-term survival of memory T cells can occur in the absence of antigen. IL-15 has been found to be important in this survival in the case of $CD8^+$ T cells. Survival of $CD4^+$ T cells, however, seems to be largely IL-15 independent, and other cytokines may play a role in their survival.

Memory T cells can be divided into two broad subsets based upon their location, proliferative responses, and activation markers. The exact relationship between these two subsets is not clear.

❑ **Effector memory cells** are in an overtly activated state and closely resemble effector cells. They have a rapid turnover and tend to express activation markers such as CD25 and CD69. Depending upon their polarization status (ie, T_{H1} or T_{H2}), they produce cytokines like IFN-γ or IL-4 respectively. Also called activated memory cells, these cells express chemokine receptors that allow them to enter non-lymphoid tissues (especially the liver, lungs, and gut). They do not express the lymph node homing receptors CD62L and CCR7 and are not found at this site.

❑ **Resting or central memory cells** have a relatively slow turnover, lack activation markers, and closely resemble naïve T cells in terms of their distribution. They produce mainly IL-2. These cells express CD62L and CCR7 and are found in lymph nodes. Though quiescent, these cells are activated more easily than naïve T cells.

8.3.5 $\alpha\beta$ T Cell Subsets

As stated earlier, $\alpha\beta$ T cells are of two types — the majority of T cells are conventional T cells that recognize antigen in the context of MHC class I or class II molecules. Only a small fraction of T cells, called NKT cells, recognize antigen in the context of CD1 molecules and express NK cell markers. Conventional T cells fall into three functional subsets — $CD4^+T_H$ cells, $CD4^+$ T_R cells, and $CD8^+$ CTLs.

8.3.5.1 T_H Cells

Upon antigenic stimulation, naïve $CD4^+$ T cells clonally expand and differentiate to effector cells. Based on their cytokine-secreting patterns and functions, currently **three broad subsets of T_H cells have been recognized — T_{H0}, T_{H1}, and T_{H2}. The** key word is *broad*. Not all T cells belong to one of these categories; instead they produce a mixed cytokine profile. **T_{H0} cells resemble non-polarized naïve T cells** that have yet not decided which way to go; the T_{H1} and T_{H2} subsets represent the two extremes of polarization. Type 1 responses are typically CMI responses against intracellular pathogens such as *Listeria monocytogenes* or *Mycobacterium* spp., ie, T_{H1} cells orchestrate responses against pathogens that have breached the epithelial

---

Tн CELLS

❏ They express αβTcR and CD4 coreceptors; they therefore recognize antigen in the context of MHC class II molecules.

❏ Three broad subsets of Tн cells are recognized on the basis of their cytokine profile.
- Tн0 subset resembles naïve T cells and produces mainly IL-2.
- IFN-γ, TNF-α/β, and IL-2 are considered signature cytokines of Tн1 cells.
- IL-4, IL-10, and IL-13 are considered the hallmark of Tн2 cells.

❏ T cells get committed to Tн1 lineage because of the action of IFN-γ and IL-12 produced by cells of the innate immune system.
- Exposure to these cytokines results in the expression of transcription factor T-bet.
- T-bet results in the remodelling of IFN-γ gene to an active status.
- IL-12 aids in the process by inducing the transcription factor STAT-4 which further augments T-bet and IFN-γ transcription.
- Tн1 cells are pro-inflammatory cells that augment CMI by activating macrophages; they may also have a role in maintaining T cell homeostasis. Uncontrolled Tн1 responses may result in DTH and organ-specific autoimmunities.

❏ Tн2 type cells develop in response to extrinsic IL-4 or as a default pathway in the absence of inhibitory signals from cells of the innate immune system.
- IL-4 induces expression of GATA-3 via the transcription factor STAT-6.
- GATA-3 induces heritable remodelling of the IL-4 locus and promotes the expression of Tн2 cytokines such as IL-4, IL-5, IL-9, and IL-13.
- Tн2 cells are associated with strong allergic and antibody responses; IL-4, IL-5, and IL-6 are important in B cell maturation and differentiation.
- Hyperactivation of Tн2 responses results in allergic responses and asthma.

---

barrier and attack internal tissues. If unchecked, type 1 responses result in **Delayed-Type of Hypersensitivity (DTH)** and organ-specific autoimmunity (described in chapters 15 and 14 respectively). In contrast, type 2 responses favour the elimination of parasites and helminths. Tн2 cells arm epithelial and mucosal sites against pathogens. If gone awry, type 2 responses culminate in immediate type of hypersensitivities (eg, allergies and asthma; chapter 15). It is important to note that the distinction between the two subsets is essentially phenotypic and is based on the profile of cytokines expressed — IFN-γ, TNF-α, TNF-β, and IL-2 are considered signature cytokines of type 1 cells. IL-4, IL-9, IL-10, and IL-13 are considered the hallmark cytokines of Tн2 cells although they also produce IL-5 and IL-6 (Table 8.5).

In spite of extensive research, marker molecules that can distinguish the two subsets have proven difficult to identify. A quantitative difference in the expression of some molecules has been reported for the two subsets. Thus, CCR5 and CXCR3 seem to be expressed more in Tн1 cells, whereas CCR3, CCR4, CXCR4, CCR8, and ICOS are thought to be expressed more in Tн2 cells. Recently, the neuropeptide **Vasoactive Intestinal Peptide (VIP)** has been added to this list. It is produced mainly by Tн2 cells following antigenic stimulation and seems to promote Tн2 pathways and inhibit Tн1 pathways. In the last few years, two molecules have finally been reported to be expressed only by Tн1 and not Tн2 cells. The first is Chandra, a transmembrane molecule of unknown function. The second is TIM-3 (**T** cell **I**mmunoglobulin- and **M**ucin-domain-containing molecule-**3**), a molecule belonging to the TIM family of proteins that seems to have multiple functions in immune regulation. The role of these molecules in the development and/or functioning of the Tн1 subset is under investigation.

The two subsets cross-regulate each other's expansion and functions. *In vitro*, the type of Tн cell generated has been shown to be influenced by the cocktail of cytokines present in the microenvironment of the T cell. These effects are reversed to some extent by antibodies against the cytokines. **Tн1 cells are preferentially obtained** when CD4⁺ T cells are cultured in the presence of IFN-γ or IL-12 (an IFN-γ inducing cytokine produced by activated macrophages). **IL-4 is required for the generation of the TH2 phenotype**. When both IL-12 and IL-4 are present in the same environment, the effect of IL-4 is dominant over that of IL-12. IL-4 partly induces this effect by reducing IFN-γ production. IL-13 is also a very powerful inducer of TH2 cells *in vitro*.

i. Development of TH1 and TH2 subsets: Recognition of peptide:MHC class II complexes by TcR along with the engagement of costimulatory molecules activates naïve CD4⁺ T cells and results in their proliferation. Naïve T cells are uncommitted cells (ie, are TH0) that can develop into TH1 or TH2 cells depending upon the type of antigen being presented, the strength of the signal, the presenting cell, costimulatory molecules engaged, and cytokine milieu (fig. 8.6). It seems probable that the naïve T cells undergo a few rounds of proliferation before commitment to a particular phenotype by the cytokine milieu.

TH1 responses seem to be driven primarily by active signals derived from pathogen-activated innate immune sources and there are indications that a strong TH1 response might be maintained only in the presence of such signals. Major stages of TH1 commitment and development are given below (fig. 8.7).

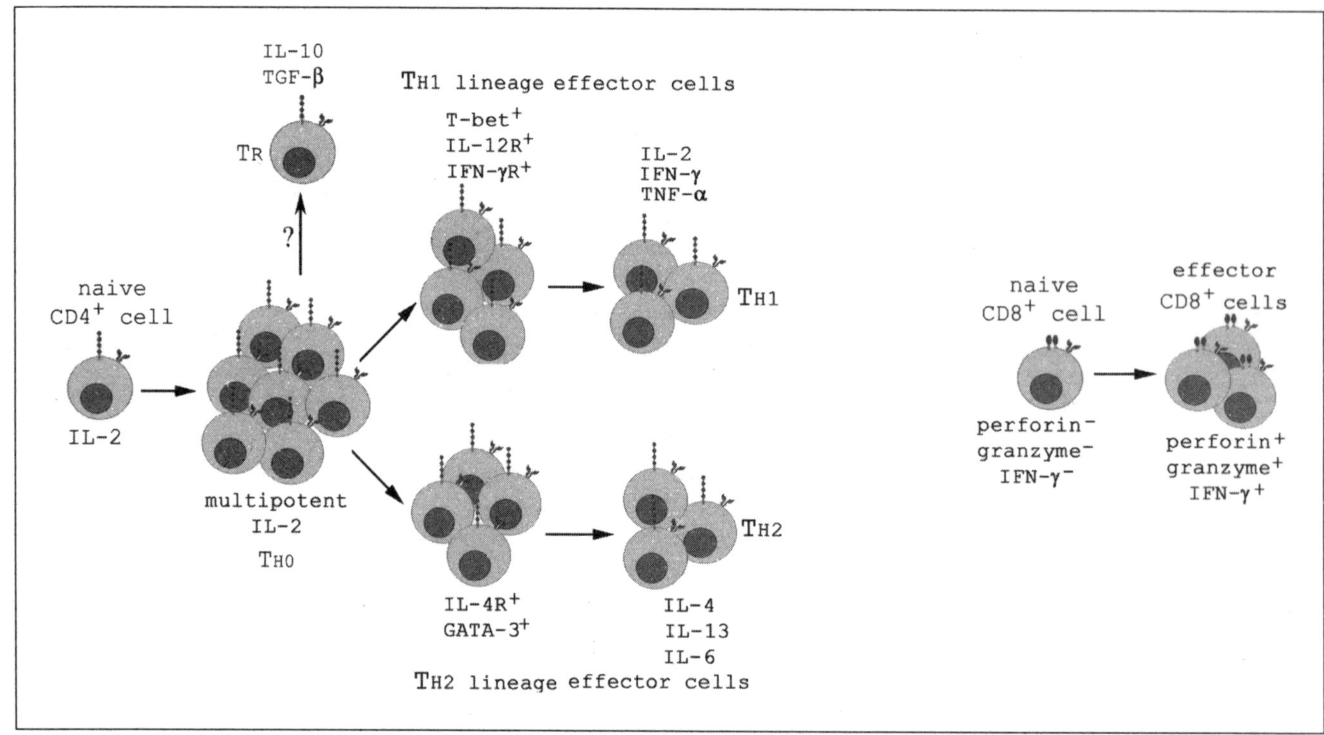

Figure 8.6 Antigen recognition, costimulation, and appropriate cytokine signalling triggers the formation of effector T cells. Effector T cells are formed after repeated rounds of proliferation of naïve T cells whether CD4⁺ or CD8⁺. The naïve CD4⁺ T cells are uncommitted multipotent cells and give rise to TH0 cells that resemble naïve cells and can produce copious amounts of IL-2 (left panel). Commitment to TH1 or TH2 lineage is dependent upon the cytokine milieu of the cells. IFN-γ and IL-12 promote TH1 pathway by inducing the transcription of T-bet. The responding cells start expressing receptors for these cytokines (IFN-γR and IL-12R). Conversely, the T cells enter the TH2 lineage if exposed to IL-4. The cells express IL-4 receptor (IL-4R). IL-4 upregulates GATA-3, the master regulator of TH2 pathway. The TH1/TH2 polarization is not absolute in the initial stages of differentiation and the cells continue to have the capacity to secrete signature cytokines of both the pathways. They eventually differentiate to produce IFN-γ, TNF-α, and IL-2 (TH1) or IL-4, IL-13, and IL-6 (TH2) immediately upon stimulation. It is not clear if and how the commitment to TR lineage occurs (denoted by a question mark). The TR cells exert their effect by producing immunosuppressive cytokines such as TGF-β and IL-10. Naïve CD8⁺ T cells do not have cytotoxic capacity (right panel). They differentiate to cells with cytotoxic and cytokine capacity upon appropriate antigenic stimulation.

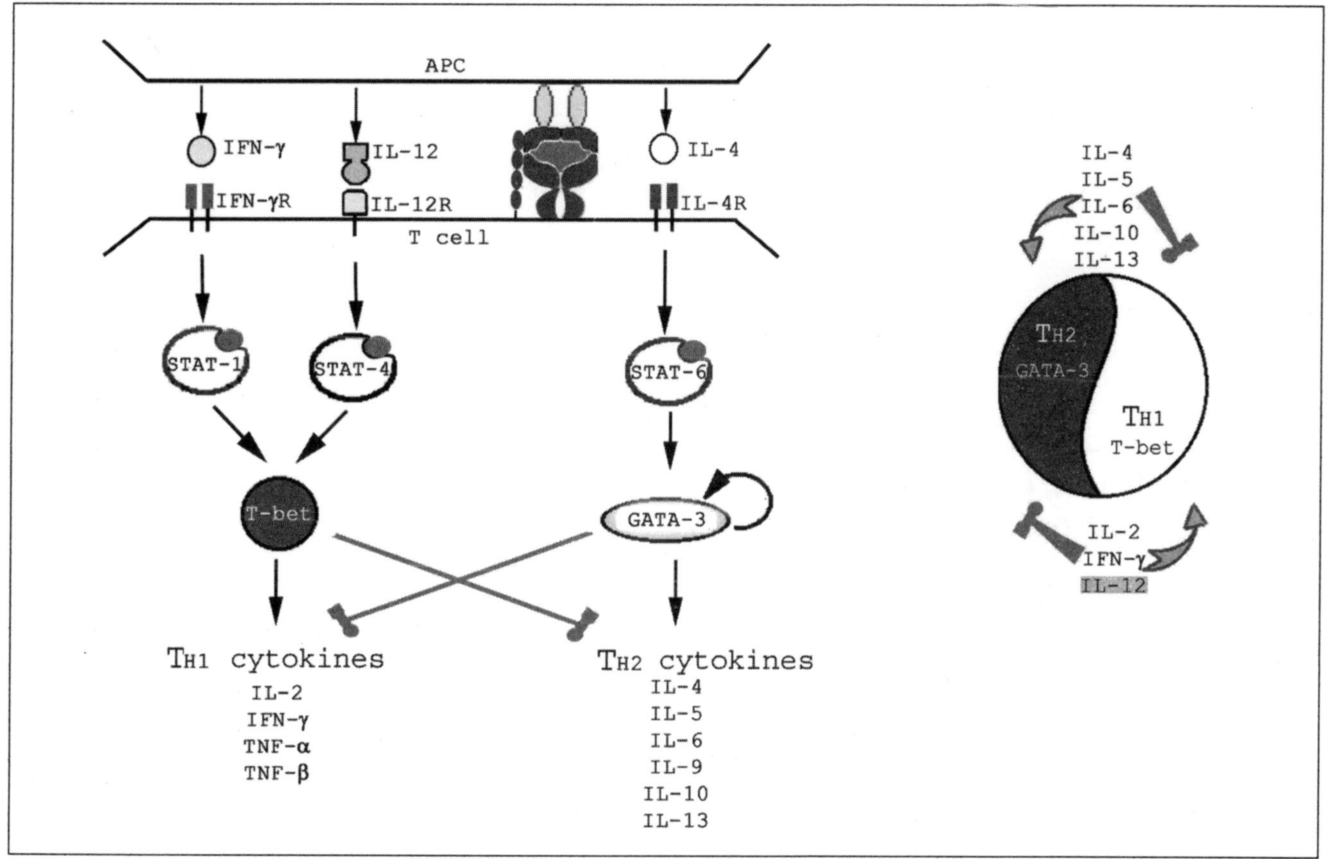

Figure 8.7 Naïve T cells exposed to IFN-γ and IL-12 get committed to the T**H1** ***lineage whereas exposure to IL-4 results in commitment to the*** T**H2** ***lineage****. Antigen recognition along with appropriate costimulation activates naïve T cells. Further development and lineage commitment is determined by cytokines present in their microenvironment. IFN-γ secreted by APCs acts through STAT-1 and results in increased expression of transcription factor T-bet (left panel). IL-12 acts through STAT-4 to increase T-bet expression. T-bet increases both IL-12R expression and remodels IFN-γ gene, allowing its stable expression. Conversely, IL-4 secreted by APCs induces the expression of* T*H2-cell specific factor GATA-3 through STAT-6. GATA-3 induces heritable remodelling of the IL-4 locus and promotes the expression of several* T*H2 cytokines (IL-4, IL-5, IL-9, and IL-13) because of the co-ordinate expression of linked genes. The two subsets are antagonistic, suppressing cytokine induction in each other. This cross-regulation is due to the action of T-bet and GATA-3 (right panel). Naïve T cells are capable of expressing both T-bet and GATA-3. Induction of one extinguishes the expression of the other.* T*H2-inducing GATA-3 is extinguished in* T*H1 cells by IL-12/STAT-4 signalling. Conversely,* T*H1-inducing T-bet is extinguished in* T*H2 cells by IL-4-STAT-6 mediated signalling. With the loss of one of these master regulators, the lineages become established in response to the remaining regulator. The so-called signature cytokines of the two subsets are shown in the right panel. Although IL-12 is important in the development of* T*H1 pathway, it is not produced by T cells and is placed in a grey box.*

❑ Cells of the innate immune system get activated by the invading pathogen to secrete IFN-γ and IL-12.
- IFN-γ secreted by macrophages or NK cells has been shown to commit naïve cells to TH1 phenotype.
- IFN-γ acts through the STAT-1 (**S**ignal **T**ransducer of **A**ctivation and **T**ranscription-**1**) signalling pathway to increase expression of the transcription factor T-bet in proliferating cells.

❑ T-bet (**T-box** family transcription factor) is expressed in developing and committed TH1 cells. It has been shown to have a central role in TH1 development.
- The gene for IFN-γ expression is normally repressed in T cells; T-bet expression results in the remodelling of the gene encoding IFN-γ to an active status.
- T-bet also increases the responsiveness of activated T cells to IL-12 by inducing the expression of IL-12 receptor.
- Subsequently, T-bet also stabilizes its own expression.

Table 8.4 T$_{H1}$ and T$_{H2}$ cytokine profile.

Cytokine	T$_{H1}$ cells	T$_{H2}$ cells
IL-2	+	-
IFN-γ	++	-
TNF (α and β)	++	-
IL-4	-	++
IL-5	-	++
IL-9	-	++
IL-10	-	++
IL-13	-	++
IL-3	++	++
GM-CSF	++	+

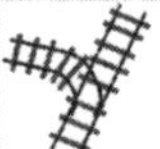

Cell to Cell SMS: Cytokines

The term 'cytokine' is employed to designate a heterogeneous group of non-enzymatic proteins produced by a wide variety of lymphoid and non-lymphoid cells. Cytokines are water-soluble, low molecular weight (<80 KD), glycosylated proteins generally secreted by one type of cell to alter either their own functions (autocrine effect), or the functions of other types of cells (paracrine effect). Originally discovered thanks to their role in immunological phenomena like inflammation and hypersensitivity, cytokines have now been shown to be soluble mediators of inter- and intra-cellular communications. They regulate development, tissue repair, haematopoiesis, inflammation, and innate and adaptive immune responses. In many respects, cytokines behave like classical hormones. They act on a systemic level, affecting the neuroimmune network, growth, and development. Classical hormones are produced by specialized glandular tissues and have a relatively small spectrum of target cells. Unlike them, cytokines are produced by a wide variety of cells that are dispersed in the body, and they are effective on an equally wide spectrum of cells. Cytokines were originally isolated and named on the basis of their functions, with the result that the same cytokines have been given different names. To further add to the confusion, cytokines were also referred to as lymphokines, monokines, etc to indicate their cellular source. The terms 'interleukin' and 'chemokine' are a hangover of the same system. Interleukin was the name given to cytokines of leukocytic origin, while cytokines with chemotactic properties were called chemokines. Mercifully, a common code of nomenclature has now been adopted. For convenience, however, some of the more popular aliases have been included in Table 8.5.

Cytokines regulate both the intensity and the duration of the immune response and mediate this effect via specific receptors on target cells. Cytokines have a very short half-life and are extremely potent — they are effective in picomolar (10^{-9} M) concentrations. Not surprisingly, the expression of most cytokines is strictly regulated. Although some cytokines are produced constitutively, the majority is produced only by activated cells, and even then, only in response to specific activation signals. Expression is normally transient and can be regulated at all levels of gene expression (transcriptional and/or translational). Expression may also be differentially regulated, depending upon cell type and developmental stage. Cytokines have multiple overlapping effects on cells, ie, they are pleuripotent. They are also redundant, since more than one cytokine can generate the same effect. Together, they form an intermingling network wherein one cytokine can influence the production of and response to many other cytokines. Some cytokines are synergistic/additive in their action, eg, IL-4 and IL-6 and IL-5 and IL-6. The presence of one induces receptors for the other or may even induce production of the other. Others, like IL-4/IFN-γ and IL-12/IL-4, are antagonistic. The type, duration, and extent of cellular activities induced by a particular cytokine are considerably influenced by the concentration of that cytokine, the microenvironment and developmental stage of the target cell, other cytokines present in the microenvironment of that cell, etc. Table 8.5 gives a brief overview of some important cytokines but is not by any means an exhaustive list.

Cytokines exert their effect by binding to specific receptors expressed by the target cells. Many of these receptors share a number of characteristics and even subunits. They also share common signal transducing components, explaining, at least partially, the redundancy of cytokines. Five broad classes of receptor families have been recognized.

- ❑ The type 1 receptor family (no relation of the T_H type 1 and 2 subsets!) includes IL-2, IL-3, IL-4, IL-5, IL-6, IL-7, IL-9, IL-11, IL-12, and GM-CSF and has a conserved extracellular domain that shares sequence motifs.
- ❑ Prominent members of the type 2 cytokine receptors are IFN-α, IFN-β, IFN-γ, and IL-10. For both type 1 and type 2 cytokine receptors, the cytokine binding subunit (called α subunit) is often different from the signal transducing unit (referred to as β or γ subunit). For example, receptors for IL-2, IL-4, IL-7, IL-9, and IL-15 share the same γ subunit. From a cell's point of view, this system is economical, since the same signal transducing subunit can associate with different α (cytokine recognizing) subunits, and it allows the same machinery to be used for different stimuli.
- ❑ The Ig superfamily receptors have at least one Ig domain. Receptors for IL-1, M-CSF, and c-kit belong to this category.
- ❑ The TNF family of receptors consists of receptors for TNF-α, TNF-β, CD40, and Fas.
- ❑ Chemokine receptors bind exclusively chemokines. Their unique feature is a transmembrane domain that transverses the membrane seven times (see sidetrack 'Instant Chemistry').

Receptors of most of the cytokines secreted by T_H cells belong to the type 1 or type 2 categories. Signal transduction via these receptors occurs by the same generalized pathway (often called the Jak/STAT pathway).

- ❑ Docking of the cytokine to its receptor causes the cytokine induced di/trimerization of the receptor.
- ❑ Intracellular domains of receptor subunits are often associated with different tyrosine kinases. Janus kinases are perhaps the most important of these. Named after the two-headed Greek God Janus*, kinases of this family have two sites — one that associates with the receptor and the other that acts as a tyrosine kinase when activated.
- ❑ Upon docking, **Ja**nus **k**inases (Jaks) phosphorylate the receptor subunits.
- ❑ Members of a family of transcription factors called STATs bind to the phosphorylated tyrosine residues — STAT-1 is involved in IFN-γ signal transduction and STAT-4 in IL-12 signal transduction. STAT-6 transduces IL-4 signal.
- ❑ Docked STATs undergo phosphorylation at a tyrosine residue.
- ❑ Phosphorylated STATs dissociate from the receptor docking sites, dimerize, and undergo further phosphorylation at a serine residue.
- ❑ STAT dimers translocate to the nucleus where they initiate the transcription of specific genes.

Cytokine inhibitors are found in the blood and extracellular fluids of healthy individuals. These proteins interfere with cytokine activity by binding either the cytokine itself or its receptor and are being investigated for their therapeutic potential. The best characterized inhibitor is the **IL-1R** **a**ntagonist (IL-1Ra) that binds to the IL-1 receptor without activating the signalling cascade. It is thought to play a role in regulating the intensity of the inflammatory response. Many antagonists arise from the enzymatic cleavage of cytokine receptors. The released extracellular domains act as soluble receptors. The soluble receptor binds to the cytokine's receptor-binding site, thereby inhibiting its binding to membrane anchored receptors. Examples include IL-2, IL-4, IL-6, IFN-γ, TNF-α, and TNF-β receptors.

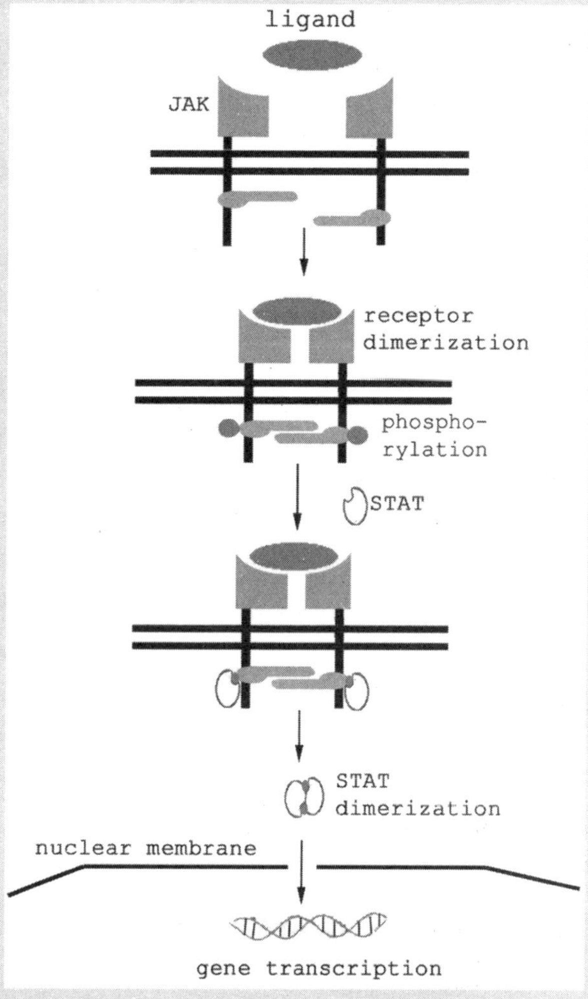

Figure 8.S4 *The Jak/STAT pathway is a general pathway for cytokine signal transduction.*

*These were originally named JAK (for Just Another Kinase), because this family of tyrosine kinases was isolated in a random screen and the function remained unknown. Later, it was revealed that these kinases are critical messengers in cytokine responses and were recast as Janus Kinases as a reference to the double-headed Greek God of gates and doorways.

Table 8.5 Functions of some important cytokines

Cytokine	Major source	Aliases	Function
IL-1	Monocytes and macrophages, epithelial and endothelial cells, DCs, T and B cells, NK cells	Catabolin	– Is pleiotropic – Is a growth and stimulatory factor for macrophages and T cells – Systemically causes fever, hypertension and shock; induces acute phase proteins
IL-2	T cells, DCs	TCGF (T Cell GF)	– Stimulates growth and differentiation of T cells, B cells, NK cells, monocytes, macrophages, etc.
IL-3	T cells, thymic epithelial cells, mast cells, eosinophils	Multi-CSF, MCGF (Mast Cell GF)	– Induces early cell differentiation antigens – Acts synergistically in haematopoiesis
IL-4	NKT cells, T_{H2} cells, mast cells, bone marrow cells, thymic stromal cells	IgE Inducing Factor	– Activates B cells – Induces isotype switching to IgG4 and IgE in humans or IgG1 and IgE in mice – Induces differentiation of naïve $CD4^+$ T cells to T_{H2} type
IL-5	T_{H2} cells, mast cells, eosinophils	EoCSF (**Eo**sinophil **CSF**)	– Induces proliferation and differentiation of eosinophils
IL-6	T and B cells, monocytes and macrophages, fibroblasts, endothelial cells, bone marrow cells, thymic stromal cells	BSF-2 (**B** cell **S**timulating **F**actor-**2**)	– Is pleuripotent – Regulates T and B cell growth – Regulates acute phase reaction
IL-7	Stromal cells of thymus, bone marrow, spleen	Lymphopoietin-1	– Is a growth factor for pre-B and pre-T cells – Stimulates proliferation and differentiation of mature T cells
IL-8	Monocytes and macrophages, T cells, and a variety of other cells	NAF (**N**eutrophil **A**ctivating **F**actor)	– Is chemotactic for neutrophils – Activates neutrophils – Promotes angiogenesis
IL-9	T_{H2} cells	TCGF-III (**T C**ell **G**rowth **F**actor-III)	– Induces erythropoiesis – Is an important growth factor for and stimulator of numerous cell types involved in the pathogenesis of asthma
IL-10	T cells, B cells, macrophages	Cytokine synthesis inhibitor factor	– Inhibits cytokine synthesis by T_{H1} cells – Suppresses macrophage and NK cell functions – Stimulates proliferation of B cells, thymocytes, and mast cells
IL-12	Monocytes and macrophages, B cells	NK cell stimulatory factor	– Is obligatory for development of T_{H1} pathways – Induces IFN-γ – Activates NK cells
IL-13	T_{H2} cells		– Inhibits pro-inflammatory cytokine production by macrophages – Induces B cell growth and differentiation – Synergizes with IL-4 in isotype switching to IgE
IL-15	Monocytes and macrophages, DCs, bone marrow stromal cells, epithelial cells		– Promotes NK cell and T_{H1} cells differentiation – Promotes NK cell and CTL cytotoxicity – Activates neutrophils
IL-18	Macrophages, Kupffer cells, DCs, B cells, intestinal and airway epithelial cells		– Accelerates differentiation to T_{H1} type – Activates cytotoxic activity of NK cells and CTLs – Inhibits angiogenesis
IFN-α/β	T and B cells, monocytes and macrophages, fibroblasts, epithelial cells		– Are important in antiviral and antitumour defence – Increase MHC class I expression on APCs – Activate NK cells – Promote differentiation of human T_R cells

IFN-γ	Monocytes and macrophages, T$_{H}$1 cells, NK cells		– Is a pro-inflammatory cytokine – Activates macrophages – Induces T$_{H}$1 pathways – Potentiates action of IFN-α and -β
TNF-α	Monocytes and macrophages, NK cells, B and T cells, neutrophils, endothelial cells	Catchectin	– Is pro-inflammatory cytokine – Induces acute phase reaction – Regulates growth and differentiation of a wide variety of cell types
TNF-β	B and T cells	Lymphotoxin	– Functions in a manner similar to TNF-α
GM-CSF	Monocytes and macrophages, T cells		– Induces growth and differentiation of granulocytes and DCs

Legend: CSF — colony stimulating factor, GF — growth factor

❑ IL-12 induces the transcription factor STAT-4. Engagement of IL-12R by IL-12 causes phosphorylation of STAT-4 and results in further augmentation of T-bet and IFN-γ transcription.
- Activated macrophages, DCs, and NK cells are a major source of IL-12. They can thus influence the polarization of the T cell response.
- Human (but not mouse) type I IFNs elaborated by DCs activate STAT-4 and hence augment T-bet and IFN-γ transcription.
- IL-12 acts both directly on T$_{H}$1 cells and their precursors and, in part, indirectly by inducing IFN-γ production by T cells and NK cells in co-operation with TNF-α and IL-1.
- IFN-γ in turn has a positive feedback effect on IL-12 production by monocytes and macrophages.

❑ In T cells that have already undergone differentiation to the T$_{H}$1 type, IFN-γ production can occur via TcR engagement or through the combined stimulus of IL-12 and IL-18. These cytokines can induce IFN-γ synthesis even in the absence of TcR engagement. Such IFN-γ induction has been shown to be strongly dependent on STAT-4.

❑ Recently, three other cytokines — IL-18, IL-23, and IL-27 — have been shown to be T$_{H}$1-promoting factors.
- IL-12 induces the expression of IL-18R, making the cell responsive to IL-18. IL-18, produced primarily by mononuclear phagocytes, synergizes with IL-12 in committed T$_{H}$1 cells to increase IFN-γ production. Interestingly, IL-18 and IL-12 can induce IFN-γ production from T$_{H}$1 cells in the absence of TcR signalling.
- IL-23, an IL-12 related cytokine, seems to increase the antigen presenting capacity of DCs. It also promotes IFN-γ production and proliferation in memory T$_{H}$1 responses via the STAT-4 pathway.
- IL-27, produced by APCs, acts in conjunction with IL-12 in promoting IFN-γ production and is thought to be involved in early T$_{H}$1 development.

Commitment and development to the T$_{H}$2 phenotype is less dependent upon signals from the innate immune system. It is still uncertain if any active innate signal drives this process, and it is currently thought that T$_{H}$2 development could occur as a default pathway in the absence of inhibition by innate immune signals or in response to an extrinsic source of IL-4. Activated DCs and NKT cells are the most likely source of external IL-4.

❑ IL-4 has been shown to be essential in the development of T$_{H}$2 subset; IL-4 induces differentiation of naïve cells to T$_{H}$2 phenotype via STAT-6.

❑ Some alternative signals such as IL-6 or IL-13 may trigger initial production of IL-4, but the identity of alternative signal is still in doubt.

❑ IL-4 rapidly induces the expression of T$_{H}$2-cell specific factor GATA-3 through STAT-6.

- GATA-3 is probably the master-regulator of T_H2 differentiation, although GATA-3 seems also to be essential in normal thymocyte development and embryonic survival.
- Naïve T cells constitutively express GATA-3 at a low level, but its expression is dramatically increased in T_H2 cells.
- GATA-3 induces heritable remodelling of the IL-4 locus and promotes the expression of several T_H2 cytokines (IL-4, IL-5, IL-9, and IL-13) because of the co-ordinate expression of linked genes.
- CD28 costimulation has been reported to augment the expression of GATA-3, whereas engagement of LFA-1 inhibits its expression.
- GATA-3 has a transcriptional autoactivating property which leads to a massive upregulation of GATA-3 gene transcription by GATA-3 protein.

❑ Several members of the NFAT family seem to regulate expression of T_H2 cytokines after the triggering of differentiated T_H2 cells through TcR.

❑ IL-5 and IL-6, produced by T_H2 cells, have been shown to act synergistically with IL-4 in potentiating T_H2 responses.

It has been known for years that the two T_H subsets act in an antagonistic fashion, suppressing cytokine induction in each other. It is now clear that this is because of the action of the transcription factors T-bet and GATA-3. These two operate intrinsically to suppress opposing cytokines. T_H2-inducing GATA-3 is extinguished in T_H1 cells by IL-12/STAT-4 signalling. Conversely, T_H1-inducing T-bet is extinguished in T_H2 cells by IL-4-STAT-6 mediated signalling. Naïve T cells are capable of expressing both T-bet and GATA-3. With the loss of one of these master regulators, however, the capacity to sustain downstream cytokine gene expression is lost, and the lineages become established in response to the remaining regulator, resulting in terminal differentiation into polarized T_H subsets. Additionally, IL-10 produced by T_H2 cells can suppress IL-12 production of the APCs, thereby inhibiting T_H1 development. IL-10 can also suppress the production of effector molecules by macrophages and downregulate their MHC class II expression. The immunosuppressive TGF-β elaborated by T_R cells (section 8.3.5.3) can suppress expression of both T-bet and GATA-3, halting the development and commitment of naïve T cells.

ii. Functioning of T_H Cells: One of the most important functions of T_H cells is to recognize peptide:MHC complexes on antigen-specific B cells and provide help for antibody production. However, naïve B and T cells are anatomically separated from each other in the secondary lymphoid organs, necessitating their movement. Antigen-specific naïve $CD4^+$ T cells rapidly express the chemokine receptor CXCR5 in response to adjuvant-activated DCs. Expression of CXCR5 is associated with the downregulation of the lymphoid homing receptors, CCR7 and CD62L. CXCR5 allows homing of naïve T_H cells to B cell areas that express its ligand BCA-1 (**B C**ell **A**ttracting chemokine-1), thus allowing the T cells to provide the required signals for B cell stimulation.

As explained, **T_H1 cells are the pro-inflammatory cells involved in augmenting CMI.** Several T_H1 cytokines activate cytotoxic and inflammatory functions as well as inducing DTH responses. These cells promote opsonizing antibody production by B cells (IgG2a and IgG2b in mice, IgG1 and IgG3 in humans), but higher T_H1 numbers may suppress B cell responses. **Activation of macrophages is the most important effector function of these cells.** Two different signals are involved in this activation. IFN-γ produced by T_H1 cells is the first signal, though $CD8^+$ T cells can also act as a source of IFN-γ. The second signal is provided by the engagement of CD154 on the surface of T_H1 cells by CD40 expressed on macrophages. There is some evidence to suggest that the second signal can also be delivered through a membrane-bound form of TNF-α or TNF-β, since antibodies to either can replace CD40 ligation in macrophage activation *in vitro*. LPS helps in the activation process by making the macrophages more responsive to IFN-γ. TH1 cells further aid CMI by recruiting fresh macrophages to the site of infection. TH1-derived IL-3 and GM-CSF are important in this process. TNF-α and TNF-β, also produced by these cells, bring about a change in the surface properties of endothelial cells, promoting adhesion of phagocytic cells to these cells. Other cytokines such as MIF (**M**acrophage **I**nhibitory **F**actor) and MCF (**M**acrophage **C**hemotactic **F**actor) promote their chemotaxis and accumulation at the site of inflammation. Activated macrophages are potent antimicrobial cells capable of secreting a variety of effector molecules (Table 2.3). Additionally, TH1 cells can induce apoptosis in target cells by the Fas-FasL pathway. They may thus have a role in maintaining T cell homeostasis.

Type 2 cells are associated with strong antibody and allergic responses. TH2 cytokines encourage antibody production, particularly non-complement fixing IgG2a, IgA, and IgE isotypes (in humans). Type 2 cytokines like IL-4, IL-6, and IL-10 are important in B cell maturation and differentiation. IL-5 and IL-6 produced by these cells also enhance eosinophil proliferation and function. Both IL-4 and IL-13 enhance IgE antibody production. IL-9, another TH2 cytokine, is a mast cell growth factor and synergizes with IL-5 in promoting eosinophil maturation. Hence, **hyperactivation of TH2 type responses leads to increased IgE antibody levels and hypersensitivity type I reactions** (fig. 8.8).

TH1/TH2 balance is found to be important in the manifestation and progression of some diseases.

❑ Balb/c mice tend to give a predominantly TH2 type response to the intracellular parasite *Leishmania major*. The consequent failure to activate macrophages results in susceptibility to the protozoal parasite. C57/Bl6 mice, on the other hand, give a predominantly TH1 response. The resultant activation of CMI protects them from infection.

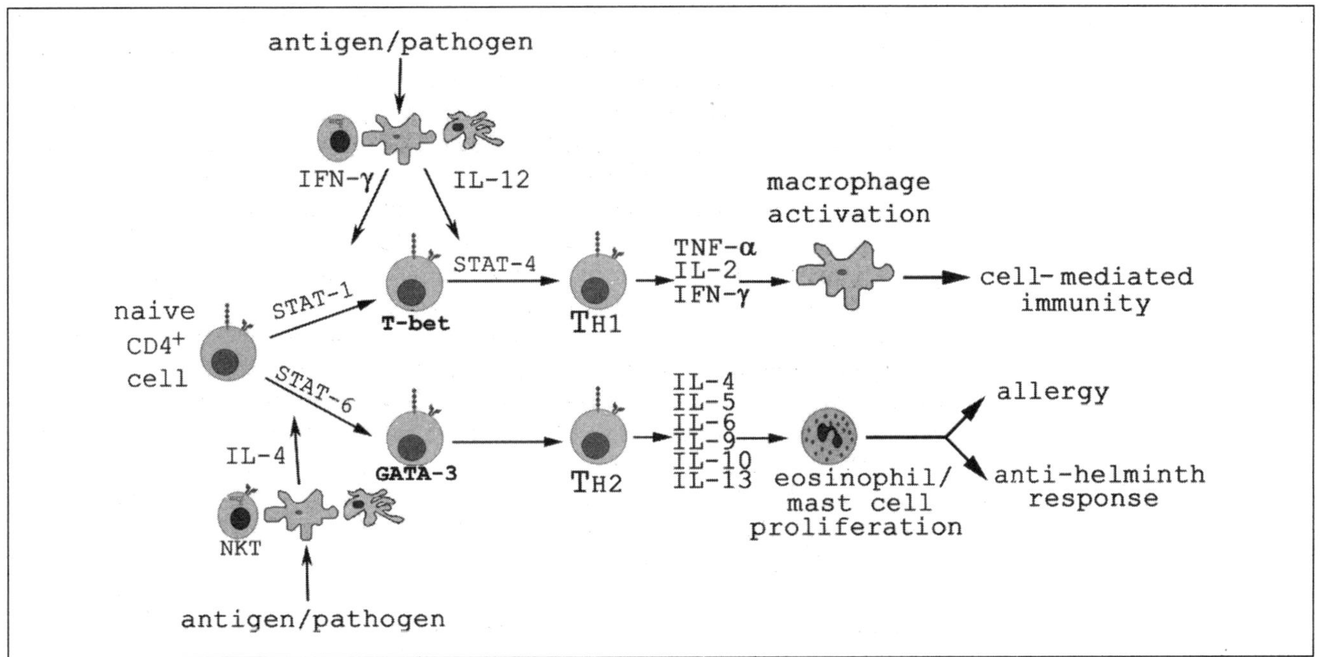

Figure 8.8 TH1 cells are pro-inflammatory cells involved in augmenting CMI, whereas TH2 cells are associated with strong antibody and allergic responses. Cells of the innate immune system such as macrophages, DCs, and NK cells are the major sources of IFN-γ and IL-12. These cytokines are instrumental in promoting naïve CD4+ T cells down the TH1 pathway. Activation of macrophages is the most important effector function of these cells — activated TH1 cells secrete IFN-γ and TNF-α, cytokines involved in activation of cytotoxic functions of macrophages. DCs, macrophages, and NKT cells are thought to be the source of IL-4 that skews the development of naïve T cells to TH2 cells. TH2 cytokines such as IL-4 and IL-13 promote IgE production. IL-5 and IL-6 produced by these cells enhance eosinophil proliferation and function, whereas IL-9 is a mast cell growth factor. TH2 cells are therefore important in anti-helminth responses, but hyperactivation of these cells can lead to allergic responses.

□ Infection by *Mycobacterium leprae* in humans results in tuberculoid leprosy if a T_{H1} type response is elicited. The infection results in tuberculoid granulomas and the growth of the pathogen is well controlled by activated macrophages. Conversely, a T_{H2} type response results in a widely disseminated bacterial response. The predominantly humoral response is unable to control the spread of the pathogen, and the infection results in widespread damage to the nervous system.

8.3.5.2 CTLs

Cytolytic lymphocytes such as NK cells and CD8 expressing T cells provide a potent defence against viral infection and intracellular pathogens which are inaccessible to antibodies. **CTLs are MHC class I restricted**, ie, they recognize the antigen only in the context of MHC class I molecules. Since virtually all nucleated cells of the body express MHC class I molecules, class I restriction of the CTL ensures that any cell infected by a virus or parasite or one that has undergone transformation (eg, tumour cell) is a potential target for the CTL. CTLs are the body's major defence against intracellular parasites.

Naïve CD8$^+$ CTL precursors lack cytotoxicity and need to be activated for maximal activity. However, naïve CD8$^+$ cells have a greater requirement for costimulation than naïve CD4$^+$ T cells. This is probably for the best, considering the tremendous destructive potential of CTLs. DCs are the most efficient activators of naïve CTLs, since they have high intrinsic costimulatory activity. In the case of other APCs that do not have the required costimulatory potential, recognition of related antigens by naïve CD8$^+$ and effector CD4$^+$ T cell on the surface of the same APC can compensate for the inadequate costimulation. The CD4$^+$ T cell is thought to act by inducing increased expression of costimulatory molecules on the APC. TcR recognition of peptide:MHC class I molecules along with the required costimulatory signals induces the expression of receptors for cytokines such as IL-2 and IL-6 and drives cytokine synthesis. Engagement of these receptors in turn leads to the synthesis of granules containing cytotoxic effector molecules. The activation process, which takes 1–3 days, also drives lymphocyte proliferation. The mechanism of the killing of infected cells by CTLs is similar to that of NK cells and is discussed in detail in chapter 11. Two major pathways of cytolysis are recognized — release of cytotoxins such as perforin and granzymes and death via the Fas pathway. Additionally, most CTLs also release IFN-γ, TNF-α, and TNF-β. These cytokines augment host defence in multiple ways. As mentioned earlier, IFN-γ directly inhibits viral replication. It also induces or upregulates MHC class I and class II expression. Increased MHC class I expression increases the possibility of infected cells being killed by CTLs; increased class II expression helps co-opt T_H cells in the response. IFN-γ also activates macrophages — augmenting their phagocytic and antigen-presenting capabilities. TNF-α and -β, on the other hand, act synergistically with IFN-γ in macrophage activation. They also induce DC maturation.

Traditionally, CD8$^+$ cells were viewed only as IFN-γ and TNF-α producing cells. However, a number of studies clearly establish the existence of T_{C1} and T_{C2} subsets (cytotoxic T cells type 1 and 2) on the lines of T_{H1} and T_{H2} types. T_{C1} produce IFN-γ and IL-2, whereas T_{C2} produce IL-4, IL-5, and IL-10. Like the T_H cells, these subsets probably represent the extremes of a whole spectrum of subsets. Once committed, the cells do not seem to be able to revert to a different phenotype. Both subsets are involved in CMI and do not provide 'help' to B cells except indirectly through the production of type 2 cytokines. Factors that determine the polarization of CTLs, their functions and role in disease, and their interplay are still under investigation.

8.3.5.3 T_R Cells

T cells which could suppress immune responses were first described in early 1970s. However, failure to clone factors that could suppress immune responses in an antigen-specific manner led to the demise of this entire field. The discovery that immunosuppressive cells occurred naturally *in vivo* and that adoptive transfer of cells suppressed immune responses in the new host rekindled interest. The realization that these T cells could suppress or enhance immune responses has led them to be renamed 'regulatory' rather than 'suppressor' T cells. Several *in vivo* and *in vitro* treatments have been shown to generate T_R cells. Many questions about them remain unanswered. **The mechanism by which T_R cells exert their effect is not clear. Both TGF-β and IL-10 have been implicated in T_R-mediated immuno- suppression.** IL-10 is known to decrease the antigen presenting capacity of APCs. It also inhibits secretion of cytokines and chemokines that influence T cell differentiation, proliferation, and migration. It has also been shown to inhibit IL-2, IL-5, and TNF-α secretion by T cells. It can induce anergy in antigen-specific T cells. TGF-β is known to suppress IFN-γ production, decrease MHC class II expression, and limit NO and ROI production by macrophages. It can also inhibit T cell proliferation, cytokine production, and cytotoxicity. However, studies in KO mice show that some autoreactive immune responses can be regulated by CD4$^+$ T cells independent of either of these cytokines. Recent evidence suggests that T_R cells may mediate suppression by direct cell-to-cell contact with CD8$^+$ or CD4$^+$ T cells. It is possible that different subsets of T_R cells are programmed to inhibit immune responses by different mechanisms. In mice, T_R cells which remain CD4$^+$CD25$^+$ seem to emerge in the thymus 2–3 days after birth, since neonatally thymectomized mice develop various organ-specific autoimmune diseases. The mechanism of selection of these cells in the thymus and their maintenance in the periphery is unclear. To summarize, there is clear evidence for the existence of T_R cells, although their nature, ontogeny, physiology, mode of action, etc are still being explored. Currently, three types of T_R cells have been described in literature, though their relation to each other is still being defined.

- ❏ **T_{R1} cells** downregulate immune responses because of their ability to produce high levels of IL-10 and TGF-β. Coculture of naïve T cells in the presence of T_{R1} cells and antigen-pulsed APCs leads to suppression of naïve T cell proliferation.
- ❏ **CD4$^+$CD25$^+$ T_R cells** constitute a minor fraction (~10%) of peripheral CD4$^+$ T cells and are found to occur naturally in both mice and humans. They have been shown to be crucial for suppression of autoreactive T cells.
- ❏ **TGF-β-secreting CD4$^+$ T_{H3} cells** are generated by the introduction of low doses of oral antigen. These cells are thought to act primarily via TGF-β, though they may secrete small amounts of IL-10.

8.3.5.4 NKT Cells

NKT cells have been shown to have cytolytic activity. TcR stimulation also results in rapid (within 90 minutes) induction of cytokine synthesis — predominantly IL-4 and IFN-γ — in these cells. The NKT-derived cytokines in turn recruit and activate several other cell types such as NK cells, conventional T cells, macrophages, B cells, and DCs. The cytokines produced by NKT cells have been suggested to help in polarizing the subsequent adaptive immune response to T_{H1} or T_{H2} type. However, experimental evidence for such a role *in vivo* is as yet unavailable. Studies aimed at establishing whether NKT cells, like T cells, polarize to the type 1 or type 2 phenotype have also proven inconclusive. **NKT cells have been shown to be involved in host defence against infections caused by a number of intracellular parasites,** eg, *Leishmania major, Plasmodium falciparum, Trypansoma cruzi,* and *Mycobacterium tuberculosis.* This protective effect has been attributed to their IFN-γ production. **They are also believed to be important in antitumour immunity** by virtue of their cytotoxicity and their production of pro-inflammatory cytokines like IFN-γ and IL-12. Studies in mice also suggest a role for NKT cells in the control and prevention of autoimmune disease like diabetes, experimental autoimmune encephalitis, and colitis. In most of these studies, the beneficial effect was due to the cytotoxic effect of perforin and secretion of IL-4 and IL-10. Their potent cytokine producing abilities and cytotoxicity has resulted in NKT cells being investigated for potential immuno-based therapies.

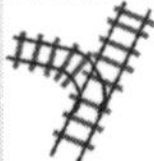

Unarmed and Defenceless: Primary Immunodeficiencies

Primary immunodeficiencies are defined as genetic or developmental defects in the immune system. They may affect both the innate and the adaptive arms of the immune system. Adaptive immune responses are impaired because of either a solely B or solely T cell immunodeficiency or a 'combined immunodeficiency' where both compartments are defective. Phagocyte or complement deficiencies, on the other hand, lead to impaired innate immune responses and will not be considered here.

B cell immunodeficiencies encompass a spectrum of diseases, ranging from a complete absence of mature recirculating B cells, plasma cells, and Ig, to selective absence of some Ig isotypes. They are characterized by recurrent respiratory and gastrointestinal bacterial infections from around three to four months of age. However, patients often display a normal immunity to most viral and fungal infections. Noteworthy deficiencies include:

❑ **BcR deficiencies**. A variety of immunodeficiencies are caused by defects in BcR. Bruton's (X-linked) agammaglobulinaemia is caused by a defect in the gene coding for Bruton's tyrosine kinase, involved in BcR signalling, that maps to the X chromosome. Consequently, the disease is almost exclusively found in males and results in a complete absence of Igs in serum. Bruton's tyrosine kinase plays a pivotal, non-redundant role in BcR signal transduction. A defect in this enzyme therefore results in severe malfunctioning of the B cell compartment of the immune system.

❑ **X-linked hyper IgM syndrome** is caused by a defect in CD40L, which also maps to the X chromosome. As a result of the CD40L defect, B cells do not receive cognate help from T cells and are incapable of responding to TD antigens. Patients are, however, capable of responding to TI antigens. The lack of T cell help results in the absence of germinal centre formation and failure of the B cells to undergo isotype switching and affinity maturation. The end result is absence of IgG, IgA, or IgE in serum coupled with very high serum concentrations of IgM (IgM concentrations of 10 mg/ml are not unusual).

❑ **Common Variable Immunodeficiency** (**CVID**) is characterized by a profound decrease in Igs of all isotypes and recurrent infections usually accompanied with enlarged lymph nodes and spleen. The underlying defect that gives rise to this disease is unknown and the condition generally manifests itself late in life.

T cell immunodeficiencies are more severe than B cell immunodeficiencies, since T cells affect both cell-mediated and humoral immunity. Defects in humoral immunity are characterized by recurrent infections with encapsulated bacteria; CMI defects result in increased susceptibility to intracellular pathogens (whether bacterial, viral, protozoal, or fungal). Opportunistic organisms seem to pose a special threat in T cell immunodeficiencies. Important deficiencies are listed below.

❑ **DiGeorge syndrome** is caused by thymic aplasia — a quantitative decrease in functional thymic mass that is associated with embryonic deletion of a region on chromosome 22. Interestingly, T cell maturation is normal in patients of DiGeorge syndrome. The syndrome is characterized by distinctive facial abnormalities, cardiac malformation, and hypoparathyroidism. Not surprisingly, the syndrome results in a profound depression in T cell numbers and absence of T cell responses. Although B cells are present in normal numbers, patients fail to respond to TD antigens. Prognosis is very poor, with long-term survival difficult even if treated for immunological deficit.

❑ **T cell receptor deficiencies** can lead to **S**evere **C**ombined **I**mmuno**d**eficiency (SCID). SCID results in a combined B and T cell deficiency. Common features of SCID include recurrent opportunistic infections, diarrhoea, paucity of lymphoid tissue, and failure to thrive. The patient shows hypogammaglobulinaemia as well as decreased or absent T and B cell responses. Lymphocytes from these patients fail to respond to mitogens. Combined immunodeficiencies are the most serious of all immunodeficiencies, with poor prognosis unless interventions to correct the defect are undertaken early in life. Mutations in the tyrosine kinase ZAP70 can result in SCID characterized by decreased serum IgG, impaired cell responses, and decreased or absent T cell function — particularly CD8$^+$ T cell function. Similarly, a defect in *RAG-1* or *RAG-2* genes results in the absence of TcR (and BcR) rearrangement, precluding the development of functional B and T cells.

❑ **X-linked SCID** is the most common form of SCID. It is caused by a deficiency in the functional common γ chain, a common subunit of receptors for IL-2, IL-4, IL-7, IL-9, and IL-15. These cytokines are crucial for normal T cell proliferation and differentiation. A defect in common γ chain receptor results in a profound perturbation in the T cell compartment. Patients show very low numbers of T cells and NK cells with low to normal numbers of B cells.

❑ **Bare Lymphocyte Syndrome** (BLS) derives its name from a lack of MHC class I or II expression on haematopoietic cells. Two types of BLS are recognized. Mutations in one of several distinct genes involved in MHC class I synthesis and loading pathways can cause BLS type I, and patients have a relatively better prognosis than type 2 BLS. Type 2 BLS patients have a mutation in one of the genes critical for the transcription of class II molecules. BLS type 2 patients have very poor prognosis and often die of progressive organ failure.

9 Humoral Immunity

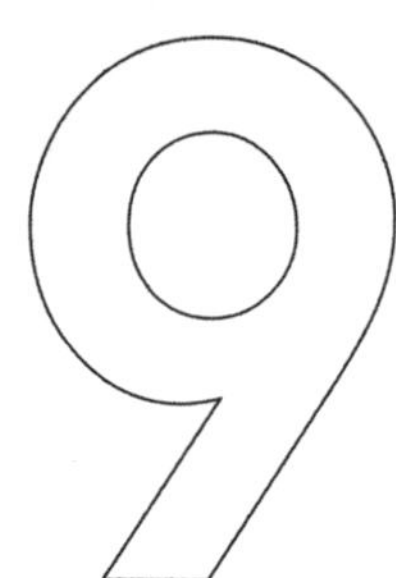

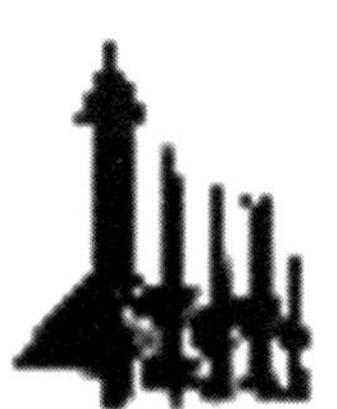

Hey baby, thought you were the one who tried to run away.
Ohh, baby, wasn't I the one who made you want to stay?
Please don't bet that you'll ever escape me
Once I get my sights on you
Got a license to kill
And you know I'm going straight for your heart.
(Got a license to kill)

—Gladys Knight, *License to Kill*

9.1 Introduction

Humoral immunity is conferred by 'body humours' (nothing to do with fun; it is an old English term for body fluids!) specifically, the Ig secreted by terminally differentiated B cells (ie, plasma cells). This Ig response is unusual in many respects.

BiP: Binding protein
Fab: Antigen-binding fragment
Fc: Fragment crystallizable
FcRn: FcR neonatal
GPI: Glycosylphosphtidylinostiol
IVIg: Intravenous Ig
mAb: Monoclonal antibody
pIgR: Polymeric Ig receptor
SC: Secretory component
SRP: Signal recognition protein

❏ Humans can produce Igs against a virtually limitless array of antigens, and each of these is specific for a particular antigen and is therefore different. These billion or more Igs are encoded by a genome consisting of about 10^5 distinct genes which are randomly rearranged to give rise to the different Igs during lymphocytic development (chapter 10).

❏ Each B cell clone can give rise to progeny that produce Igs of a single antigenic specificity but of different isotypes. Thus, naïve B cells express IgD and IgM on their cell surfaces. Upon stimulation, the progeny of these B cells can switch the class of Ig to express and secrete a different class of antibody (IgG, IgA, or IgE).

❏ A second or subsequent challenge with the same antigen generally results in a more rapid and more specific humoral response than the primary response.

❏ B cells secrete Igs while simultaneously expressing them as an integral part of their cell membrane. This is remarkable, since membrane proteins differ from secreted proteins in their primary amino acid sequences — a stretch of hydrophobic amino acids in the transmembrane region is indispensable for anchoring the protein in the cell membrane.

Certain unusual structural characteristics and genetic mechanisms are responsible for these exceptional features of the humoral response. This chapter and the next are devoted to explaining them.

9.2 Primary Humoral Response

The sequence of events leading to antibody secretion by B cells in the primary humoral response has already been discussed in the preceding chapters (chapters 6 and 8) and is summarized below.

❏ On primary challenge, the TD antigen (microbial, viral, etc) is captured and transported to the draining lymph node by DCs or macrophages.

❏ Digested fragments of the antigen are loaded on MHC class II molecules by these APCs and presented to naïve $CD4^+$ T cells.

❏ Recognition of the peptide:MHC complex (or lipid:CD1 complex) along with engagement of costimulatory molecules activates the naïve T cells. Cytokines released by APCs further help in this activation. Activated T cells proliferate and finally differentiate to the helper phenotype; they also secrete chemokines.

❏ Ligation of BcR by the antigen stimulates the B cells. They internalize antigen via pinocytosis (if it is soluble) or BcR, digest it and display parts of the antigen in the context of MHC class II molecules.

❏ B cells migrate to the edge of the B cell zone in response to T cell chemokines and in turn secrete chemokines like BCL-1 that result in migration of T cells to the edge of the B-T cell areas. The two cells engage in cognate interaction.

❏ As a result of the signals delivered by TH cells, B cells undergo blast transformation and migrate from the primary foci of proliferating cells to secondary follicles where they differentiate to plasmablasts and memory cells. Some of the proliferating B cells undergo affinity maturation and isotype switching in the germinal centre.

❏ Plasmablasts migrate to the bone marrow or medullary cords of the lymph nodes and start producing Ig. These effector cells are capable of secreting Ig at the astounding rate of about 2000 antibodies/sec!

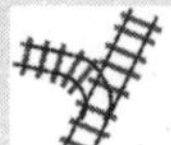

In the Footsteps of Gandhi: Passive Immunity

Adaptive immunity can be divided into two broad groups, depending upon the mode of acquisition — active and passive.

❑ **Active immunity** is acquired or gained by an individual in response to the introduction of microbes or their products into the body. The immunity is natural active immunity if it results from a clinical or subclinical infection. Artificial acquired immunity, on the other hand, results from a deliberate inoculation of microbes or their products, ie, through vaccination.

❑ **Passive immunity** is acquired passively, ie, without the active involvement of the recipient's immune system (eg, immunity transferred passively to the child via placenta or mother's milk). Artificial passive immunity results when the serum of an actively immunized animal is injected into the recipient. Antibodies in the donor's serum confer immunity to the recipient. **Adoptive immunity** is the transfer of primed (antigen stimulated) lymphocytes from an actively immunized donor to a non-immunized individual. Since actual lymphocytes are passively acquired, the recipient may show cell-mediated and/or humoral responses, depending upon the types of cells transferred.

Passive immunity is of a short duration (8–10 days), since the donor antibodies are eventually catabolized and destroyed. Passive immunization is used for various reasons.

❑ **Intravenous Ig** (IVIg) is the treatment of choice for patients with antibody deficiencies. IVIg is given at a dosage of 200–400 mg/Kg of body weight every three weeks; high dose IVIg may be given (2 gm/Kg/month) as an immunomodulatory agent in a number of immune and inflammatory disorders (eg, idiopathic thrombocytopenic purpurea).

❑ Passive immunity may be used as an emergency prophylactic measure to afford protection in the lag phase of the recipient's immune response, eg, in the treatment of diphtheria. Diphtheria is a potentially fatal infection caused by *Corynebacterium diphtheriae*. A toxin produced by the organism is responsible for the fatality of the infection. Individuals diagnosed with diphtheria are therefore given diphtherial antitoxin. The antibodies neutralize the toxin and allow survival until the patient's immune system is activated. It is for the same reason that ATS (**A**nti-**T**etanus **S**erum) is administered to patients with deep wounds likely to be infected with *Clostridium tetani*.

❑ Passive immunization may also be used to neutralize toxins introduced by snakebites or scorpion bites.

IVIg is obtained from the pooled plasma of thousands of donors, and anti-toxins are raised by the repeated immunization of animals. The collected sera are treated to ensure absence of antibody aggregates, since such aggregates can trigger massive complement activation, resulting in type III hypersensitivity, kidney damage, and severe anaphylactic shock. They are also treated with detergents and solvents to minimize the danger of transferring infectious agents. Repeated administration of heterologous antibodies (ie, from people with different genetic backgrounds or from other species) are likely to give rise to anti-isotypic or anti-idiotypic antibodies in the recipient. The anti-isotypic antibodies can result in serum sickness (chapter 15). Anti-idiotypic antibodies, on the other hand, can neutralize antibodies in the antiserum, lowering its usefulness.

The advent of **m**onoclonal **A**nti**b**ody (mAb) technology with its possibility of engineered 'humanized antibodies' has opened a new era in passive immunotherapy, and a number of mAb preparations are now approved for therapeutic use. mAbs are Igs produced by a single clone of B cells. It follows that mAbs are monospecific and homogeneous. In contrast, serum antibodies are polyclonal and heterogeneous, since they are a product of multiple clones of B cells. Kohler and Milstein introduced mAb technology in 1975. In this method, spleen cells from immunized animals are fused with myeloma cells and placed in a selective medium that allows the survival of only hybrid cells (called hybridomas). These hybridomas have the Ig producing capacity of the plasma cell and the potential for unlimited growth of the myeloma cell line. Originally, the hybridomas were injected in laboratory animals where they established tumours and produced Ig of given specificity and isotype. Refinement of the technology allowed the elimination of animals and large-scale production *in vitro*. mAb treatment is now being explored for treating tumours, autoimmune diseases, graft rejections and infectious diseases. Its potential can be judged from the fact that more than a quarter of all new biotech drugs in development are mAbs.

Because of technical difficulties (lack of suitable myeloma cells, low rates of mAb secretion, etc), initial clinical trials used murine mAbs. However, repeated administration of murine antibodies give rise to human anti-mouse antibodies. In addition, murine antibodies are hampered in their effector function because of the low affinity of human FcRs for mouse Fc. Development of chimeric antibodies, consisting of the Fab region of mouse antibodies and Fc region of human antibodies, has helped overcome some of these problems (fig. 9.S1). A further refinement was the creation of humanized antibodies produced by grafting CDRs from a mouse mAb into human IgG. An alternative approach is to create bispecific antibodies. These are non-natural antibodies created to bind two different epitopes. Often, one epitope is a tumour-associated antigen, and the other is associated with an immune effector cell. The antibodies directly link the effector cell to the tumour cells, enhancing immune response. The epitopes of choice on effector cells include $Fc\gamma RI$, expressed by granulocytes and macrophages; CD16, expressed by NK cells; and the pan T cell molecule CD3. Fusion proteins consisting of radionuclides, toxins, or chemotherapeutic agents conjugated to the Fc region of human mAbs are now being explored for therapeutics. Such immunoconjugates provide the advantage of targeting specificity. Additionally, since the toxic payload is delivered directly to the target cell, both the dosage and side effects are reduced. Radiolabelled mAbs can also be used as diagnostic tools for detecting or locating tumour antigens, permitting early diagnosis of metastatic tumours. For example, ^{131}I labelled mAbs have been used in the detection of breast cancer metastases. Below are listed some mAbs with potential clinical use.

- ❑ Muromonab, an anti-CD3 murine mAb preparation, has been shown to improve graft survival in some studies. Since it knocks out all $CD3^+$ T cells, treatment increases the risk of infection. It is therefore used only for steroid-resistant patients.
- ❑ Anti-CD25 mAbs that bind the IL-2R have the advantage of being effective against activated T cells. Basiliximab and daclizumab are chimeric humanized mAbs now in clinical trials for prolonging graft survival.
- ❑ Anti-TNF mAbs are of potential use in anti-inflammatory therapy. A human-mouse chimeric anti-TNF mAb, infliximab, has shown great promise in the treatment of rheumatoid arthritis and Crohn's disease. Similar anti-inflammatory activity has also been reported for the TNF-receptor-IgG1 fusion protein, etanercept.
- ❑ Rituximab, a chimeric anti-CD20 mAb, is the first mAb approved for treatment of low grade and follicular non-Hodgkin's lymphomas. It is an IgG1 mAb that can activate complement and aid in ADCC. CD20 is expressed on pre-B and mature B cells. Rituximab has also been shown to possess anti-proliferative and apoptosis-inducing activity against B cells expressing CD20.
- ❑ Trastuzumab is a chimeric IgG1 mAb directed against the HER2/neu receptor. It is now approved for clinical use. Also called ERBB2, this receptor is expressed on many breast and ovarian carcinomas.
- ❑ MDX-210 is a bispecific mAb directed against ERBB2 and $Fc\gamma RI$. Used to treat ovarian cancers overexpressing ERBB2, this mAb is currently in phase II clinical trials.
- ❑ Humanized anti-CD33 antibody conjugated to the toxin calicheamicin has been approved for treatment of $CD33^+$ acute myeloid leukaemia.

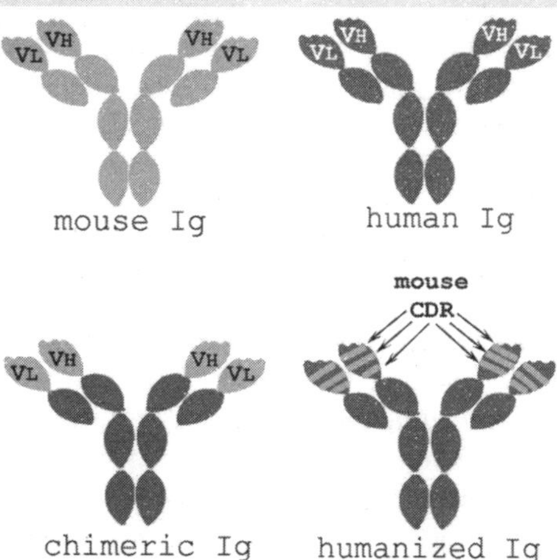

Figure 9.S1 Chimeric antibodies and humanized antibodies have helped reduce complications arising from passive immunization with murine antibodies.

❑ If the challenging antigen is of TI type, T cells do not participate in the immune response and the response primarily involves B1 and MZ B cells.

❑ The secreted Igs bind the antigen, resulting in a transient phase where the antigen exists mostly as soluble antigen-antibody complexes. Phagocytes scavenge the complexes, resulting in their elimination (this is also referred to as the phase of immune-elimination).

❑ Free antibodies appear in the peripheral blood at the end of the immune-elimination phase and remain there until eventual catabolization.

The kinetics of the primary immune response and the concentrations of antibodies reached are dependent upon the nature of the antigen; presence of adjuvants; the route of administration; and the species, strain, and age of the animal. Serum analysis for antigen-specific antibodies following antigenic stimulation reveals four distinct phases (fig. 9.1).

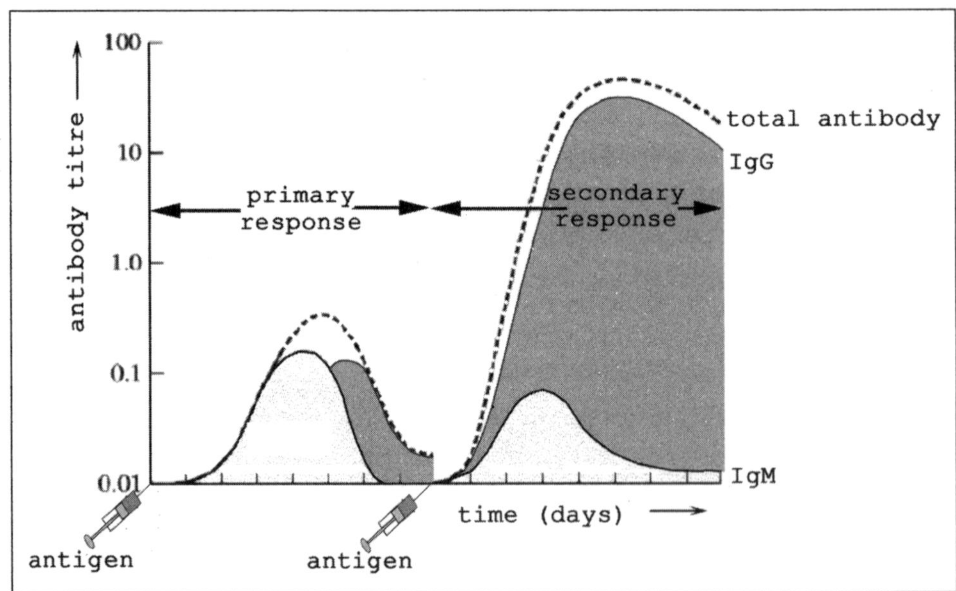

Figure 9.1 Secondary humoral responses to TD antigens differ from primary humoral responses in terms of their kinetics as well as concentration, affinity, isotype, and duration of antibody response. The time required for the appearance of free antibodies in serum is much longer in primary humoral responses. This phase, called the lag phase, represents the time required for the selection, clonal expansion, and differentiation of naïve B and T cells. It also includes the time required for immune-elimination. IgM (represented by the solid line) is the predominant antibody produced in the early stages of the primary response but changes to IgG (grey fill) in the later stages. Thanks to clonal expansion, the frequency of B and T cells capable of recognizing the antigen increases at the end of the primary response. The reprogramming of their antigen receptors also makes these cells responsive to lower concentrations of antigen. Hence, secondary responses have faster kinetics. The total antibody secreted is much greater (broken line) in secondary humoral responses; the response lasts longer and consists of predominantly IgG antibodies.

❑ An **initial lag phase** lasts for 4–7 days during which antigen-specific antibody is not detected in the serum. This is the time required for the selection, clonal expansion, and differentiation of naïve B cells to plasma cells. It also includes the time required for immune-elimination of the antigen.

❑ A **log phase** occurs when concentration of antigen-specific antibodies increases exponentially with time. Antibody production peaks within 7–10 days of antigen exposure. If the challenging antigen is of the TD type, isotype switching from IgM to IgG is observed. In this phase, the rate of antibody synthesis is far greater than its catabolization and the net result is a logarithmic increase in serum antibody concentration.

❑ The **steady state** is when the antigen-specific antibody concentration reaches a plateau. The amount of antibody secreted is balanced by the amount that is catabolized, resulting in this brief steady state. Once the antigen is eliminated, homeostatic mechanisms swing into action and the proliferating and differentiating B cells receive death signals.

❑ A **stage of decline** where the rate of antibody catabolization outstrips the rate of synthesis.

9.3 The Secondary Humoral Immune Response

Second or subsequent encounters with an immunogen are deemed 'secondary' or anamnestic immune responses (from the Greek word *anamnesis* meaning recall). TI antigens elicit secondary responses that do not differ significantly from primary responses. Secondary responses to TD antigens, however, are more rapid and aggressive than primary responses because of a variety of factors.

❑ Clonal expansion during primary immune responses results in a much larger pool of B and T cells capable of specifically reacting with the immunogen after primary immunization. A 1000-fold increase in the frequency of antigen-specific lymphocytes has been reported in experimental animals.

❑ Memory cells formed at the end of the primary immune response are reprogrammed in their signal transduction capabilities and hence are quicker in responding to immunogenic challenge.

❑ Thanks to affinity maturation, BcRs expressed by memory B cells bind the antigen with a much higher affinity than BcRs expressed by naïve B cells, hence fewer immunogenic molecules are required for activation (chapters 8 and 10).

Thus, secondary humoral responses differ from primary responses in several respects.

❑ **Secondary responses occur with faster kinetics.** The lag phase is shorter (about 1–3 days), the response peaks much faster (3–5 days), and the steady state is maintained for a much longer period in secondary responses. The decline is also slower, so secondary responses persist for prolonged periods.

❑ **They result in antibody titres** (concentration) **of much higher magnitudes.** The large pool of antigen-specific B cells formed at the end of the primary response results in an increased number of plasma cells in the secondary response with a concomitant increase in antibody titres.

❑ **Secondary responses are dominated by isotypes other than IgM** because of class switch recombination undergone by the proliferating B cells in later stages of the primary immune response.

❑ **Antibodies produced in the secondary response have a much greater affinity for the antigen.** An immune challenge, whether primary or secondary, results in a spectrum of antibodies with varying affinities for the antigen, reflecting the recruitment of multiple B cell clones in the immune response. Primary responses result in predominantly low affinity antibodies. In secondary responses, only a fraction of the antibodies continue to be of low affinity; the remainder have a much higher affinity for the antigen. This phenomenon, called affinity maturation, can be attributed to two distinct processes.

  • During proliferation of B cells in the germinal centres, the DNA coding for the V region of Ig (ie, the antigen-binding domain) undergoes point mutations. B cells expressing BcR with higher affinity for the antigen are selectively allowed to undergo clonal expansion, while those expressing low-affinity BcR are sent down the path of apoptosis. Antibodies produced later in the immune response therefore have a higher affinity for the challenging antigen (section 10.4.2).

- During primary immune responses, the antigen is in far excess of the number of cells capable of recognizing and binding it. Hence, irrespective of affinity, the entire repertoire of cells responding to the antigen is stimulated. On subsequent challenges, however, the number of cells capable of reacting with the antigenic determinants is much larger. The ensuing competition for the limited antigenic determinants results in selective stimulation of cells expressing high affinity BcR.

Secondary responses to hapten-carrier conjugates are dependent upon both hapten-primed memory B cells and carrier-primed memory T_H cells. If the secondary challenge is with the same hapten used in the primary challenge but conjugated to a different carrier (eg, dinitrophenyl conjugated to ovalbumin — DNP-OVA — used in primary challenge and DNP-bovine serum albumin — DNP-BSA — in the secondary challenge), the ensuing response to the hapten is of the primary type, not the secondary type. This phenomenon is called the carrier effect. As explained in chapter 4, hapten-carrier conjugates behave like TD antigens, resulting in an antibody response to the hapten and a T cell response to the carrier. The requirement for associative recognition necessitates that B and T cells recognize antigenic-determinants on the same molecule. DNP conjugated to BSA is therefore unable to stimulate a secondary humoral response to DNP. However, if the animal is primed with the second carrier (BSA alone) before the administration of DNP-BSA, BSA-primed memory T_H cells will be formed in the animal and result in a secondary-type humoral response to DNP.

9.4 Ig Synthesis

As explained, Igs are unique in that they are simultaneously synthesized in both the membrane and the secreted form by plasma cells. Although both secreted and membrane proteins are synthesized in the ER, the sequence of events differs for the two. A hydrophobic sequence of amino acids at the N– terminus, called the leader sequence, is present in either form of the proteins. This sequence causes the mRNA, ribosome, and translated leader sequence of the protein to bind to the pore structures in the membrane of the ER. The leader sequence causes the protein to thread through the pore and is eventually cleaved off. Membrane-bound proteins have a stretch of hydrophobic amino acids that stops the transfer through the ER membrane and causes the protein to remain trapped in the membrane. When the hydrophobic stretch is absent, the proteins pass through the pore into the lumen of the ER and are secreted. The translated proteins (whether membrane or secreted) are transported to the cell surface via the golgi apparatus and may be modified by the addition of carbohydrates. When vesicles are pinched off from the ER for transport through the golgi, membrane-bound proteins stay in the golgi membrane, whereas secreted proteins are retained in the lumen of the golgi. The golgi vesicles ultimately fuse with the plasma membrane. The proteins in the vesicle are released to the exterior, while membrane-bound proteins become a part of the plasma membrane. Thus, the fate of the protein (ie, membrane-bound or secreted) is determined by its amino acid sequence, and this decision is taken at the rough ER at the time of its synthesis. Needless to say, how the plasma cell manages to produce both the secreted and membrane-bound form of Ig was a fascinating puzzle. It is now established that it achieves this feat by differential RNA splicing. Two separate regions at the 3′ end of the C_H region code for the two different forms of Ig. One codes a stretch of hydrophilic amino acids called the S (**S**ecreted) region, whereas two other exons code for a stretch of hydrophobic amino acids called the M (**M**embrane) segment. The primary transcript encodes both segments. Alternative splicing of the primary transcript in the nucleus yields transcripts that have either the M segment or have been cut after the S segment. The M segment containing H chain gets trapped in the membrane and the Ig becomes

Trying to 'Fit In': Cross-reactivity

An antibody is said to be cross-reactive when it binds an antigen other than the one used for eliciting the immune response. This cross-reactivity could be because of chemical relatedness or the presence of identical epitopes (ie, shared epitopes) on unrelated antigens. If chemical similarity is the underlying cause of cross-reactivity, generally the cross-reacting antibody binds the homologous antigen better than the heterologous one. In the case of shared epitopes, however, the affinity of the antibody for both the antigens is similar (fig. 9.S2). Although the phenomenon of cross-reactivity is exploited in the diagnosis of infections (chapter 4), its disadvantages far outweigh this advantage. Cross-reactivity has been implicated in many autoimmune diseases (chapter 14). It is also the underlying cause of 'the phenomenon of the original antigenic sin[1]'. Also called epitope imprinting, the term is used to describe a phenomenon whereby exposure to an antigen influences subsequent responses to similar antigens. It was originally described for the influenza virus, wherein it was observed that antibodies elicited after a second infection by an antigenically different influenza strain reacted more strongly to the original infecting viral variant. Thus, the immune response to the first viral infection seems to have a dominating influence on subsequent immune responses to antigenically related viruses, and the second virus often induces a response that is directed against the original strain. Epitope imprinting is attributed to the activation of memory B cells formed at the end of the first infection by cross-reacting antigens on the second viral strain. As a result, the antibodies produced are not efficient in neutralizing the second virus and allow the virus to escape and cause infection. Antigenic variation is thus a mechanism of immune evasion observed in a variety of viral, bacterial, and parasitic infections such as those caused by the enterovirus, reovirus, paramyxovirus, togavirus, chlamydia, and *Plasmodium* spp. The phenomenon is exploited in epidemiological studies of these infections. Although initially observed for Ig responses, antigenic imprinting is found to occur for CD8[+] T cells as well. It proves especially deleterious in HIV infections. HIV is extremely prone to antigenic variation and multiple variants of HIV are found to co-exist in the same individual. As a result of epitope imprinting, antibodies able to neutralize the initial virus or CTLs active against cells infected with the initial virus continue to rise with time. However, these antibodies/CTLs are not effective against concurrent HIV isolates. Thus, continued evolution of the virus combined with the phenomenon of original antigenic sin allows HIV to escape adaptive immune responses (chapter 17). Antigenic variation is also a major obstacle in designing vaccination strategies. As a consequence of epitope imprinting, immune responses generated due to an infection will be against the strain used in the vaccination rather than against the variant causing the infection. Thus, the vaccine might help the infection rather than checking it. One way to circumvent the problem is to embark upon fresh vaccinations with newly emerging viral strains every year, as is done for the influenza virus. An alternative approach of inoculating with a cocktail of closely related viral peptides to elicit a more broadly reactive T cell response is now being investigated.

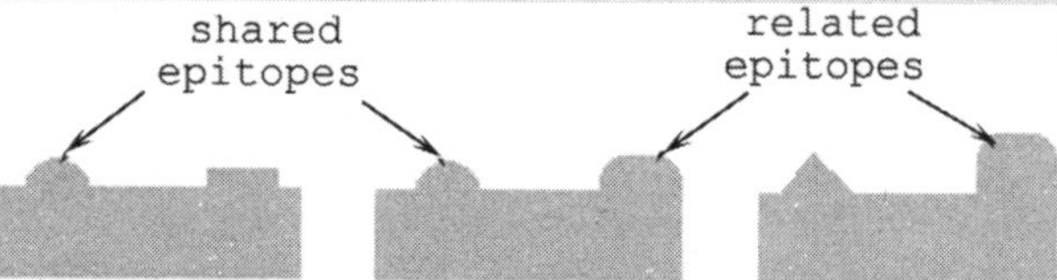

Figure 9.S2 Antibodies may cross react with heterologous antigens because of the presence of shared epitopes or chemically related epitopes.

an integral membrane protein. The S segment containing transcript encodes an Ig H chain that passes through the ER membrane into the ER lumen and becomes a part of the secreted Ig. The major steps in Ig synthesis are listed below (fig. 9.2).

❏ Ig L chains and H chains are synthesized separately; L and H chain genes are transcribed in the B cell nucleus to produce RNA transcripts. The introns are then spliced out to yield mRNA, which is translated by the ribosomes at the membrane of rough ER.

❏ Both chains are formed as larger precursors with an N− terminal sequence of about 20 amino acids, called the leader.

[1] The name is derived from a term in the Bible that refers to the human race possessing an inherent tendency to sin or do evil, just as their progenitors, Adam and Eve, did. In the immunological context, it implies that having erred once, the immune system tends to commit the same sin again.

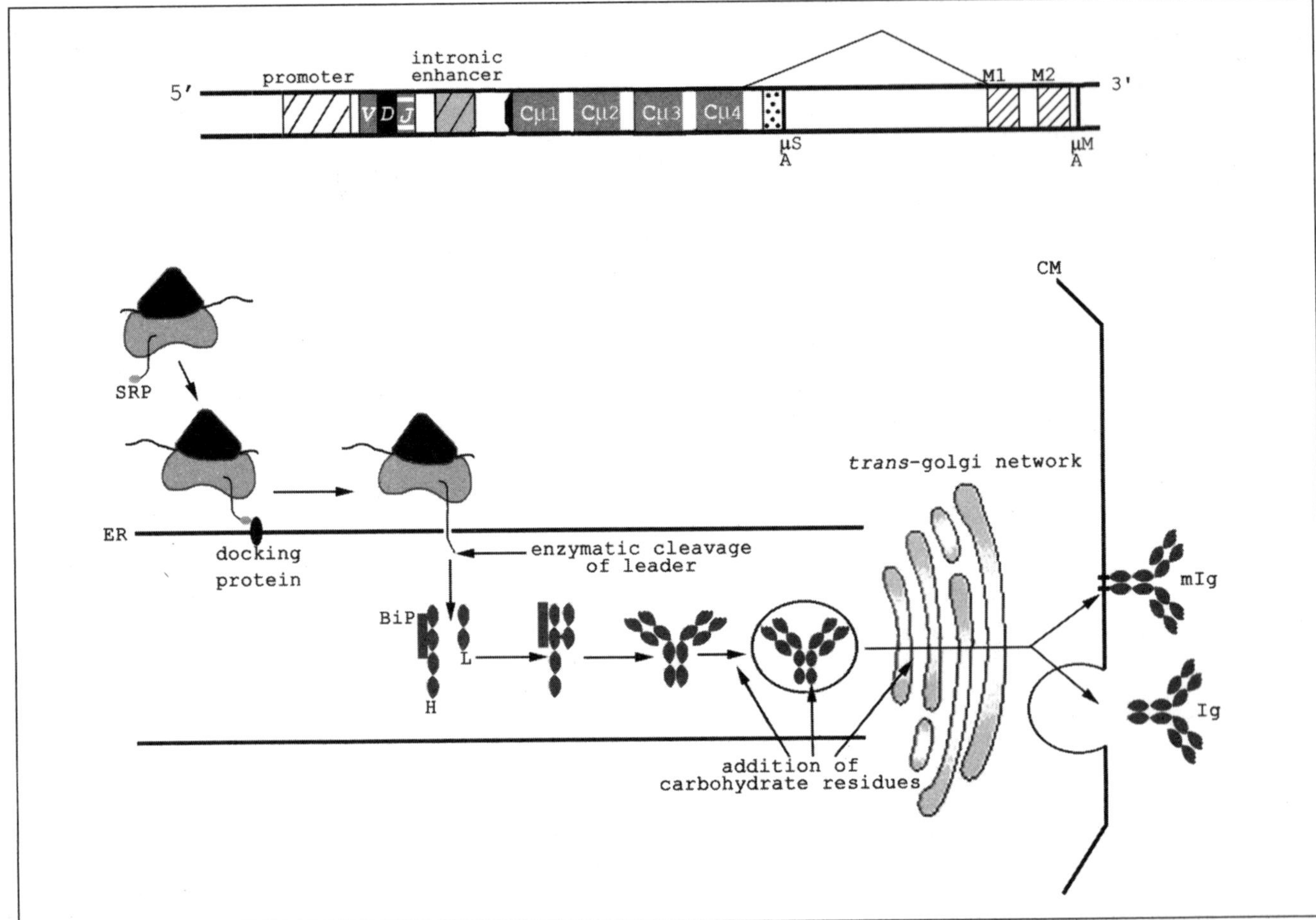

Figure 9.2 Differential splicing of the primary transcript allows plasma cells to simultaneously synthesize membrane and secreted forms of Ig. *The organization of human μ chain locus on the chromosome 14 is shown in the top panel and is not to scale. The assembled V region (consisting V, D, J subexons) lies downstream of the promoter. Regions encoding the four constant domains (Cμ1 to Cμ4) lie 3' to the intronic enhancer. Downstream to Cμ4 is the region encoding the tail-end (Carboxy–terminus) of secretory IgM. This region has a polyadenylation site (μSA) that allows chain termination. Two separate regions encode the transmembrane region of mIgM (M1 and M2). They too have their own polyadenylation site (μMA). The primary transcript encodes both segments. Alternative splicing of the primary transcript in the nucleus yields transcripts that end at μSA or have Cμ4 joined to M1/M2 and μMA. Transcripts of membrane and secreted forms of other isotypes are produced on similar lines. Both the H and L chains (whether of secretory or membrane Ig) are synthesized as larger precursors with an N– terminal leader sequence. Translation of the leader sequence occurs in the cytoplasm (bottom panel), but further translation is blocked by the binding of the leader sequence to the Signal Recognition Protein (SRP). Docking of SRP to its binding protein on the ER membrane permits further translation. The leader is cleaved during the translocation of the growing chain in the ER lumen. The elongating H chain binds to BiP (Binding Protein) and eventually combines with other H and L chains to form the complete Ig. Post-translational modifications, such as addition of carbohydrate residues, occur both in the ER and during transport through the trans-golgi network. The newly synthesized secretory Igs are released to the external environment by reverse pinocytosis, whereas the membrane Igs are expressed on the cell surface by fusion of the transporting vesicle membrane with the cell membrane.*

- ❑ The leader sequence is translated by the ribosome in the cytoplasm; the translated leader sequence binds to a Signal Recognition Protein (SRP). SRP binding blocks further translation.
- ❑ The complex consisting of the mRNA, translated leader sequence, SRP, and the ribosome is translocated to the ER membrane.
- ❑ SRP binds to a protein called the 'docking protein' at a vacant site on the ER. If SRP is the lock that stops further translation, the docking protein is the key that permits further translation.
- ❑ The leader is cleaved during the process of chain transfer in the lumen of the ER.

❑ The new chain being synthesized at the ER traverses the membrane of the ER; as the chain elongates, it complexes with Binding Protein (BiP) at the C_{H1} domain. BiP is a chaperone molecule that catalyzes the folding of the growing H chain.

❑ The newly synthesized chain combines with other H and L chains to form the complete Ig unit. BiP is progressively displaced in this process.

❑ In the lumen of the ER, enzymes add carbohydrate units to the newly formed Ig molecules.

❑ Ig molecules are transported to the cell surface via the *trans*-golgi network; further post-translational enzymatic modification occurs during this transport.

❑ Igs are released in the external environment by reverse pinocytosis; the transporting vesicle's membrane fuses with the cell membrane to release Ig molecules.

❑ mIgs are inserted into the membrane of the ER by its hydrophobic sequences as it is being synthesized. They are expressed on the cell surface after fusion of the vesicle membrane with the cell membrane.

9.5　Ig Structure

Igs are characterized by their specificity and sensitivity. Specificity is defined as the ability of antibodies to discriminate between homologous epitopes (ie, epitopes against which the antibody was raised) and heterologous (ie, related) epitopes. As explained in chapter 4, antibodies can differentiate between the three-dimensional conformations of closely related structures. This does not imply that antibodies cannot react with related ligands, ie, display cross-reactivity. However, the reaction between the antibody and the related ligand is generally weaker than that between the antibody and its homologues antigen[2]. Thus, specificity depends upon the relative affinity of the antibody for two closely related structures. The greater this difference, the more specific the antibody. Sensitivity refers to the ability to detect a variable (ie, the antigen) in the presence of large amounts of other extraneous substances. Ig sensitivity is thus a consequence of Ig specificity.

9.5.1　Elucidation of Ig Structure

When Tisselius and Kabat electrophoresed[3] serum at pH 8.5, they discovered that IgG is positively charged and lies in the fraction closest to the anode (called the γ fraction; Igs are therefore called γ-globulins). They found that albumin, having the greatest negative charge, moves rapidly towards the positively charged cathode and is followed by three globulin fractions (called α, β, and γ respectively). Although majority of the IgG lies in the γ fraction, significant amounts of Igs can be found over the entire spectrum, extending from α to γ fractions.

Elegant experiments by Porter, Nisonoff, and Edelman helped establish Ig structure (and earned Porter and Edelman a Nobel Prize). Their approach, consisting of digestion by proteinases and the use of reducing agents, has been extensively used to establish the structure of many proteins.

❑ Porter subjected the low MW fraction of globulins containing a γ globulin (known to possess antibody activity) with MW 150 KD to brief papain digestion. Prolonged digestion with this protease will completely digest practically any protein. On brief exposure, however, papain digests only the most susceptible bonds of IgG, yielding two identical 45 KD **Fragments** that retain their **antigen-binding** property (therefore called **Fab**) and one **Fragment** of 50 KD that **c**rystallizes during low temperature storage (hence called **Fc**), but cannot bind antigen. Unlike whole Ig, the Fab fragments cannot precipitate or aggregate antigen molecules, suggesting that the two Fab fragments need to be joined together to participate in visible reactions (fig. 9.3).

[2] Heteroclitic antibodies (Greek, *heteros* — other, *klinein* — inclined) are an exception in that heteroclitic antibodies bind heterologous antigens better than homologus antigens.

[3] Electrophoresis allows the separation of molecules on the basis of their electric charge and is explained in Appendix III.

- Nisonoff treated IgG to brief digestion with pepsin and ended up with one single fragment of 100 KD that could bind antigen and yield a visible reaction. Treating this fragment with very mild reducing agents gave two identical fragments that, like Fab, reacted with the antigen but did not give a visible reaction. The large fragment was therefore called F(ab')$_2$.
- Porter and Edelmen also treated IgG with the reducing agent β-mercaptoethanol and separated the fragments by chromatography. β-mercaptoethanol irreversibly cleaves disulphide bonds. The experiment revealed that 150 KD IgG consisted of two H chains of 50 KD and two L chains of 25 KD.
- Porter established the relation of the Fab and Fc fragments to the H and L chains by raising antisera against Fab and Fc fragments. Antisera raised against Fab reacted with both H and L chains but that against Fc reacted only with the H chain.
- On the basis of these experiments, Porter suggested a four-chain Y shaped structure for IgG that was later confirmed by X-ray crystallographic studies.

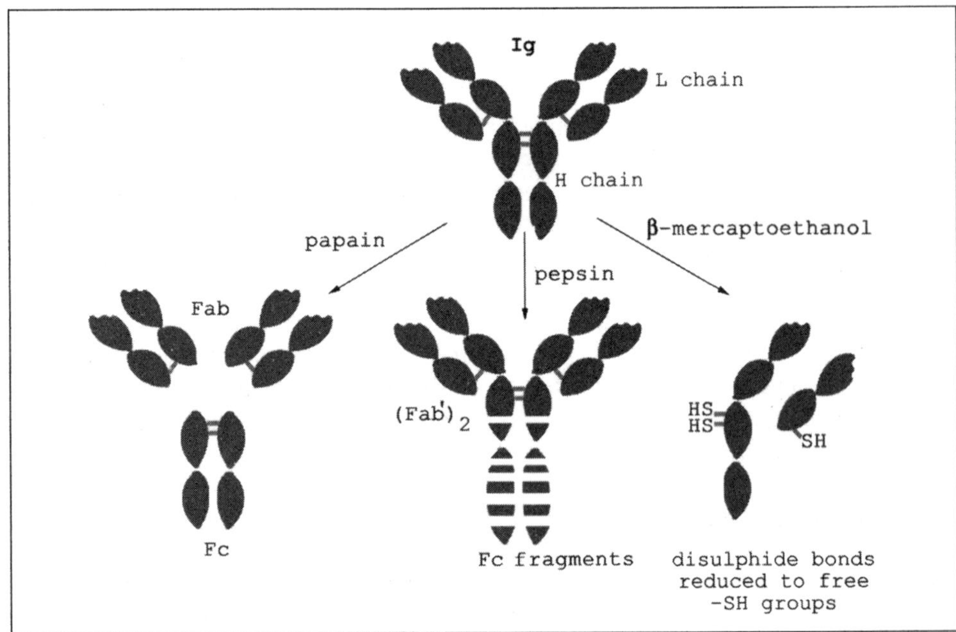

Figure 9.3 The four-chain structure of Igs was proposed on the basis of the experiments of Porter, Nisonoff, and Edelman. They treated Igs by two proteases (papain and pepsin) and a reducing agent (b-mercaptoethanol). Papain digestion yielded two identical fragments (Fab) capable of antigen binding but incapable of visible reaction. It also yielded another fragment that crystallized on low temperature storage (Fc). In contrast, pepsin digestion yielded a single fragment capable of both antigen binding and precipitation and multiple low MW fragments. On treatment with mild reducing agents, the large fragment generated two identical fragments that had higher MW than Fab fragments and were capable of antigen binding but incapable of producing a visible reaction. Hence, the fragments were called Fab' and their dimer, (Fab')$_2$. b-mercaptoethanol treatment resulted in the formation of two identical fragments consisting of H and L chains.

9.5.2 IgG Structure and Function

The prototypical Ig, IgG, has a sedimentation coefficient of 7S. Chapter 6 explains how it consists of a pair each of two distinct types of polypeptide chains — L and H. The predicted MW of this four-chain structure is between 150–200 KD. However, addition of carbohydrates at various sites on the H chains results in the actual weight of the molecule being greater than this predicted weight. Each L chain is bound to the H chain by a disulphide bond and non-covalent interactions, eg, salt linkages,

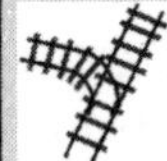 ## Making the Heavy Burden Light:
Tylopoda IgG

It is generally accepted that antibodies are tetrameric molecules consisting of two H and two L chains. Ig molecules of camels are exceptional in that 75% of serum antibody (IgG2 and IgG3) molecules in camels are devoid of L chains. Llamas and dromedaries also have these L chain lacking antibodies, but they form a smaller percentage (< 45%) of the total serum Ig. These two-chain antibodies, called heavy chain antibodies, are nonetheless *bona fide* antibodies that can bind complement, are capable of agglutination, and have a comprehensive binding repertoire. They bind homologous antigens with high specificity and high affinity. The antigen-binding site of these antibodies consists only of a single domain called V_{HH}. The V domain of naturally occurring heavy chain antibodies is very similar to conventional Ig and consists of three CDR regions. However, these antibodies have a mutation in key residues in the region corresponding to the side of V_H region that interacts with V_L region. The normal hydrophobic amino acids are substituted by hydrophilic amino acids. Consequently, V_{HH} domains and heavy chain antibodies are highly soluble. V_{HH} domains also have additional cysteine residues which allow the formation of an interloop disulphide bond that stabilizes this domain. The V_{HH} region otherwise adopts a typical Ig-fold and superimposes perfectly on conventional V_H structure. Heavy chain antibodies differ from conventional Ig in one more respect — they lack a C_{H1} domain (fig. 9.S3).

Immunization studies indicate that the type of Ig response (whether normal or heavy chain) is dictated by the type of antigen. Heavy chain antibodies seem to be preferentially formed against active sites of enzymes or small haptens. For example, in llamas, administration of hapten-carrier conjugates gives rise to conventional anti-carrier IgG but anti-hapten heavy chain IgG. This preferential binding to haptens or active site of enzymes reflects a propensity of heavy chain IgG to bind to grooves or cavities of proteins. It is thought to be due to an inherent structural property of the single domain V_{HH}.

The occurrence of heavy chain antibodies raises many questions regarding the function of the L chains, isotype switching, and the role of various domains of conventional antibodies. It also helps to drive home the point that there is no room for complacency in immunology — no tenet of immunology can be regarded as absolute and unquestionable. Surprising and fundamental discoveries are constantly being made, and immunologists may be justified in expecting a life of excitement and adventure (!).

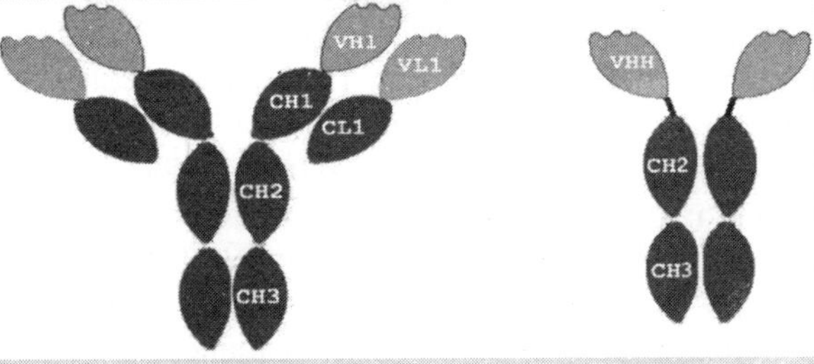

Figure 9.S3 Heavy chain Igs found in camels are devoid of L chains (depicted schematically in the right panel) unlike normal Ig molecules that consist of two H and two L chains each (left panel) (Adapted from Trends in Biochemical Sciences (2001) 26:230).

hydrogen bonds, and hydrophobic interactions (Table 4.1). Similar disulphide bridges and non-covalent interactions link the two H-L subunits together to give a four-chain structure. The Ig molecule is thus a dimer $(H-L)_2$ of a dimer (H-L). The whole molecule may be visualized as a Y shaped structure (fig. 9.4). Each arm of the Y consists of a dimer comprising the entire L chain and half H chain. The tail of the Y is formed by a dimer of the remaining half of the H chains. The arms of the Y contain the antigen-binding site, whereas the tail is involved in effector functions. The Ig molecule is flexible and changes its tertiary structure upon antigen binding. When not bound to the antigen, the arms of the Y lie relaxed, covering the C_{H2} domain. When in contact with the antigen, the arms swing out. The disulphide bonds

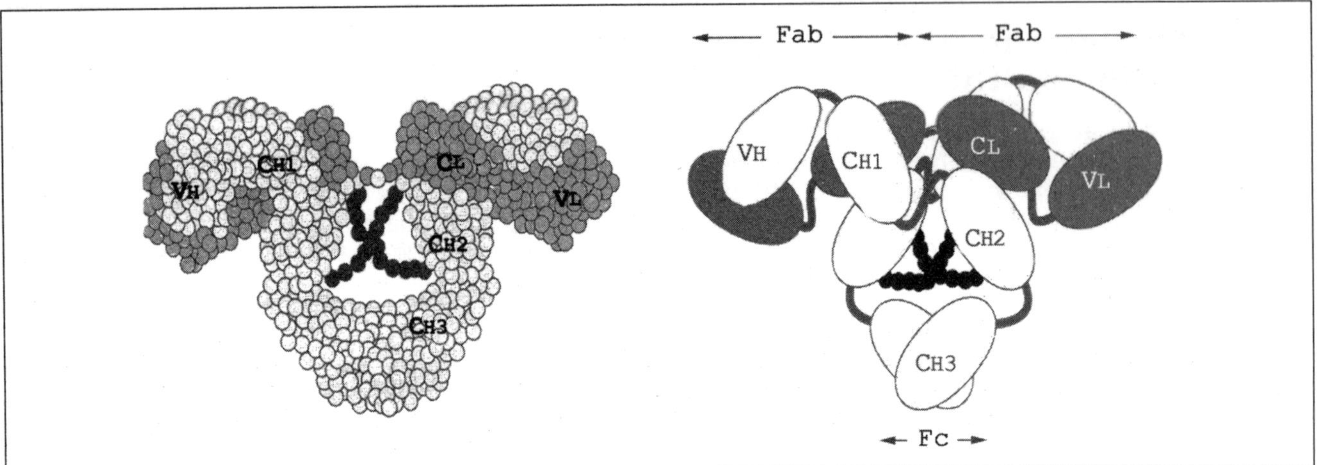

Figure 9.4 *The four chains of IgG are linked by inter- and intra-chain disulphide bonds to yield a Y shaped molecule. The panel on the left is a space-filled model of IgG based on X-ray crystallography. The two antigen-binding sites (Fab) lie at the tips of the arms of the Y; both H and L chains contribute to the antigen-binding. The main stem of the Y is formed by the H chains (Fc). The two arms of the Y are attached to the stem by a flexible hinge region. Note that when not bound to the antigen, the arms of the Y lie relaxed, covering the C_{H2} domains. The panel on the right is a schematic depiction of the molecule showing the different Ig folds (courtesy the Department of Immunology, Erasmus MC, Rotterdam, The Netherlands).*

between the two H chains facilitate this movement, and hence, this region is called the hinge region.

The determination of the amino acid sequence of IgG was delayed because of the unavailability of sufficient amounts of homogenous IgG. The discovery of IgG in the blood and urine of multiple myeloma patients finally made IgG sequence determination possible. As explained in chapter 6, amino acid sequencing of L and H chains revealed the presence of a NH_2– terminal V region that differed considerably in amino acid sequences between different IgG samples and a COOH– terminal C (for **C**onstant) region with much less variability. Consequently, the Carboxy-terminal 110 amino acid region of the L chain is denoted C_L (**C**onstant **l**ight) and the Amino– terminal half V_L (**V**ariable **l**ight) region. Similarly, the 110 amino acid domain at the NH_2– terminal of H chain is called the V_H region and the rest (around 330 amino acids) the C_H region. The C_H region consists of three separate domains — C_{H1}, C_{H2}, and C_{H3}. C regions of both H and L chains can be further subdivided into different groups, called isotypes, on the basis of their amino acid sequences. The C_L region consists of two groups, κ and λ. The C_H regions revealed five basic sequence patterns μ, δ, γ, ε, and α, giving the five isotypes IgM, IgD, IgG, IgE, and IgA.

Examination of amino acid sequences of a large number of Ig molecules has established that the variability is not evenly distributed within the V domains[4]. Some short segments show a high degree of variability and are called hypervariable regions. These hypervariable segments are located near amino acid positions 30, 50, and 95 in both the H and the L chains and together constitute about 15–20% of the human and murine V domjain. These regions are directly involved in the formation of the antigen-binding site and are referred to as CDRs. The intervening peptide segments are called the FRs — **F**ramework **R**egions — and are responsible for maintaining the architecture of the molecule. Each Ig chain (whether L or H) contains three CDRs (CDR1, CDR2, and CDR3) and four FRs (FR1- FR4). The FRs form the basic β-pleated sheet structure of the Ig fold of the V region (chapter 6), whereas the H and L CDRs are located on the loops that connect the β-sheets of the V_H and V_L domains. The hypervariable regions are thus exposed in three separate but closely disposed loops because of the folding of the V domain, much like three fingers of a hand and the FRs form the scaffold that holds these loops. The six hypervariable loops (three each of the V_H and V_L domains) together contribute to

[4] In hindsight, this distribution of variability seems perfectly logical. Since Igs can react with a virtually unlimited number of epitopes of different shapes and since a close fit is a pre-requisite for epitopes and paratope inter-action, antigen-binding sites of different Igs had to have different shapes. In other words, to allow for the different configurations needed to interact with different antigens, the amino acid sequence of the Fab region of the molecule had to be highly variable. However, since the basic architecture of the molecule has to be maintained, the V region had to have portions that were relatively less variable.

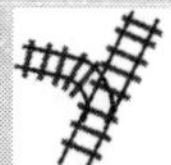

Milk and Tears

(No, this is not about how hard those early years are on mothers, but about the role these secretions play in immunity!)

Lachrymal glands, responsible for tear secretion, play a crucial role in the immunological protection of the ocular surface. These glands are the predominant source of sIgA in tears. They contain T cells, B cells, DCs, and macrophages along with an extraordinarily high density of IgA+IgD+ plasma cells. Once produced, sIgA antibodies are secreted into the tear film. The defensive role of sIgA seems to be especially important during prolonged eye closure and at night, when sIgA represents almost 80% of the total tear protein. Contact lens usage is found to be associated with decreased sIgA, IL-8, and PMN levels in the tear film, and it may predispose the wearer to eye infections.

The capability of producing milk has a major survival advantage for mammals. Apart from providing balanced nutrition for the newborn, breast milk is important in the defence, growth, and development of the newborn. Important components of breast milk include:

❑ **IFNs.** Colostrum — the scant, sometimes yellowish milk produced in the first few days after birth — is particularly rich in IFNs and provides strong antiviral defence.

❑ **Leukocytes.** During the first ten days after birth, there are more leukocytes per mililitre of breast milk than blood.

- Macrophages and neutrophils are the most common leukocytes in human milk and confer immunity by virtue of their phagocytosing capabilities.
- Macrophages also secrete lysozyme, an enzyme that can disrupt the cell walls of Gram-positive bacteria.
- Breast milk has both B and T cells. Milk lymphocytes seem to behave differently from blood lymphocytes in that they proliferate in response to bacteria like *E. coli* that cause life-threatening illnesses in babies but are less responsive to other non-threatening organisms. Milk lymphocytes also secrete chemokines and cytokines like IFN-γ that help strengthen the infant's immune response.
- HIV positive mothers show the presence of CD8+ T cells in their breast milk. This adoptive transfer of cells to infants helps reduce the viral load and may help in controlling transmission of the virus from the mother to the infant.

❑ **Igs.** Although IgM, IgD, IgG, and IgA are all found in milk, sIgA is by far the most abundant. sIgA is synthesized and stored in breast tissue. sIgA antibodies are produced by the mother in response to pathogens present in her (and hence the child's) immediate environment and are especially useful in protecting the child. Since the mother's immune system is tolerized to normal gut flora, the antibodies are not directed against this flora and therefore, do not interfere with colonization of the infant's gut. Being a complement non-fixing antibody, binding of sIgA to the antigen does not trigger inflammation and avoids damaging the delicate mucosal membranes of the infant gut.

❑ **Oligosaccharides and mucins.** Both oligosaccharides and mucins intercept bacteria and form harmless complexes which are then excreted. They thus prevent micro-organisms from attaching to mucosal surfaces.

❑ **Lactoferrin and B12 binding factor.** These factors bind iron and vitamin B12 respectively, making them unavailable to micro-organisms.

❑ **Bifidus factor.** This is one of the oldest known components of human milk. It promotes the growth of *Lactobacillus bifidus* in the infant gut, helping to crowd out potential pathogenic varieties.

❑ **Erythropoietin.** Mammary epithelial cells secrete this erythropoiesis-regulating hormone. It is thought that milk erythropoietin may play a role in erythropoiesis, neurodevelopment, gut-maturation, apoptosis, and immunity in the infant.

❑ **Hormones and growth factors.** The gut membrane of newborn babies is called 'leaky', since it allows easy access to potentially harmful agents. Breast milk contains hormones that stimulate the baby's digestive tract to mature quickly. Hormones like cortisol and growth factors such as epidermal growth factor, nerve growth factor, insulin-like growth factor, and somatomedin C, present in breast milk, help in the maturation of this mucosal lining so that it becomes relatively impermeable to pathogens or harmful agents. Some hormones are thought to stimulate the production of lactoferrin, lysozyme, and sIgA by the mucosal lining of the baby's urinary tract, inducing local immunity.

the conformation of the antigen-binding site (fig. 6.1). It may seem surprising that these small hypervariable regions are responsible for generating the enormous variety of antigen-binding specificities. However, a little reflection will show why this is possible. Variation in both the length and the amino acid sequences is responsible for the wide range of specificities of antibody molecules. There are three CDRs each in the V_H and V_L region. Even if each hypervariable region was assumed to consist of a stretch of 12 to 15 amino acids, a large repertoire of possible combinations is available, since a change in a single amino acid position can change the conformation of the antigen-combining site.

Recognition of individual domains in the IgG molecule led to the suggestion that each of these domains had evolved for some particular function.

❑ V_L and V_H domains together constitute the antigen-binding site (also called the paratope of the antibody).
❑ Both C_{H1} and C_L domains help to hold the V domains together by virtue of their disulphide linkages; they also serve to extend the antigen-binding arms of the molecule, facilitating interaction with the antigen and increasing the maximum rotation of the arms.
❑ C_{H1} domain binds the complement component C4b.
❑ The hinge region, an extended peptide sequence between the C_{H1} and C_{H2} domain of IgG (also IgD and IgA), is a proline-rich region that has no homology with other domains. It is responsible for the flexibility of these molecules and allows them to assume various angles with respect to each other upon antigen binding.
❑ The C_{H2}-C_{H3} interface contains the binding sites for FcRs.
❑ The C_{H2} region interacts with the C1q component of complement.
❑ A site for binding to FcRn (FcR neonatal; section 9.8) lies at the C_{H2}-C_{H3} interface; this interaction is thought to determine the half-life of serum IgG.
❑ The C_{H3} domain is thought to be necessary for optimal complement activation.

9.6 Classes of Antibodies

Igs, being large glycoproteinic molecules, are by themselves good antigens and can induce a potent immune response. Such anti-Ig antibodies are powerful tools used to dissect and understand B cell development and humoral responses. Antigenic determinants are found on the entire molecule, and differences in antigenicity reflect differences in amino acid sequences of these molecules. Depending upon the location of these epitopes, Igs are classified as isotypes, idiotypes, and allotypes.

9.6.1 Isotypes

Isotypic determinants are present in the C regions of H and L chains. They are used to define H or L chain subclasses. As explained, five major classes of Igs are recognized on the basis of the amino acid sequences of the H chains (IgM, IgD, IgG, IgA, and IgE; fig. 9.5) and two classes on the basis of L chains (κ and λ). Either type of L chain can pair with any of the H chains. However, in a single molecule, both the L chains are identical, ie, Igs have either two κ or two λ chains. Hybrid molecules having one Lκ and one Lλ chain do not occur naturally. A separate C region gene encodes each isotype. All individuals of a species carry the same C region genes, and all isotypes are expressed in normal individuals. This implies that isotypic determinants are species specific and the administration of antibodies of a particular isotype in an unrelated species will elicit an immune response. Antisera raised against isotypes of various species are routinely used as diagnostic and research tools. The various human H chain isotypes are discussed below (Table 9.1).

Table 9.1 Properties of human Ig isotypes

Property	IgM	IgD	IgG	IgE	IgA
MW (KD)	900	150	150	190	150–600
Form	Pentamer mIg – monomer	Monomer	Monomer	Monomer	Monomer/polymer
Carbohydrate content (%)	12	11	3	13	7
Subclasses	–	–	4 (IgG1–IgG4)	–	2 (IgA1, IgA2)
Adult serum conc (mg/ml)	1.5	0.04	13	0.0003	2.5
Biological Functions					
Opsonization	+	may bind to microbes	+++	–	++
Virus neutralization	+	–	++	–	+++
ADCC	–	–	+++	–	–
Degranulation of mast cells, basophils and eosinophils	–	–	–	+++	–
Complement activation pathway	Cls	–	Cls/Alt	Alt	Alt
Transcytosis	+	–	–	–	+
Placental transfer	–	–	IgG1 + IgG2 +/– IgG3 +++ IgG4 –	–	–

Legends: +++ – high, ++ – medium, + – low, – – negative, +/– – negligible, ? – unclear, Cls – classical, Alt – alternative

❑ **IgM.** Accounting for about 5–10% of the serum Ig (mean serum concentration about 1.5 mg/ml), **IgM is the predominant antibody produced early in primary immune responses**. Monomeric IgM is an integral part of BcR of naïve B cells. Serum IgM is a 19S pentamer with a MW of about 970 KD. It consists of five monomers held together by disulphide bonds at the Fc region; the Fc regions are placed at the core of the pentamer and the ten Fab regions at the periphery. Each Fab can bind antigen so that IgM has a theoretical valency of ten. However, steric hindrance can cause IgM to simultaneously bind only five or fewer molecules of large antigens. Its multivalency makes IgM highly efficient in complement activation, opsonization, etc. Its large size hinders its diffusion in intercellular tissue fluids, and **IgM is largely confined to the intravascular pool.**

The pentamer dissociates to monomers upon treatment with mild reducing agents. The H chain of monomeric IgM is longer and heavier than that of IgG. It has a MW of around 65 KD because of the presence of an extra domain of about 130 amino acids. The IgM H chain thus has five domains — V_H and $C_{H}1$ through $C_{H}4$. Amino acid sequencing shows that the additional domain is placed at the $C_{H}2$ position (ie, it follows $C_{H}1$ domain). The $C_{H}1$, $C_{H}2$, and $C_{H}3$ domains of the γ chain thus correspond to the $C_{H}1$, $C_{H}3$, and $C_{H}4$ domains of the μ chain. In addition, the μ chain contains a C– terminal, 18 amino acid long, secretory tailpiece. Pentameric IgM antibodies have a small polypeptide unit (15 KD, 129 amino acids) called the J (Junction) chain bound to the first and fifth μ chain. The J chain forms disulphide linkages with cysteine residues on the secretory tailpiece. The J chain is not mandatory for polymer formation but regulates the structure and function of polymers formed. Similar J chains are also found in dimeric IgA antibodies. The J chain is synthesized by IgM– (or IgA–) secreting plasma cells in secretory

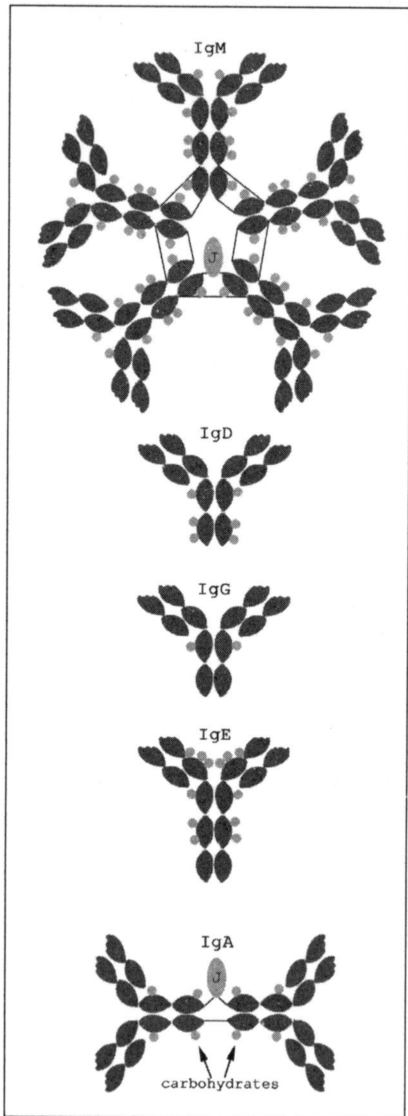

Figure 9.5 Five classes of Igs are recognized on the basis of their H chain amino acid sequences. *These classes also differ from each other in their fine structure, carbohydrate content, and functions. Serum IgM is a pentamer that can dissociate to monomers on treatment with mild reducing agents. The μ chain consists of five Ig domains (four CH and one VH). The first and fifth μ chains of pentameric IgM are bound by the J chain. IgD, IgG, and IgE are monomers having the prototypical four-chain structure. Like the μ chain, the ε chain also consists of five Ig domains. IgA is found both as a monomer and a dimer. Dimeric IgA is present predominantly in exocrine secretions. The two monomers of dimeric IgA are linked to each other by the J chain.*

tissues. By contrast, antibody-secreting cells in the bone marrow, lymph nodes, or spleen do not secrete the J chain. The gene for the J chain does not lie on the same chromosome as those for antibodies. The presence of the J chain enables IgM to bind to receptors on secretory cells that facilitate its transport across the epithelial lining to mucosal secretions (see IgA described further).

❑ **IgD.** A 7S monomer of 184 KD (serum concentration–0.04 mg/ml) the structure of IgD differs from IgG in two respects — a longer hinge region consisting of about 64 amino acids and an unusually high carbohydrate content that is responsible for its high MW. **mIgD, along with mIgM, is found on all naïve B cells and is the major component of BcR expressed by mature B cells.** Curiously, by mechanisms not yet understood, the L chain of mIgD is of the κ type but that of serum IgD is λ type. Like other isotypes, the majority of mIgD is anchored in the plasma membrane via a transmembrane domain (chapter 6). However, a small fraction of mIgD is linked to the plasma membrane by a **g**lycosyl**p**hosphatidyl**i**nostiol (GPI) anchor. The function of this form of mIgD is not known.

IgD forming plasma cells are very rare in the bone marrow or digestive mucosa. They are much more numerous in the lymphoid tissue of the upper respiratory tract such as nasal mucosa, salivary glands, lachrymal glands, adenoids, and tonsils. As much as 20% of tonsil plasma cells produce IgD, suggesting a role in defence against upper respiratory tract infections.

❑ **IgG** is the major Ig in serum, constituting 70–75% of the total Igs (mean adult serum concentration of about 13 mg/ml). **It is the major serum antibody in secondary immune responses.** Found in intra- and extra-vascular pools, IgG is important in defending the internal milieu. IgG has a very low carbohydrate content (2–3% compared to 7–14% found in other isotypes). On the basis of amino acid sequences, four subclasses of IgG antibodies are recognized in humans (IgG1 to IgG4). They differ from each other in the size of the hinge region and the number of inter-H chain bonds. IgG1 is the most common Ig, accounting for 70% of the serum Ig, whereas IgG4 is the least common (3%). The four subclasses also differ in their functions.

- Except for IgG2, all other IgG isotypes cross the placenta and protect the new-born in the first few months after birth.
- IgG3, IgG1, and IgG2 can fix complement (in that order of efficiency). IgG4 cannot fix complement. The complement fixing isotypes are responsible for causing lysis of microbes that have breached the physical barriers and gained entry into the body.
- IgG1 and IgG3 can opsonize microbes, since they can bind to high affinity FcRs (FcγRI) expressed on phagocytic cells. Comparatively, IgG4 is not as efficient in opsonization, since it binds the receptor with intermediate affinity. IgG2 has very low affinity for (FcγRI) and hence a negligible role in opsonization.

❑ **IgE.** Although it is present at extremely low concentrations in normal serum (0.03–0.05 μg/ml), IgE has potent biological activity. **It is responsible for immediate hypersensitivity disorders** such as asthma, hayfever, and urticaria. Basophils, mast cells, and eosinophils express a high affinity receptor (FcεRI) for the Fc region of IgE antibody. Ligation of the receptor-bound IgE by homologous antigen causes the degranulation of these cells. Pharmacological mediators released by the cells are responsible for symptoms of allergic diseases (eg, coughing, sneezing, and vomiting; chapter 15). IgE has a sedimentation coefficient of 8S and a MW of 188 KD. It is heat labile and is destroyed by heating at 56°C for 30 min. Like the μ chain, the ε H chain also has five domains — the additional domain being C$_{H2}$. IgE is thought to confer immunity against intestinal parasites.

❑ **IgA.** It accounts for 15–20% of serum Ig with a mean serum concentration around 2.5 mg/ml. **It is the main Ig in exocrine secretions** such as saliva, tears, colostrum, milk, genito-urinary, and tracheobronchial secretions. The fact that it is the major antibody isotype on a biosynthetic basis is often missed, because it is not the major isotype in serum. The bulk of the body's Ig-producing plasma cells are concentrated along mucosal and exocrine sites, especially along the intestinal tract and most of them produce IgA against environmental antigens.

In human serum, more than 80% of the IgA antibodies occur as monomers; the rest are dimers or even higher polymers. In human external secretions, however, polymers predominate. In other mammals, IgA antibodies are mainly dimeric (whether in serum or secretions). **IgA does not bind complement and hence protects mucosal surfaces without triggering an inflammatory response.** Two subclasses of IgA antibodies are recognized in humans — IgA1 and IgA2. About 80% of the serum IgA antibodies are IgA1 type, whereas both subclasses are equally represented in exocrine secretions. Secretory IgA antibody is 11S dimeric form with a MW of about 385 KD. The Cα chain, like the Cμ chain, has a secretory tailpiece and a J chain. Two IgA monomers are linked via disulphide linkages between the J chain and cysteine residues on the secretory tailpiece to give the

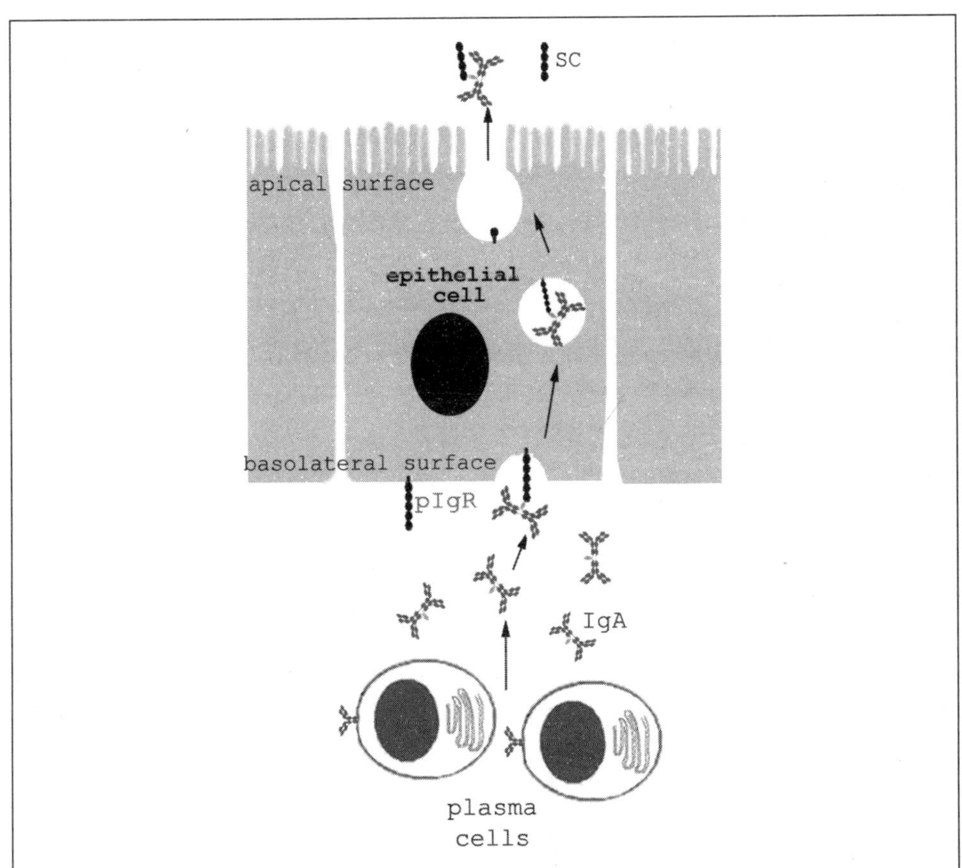

Figure 9.6 Receptor-mediated endocytosis via pIgR-J chain interaction enables transcytosis of polymeric IgA or IgM. Secretory epithelial cells produce and express pIgR, a receptor for the J chain of polymeric Igs, on their cell surface. Polymeric Igs bind to pIgR expressed on the basolateral surface of the epithelial cells and are internalized and transported to the apical surface of these cells. The antibodies eventually get released at the apical surface by cleavage of pIgR. Free, soluble pIgR, called SC (secretory component), is also secreted by the epithelial cells.

dimer. Cysteine residues in the two α C$_{H3}$ regions are also directly linked by disulphide bonds, resulting in tail to tail dimers with Fab regions that are free to react with the antigen (fig. 9.6). A glycoprotein called the **S**ecretory **C**omponent (SC) was originally found to be associated with IgA from exocrine secretions. Later, it was established that SC occurred in the free, unassociated form as well. Secretory epithelial cells were found to express the molecule on their cell surface and secrete it into the surrounding milieu. SC is now known to be a transmembrane epithelial receptor for the J chain containing dimeric IgA and pentameric IgM and is now called by its functional name, **p**olymeric **Ig R**eceptor (pIgR). Dimeric IgA or polymeric IgM bind to pIgR on the surface of epithelial cells via the J chain. The pIgR-antibody complexes get internalized by endocytosis at the basolateral surface of the cell and are eventually released to the apical surface[5]. Thus, receptor-mediated endocytosis via pIgR-J chain interaction enables the antibodies to be transcytosed across epithelial cells and released in exocrine secretions (fig. 9.6).

9.6.2 Allotypes

Allotypes are allelic variants of isotypes that are found in some members of a species but not others (from the Greek *allos*, meaning others).

All individuals of a species inherit the same set of C region genes. However, multiple alleles for these genes code for subtle amino acid differences, called allotypic determinants, which occur in some but not all individuals of the species. Allelic variation is caused by mutations in the corresponding structural genes that occur mainly in the C regions of the molecule. Each allotypic determinant represents a difference of between one to four amino acids that are encoded by the different allele. In the case of a heterozygote, it is possible to find multiple allotypes in the same individual but not on the same Ig molecule. Most Ig allotypic variations do not seem to affect the antigenic specificity or the effector functions of the Ig. Allotypes have been identified in both the L and H chains and are designated by the class and subclass followed by the allele number, eg, G1m(1) is a IgG1 allotype number 1. In humans, 25 γ chain allotypes, 2 α2 allotypes, and 3 κ chain allotypes have been identified to date. Antibodies to allotypic determinants can be produced by injecting antibodies from one member of a species into another member of the same species, provided they differ in their allotypic determinants. Such antibodies can arise during blood transfusions or during pregnancy, when the mother produces antibodies to paternal allotypic determinants on foetal Ig.

9.6.3 Idiotypes

An individual can produce antibodies to a virtually limitless number of antigenic determinants. These antibodies differ in their antigen-binding sites because of subtle differences in the amino acid sequences of the V region. These unique amino acid sequences in the antigen-binding region of the molecule also give rise to unique antigenic determinants and are called idiotypic determinants (fig. 9.7). Both L and H chains contribute to the conformation of the antigen-binding site and therefore to the idiotype. The actual antigen-binding site and V region sequences outside this site can also contribute to idiotypic determinants. Since a clone of B cells gives rise to Igs with identical V regions, they will all have the same idiotype. A single determinant is called the idiotope, and the sum of the idiotopes on a single V region is an idiotype. As it is difficult to determine if a given antiserum detects one or more idiotopes, such antisera are referred to as anti-idiotypic antisera. Anti-idiotypic reagents can be used to follow the inheritance of genetic markers on Ig V regions, to map V region genes, and to measure the regulation of V gene expression.

[5] Epithelial cells have an apical surface that faces the outside world (that is the lumen) and a basolateral surface that contacts adjacent cells and the underlying connective tissue.

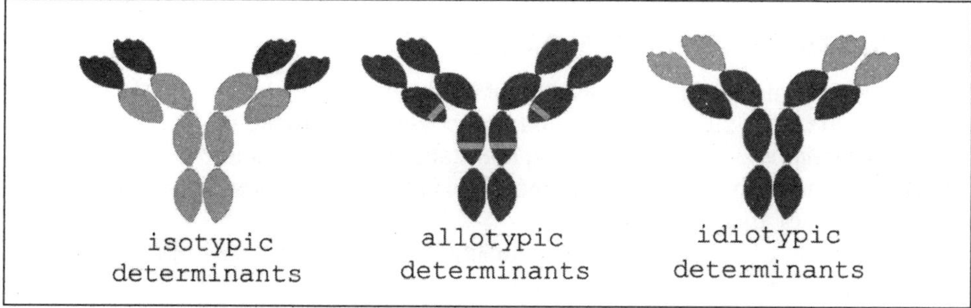

Figure 9.7 Antibodies can be divided into three broad classes depending upon the location of the antigenic epitopes (shown by the grey areas). Isotypic determinants are present on the C regions of the H and L chains. Differences arising from different alleles of same C genes result in allotypic determinants. Antigenic determinants arising from the differences in rearranged V_H and V_L genes are the idiotypic determinants.

9.7 Role of Ig in Immunity

Igs bind antigen via their Fab regions. This binding is in some instances sufficient to confer a degree of resistance to the host. For example, binding of Ig to viral epitopes interferes with attachment to their receptors on target cells and helps in antiviral resistance. Additionally, an antibody may act by disrupting the virus structure, preventing its interaction with cell surface receptors or interfering with the fusion of the virus membrane with the cell surface after the virus has engaged its cell surface receptors. In either case, since the antibody interaction neutralizes the infecting potential of the virus, the process is termed virus neutralization. Similarly, antibodies can neutralize the action of toxins or enzymes. However, mere binding of Igs to the pathogen is not sufficient to kill it or remove it from circulation. **To be effective instruments of defence, antibodies must not only bind the target antigen but also invoke effector functions that will result in the removal of the antigen and/ or death of the pathogen.** The Fc region of the antibody is important in invoking these effector functions. It is responsible for interactions with proteins or cells that result in effector functions of humoral immunity.

Tissues and cells of the body express specific receptors (FcRs) for the Fc region of different isotypes of antibodies. Ig-FcR interaction results in the triggering of different effector functions depending upon the type of FcR and the isotype of the antibody.

❑ **Opsonization.** Macrophages and neutrophils express FcRs that can bind the Fc region of most IgG subclasses with a high affinity. Particulate antigens or pathogens coated by IgG bind to these FcRs. Although the strength of interaction between individual FcR and IgG is weak, the simultaneous binding of multiple Ig molecules attached to the same target results in a signal of considerable strength. These interactions immobilize the pathogen to the surface of the phagocyte. The signal generated by cross-linking of FcRs by IgG antibodies bound to the same antigen results in activation of the cell, phagocytosis of the immobilized pathogen-antibody complex, and its eventual destruction. Antigen internalized via FcR is loaded more efficiently on MHC molecules than that internalized by other receptors and is therefore more efficient in triggering the immune response.

❑ **Complement activation.** Interaction of IgM and most IgG isotypes with homologous antigen activates complement. Activated complement components are multifunctional molecules, having powerful immunomodulatory and effector functions (chapter 3). For example, the complement component C3b and its products promote opsonization, virus neutralization, B cell activation, etc.

Ig STRUCTURE AND FUNCTION

❑ The prototypical Ig molecule has a four-chain structure consisting of two H and two L chains.
  - Each L chain is bound to the H chain by a disulphide bond and non-covalent interactions.
  - The two H-L dimers are linked by disulphide linkages, yielding the Y shaped Ig molecule.
  - Presence of disulphide linkages in the hinge region binds the two H chains and allows the molecule to change its conformation upon antigen binding.
  - The H chain consists of one Ig domain of high sequence variability (V_H region) and three Ig domains of lesser variability (C_{H1}, C_{H2}, and C_{H3} regions).
  - The L chain has one Ig domain each of variable and constant sequences (V_L and C_L respectively).
  - The V region contains three hypervariable CDRs that form the antigen-binding pocket and four FR regions of less variability responsible for maintaining the architecture of the molecule.

❑ Five classes of Igs, called isotypes, are recognized on the basis of immunogenicity of H chains; two classes are recognized on the basis of immunogenicity of the L chains.

❑ Allelic variants of isotypes that are found in some members of a species but not others are called allotypes.

❑ Immunogenicity of the antigen-binding site of the antibody gives rise to Ig idiotypes.

❑ Igs have a role in neutralization of toxins, enzymes, and viruses, as well as opsonization, complement activation, and degranulation of mast cells and ADCC.

C3a and C5a are chemotactic agents that attract neutrophils and macrophages to the site of antigen-antibody interaction and promote inflammatory responses. C5b6789 is responsible for lysis of target cells.

❑ **ADCC.** Ligation of FcRs on K cells and phagocytes by pathogen- (or antigen-) bound antibodies results in their activation. Activated cells release cytotoxins that bring about the lysis of the target cell, and the process is called ADCC (chapter 11).

❑ **Degranulation.** Ligation of FcεRI on the surface of mast cells, basophils, and eosinophils by parasite- (or antigen-) bound IgE results in the release of pharmacological mediators that can cause the death of the parasite. These mediators are also responsible for the unpleasant effects of immediate-type of hypersensitivity.

❑ **Trancytosis.** IgA (and IgM) is transported across the epithelial cell barrier because of pIgR-mediated endocytosis; IgA, present in exocrine secretions, defends the mucosal surfaces against pathogenic invaders.

9.8 Ig Receptors

Physiologically, antibody molecules are adaptors that link the target (antigen) to effectors and hence mediate elimination of the target. By definition then, receptors for Ig molecules must be expressed by a variety of effector cells. These receptors comprise a family of molecules that bind the Fc region of Ig, each member of the family recognizing Igs of one or few closely related types. FcRs are expressed by many cells of the immune system, eg, macrophages, neutrophils, basophils, mast cells, eosinophils, lymphocytes (K cells, T, and B cells), DCs, and FDCs.

Most FcRs are members of the Ig superfamily. **FcRs are membrane-associated glycoproteins that mediate a vast array of functions,** including positive and negative regulation of immune cell responses, triggering internalization of opsonized cells, transcytosis, etc. FcRs have been identified for all Ig istoypes except IgD (fig. 9.8). Different types of FcRs are found for a single Ig isotype, and these differ in their functions as well. Generally, type I receptors bind Ig with high affinity and type II or III receptors bind Ig with low affinity. Thus, of the three different types of FcRs that bind IgG, FcγRIs are high affinity receptors that bind monomeric IgG, whereas type II and III are low affinity receptors that can only bind antigen-IgG

Ig RECEPTORS

❑ They bind Fc regions of Ig molecules.

❑ Many receptors act as adaptors that link Ig to the target cell.

❑ Multiple types of receptors can bind Ig of a single isotype; those that bind Ig with high affinity are called type I; those with low affinity are called type II FcRs.

❑ The presence of ITAMs or ITIMs in their cytoplasmic tails determines whether the coligation of FcRs delivers an activatory or inhibitory signal.

❑ Important Ig receptors include:
- FcεRI, involved in the degranulation of mast cells, activated eosinophils, and basophils
- FcγRIIB, which acts as a negative regulator of B cells
- Isoforms of FcεRII expressed on B cells, T cells, macrophages, monocytes, DCs, etc.
- FcRn, involved in the transfer of maternal IgGs and possibly IgG catabolization
- pIgR, responsible for the transcytosis of IgA and IgM

---

complexes. Similarly, the FcεRI present on eosinophils and mast cells is a high affinity IgE receptor, whereas FcεRII present on a variety of cells binds IgE with low affinity.

Whether FcRs deliver an activatory or an inhibitory signal depends upon the type of motifs in their cytoplasmic domains. In mice, FcγRI, FcγRIIA, FcγRIIC, and FcγRIIIA deliver activating signals. Most activatory FcRs are multi-component units. The component chains of these receptors are named α, β, γ, etc. The α chain is involved in specific recognition and is unique to each receptor. The other chains are involved in signal transduction or intracellular transport. The γ chain, called FcR common γ chain, is related to the TcR ζ chain and contains an ITAM. Interestingly, this common γ chain is also necessary for the assembly and surface expression of FcγRI, FcγRIII, FcαRI, and FcεRI. Clustering of the activating receptors results in

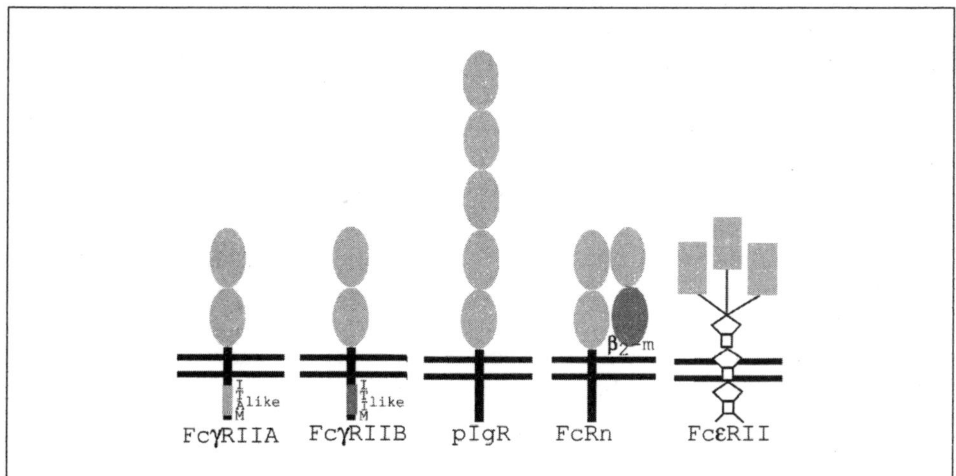

Figure 9.8 FcRs are membrane associated glycoproteins that differ greatly in terms of the structure and functions they mediate. *Most FcRs have an Ig fold and belong to the Ig superfamily. Some FcRs can activate or inhibit cellular functions when Igs bound to them are ligated by the antigen. FcRs having an ITAM (or ITAM-like motif) in their cytoplasmic tail deliver activatory signals whereas those having an ITIM (or ITIM-like motif) deliver negative signals. Others, like pIgR, trigger the internalization and transport of bound Igs from basolateral to apical surfaces. FcRn is unique in that it is structurally similar to MHC class I molecules. It is thought to be involved in the transfer of maternal IgG across neonatal intestinal epithelium and IgG homeostasis in adults. Unlike other FcRs, the low affinity receptor for IgE, FcεRII does not have the Ig fold. It is a C-type lectin adhesion molecule expressed in different isoforms on different cells.*

the phosphorylation of tyrosine residues in the ITAMs by Src family kinases. Further phosphorylation events result in the phosphorylation of Syk and activation of PLCγ, PI3-kinase, etc resulting in the activation of MAP kinases, Ca^{2+} mobilization, and cytoskeleton reorganization (these signalling pathways are explained in chapter 6). Signalling through ITAM-containing FcRs leads to an oxidative burst, cytokine release, and phagocytosis by macrophages, ADCC by K cells, and degranulation in mast cells.

Conversely, FcγRIIB (incidentally, the only FcγR expressed by B cells) is a single chain molecule that has an ITIM in its cytoplasmic domain. Although it has been studied most extensively in B cells, it is also expressed on myeloid and monocytic cells. It acts as a negative regulator of immune complex triggered activation. Coligation of BcR with FcγRIIB by antigen-IgG complexes blocks downstream biological responses of B cells (including activation, antigen presentation, proliferation, and antibody production). The initial event in this inhibitory signalling is the phophorylation of tyrosine in the ITIM by the Src family kinase Lyn. This signalling interferes with the translocation of Btk that is essential in BcR signalling. It also suppresses anti-apoptotic signals that are necessary for the proliferation and survival of activated B cells. Additionally, cross-linking of FcγRIIB by IgG is thought to deliver an apoptotic signal to germinal centre B cells. Thus, when the concentration of serum IgG exceeds a certain threshold, FcγRIIB seems to switch off Ig synthesis and downregulate the humoral response.

FcϵRI is of special interest because of its importance in type I hypersensitivity reactions (chapter 15). It binds IgE with very high affinity and has very limited distribution. The classical tetrameric form of this molecule is constitutively expressed on effectors of anaphylaxis (ie, mast cells and basophils as well as activated eosinophils); a trimeric form of the molecule is found on APCs such as monocytes, DCs, and Langerhans cells. It is one of the earliest markers expressed on mast cells. The α chain is responsible for IgE binding, the β chain increases stability and signalling capacity, and the shared γ chain dimer has ITAMs that are responsible for downstream signalling. Binding of polyvalent antigens by receptor-bound IgE causes receptor aggregation and triggers cellular activation, resulting in the release of pharmacological mediators by mast cells and basophils. Activation of eosinophils by FcϵRI provides defence against parasitic infection, whereas on APCs, the receptor delivers IgE-bound antigen to MHC class II presentation pathways. FcϵRII (CD23) is the low affinity receptor for IgE. CD23a is expressed constitutively on B cells, whereas the IL-4 induced CD23b isoform is found on T cells, macrophages, monocytes, DCs, platelets, eosinophils, etc. Unlike other FcRs, CD23 is a C-type lectin adhesion molecule that can bind CD21 (CR2). Proteolysis of CD23 leads to the release of a soluble form of FcϵRII that can be further degraded. All except the smallest 12 KD fragment retain IgE binding capacity. In rats, CD23 has been shown to be involved in transepithelial transport of IgE and a similar role is suspected in humans. CD23 has been implicated in IgE synthesis and IgE-mediated immune and inflammatory functions.

Neonatal FcR (FcRn) is structurally similar to the MHC class I molecule except that its peptide groove is closed. It is involved in the transfer of maternal IgGs to the young via the neonatal intestine in rodents. It may have a similar role in the early days after human childbirth, when colostrum has a high percentage of IgG. Interestingly, adult human enterocytes express high levels of FcRn and have been shown to be involved in bi-directional transcytosis of IgG across intestinal epithelial monolayers *in vitro*. FcRn is also thought to have a role in IgG homoeostasis through its regulation of the rate of IgG catabolization by endothelial cells. These cells are postulated to take up IgG via non-specific pinocytosis, since the pH of the blood is not permissive for FcRn-IgG interaction. The internalized IgG enters the acidic

Historical Perspective:
Theories of Antibody Formation

As the knowledge of immunology developed, a theoretical framework was needed to explain antibody formation. In these early years, theories focused entirely on antibodies, as the two types of immune responses (cell-mediated and humoral) were not recognized or distinguished. Two broad schools of thought emerged, and each had its own adherents.

☐ **The instructive theorists** proposed that antibody formation could occur only after the antigen provided the necessary information for antibody synthesis.

☐ **The selective theorists** hypothesized that information required for antibody synthesis pre-existed in the cell, and the immunogen merely selected and stimulated the appropriate cell.

The Instructive Theories: Template Hypothesis

The best known of the instructive theories was the template hypothesis. It was formulated by Haurowitz, Mudd, and Alexander in the early 1930s and was later modified by the renowned scientist Linus Pauling. It postulated that the antigen acts as a mould or template which can enter any Ig producing cell and cause the pattern of amino acids laid down to be modified to fit the template, resulting in the synthesis of a molecule with a spatial configuration complementary to that of the antigen molecule. Thus, the template hypothesis suggests that the specificity of the Ig molecule is determined not by the primary amino acid sequence but by the process of moulding the nascent molecule around the antigenic determinant. The immunogen was suggested to be a template at the level of protein synthesis. To account for the continued production of antibodies, it was further assumed that the antigen, or a part thereof, remains in the cell to direct the configuration of future antibody production. A modified form of the theory proposed that the antigen modifies the genetic information in the DNA of the cell so that the cell and its progeny continue to produce immunoglobulins of a particular specificity.

These theories gained popularity because they seemed to fit in so well with immunochemical discoveries of the specificity of the immune response, especially Landsteiner's experiments, outlined in chapter 4. Also, little was known about macromolecular synthesis then. Once it became evident that the shape as well as activity of a protein is determined by its amino acid sequence, which in turn reflects the DNA sequence, the template theory was abandoned. The fact that the three dimensional structure of antibodies is reversible, ie, the molecule unfolds on denaturation but refolds under appropriate conditions, rang the death knell of the template hypothesis. The idea of the template hypothesis may sound ridiculous today, but countless number of papers were published and tempers frayed over these postulates in the early 1940s.

The Selective Hypothesis: Clonal Selection Theory

Proposed by Jerne and Talmage, the clonal selection theory states that an individual possesses an immensely diversified pool of cells, each capable of responding to only one antigen or a few related antigens. When an immunogen penetrates the body, it selects only those few cells that already possess the Ig specific for the antigen from this population of cells. The antigen is only a trigger that induces the cells to produce antibodies.

Burnet proposed in 1959 that cells of the antibody forming system arise from random mutations, resulting in the emergence of a small number of cells or clones of differentiated cells capable of producing one or a very small number of specific antibodies. He further postulated that contact of such differentiated cells with self- or foreign immunogens during foetal life — before the cells reached maturity — led to suppression rather than stimulation of antibody formation, possibly because of clonal abortion. He later suggested that this censoring of the clones could occur in the thymus. In an immunocompetent individual, however, the contact was stated to trigger proliferation and generation of clones of effector cells that were capable of antibody secretion. Some of these lymphocytes were said to circulate in the body and give rise to an increased response on secondary immunization. The clonal selection theory explained most of the phenomena known at the time and was generally accepted. Reality, as we now know, although very close to the proposed theory, is much more complicated.

Historical Perspective:
The Network Hypothesis

Jerne propounded the network hypothesis to explain self-tolerance in 1974. He proposed that the immune system is a network of idiotypes and anti-idiotypes. It was suggested that when an antibody is produced in response to an antigen, its V region — consisting of many idiotopes — can itself act as an antigen and in turn stimulate the production of an antibody, the anti-idiotype. The idiotopes on the anti-idiotype can lead to production of anti-anti-idiotype and so on until a network of idiotypes and anti-idiotypes is produced. Some of these anti-idiotypes will be internal images of the idiotypes, ie, internal images of the antigens. The original hypothesis postulated that the network is multi-branched, with each idiotype-producing cell being controlled by several anti-idiotypes. The whole network is thus dependent on all its parts for control. When an external antigen is added to the network, the equilibrium is disturbed and appropriate cells are stimulated to produce antibodies to the antigen, the idiotype, etc to regain balance. Thus, antibody production will continue until equilibrium is once again established.

The concept of the theory is very attractive and even seems within the realms of possibility. However, experimental proof — the real test of any hypothesis — is still elusive. Any experiments designed to prove the existence of networks have to be conducted under conditions so far removed from normality that there are theoretical objections to extrapolating the evidence to *in vivo* physiological conditions. It seems certain that anti-idiotypes are produced in normal immune responses and co-exist in serum with their specific idiotype, probably in the form of immune complexes. However, presence of an extensive network of idiotypes-anti-idiotypes has not been proven to date. In support of the theory is the fact that anti-idiotypes can modulate (transiently suppress or enhance) immune responses. This modulation is observed even when the anti-idiotype is injected in amounts that are likely to be present in normal serum. Moreover, T_R cells that are idiotype — and not antigen-specific — have been found in normal immune responses. There is also some evidence to show that idiotypic T_H cells are formed and needed in the development of normal immune responses.

The hypothesis continues to generate a lot of heat and raise the passions of immunologists. It appears that the antigen is of prime importance in stimulating and regulating an immune response, but it is conceivable that idiotypic regulation may direct the response towards a particular spectrum of idiotypes. In the resting stage, before the immune system comes in contact with the antigen, idiotype-anti-idiotype regulation is probably important in determining the initial state in which the immune system encounters the antigen.

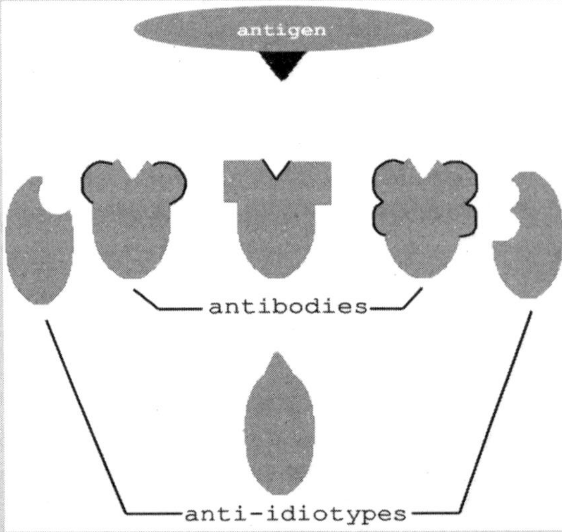

Figure 9.S4 The network hypothesis proposes that antigenic challenge gives rise to a network of antibodies, consisting of idiotypes and anti-idiotypes, so that the whole network is dependent on all its parts for control.

endosomal/lysosomal pathway, where it can bind FcRn and get rescued from catabolization. IgG that fails to bind to FcRn is thought to be destroyed. Support for this theory comes from work in KO mice deficient in β_2-m (required for FcRn assembly). These mice show dramatically reduced levels of serum IgG despite an apparently normal B cell compartment, suggesting abnormally high degradation of IgG.

pIgR, like FcRn, is responsible for transcytosis of polymeric IgA (and IgM, if present) across the epithelial cells. Interestingly, non-IgA bound pIgR is also efficiently transcytosed, leading to the release of the free cleaved extracellular domain of pIgR, called SC, in the lumenal secretions. Recent evidence suggests that the carbohydrate-rich SC may act as a scavenger molecule in its own right, helping mop up enteric pathogens in the lumenal secretions. Thus, pIgR seems to have a dual function — it can behave as a FcR and as a PRR.

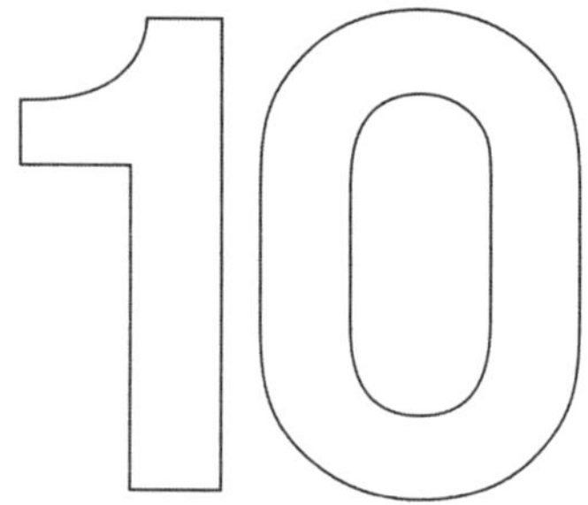

10 Genetic Mechanisms of Immune Diversity

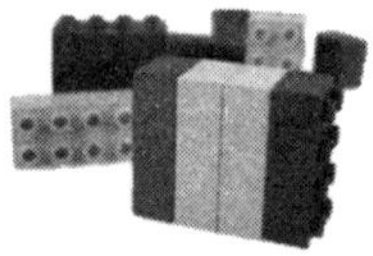

The line, it is drawn
The curse, it is cast
The slow one now
Will later be fast
As the present now
Will later be past
The order is
Rapidly fadin'.
And the first one now
Will later be last
For the times they are a-changin

— Bob Dylan, *The Times They Are A-Changin*

10.1 Introduction

The immune system's efficiency in defending the body against a world of forever evolving pathogens and transformed cells is due to its ability to specifically recognize and respond to an enormously diverse spectrum of antigens. This immune recognition and interaction is mediated by antigen receptors expressed on the surface of B and T lymphocytes. The number of different Ig molecules that the individual's immune system can produce is known as its antibody-specificity repertoire or B cell repertoire. Similarly, the diversity of epitopes recognized by T cells is the T cell repertoire. This chapter describes the molecular and genetic mechanisms which result in the diversity of these repertoires. Familiarization with BcR, TcR, and Ig structure (chapters 6 and 9 respectively) are necessary to understand this chapter. It also requires some knowledge of the principles of protein synthesis and genetics. Admittedly, this is a difficult chapter to follow; some students may find the details too extensive. To facilitate comprehension, the essentials of the processes have been summarized in main bullets (❑) and the details appear as sub-bullets (●).

Faced with the dilemma of generating a virtually unlimited repertoire from a limited number of genes, nature evolved an elegant solution that utilized some unusual mechanisms to achieve diversity.

AID:	Activation-induced cytosine deaminase
CSR:	Class switch recombination
DNA-PK:	DNA-dependent protein kinase
HMG:	High mobility group
NHEJ	Non-homologous DNA end-joining
RAG:	Recombinase activating genes
RSSs:	Recombination signal sequences
TdT:	Terminal deoxynucleotidyl transferase
TSE:	Transmissible spongiform encephalopathies

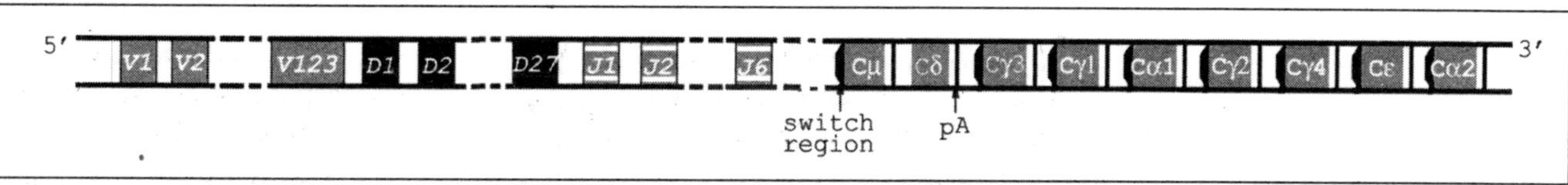

Figure 10.1 The germline locus of human Ig H chain contains several $\mathcal{V}$, $\mathcal{D}$, $\mathcal{J}$ subexons and multiple C region gene segments encoding different isotypes. *This panel is a schematic organization of the human Ig H chain locus on chromosome 14 and is not to scale. Each C region is flanked by a switch region (except of Cδ) on the 5′ end and a polyadenylation site that allows termination of transcription on the 3′ end. For simplicity, exon details within each C region and pseudogenes have not been shown.*

❑ BcR and TcR genes are assembled from separate (randomly chosen) gene segments, much as a child assembles a structure from Lego pieces (fig. 10.1).

❑ The antigen-binding sites of BcR or TcR are also not preformed in the cell but require some assembly. Variable (V) regions of the Ig H chain (V_H) and TcR β and δ chains (Vβ and Vδ respectively) are assembled from three separate segments — $\mathcal{V}^1$ (coding for first ~97 amino acids), $\mathcal{D}$ (coding for the next 2–3 amino acids) and $\mathcal{J}$ (coding for the remaining 10/11 amino acids). Similarly, Ig L chain (V_L) and TcR α and γ chains (Vα and Vγ respectively) are put together from two segments — $\mathcal{V}$ (encoding the first 97 amino acids) and $\mathcal{J}$ (encoding the remaining 13 amino acids). As the germline genome contains several $\mathcal{V}$, $\mathcal{D}$, and $\mathcal{J}$ segments, there are multiple choices for each segment (Table 10.1). Since random selection of $\mathcal{V}$, ($\mathcal{D}$), and $\mathcal{J}$ regions during recombination generates the antigen receptors, the resultant diversity is called combinatorial diversity (Table 10.2).

❑ The joining of the $\mathcal{V}(\mathcal{D})\mathcal{J}$ segments is imprecise, allowing for addition or deletion of nucleotides and further increasing the potential diversity of the repertoire. Since this diversity is generated through alterations at $\mathcal{V}$-$\mathcal{D}$, $\mathcal{D}$-$\mathcal{J}$, or $\mathcal{V}$-$\mathcal{J}$ junctions, it is called junctional diversity.

❑ The assembled V region couples with the C (constant) region, coding for the final segment of amino acids (equal to one Ig fold ~110 amino acids in the case of Ig L and TcR α (or γ) chains, or three Ig folds ~330 amino acids in the case of Ig H and TcR β (or δ) chains), to yield the complete Ig L, Ig H, TcR α, γ, β, or δ genes.

❑ The functional heterodimeric B cell antigen receptor is formed by random pairing of the L chain with the H chain; similarly, the random pairing of α (or γ) with the

[1] To avoid confusion between the V region of the antigen receptor and the V gene segment that codes for only a part of the assembled V region, the latter, ie, gene segments, are represented by $\mathcal{V}$, $\mathcal{D}$, and $\mathcal{J}$ in this chapter.

Table 10.1 Elements of human $V(D)J$ recombination

	Ig H chain	Ig L chain		TcR chain			
		κ	λ	α	β	γ	δ
Chromosome	14	2	22	14	7	7	$14^{\$}$
V region subexons	3 (V-D-J)	2 (V-J)	2 (V-J)	2 (V-J)	3 (V-D-J)	2 (V-J)	3 (V-D-J)
Number of subexons*	V–123 D–27 J–6	V–76 J–5	V–31 J–4	$V \sim 70$ J–61	V–52 D–2 J–13	V–14 J–5	V–4 D–3 J–3
Minimum recombination events required for V region assembly	3	2	2	2	3	2	3
Order of recombination events	D joins J; D-J joins V	V joins J	V joins J	V joins J	D joins J; D-J joins V	V joins J	V joins D; V-D joins J

* These numbers are derived from the exhaustive cloning and sequencing of DNA from one individual. Thanks to polymorphism, the number will not be the same for all individuals. Also, the numbers do not include pseudogenes, which are essentially mutated and non-functional versions of a gene sequence.

$\$$ The δ gene cluster lies within the α gene cluster, and hence, rearrangement of the α chain genes inactivates genes encoding δ chain; the exact number of Vδ genes is not clear.

β (or δ) chains yields the $\alpha\beta$ (or $\gamma\delta$) TcR. This further increases diversity and gives rise to the large and varied repertoire of the primary immune response. This primary B (or T) cell repertoire is achieved through combinatorial and junctional diversity. It does not require exposure to antigen, ie, it is shaped during the process of B (or T) cell maturation. In this way, the immune system is prepared to recognize and deal with antigens it has not yet encountered.

❑ Two additional processes increase only the B cell repertoire following antigenic challenge, viz, hypermutation and **C**lass **S**witch **R**ecombination (CSR).

- Locus-specific somatic hypermutation alters the affinity of the antibody for the antigen following antigen challenge.
- Ig H CSR allows the fully assembled and expressed V$_H$ region gene to be coupled to a new C$_H$ region gene so that the antigenic specificity of the antibody remains unchanged while effector functions vary.

10.2 $V(D)J$ Recombination

As explained above and summarized in Table 10.1, V region exons of BcR and TcR are assembled from subexons. Separate chromosomes encode the BcR (and Ig) H and L chains. Similarly, gene segments encoding TcR α, β and γ chains also lie on different chromosomes. The TcR δ chain locus lies within the α chain locus and hence, rearranging the α locus results in the deletion of the entire δ locus. The respective C regions are encoded by separate exons downstream of the V gene segments. DNA recombination events that occur at the three Ig (H, Lκ, and Lλ) and four TcR (α, β, γ, and δ) loci to yield productive V genes are similar. The Ig H, TcRβ, or TcRγ chains rearrange before the Ig L, TcRα, or δ chains, and the recombination process assembles the complete (and unique) V$_H$/Vβ/Vδ exon from linear gene arrays of V, D, and J gene segments. Assembly is tightly regulated, occurring in a preferred temporal order in the case of Ig H and TcRβ chains — D joins J and combined DJ is joined to the V subexon. In the case of TcRδ, however, the order is different, with $V D$ joining preceding DJ joining. In the case of the light chains (whether Ig L, TcRα, or TcRγ), the question of order does not arise — V joins J. The main features of $V(D)J$ recombination are given below.

Understanding Terminology

Exons and introns: The coding sequences in genes are called exons. Exons have intervening, non-coding nucleotide sequences called introns. Both, the exons and introns are transcribed into RNA. The primary RNA transcripts are converted to mature mRNA molecules by the excision of the introns and splicing together of the exons.

Promoters: Relatively short nucleotide sequences extending up to 200 base pairs upstream from the transcription initiation site (ie, 5′ region of the DNA) that promote initiation of the RNA transcription in a specific direction are called promoters. Promoter regions facilitate the binding of RNA polymerase to the DNA and orient it for the proper transcription of the gene.

Enhancers: These are the nucleotide sequences, situated some distance upstream or downstream from a gene, that activate transcription from the promoter sequence in an orientation-independent manner. Enhancers activate nearby promoters, probably by binding a regulatory protein that can also bind the promoter and RNA polymerase.

Silencers: Nucleotide sequences that downregulate transcription in both directions over a distance are called silencers.

Recombination: This is the reciprocal exchange of genetic material between DNA fragments. The process involves the breaking and rejoining of DNA pieces to generate new DNA pieces, and it can occur between two different double stranded DNA molecules or between two parts of the same DNA molecule.

❑ Homologous recombination occurs between DNA strands that have long stretches of homology. Double stranded breaks can be repaired if a chromosome or chromatid that is homologous to the broken DNA is available in the cell.

❑ **N**on-**H**omologous DNA **E**nd-**J**oining (NHEJ) is a pathway that rejoins DNA strand breaks without relying on marked homology. The main known pathway uses the Ku protein binding complex and is regulated by the DNA protein kinase. This pathway is often used in mammalian cells to repair strand breaks that are caused by DNA-damaging agents.

❑ Site-specific recombination occurs at a specific sequence of DNA due to targeting by a specific enzyme called recombinase. V(D)J recombination is an example of site-specific recombination that occurs between DNA regions of a single chromosome.

Mutations: A mutation is a change in the DNA sequence. Transition is the swapping of one pyrimidine base (cytosine, thymine, or uracil) for another pyrimidine base or one purine base (adenine and guanine) for another purine base. Transversions occurs when one pyrimidine base is swapped for a purine base or vice versa.

Error-prone DNA polymerases: DNA polymerases that copy templates inaccurately are termed error-prone. Examples include POLζ, POLν, POLμ, and POLι. Some of these are candidates for enzymes that introduce base changes during somatic hypermutation.

❑ $\mathcal{V(D)J}$ **recombination occurs at conserved non-coding Recombination Signal Sequences (RSSs) that lie adjacent to each** $\mathcal{V}$**,** $\mathcal{D}$**, and** $\mathcal{J}$ **segment.**

- An RSS consists of a palindromic[2] heptamer (seven DNA base pairs) and an A/T-rich nonamer (nine DNA base pairs; fig. 10.2) separated by intervening spacers of either 12 base pairs (one turn of the DNA helix) or 23 base pairs (two turns of the helix).

- The length of the spacer is important in determining the functionality of the RSS; efficient recombination can occur only between RSS with 12- and 23-base pair (called the 12/23 rule) spacers. Thus, for the Ig κ locus, all $\mathcal{V}$ segments are attached to 12-spacer RSSs, whereas all $\mathcal{J}$ segments are attached to 23-spacer RSSs, ensuring that $\mathcal{V}$-$\mathcal{J}$ joining is much more efficient than $\mathcal{V}$-$\mathcal{V}$ or $\mathcal{J}$-$\mathcal{J}$ joining. Whenever the V region is assembled from three subexons (ie, H/β/δ), both $\mathcal{V}$ and $\mathcal{J}$ segments must join $\mathcal{D}$, so the $\mathcal{D}$ segments are flanked by RSSs of appropriate spacer lengths on each side (fig. 10.2). For Ig H chains, both $\mathcal{V}$ and $\mathcal{J}$ segments have 23-spacer RSSs, whereas the $\mathcal{D}$ segment is flanked by 12-spacer RSS on both sides.

[2] A palindrome is a word, verse, sentence, or numerical which reads the same backwards or forwards. 'Madam I'm Adam' is a classic example.

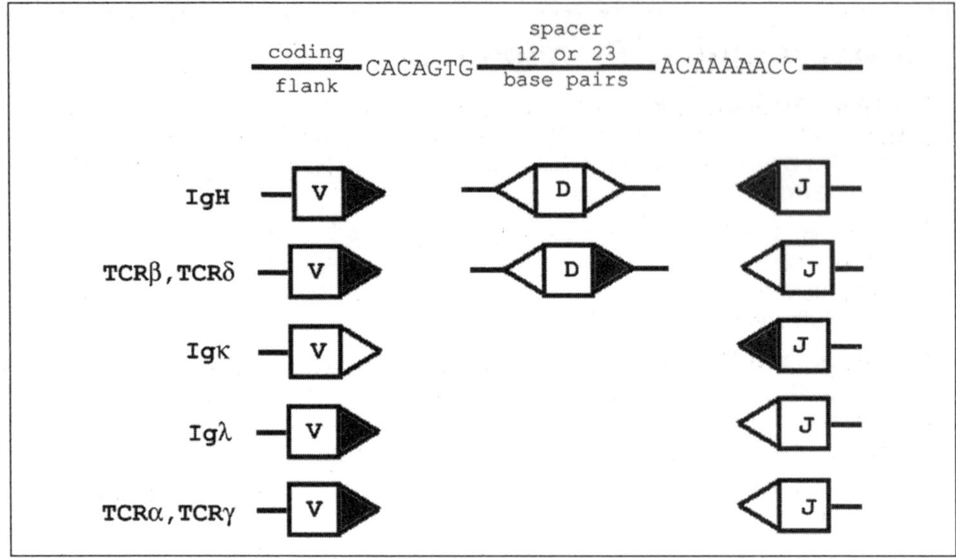

Figure 10.2 𝒱𝒟𝒥 recombination occurs at Recombination Signal Sequences (RSSs) that are adjacent to each 𝒱, 𝒟, and 𝒥 segment. *Each RSS contains moderately well conserved heptamer and nonamer sequences (represented here by consensus sequences CACAGTG and ACAAAAACC) separated by an intervening stretch of 12 or 23 base pairs, non-conserved DNA called the spacer (upper panel). The bottom panel shows the arrangement of 12 (open triangle) or 23 (closed triangle) base pair spacers in the three Ig (H,κ,λ) and four TcR (β,δ,α,γ) loci (Adapted from Annual Review of Biochemistry (2002) 17:101).*

- Distances between the RSSs does not seem to affect efficiency of the 𝒱(𝒟)𝒥 recombination. For example, human Ig κ and Ig H loci have 𝒱 subexons extended over 2300 kilobases, and distal 𝒱 segments are still utilized with reasonable frequency. How RSS pairs locate each other over such large distances is not clear. However, recombination within a single chromosome is strongly preferred. Thus, recombination between κ and λ loci (lying on different chromosomes) is 1/1000 as frequent as 𝒱-𝒥 recombination within the same loci.
- RSSs are generally arranged such on the antigen receptor loci that the joined coding segments remain in the chromosome and the junction of the RSSs (called the signal joint) is excised on a circular DNA that is eventually lost from the cells.

❑ **𝒱(𝒟)𝒥 recombination has two distinct stages — DNA breakage and strand break repair.**
- In the first stage, the lymphoid-specific proteins RAG-1 and RAG-2 (**R**ecombinase **A**ctivating **G**enes-1 & -2) recognize the RSSs, ensure their correct 12/23 pairing, and break the DNA between each heptamer and the neighbouring coding sequence.
- The second stage of the process is the joining phase and has many aspects in common with general DNA double strand break repair. Ubiquitously expressed **N**on-**H**omologous DNA **E**nd-**J**oining (NHEJ) proteins process and link the ends into coding joints and signal joints. At the end of the process, two (or three) separate segments of DNA recombine to yield a single V region.

❑ **RAG-1 and RAG-2 are highly conserved genes that are expressed in early lymphoid cells undergoing 𝒱(𝒟)𝒥 recombination and are indispensable for this process[3].**
- All known RAG activities require the presence of both proteins. By themselves, they seem to preferentially bind RSS with 12 spacers. However, in the presence of HMG-1 & 2 (**H**igh **M**obility **G**roup Proteins; one of a group of non-specific, DNA-binding and -bending proteins), the RAG proteins bind coding sequences flanked by either 12- and 23-spacers.

[3] The indispensability of RAG proteins in the process of antigen-receptor generation can be judged from the fact that RAG KO mice lack mature functional T and B cells.

$\mathcal{V(D)J}$ **RECOMBINATION**

❑ It is the process by which antigen receptors of B and T lymphocytes are assembled.
❑ The antigen-binding regions of the receptors are assembled from separate subexons.
  • Three separate subexons ($\mathcal{V}$, $\mathcal{D}$, and $\mathcal{J}$) code for Ig VH region and TcR β, δ chains.
  • The assembling occurs in a temporal fashion; $\mathcal{D}$ joins $\mathcal{J}$ and $\mathcal{DJ}$ is joined to $\mathcal{V}$.
  • Ig VL region and TcR α, γ chains are encoded by two subexons $\mathcal{V}$ and $\mathcal{J}$.
❑ $\mathcal{V(D)J}$ recombination occurs at conserved non-coding Recombination Signal Sequences (RSSs) that lie adjacent to each $\mathcal{V}$, $\mathcal{D}$, and $\mathcal{J}$ segment.
  • Each RSS consists of a palindromic heptamer and A-T-rich nonamer separated by a spacer of 12- or 23-base pairs.
  • The nonamer and heptamer come together during recombination.
  • Efficient recombination occurs only between RSSs with 12- and 23-base pair spacers.
❑ RAG-1 and RAG-2 proteins are involved in the recombination reaction.
  • They recognize the RSSs, ensure their correct 12/23 pairing, and introduce a double strand break between the target heptamer and flanking coding sequence.
  • The breakage yields two types of termini — a blunt 5′-phophorylated signal end and an hairpin coding end that retains the full coding sequence.
  • Two blunt signal ends are joined to yield a signal joint on a circular DNA.
  • The two coding joints are ligated by nucleocide modification, ie, either addition or deletion.
❑ Those cells that successfully recombine their Ig H or TcR β, δ chains express these chains as a part of the prereceptor complex and start rearranging Ig L or TcR α, γ chains.
❑ Cells that make non-productive rearrangements go on to rearrange their second allele; if they fail to rearrange the second allele they apoptose.

  • The complex consisting of RAG-1, RAG-2, HMG-1, and 12- and 23-spacer DNA is highly stable. It is also resistant to other non-specific DNA present in the vicinity.
❑ **RAG (1&2) proteins bind DNA and introduce DNA double strand breaks between the target RSS heptamer and the flanking sequence of $\mathcal{V}$, $\mathcal{D}$, or $\mathcal{J}$ coding segments**, yielding two types of termini — a blunt 5′-phophorylated signal end and a hairpin coding end that retains the full coding sequence. The four RAG-liberated DNA ends remain associated with RAG proteins in a stable, post-cleavage synaptic complex.
  • The cleavage occurs in two steps and seems to require Mg^{2+}; first, a nick is introduced at the 5′ end of the signal heptamer of the two participating coding sequences, leaving a 5′-phosphoryl group on each RSS and a 3′-OH group on the coding end (fig. 10.3).
  • The second step is a transesterification reaction catalyzed by RAG proteins; the 3′-OH group of the coding strand invades and joins the phosphoryl group at the same nucleotide position on the opposite strand, yielding the DNA hairpin coding end and a blunt, 5′-phosphorylated signal end.
❑ **The two blunt signal ends are joined to yield a signal joint on a circular DNA**; this signal joint has no further role and is eventually lost[4].
  • Signal joints are relatively simple, usually precise, end-to-end fusions of the two heptamer sequences.
  • DNA-ligase IV and XRCC4 along with the heterodimeric subunit of the **DNA-dependent protein kinase (DNA-PK)[5]** are required for this ligation.
❑ **Joining the coding ends is a more complex process.** The coding ends undergo nucleotide addition or deletion before ligation.
  • The hairpin ends produced by RAG cleavage must be reopened before the end-joining pathway can process and join them.
  • Hairpin coding ends are opened at the apex or points nearby; RAG proteins along with (a newly discovered protein) artemis seem to be involved in this opening though other DNA repair proteins may also be involved.

[4] Thus, $\mathcal{V(D)J}$ arrangement results in *loss* of genetic information. Incidentally, this is a unique process involving destruction of genetic information rather than regulation of gene expression.

[5] DNA-PK is a multimeric protein consisting of a catalytic unit (DNA-PKcs) and a heteromeric binding subunit Ku (consisting of Ku70 and Ku80). As explained in chapter 5, loss of DNA-PK results in SCID, since developing lymphocytes fail to rearrange their antigen receptors.

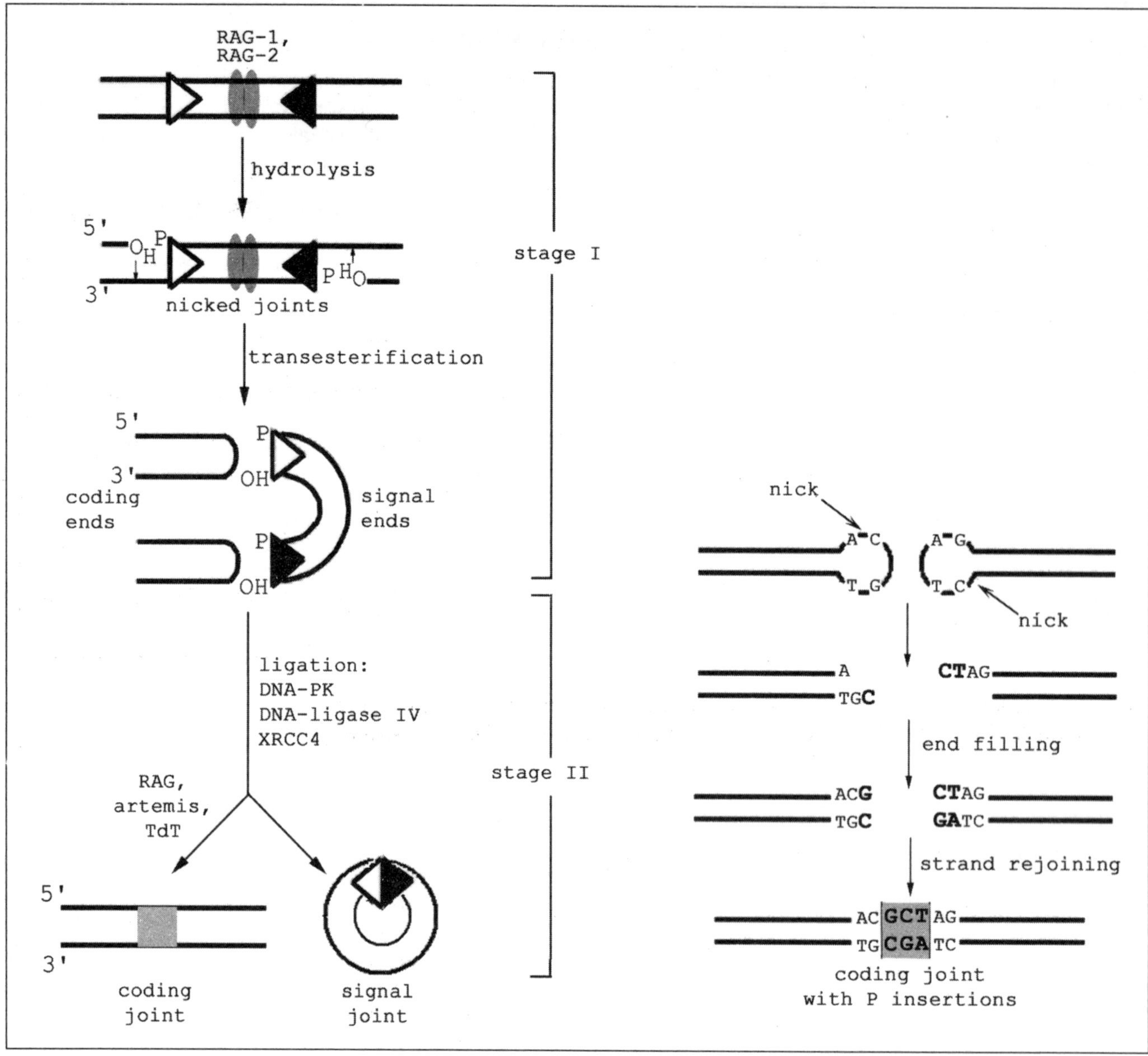

Figure 10.3 V(D)J recombination occurs in two stages — DNA breakage catalyzed by RAG proteins and DNA double strand break repair catalyzed by NHEJ proteins. RAG-1 and RAG-2 recognize the RSSs and ensure their correct 12/23 pairing (open and closed triangle; left panel). They bind to the DNA and introduce double strand breaks between the target RSS heptamer and the flanking sequence of the coding segments to yield a 5′-phosphoryl group on each signal end and a 3′-OH group on the coding end. Transesterification catalyzed by RAG proteins results in the 3′-OH group of the coding strand invading and joining the phosphoryl group at the same nucleotide position on the opposite strand to generate a hairpin coding end and a blunt signal end. The two blunt signal ends are joined to yield a signal joint — usually end-to-end fusion of the two heptamer sequences catalyzed by NHEJ enzymes such as DNA-PK, DNA ligase IV, and XRCC4. The coding ends undergo nucleotide additions or deletions (grey area) before ligation and require RAG proteins, TdT, and artemis, in addition to the NHEJ machinery. The right panel depicts the process of P insertions in the coding joints. For simplicity, the two coding ends are shown adjacent to each other. The hairpin coding ends are opened by introducing nicks that are a few bases off each other, leaving self-complimentary single strand extensions (bold letters). End-filling using the overhang as template results in P insertions.

- The opened coding ends undergo nucleotide excision or nucleotide addition; the junctional sequences lie within the antigen-binding site (in the CDRs), so alterations in coding joints are responsible for increasing the diversity of the antigen receptors beyond that generated by combinatorial joining of gene segments.

- The mechanism of nucleotide deletion at the coding junctions is not clear; it is generally believed that exonucleases may be involved.
- Two types of nucleotide additions are observed in the coding joints, non-templated and templated.
  - Non-templated addition may result in an addition of up to 15 nucleotides at the coding joint. This template-independent addition is due to the enzyme **T**erminal **d**eoxynucleotidyl **T**ransferase (TdT) that is normally expressed only in early lymphoid cells where $\mathcal{V}(\mathcal{D})\mathcal{J}$ recombination is active. TdT adds deoxynucleotides without a template to the ends of DNA chains but has a preference for G residues that results in N regions being generally G-C rich.
  - Templated nucleotide additions occur because of the off-centre nicking of hairpin DNA intermediates, which results in a self-complementary overhang. These nucleotide additions are called P (for **P**alindromic) insertions.
  - The catalytic subunit of DNA-PK along with DNA-ligase IV and XRCC4 seems to be important in the formation of the coding joint.
- ❑ All V regions have a weak promoter. Proper ligation places the weak promoter adjacent to the assembled V region into close proximity of enhancers present downstream of the J region or upstream of the C region. These enhancers activate transcription from the particular promoter, enabling the cell to make complete Ig (H or L) chains.

Table 10.2 Combinatorial diversity

BcR V region subexons	Number	Combinations generated
$\mathcal{V}$κ	40	200 κ chains
$\mathcal{J}$κ	5	
$\mathcal{V}$λ	31	124 λ chains
$\mathcal{J}$λ	4	
$\mathcal{V}$H	65	1.05×10^4 H chains
$\mathcal{D}$H	27	
$\mathcal{J}$H	6	
Random association of H and L chains		4.96×10^6

10.3 Regulation of $\mathcal{V}(\mathcal{D})\mathcal{J}$ Recombination

As explained, lymphocyte-specific RAG protein expression limits $\mathcal{V}(\mathcal{D})\mathcal{J}$ recombination activity to non-proliferating stages of developing lymphocytes. The randomness and imprecision of $\mathcal{V}(\mathcal{D})\mathcal{J}$ recombination results in only about one in three $\mathcal{V}(\mathcal{D})\mathcal{J}$ rearrangements being in frame and therefore, productive. Those cells that make non-productive rearrangements go on to rearrange their second allele so that majority of differentiating lymphocytes eventually achieve productive rearrangements. V-J joining affords even more chances of corrections, since recombination may be tried again on the same allele by the use of a $\mathcal{V}$ region upstream and a $\mathcal{J}$ region downstream of the erroneous junction. If a lymphocyte fails to rearrange its receptor productively, it is pushed down the path of apoptosis. Upon productive rearrangement, the newly synthesized Ig H (or TcRβ) chains associate with surrogate L (or TcRα) chains to form pre-receptor complexes. Expression of these surrogate pre-receptors results in the cessation of further rearrangements, ensuring allelic exclusion (fig. 10.4). It also activates rearrangement of the Ig L or TcRα genes.

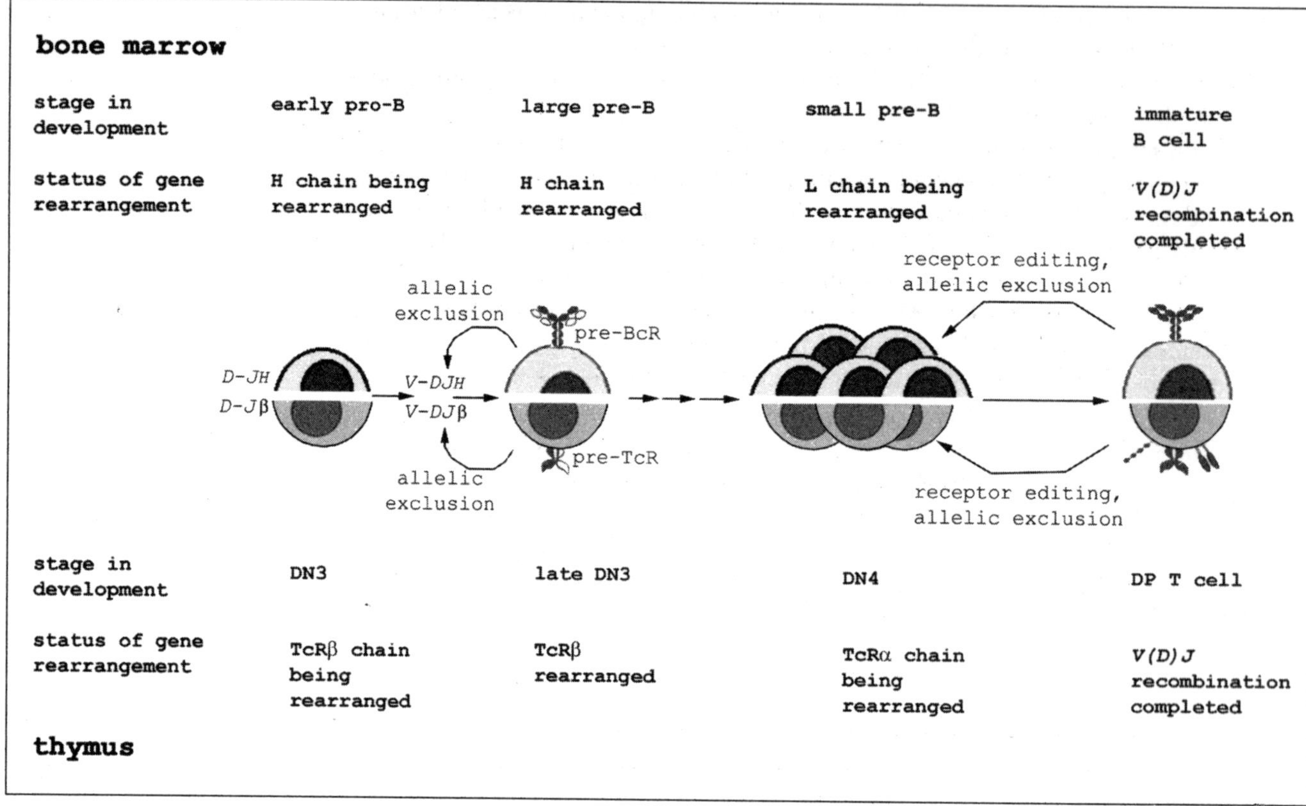

Figure 10.4 The developing B and T lymphocytes undergo similar ordered $V(D)J$ gene rearrangements; feedback mechanisms link appropriate antigen receptor expression to further development. V region genes of the H chain and TcRβ chain are the first to undergo recombination in the developing lymphocytes. The D-J rearrangement occurs first and the assembled DJ is joined to the V subexon. Productive rearrangement results in gene expression. The newly synthesized Ig H or TcRβ chain associates with its surrogate partner (indicated by open symbols) and is expressed at the cell surface. Pre-receptor expression is a major check point in the life of the developing lymphocyte. Signalling through the pre-receptors ensures allelic exclusion, allows clonal expansion, and further progression on the developmental pathway. Ig L or TcRα chain rearrangement is also activated. Productive rearrangement causes cessation of rearrangement of these chains and enforces allelic exclusion. Cells that fail to undergo productive rearrangement may undergo receptor editing. Only those cells that have undergone productive rearrangement express the antigen receptors on their cell surface and become immature (B or T) lymphocytes.

Allelic exclusion makes certain that only a single allele at a particular locus is expressed in a single B/αβ T cell; since the second allele does not undergo productive rearrangement, it is automatically excluded from expression. Allelic exclusion is an actively regulated process that occurs at the progenitor to precursor transition via feedback control of the V- to -DJ joining step, possibly by the surrogate light chain. The exact mechanism that enforces allelic exclusion is not clear. If the receptor generated after gene rearrangement recognizes self-antigens, the lymphocytes get one more chance at gene rearrangement in the process of receptor editing. Receptor editing allows a secondary rearrangement of the antigen receptor locus and avoids clonal deletion of the newly formed immature B or T cells. It is relatively easy to understand such rearrangements at the Ig Lκ and TcRα loci; the genomic organizations of these loci, consisting of only V and J subexons, permit successive rearrangements. However, the mechanism of the receptor editing of the Ig H/TcRβ is not clear. Receptor editing is possible only because of continued expression of RAG proteins in immature lymphocytes.

10.4 Somatic Hypermutation and Class Switch Recombination

Following productive rearrangement, the lymphocytes undergo selection in the primary lymphoid organs before leaving. T cells do not undergo any further recombination events at their antigen receptor locus, ie, they (and their progeny) are stuck with the TcR assembled in the primary lymphoid organs. B lymphocytes, on the other hand, are subject to further recombination events. This happens in the later phases of the primary immune response to TD antigens, when proliferating B cells differentiate to memory cells and plasma cells. B cells undergo a second wave of genetic alterations — somatic hypermutation and CSR at the Ig gene loci — at this stage. Somatic hypermutation involves a change in the nucleotide sequences of genetic loci of the antigen-binding pocket of the antibody V regions, and it results in an increased affinity of the antibody for the antigen. Conversely, CSR allows the switching of the C_H region expressed from $C\mu$ to $C\gamma$, $C\alpha$, or $C\varepsilon$, resulting in the expression and secretion of IgG, IgA, and IgE respectively, without changing antigen-specificity[6]. The different Ig isotypes use the same set of V genes and only the C regions of the H chains are shuffled so that the effector functions of the Ig vary, but their antigenic specificity remains unchanged. Although CSR may be observed in B1 or MZ cells responding to TI antigens, somatic hypermutation is generally not observed for TI antigens.

Table 10.3 Genetic changes observed in B and T cells

Event	B cells			T cells		
	Stage in development	*Site*	*Nature of event*	*Stage in development*	*Site*	*Nature of event*
Heavy chain rearrangement Ig H/TcRβ* chain $\mathcal{D}$-$\mathcal{J}$ / $\mathcal{V(D)J}$	Early pro-B Late pro-B	Bone marrow	DNA recombination	DN3 DN3	Thymus	DNA recombination
Light chain rearrangement Ig L/TcRα chain $\mathcal{V}$-$\mathcal{J}$	Small pre-B	Bone marrow	DNA recombination	DP	Thymus	DNA recombination
Receptor editing	Immature cells	Bone marrow	DNA recombination	Immature cells	Thymus	DNA recombination
Somatic hypermutation	TD antigen-activated mature cells	Germinal centre	Point mutations	–	–	–
Class switch recombination	Antigen-activated mature cells	Germinal centre	DNA recombination	–	–	–

* TcRγ and TcRδ gene segments rearrange ($\mathcal{V}\gamma$ to $\mathcal{J}\gamma$ and $\mathcal{V}\delta$ to $\mathcal{D}\delta$ to $\mathcal{J}d$) without any strict order and without the clonal expansion and selection observed after Ig H, L, TcRα, and TcRβ rearrangements.

10.4.1 Site of Somatic Hypermutation and Class Switch Recombination

Mature B cells that have completed functional $\mathcal{V(D)J}$ recombination of both H and L chain genes express IgM at their cell surfaces and get negatively selected for self-antigens. Those that do not express BcR capable of reacting with self-antigens survive this selection, express mIgD, and migrate to the secondary lymphoid organs (eg, spleen and lymph nodes). Here, they compete for survival signals. Those B cells that receive these survival signals enter the pool of circulating lymphocytes and remain quiescent until an encounter with TD antigens. When these B cells encounter a TD antigen recognized by their BcR and receive appropriate signals from T cells, they proliferate vigorously in the lymphoid follicles in special

[6] This is similar to your dressing up for an evening by keeping your workplace trousers and substituting your shirt for a more glamorous option. A similar trick is used in languages. For example, in English prefixes to the word *logy* (meaning 'study of') are switched to describe various fields of study — zoology, biology, sociology, etc.

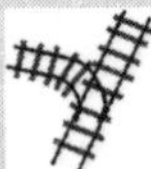

Aging AIDS Mad Cows: FDCs in Health and Disease

FDCs derive their name from their morphology and geography — they have long, slender protrusions (dendritus) and are found in the follicles (germinal centres) of secondary lymphoid tissues. In spite of their having dendritic projections, FDCs are both morphologically and functionally distinct from DCs. They are non-phagocytic cells that do not express MHC class II molecules and hence are not involved in antigen presentation. Additionally, they have one unique cardinal feature — they can trap native antigen in the form of immune complexes. Surprisingly, antigenic epitopes in these complexes are not masked by the antibodies and the epitopes are accessible and recognizable by BcRs. The nature and ontogeny of the FDCs are yet to be defined. FDC precursors remain elusive; it is not clear whether they develop from haematopoietic precursors or stromal precursors. There is some data to suggest that human FDCs may be of fibroblastic origin. The differentiation pathway that leads to their formation is also poorly defined. TNF-α and membrane lymphotoxin (LT-α/β) are two key B cell derived cytokines important to maintaining FDCs in their differentiated state. FDCs are potent accessory cells for B cell functioning.

❑ FDCs trap and retain antigens in the form of immune complexes formed with specific antibody and/or complement proteins; this ability to trap and retain antigens stems from the expression of FcγRIIB and CR2 (CD21) receptors on their cell surface. Incidentally, since the antigen trapping is dependent on the presence of Ig, FDCs do not have a role in early phases of the primary immune responses.

❑ Engagement of the intact antigen in the immune complex by the BcR delivers a survival signal to B cells. The effect of this survival signal is enhanced by the coligation of CD21 in the BcR complex by C3b or its fragments present in immune complexes. Blocking of this interaction has been shown to dramatically reduce antibody responses and memory B cell generation.

❑ Coligation of BcR with FcγRIIB, expressed by B cells, is known to deliver a negative signal to B cells as a consequence of the phosphorylation of ITIM in the cytoplasmic tail of the receptor; however, the high density of FcγRIIB expressed by FDCs bind all the available FcRs of Igs in the immune complexes, ensuring the absence of such coligation.

❑ FDCs convert immune complexes to iccosomes (immune complex coated bodies). These are antigen-coated liposome-like particles of about 0.25–0.38 μm diameter derived from FDC membranes. Iccosomes consist of antigen, C3b or its fragments, and Ig attached to FDC membranes. Iccosomes are released from FDC dendrites and are rapidly endocytosed by germinal centre B cells. The presence of C3b (or its fragments) is thought to aid this rapid endocytosis. Antigen in the iccosomes is efficiently processed, loaded on MHC class II molecules, and presented to follicular T_H cells. The ensuing cognate interaction is indispensable for survival and differentiation of germinal centre B cells.

FDCs and aging: Aging is known to affect the development of memory B cell responses and is closely related to the presence of fewer germinal centres. Experimental data suggests that FDCs, rather than B or T cells, are the reason for the impaired humoral responses observed in the aged. DCs normally trap and transport the antigen to the draining lymph node. Some of them eventually join the FDC network and augment the formation of iccosomes. Recent data suggests that antigen transport is less efficient in the aged. This defect in antigen transport leads to a reduction in the formation of immune complexes and hence, poorly developed FDC networks. Furthermore, FDC accessory activity also seems to be affected in aging animals. Expression of FcγRIIB and CD21 seems to be downregulated in FDCs of the old. Consequently, markedly fewer iccosomes are found on the surface of these cells and may contribute to poor humoral responses.

FDCs, HIV, and TSE (**T**ransmissible **S**pongiform **E**ncephalopathies)**:** The ability of FDCs to trap and hold the antigen in its native form for prolonged periods has devastating consequences in the case of two infections — HIV and TSE.

FDCs appear to play a role in the pathogenesis of HIV/AIDS after the initial infection and seeding of secondary lymphoid tissues has occurred. The lymphoid tissues represent a major reservoir of

HIV; it is estimated that about 1.5×10^8 copies of viral RNA can be found per gram of lymphoid tissue. Throughout clinical latency, active HIV infection is largely confined to germinal centres. The majority of trapped viruses exist on the surface of FDCs. This trapping is advantageous to the virus because of the close proximity of activated CD4+ T cells and a microenvironment that facilitates both transmission of infection and maintenance of virus infectivity. This association of the retrovirus with FDCs has profound consequences for the host.

❑ Experimental data establish both the longevity and potency of FDCs as HIV reservoirs and indicate that FDCs need not be infected to transmit infection; mere trapping of the virus on their surface is enough.

❑ The trapped virus continues to be infectious even in the presence of high quantities of neutralizing antibodies; ironically, the antibodies are found to lead to a slightly better preservation of the virus infectivity *in vitro*.

❑ CD4+ T cells trafficking through germinal centres become infected by the trapped virus and further replenish the FDC-HIV reservoir; latent infection in these cells may also get activated because of the activatory signals in the germinal centre.

❑ HIV is known to mutate throughout the course of infection. The mutated forms (called quasi species) co-exist in the host. FDCs may trap and maintain these quasi species in an infectious state, allowing one or the other quasi species to outgrow whenever conditions are favourable. Thus, FDCs may indirectly help in the emergence of drug-resistant strains of the virus.

❑ As a consequence of virus trapping, previously trapped antigens are lost from the FDCs, leading to a marked impairment of overall antibody responses.

TSEs are chronic neurodegenerative diseases thought to be caused by prions that affect humans and wild and domestic animals. Prions (pronounced pree-ahns) are intriguing in that they enter cells and apparently convert normal proteins found within the cells into prions just like themselves. The normal cell proteins have all the same 'parts' (ie, the same amino acids) as the prions, but they fold differently, that is, have a different tertiary structure. They are much like the 'Transformer' toys of the 1980s where a locomotive engine could become a robot without any addition or subtraction. Most TSEs (scrapie in sheep, BSE or mad cow disease in cattle, and **v**ariant **C**reutzfeldt-**J**akob **D**isease — vCJD — in humans) are thought to be acquired peripherally by ingestion or accidental inoculation, eg, via contaminated surgical instruments. Following entry, high levels of disease specific isoforms of host prion protein (PrP^{SC}) usually accumulate in lymphoid tissues prior to their detection in the CNS. Accumulation in lymphoid tissue appears to be critical for efficient neuroinvasion. Germinal centres, especially FDCs, have long been suspected to be involved in peripheral prion pathogenesis. FDCs are an ideal target for invasion, since they express the cellular form of the prion protein (PrP^{C}), a prerequisite for susceptibility to TSE infection. Additionally, they are long-lived cells that trap antigens in an unaltered state for prolonged periods. Soon after inoculation, TSE agents are thought to become rapidly opsonized by complement components like C1q and C3. This allows their localization on FDCs and helps in evading early destruction by macrophages. Subsequent to replication of infectivity on FDCs, neuroinvasion appears to follow the dissemination of infection along fibres of sympathetic nervous system. Exactly how infectivity passes from FDCs to sympathetic nerve endings is not known. Neuroinvasion is significantly impaired in the absence of mature FDCs and therapies targeting FDCs are currently under investigation for the treatment of TSEs.

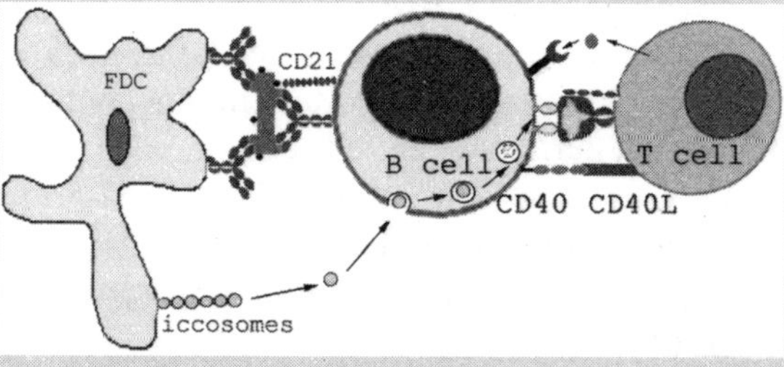

Figure 10.S1 FDCs are vital for affinity-based selection of germinal centre B cells.

microenvironments called germinal centres. **Germinal centres are thus the sites for B cell differentiation and secondary genetic alterations in the BcR.**

The principle of affinity-based selection operates right from the earliest stages of the immune response. Thus, of all the B lymphocytes available in circulation at the time of contact with antigen, only those cells with an affinity high enough to permit the molecules to remain bound together until internalization will be recruited into the immune response. By the second day after primary immunization with a TD antigen, antigen-specific T cells are found within PALS of the spleen and lymph nodes. By the fourth day, antigen-specific B cells migrate to lymphoid follicles. There, they proliferate exponentially; within 72 hours their numbers increase 10,000-fold. The resting B cells not taking part in the immune response are pushed to the periphery and make up the mantle zone around the proliferating B cells. The proliferating lymphoblasts begin to fill the FDC network of the lymphoid follicle and give rise to an organized structure called the germinal centre[7]. The main constituents of the germinal centre are activated B lymphocytes, FDCs, macrophages, and CD4[+] T lymphocytes. Germinal centres are made of three distinct zones.

❏ **The dark zone.** In forming the germinal centre, B cell blasts cluster in the part of the follicle nearest to the T cell zone, and this area is called the dark zone. The proliferating B cells, called centroblasts, undergo a number of changes in the dark zone. BcR expression is downregulated so that the centroblasts appear to be mIg[−]. They proliferate vigorously and undergo diversification of their antibody repertoire through somatic hypermutation of their Ig V region genes. Although centroblasts continue to proliferate, they do not increase in numbers, since they give rise to non-dividing cells, called centrocytes, which express surface Ig and migrate to the light zone.

❏ **The light zone.** Although it appears as a single zone under the microscope, the light zone consists of two distinct regions — the basal light zone that is adjacent to the dark zone and the apical light zone. The light zone is the site of isotype switching and the positive and negative selection of B cells — positive selection for cells expressing high affinity receptors for the antigen eliciting the immune response and negative selection of those cells that have lost their capacity to recognize that antigen. B cells that receive the necessary survival signals eventually differentiate to plasmablasts (that give rise to plasma cells) and memory cells and leave the germinal centre.

- FDCs are specialized cells present in the basal light zone. These cells can be distinguished by their long protrusions and relatively high expression of FcγRIIB and CR1 and CR2 (CD35 and CD21 respectively). These receptors trap antigen in the form of immune complexes on FDC cell surfaces; antigen-antibody complexes can be detected on the FDCs months after immunization.

- FDCs are thought to be instrumental in the selection of B cells on the basis of their affinity for the antigen; competition for the limited antigen results in only those B cells expressing high affinity BcR binding antigen present on the FDCs. Adhesion molecules on B cells (eg, LFA-1 and Very Late Antigen-4) and FDCs (ICAM-1 and VCAM-1) are crucial for intimate contact between the two cells. In humans, interaction between CD23 expressed on B cells and CD21 on FDCs is also found to be important in this context.

- Human germinal centre B cells show a typical apoptosis sensitive phenotype; they express low levels of the anti-apoptotic Bcl-2 and high levels of pro-apoptotic Fas and Bax. These cells are thought to contain preformed DISC that causes rapid activation of enzymes involved in apoptosis (chapters 8 and 11).

- FDCs deliver anti-apoptotic signals to the bound B cells, rescuing them from apoptosis and enabling their migration to the apical light zone. The exact

[7] In 1885, Flemming observed strong proliferation of lymphocytes in the follicles of peripheral lymphatic organs. He thought that leukocytes germinated in these follicles and therefore named the structures germinal centres.

nature of the anti-apoptotic signal is not clear, but it seems to prevent rapid activation of two enzymes involved in apoptosis — caspase-8 and caspase-3.

- Centrocytes with low-affinity receptors are less likely to bind the antigen and hence fail to get survival signals from FDCs. They are pushed on the road to apoptosis or may re-enter the dark zone. Thus, a large proportion of centrocytes that arrive in the light zone die there.
- Macrophages present in the light zone phagocytose dead or dying cells. They are called tingible body macrophages, because they contain dense nuclear fragments of cells undergoing apoptosis.
- Engagement of BcR by the antigen results in internalization of the antigen. As B cells migrate to the apical light zone, they process and load the antigen on MHC class II molecules.
- In the apical light zone, B cells encounter and present antigen to CD4$^+$ T cells. These T cells, called follicular helper T cells, are found at the outer edge of the light zone. They express the chemokine receptor CXCR5 and costimulatory molecule ICOS.
- Antigen presentation by B cells along with engagement of ICOS induces T cells to express CD154. Follicular helper T cells have an intracellular store of CD154 which is expressed on the cell surface upon stimulation. Engagement of CD40 on B cells by CD154 delivers a second survival signal to the B cells. The ensuing cognate interaction results in cytokine secretion by T cells.
- B cells that express MHC:peptide complexes not recognized by T cells (eg, B cells expressing self-antigens) fail to engage in CD40-CD154 interaction and undergo apoptosis.
- Centrocytes expressing high affinity BcRs for the antigen undergo clonal expansion and isotype switching; they also differentiate to memory cells and plasmablasts.
- The plasmablasts leave the germinal centre and migrate to the site of Ig production; those formed in GALT germinal centres migrate to the lamina propria of the gut, those formed in lymph nodes or spleen migrate to various sites (eg, bone marrow, medullary cords of the lymph nodes, or red pulp of spleen).
- The memory cells may leave the germinal centre and re-enter circulation or migrate to other sites (marginal zone of spleen, sub capsular sinus of lymph node, intestinal epithelium under Peyer's patches, etc). Alternatively, they may even re-enter the dark zone for a further round of mutations. Figure 10.5 summarizes the events in the germinal centre.

❑ **The outer mantle.** The outer follicular mantle is the place where the migrating B cells briefly reside before leaving the germinal centre.

10.4.2 Somatic Hypermutation

BcR diversity in uncommitted B cells arises through combinatorial usage of $\mathcal{V}(\mathcal{D})\mathcal{J}$ gene fragments to form functional H and L chains and through junctional diversity generated because of the imprecision of the joining process. Antigen-stimulated (selected) cells show further diversification as a result of somatic point mutations in their V regions. The frequency of such mutations is extraordinarily high. A mutation rate of 1×10^{-3} per base pair per generation is achieved. Since this rate is 10^3 times higher than spontaneous mutations, the process is referred to as hypermutation. This increase in affinity observed in latter phases of the primary response and especially in the secondary response is called affinity maturation and it can be directly correlated to a steady increase in the total number of mutations. Hypermutation seems to occur specifically on the rearranged V gene, independent of whether this gene is translated into a functional H or L chain or whether it is on the non-active chromosome. Even an unrelated sequence introduced on the V region undergoes hypermutation.

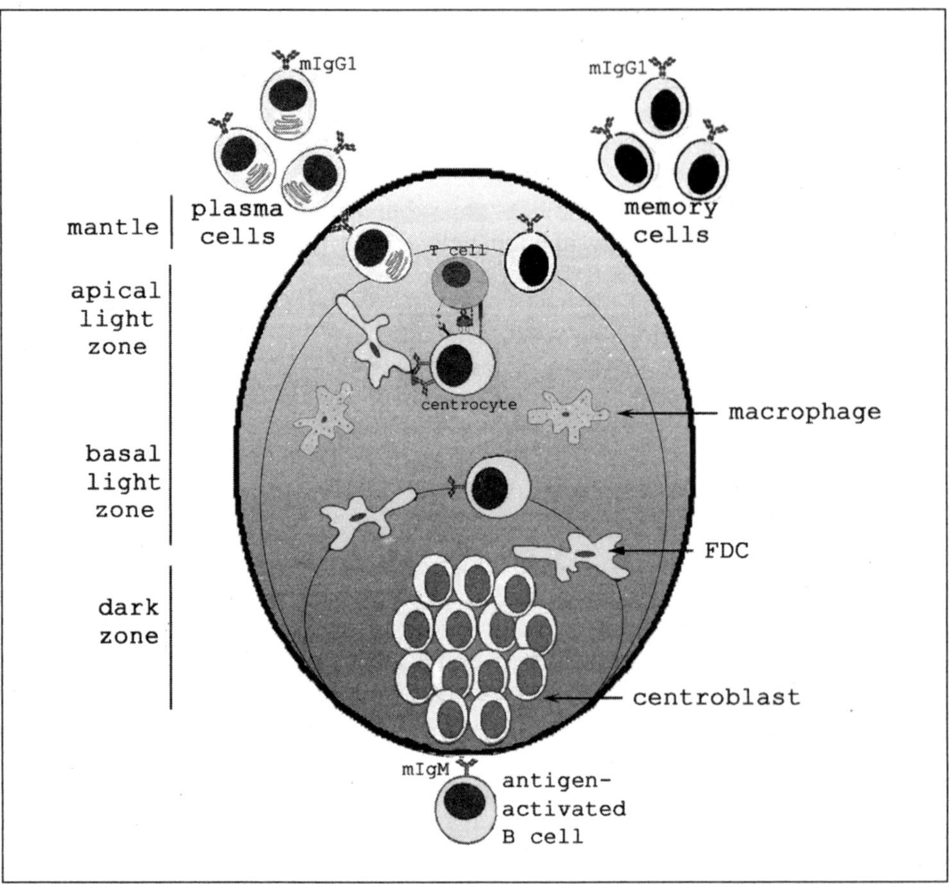

Figure 10.5 Germinal centres are the discrete lymphoid compartments where antigen-activated B cells divide, switch the isotype of Ig expressed, and differentiate. Germinal centres can be divided into three distinct zones — the dark zone, the light zone, and the mantle. Antigen-activated B cells enter the germinal centre and undergo proliferation in the dark zone. The rapidly proliferating cells do not express mIg and are called centroblasts. The centroblasts undergo hypermutation in their Ig V region genes and give rise to non-dividing centrocytes that express mIg and migrate to the light zone. The centrocytes have an apoptosis sensitive phenotype. They are rescued from apoptosis by signals delivered by FDCs. FDCs trap antigen-Ig complexes on their cell surface and are instrumental in selecting B cells with increased affinity for the antigen. FDCs deliver a survival signal to such B cells; the rest undergo apoptosis. Macrophages present in the light zone phagocytose the dead or dying cells. The centrocytes receiving survival signals migrate to the apical light zone. The migrating centrocytes internalize, process, and present the antigen to CD4+ T cells. This cognate interaction results in stimulating the B cells and promotes their clonal expansion, isotype switching, and differentiation to memory cells and plasmablasts. The differentiated cells eventually enter the follicular mantle and leave the germinal centre.

To understand how hypermutation increases affinity, it is necessary to look at antigen-antibody interaction at the molecular level. Complexes between proteinic antigens and homologous antibodies involve contacts between multiple amino acid residues on both the molecules. Multiple non-covalent bonds formed between these residues determine the strength of the reaction (Table 4.1). Bond formation is critically dependent on the distance between interacting groups. The closer the groups, the stronger the forces between them, and the higher the affinity of the antibody for that antigen. For example, in an antibody-hen egg lysozyme complex, 17 residues of the antibody interact with 16 residues of lysozyme. A change in a single amino acid at or around these residues may permit additional salt links, hydrogen bonds, etc, resulting in firmer binding. Obviously, a maturation system based on a process of random mutation is a game with few winners and many losers. Most point mutations

---

AFFINITY MATURATION

- ❏ Affinity maturation is the phenomenon of increase in affinity of the antibodies for their homologous antigen with respect to time. Thus, antibodies produced later in the immune response have a much greater affinity for the antigen than those produced earlier.
- ❏ Affinity Maturation
  - Is observed only for TD antigens,
  - Occurs in germinal centres, and
  - Is the result of hypermutation in the rearranged V gene.
- ❏ Hypermutation occurs during a small window in the proliferative stage of B cells in the germinal centre.
  - It occurs in a step-wise manner — brief bursts of high mutation rates interspersed with mutation free growth.
  - The process of hypermutation is non-random; the RGYW motif is the preferred target of the hypermutation machinery.
  - Most of the accumulated mutations are point mutations that alter antibody CDRs.
  - AID, an RNA-editing enzyme specific to germinal centre B cells, seems to be important in the process.

---

do not result in an increased affinity for the antigen; they may either result in a lowered affinity for the antigen, early termination of the protein chain, or recognition of self-antigens. Such B cells are the 'losers' and are eliminated by apoptosis. Only a few B cells will show an increased affinity for the challenging antigen and they are permitted to expand and differentiate. Selection thus has a major role in affinity maturation. A short burst of somatic hypermutation, followed by selection and clonal expansion, forms the basis of the maturation process.

Although the process of hypermutation has been recognized since the early 1960s, the actual mechanism is still unclear. The nature of the DNA breaks and the mutator enzyme(s) involved in the process are still being elucidated. The postulated mechanism of hypermutation is summarized below.

- ❏ The process of hypermutation is non-random, with distinct areas showing a high frequency of mutations (therefore called hotspots). Mutations seem to be confined to a region spanning about two kilo base pairs downstream of the Ig promoter region.
  - The frequency increases from 5′ to 3′ along the leader exon, peaks over the rearranged $\mathcal{V(D)J}$ exon, and decreases in the J-C intron of the Ig genes.
  - Majority of the mutations are point mutations, with transitions more frequent than transversions and A nucleotides in the coding strand being replaced twice as frequently as T nucleotides. Certain nucleotide motifs have been shown to be the preferred targets of the hypermutation machinery. These are the RGYW (where R – A or G, Y – C or T, W – A or T) or its complement, WRCY motifs. They were identified by establishing and analyzing a large database of somatically mutated Ig genes. The surrounding sequences seem to be important in deciding whether the RGYW motif becomes a substrate of the mutation machinery. These mutational properties probably reflect the specificities of the mutator enzyme(s).
- ❏ Somatic hypermutation seems to be dependent on transcription; whether transcription enables hypermutation because of the opening of chromatin or whether the mutator enzyme(s) physically interacts with components of the RNA-polymerase complex involved in transcription is not clear.
- ❏ Hypermutation of the targeted region appears to be under the direction of transcription-related elements, including the promoter and enhancer regions. Experimental data suggests that the transcriptional promoter determines the precise region that will mutate and specific enhancers allow mutations at particular loci.
- ❏ Analogous to $\mathcal{V(D)J}$ recombination and RAG proteins, a hypermutator is believed to start the process of somatic mutation and use pre-existing DNA repair and synthesis machinery to complete mutagenesis.

❑ The nature of the DNA lesion is not clear. Whether single- or double-stranded breaks precede hypermutation or are caused secondarily is still under debate.

❑ Like $\mathcal{V}(\mathcal{D})\mathcal{J}$ recombination, TdT is thought to have a role in somatic hypermutation.

❑ It is believed that one or more of a growing family of error-prone DNA polymerases are involved in the repair of the DNA lesion; this error-prone repair is thought to result in the high frequency of mutations (fig. 10.6).

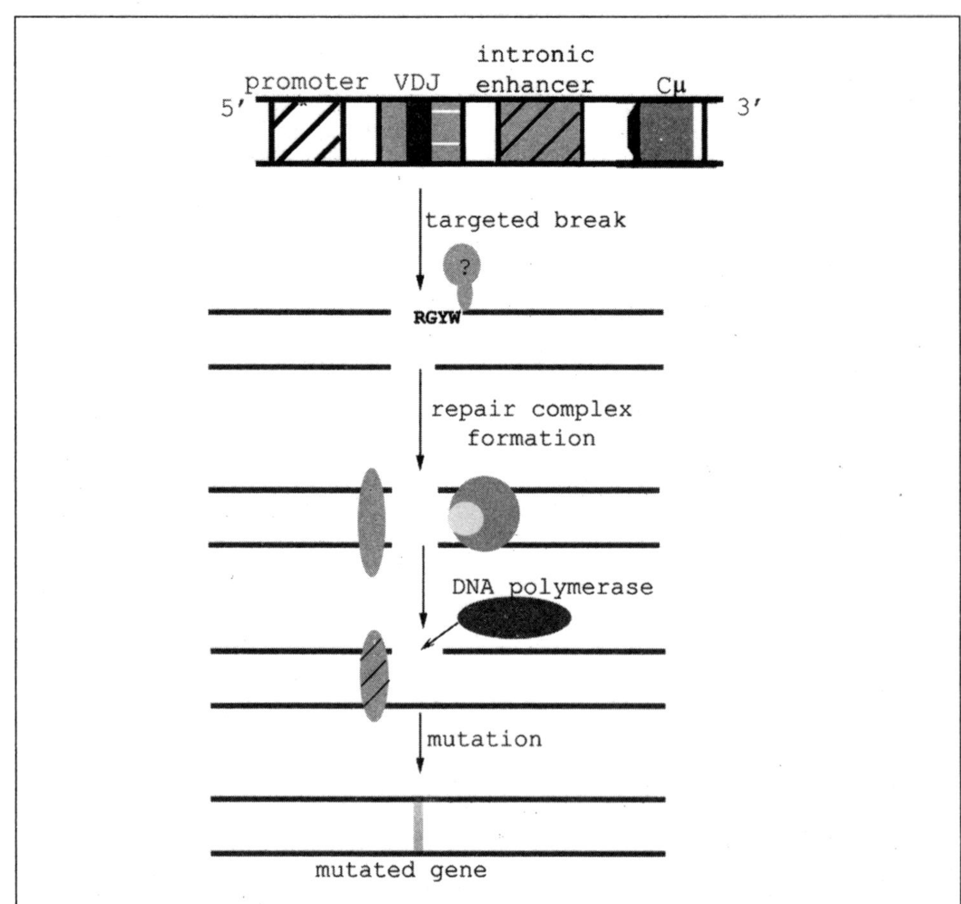

Figure 10.6 B cells activated by TD antigens undergo diversification of their antibody repertoire as a result of somatic hypermutation in their V region genes. *The figure depicts the proposed model of hypermutation. The uppermost panel is a schematic of Ig H chain genes of a B cell that has undergone VDJ recombination. Also shown are the promoter and enhancer regions that seem to permit hypermutation at particular loci and the preferred targets (RGYW nucleotide motif) of the hypermutation machinery. The putative mutator enzyme(s) (shown with a question mark) introduces a DNA lesion at the target motif, resulting in a double stranded break. A repair complex is formed at the site and leaves a gap in one strand that is filled in by error-prone DNA polymerases. This results in a mutated gene (grey box) upon strand replication. For simplicity, only the mutated strand is shown in the figure (Adapted from Nature Reviews in Immunology (2001) 1:187).*

❑ A newly discovered RNA-editing enzyme, AID (Activation-Induced cytosine Deaminase), specific to activated germinal centre B cells, is thought to be important in both CSR and hypermutation.

● Hypermutation is postulated to start as a result of the deamination of DNA by AID; such deamination converts cytosine in DNA to uracil.

● Replication of a mismatch causes uracil to be read as adenine, resulting in the addition of thymidine, ie, a transition of the deaminated strand.

● Alternatively, uracil glycosylases may remove uracil before replication, leaving a gap which may be filled during replication or via DNA repair pathways.

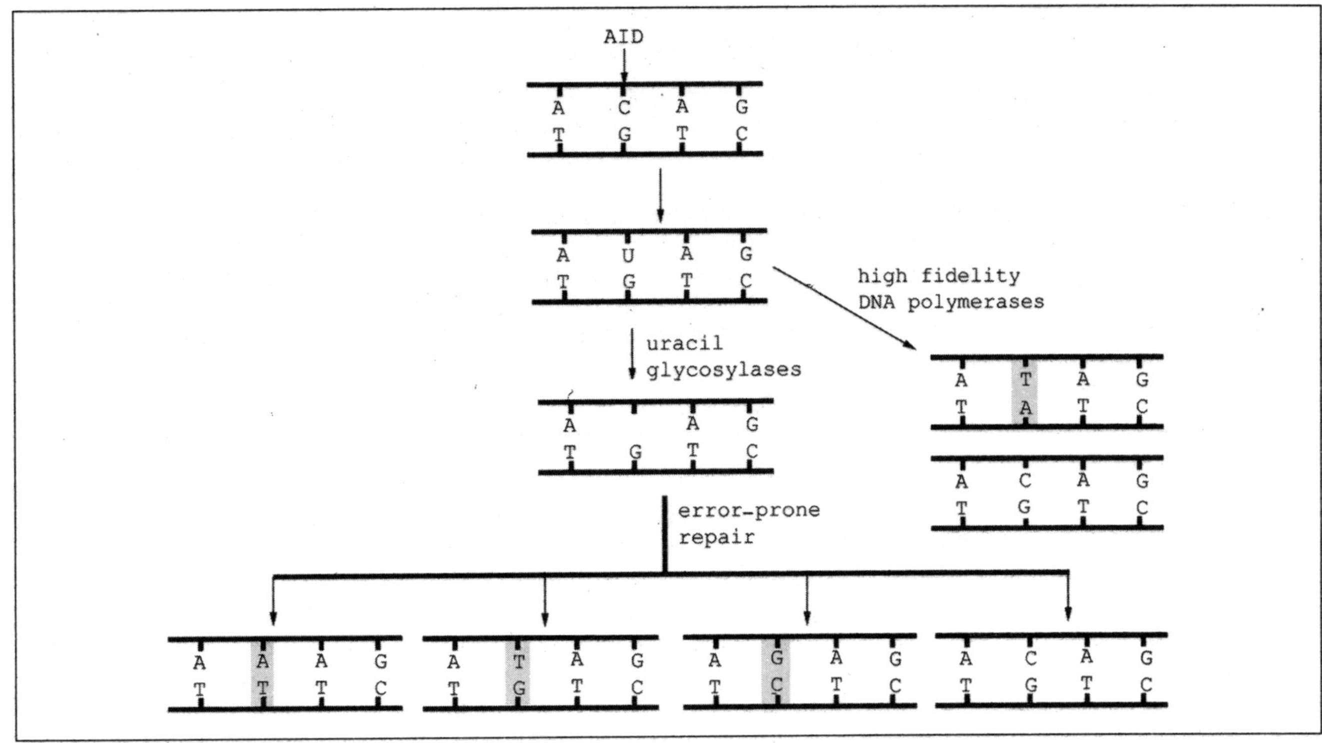

Figure 10.7 AID (Activation-Induced cytosine Deaminase), found in germinal centre B cells, is postulated to start hypermutation by deamination of DNA. *AID is thought to convert cytosines (C) in the rearranged V regions of Ig chains to uracil (U). High fidelity DNA polymerases read U as T (thymine) and pair it with A (adenine), resulting in a mutation (grey box). Removal of U by uracil glycolases leaves a gap at the site, and low fidelity polymerases fill the gaps more or less at random. For simplicity, only the mutated strand is shown in the low fidelity DNA repair (Adapted from Nature (2002), 419:29).*

Mutations have been postulated to occur when error-prone DNA polymerases (especially POLι) try to correct the error (fig. 10.7).

- Although many recent experiments support the role of AID in hypermutation, many questions remain unanswered. It is unclear how AID targets the rearranged V genes. Also unclear is how and why error-prone polymerases are involved in the DNA repair. DNA repair is usually carried out by the more accurate DNA polymerase β. Thus, factors that subvert DNA polymerase β usage and promote error-prone polymerase usage also need to be identified.

10.4.3 Class Switch Recombination

The murine Ig H locus consists of eight different C$_H$ genes located downstream of the $\mathcal{V}(\mathcal{D})\mathcal{J}$ locus. The *C*μ gene is located at the V$_H$ proximal end of the C$_H$ gene cluster; *C*α is at the distal end (fig. 10.8). Each C$_H$ gene (except that of *C*δ) is flanked at its 5′ by the Switch (S) region, a one to ten kilo base pairs repetitive region composed of tandem (ie, one behind the other) sequences with many palindromes. Although their exact primary sequences are not similar, all S regions contain G-rich pentameric sequences that are major repeat units of Sμ. These S regions are the sites of CSR. Since the *C*δ gene is not flanked by an S region, an isotype switch to IgD cannot occur. Instead, the entire $\mathcal{V}\mathcal{D}\mathcal{J}C$μ*C*δ region is transcribed into a long primary RNA transcript and then differentially spliced to yield $\mathcal{V}\mathcal{D}\mathcal{J}C$μ (ie, to code for IgM) or $\mathcal{V}\mathcal{D}\mathcal{J}C$δ (yielding IgD). The formation of this long primary transcript is feasible because of the proximity of *C*μ and *C*δ genes (only five Kb apart). This differential splicing results in naïve B lymphocytes expressing both mIgM and mIgD on their cell surfaces. Upon activation, naïve B cells initially produce the μ heavy chain and

---

CLASS SWITCH RECOMBINATION

❏ CSR allows the B cells to produce Igs with the same antigenic specificity but different isotypes.

❏ Isotype switching is feasible because the V region and C region of Ig molecule are encoded by different genes.
  - The murine (and human) Ig H locus consists of eight different C_H genes located downstream of the V(D)J locus.
  - The $C\mu$ gene is located at the V_H proximal end of the C_H gene cluster, whereas $C\alpha$ is at the distal end.

❏ S regions flank each C_H gene (except of $C\delta$) at its 5′ region.

❏ CSR occurs within two S regions, resulting in the looping out and deletion of intervening DNA segments as circular DNA.

❏ Transcription through the S region plays a primary role in targeting CSR; CSR is preceded by transcription of the two S regions undergoing CSR.

❏ Cytokines can influence the outcome of CSR.

---

hence IgM[8]. Activation also starts the process of CSR. CSR occurs within two S regions, resulting in the looping out and deletion of intervening DNA segments as circular DNA; the $\mathcal{V(D)J}$ exon is juxtaposed to a downstream C_H gene, allowing the generation of a different isotype. As shown in fig. 10.8, CSR between the $S\mu$ and $S\gamma_1$ region 5′ to the C_H gene brings the $C\gamma_1$ gene adjacent to the V_H exon, resulting in isotype switching to IgG1. Subsequent switching to other isotypes may occur at the recombinant switch region. Thus, CSR could result in direct isotype switching from IgM to IgE or sequential isotype switching — from IgM to IgG1 to IgE. CSR has been shown to generate two products — the rearranged chromosome and extrachromosomal circles containing the deleted intervening circles. Although CSR is a key process in humoral immunity and has been investigated for many years, the actual events and molecules mediating this process remain largely elusive. Enzymes involved in CSR have not been identified. It is not yet clear if there is a single CSR recombinase that recognizes all S regions or if multiple recombinases are involved. Additionally, the S region joining mechanisms are also largely unknown. The importance of AID in CSR is apparent from the fact that AID-deficient mice generated by gene-targeted mutations completely lack the ability to undergo CSR. Similarly, some hyper-IgM syndrome patients with impaired CSR have been shown to have mutations in the human gene encoding AID. The exact function of AID is however still speculative.

Based on the current knowledge, the molecular mechanism of CSR can be divided into four steps.

❏ **Selection of target S region.** Germline C_H genes are organized into germline transcription units in which transcription initiates from a promoter 5′ of the I exon[9], runs through the S region, and undergoes polyadenylation downstream of the C_H exon (fig. 10.8). A 3′ enhancer complex located 40 kilo base pairs downstream of the last C_H gene ($C\alpha$ in the case of the murine Ig H locus) can affect germline transcription and therefore CSR. RNA splicing generates a processed germline transcript by fusing the I exon to the C_H exons and deleting the intervening S region derived sequences. Gene-targeting studies have demonstrated the necessity of promoter integrity of the I exon for efficient CSR. Transcription through the S region plays a primary role in targeting CSR; CSR is preceded by transcription of the two S regions, starting from the I promoter located 5′ to each S region. Cytokines can influence CSR in multiple ways.

  - Cytokines influence the outcome of CSR. Thus, IL-4 is known to promote isotype switching to IgG1 and IgE in mice (IgG4 and IgE in humans). IFN-γ has been shown to promote isotype switching to IgG2b/IgG2a in mice and IgG1 in humans, whereas TGF-β induces germline transcripts and subsequent switching to IgA.

---

[8] Although most B cells do express IgM and then switch to a different isotype in the microenvironment of germinal centres, CSR can also occur outside germinal centres and, in the case of IgA, occur without prior expression of mIgM.

[9] Ig H μ gene, like other CSR-capable C_H genes, has Ig H Intronic enhancer — a two kilo base pairs DNA sequence that lies between the V region and the $S\mu$ region. Immediately downstream of the I enhancer lies the I exon that serves as a promoter of the $C\mu$ gene and regulates the transcription of the Ig H gene. This non-coding I exon is spliced onto the first exon of the C_H region being transcribed. Disruption of I promoter or I exons prevents CSR.

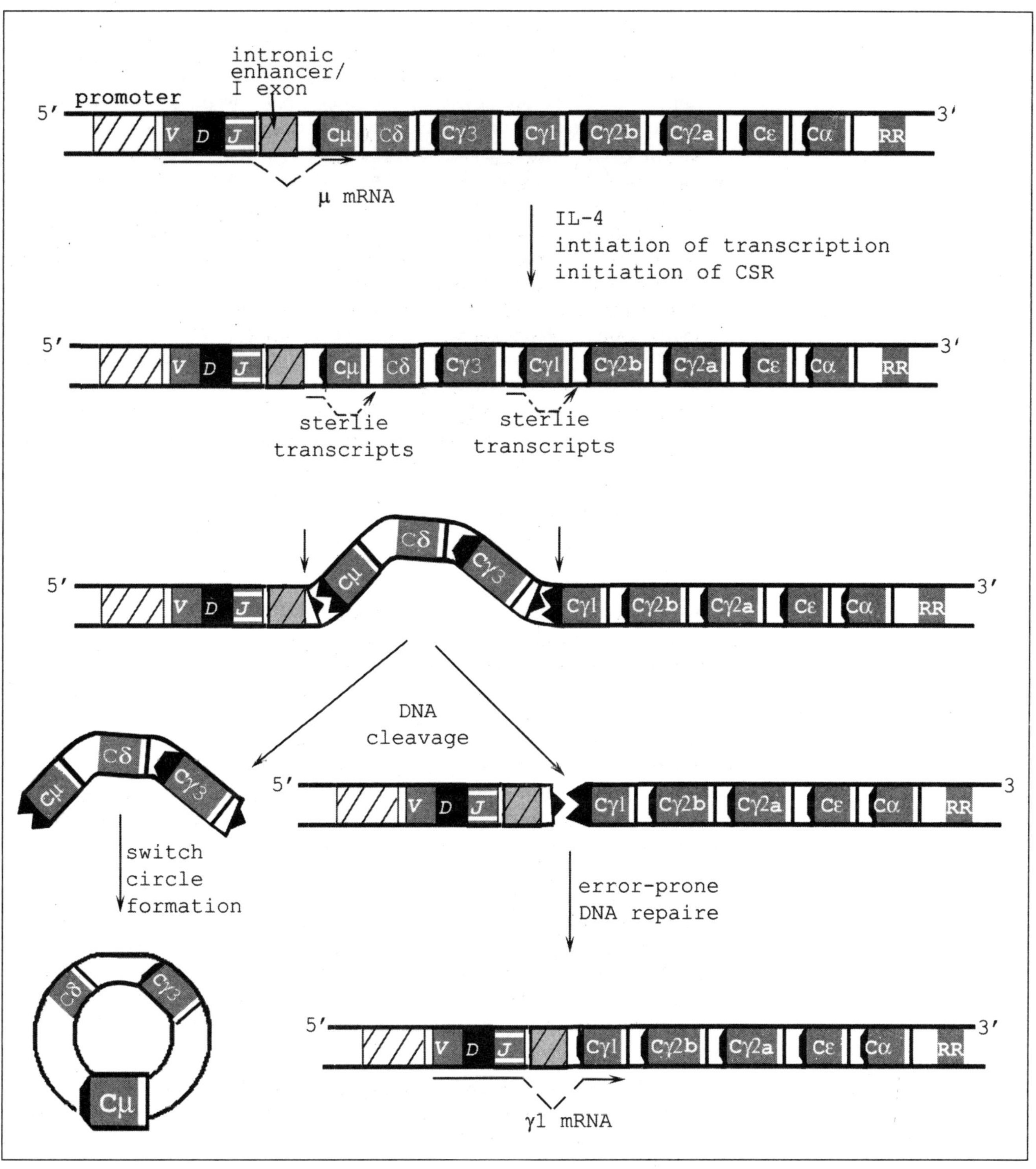

Figure 10.8 DNA recombination in the switch regions of the Ig CH genes allows isotype switching in antigen-activated B cells. *The figure depicts a simplified schematic of the germline murine Ig H chain on chromosome 12. Each CH gene (except that of Cδ) is flanked at its 5′ end by a Switch (S) region that is the site of CSR. Transcription is initiated from a promoter 5′ of the I exon, runs through the S region, and undergoes polyadenylation downstream of the CH exon. In the cells that have not switched their isotype, this yields a μ chain transcript. Downstream of the last CH gene (Cα) lies a Regulatory Region (RR) that can influence class switching. CSR is preceded by transcription of the two S regions and is influenced by cytokines such as IL-4. The putative recombinase enzyme introduces nicks in the two S regions, resulting in the looping out and deletion of intervening DNA segments as circular DNA. Error-prone repair enzymes then ligate the DNA so that the rearranged V region is juxtaposed to a new CH region (here Cγ1). For clarity, the switch regions and the intervening segments have been magnified.*

- One of the ways cytokines influence CSR is by the regulation of expression of germline transcripts. Segments of DNA located 5′ (or upstream) of the I exons contain promoters/enhancers which regulate transcription of germline transcripts. These promoters have elements responsive to cytokine-induced transcription factors and hence, cytokines influence the product of isotype switching by promoting the transcription of a particular S region.
- Docking of the cytokine to its receptor on the cell surface results in the induction of specific transcription factors (eg, NFκB induction by IL-4). These transcription factors promote the transcription of I region promoters, that is, the selection of target S regions among many is mediated by transcription from the particular I promoter of that S region.
- Four enhancer elements downstream of $C\alpha$ are thought to influence germline transcription of distal genes. Cytokines may influence CSR to a particular C_H gene by inducing its transcription and influencing interaction with the downstream enhancer elements.
- Cytokines accompanied by appropriate costimulatory signals (eg, via CD40-CD154 interaction) induce the production of sterile transcripts[10] from promoters that are upstream of the targeted switch regions. Although the exact function of these sterile transcripts is not known, transcription through the switch region is thought to be important for CSR. One possibility is that germline transcription and associated chromatin opening makes the Ig locus accessible to *trans*-acting factors, allowing the CSR recombinase machinery access to S regions, thereby initiating CSR.
- Cytokines also induce *de novo* synthesis of CSR recombinase or its activator.

❑ **Recognition of target sequence.** Experiments suggest that the primary S region structure is not important to CSR, but the palindromic nature of the S region primary sequence is. It is thought that such palindromic sequences can transiently form stem-loop structures when denatured during transcription. These stem-loop structures are proposed to be the recognition targets of CSR recombinase.

❑ **Cleavage by a putative recombinase.** It is well established that two double stranded cleavages occur in CSR. The exact mechanism of how and where these nicks are made is unclear. Experimental evidence supports the theory that two successive nicks are made in each S region, generating staggered double stranded cleavages. The NHEJ pathway may then process the single stranded tail of the staggered cleavage product.

❑ **Repair and ligation.** The enzymes involved in the ligation of the four DNA strands are yet to be established. Constituents of NHEJ pathway, viz., Ku complex and DNA-PKcs, have been shown to be involved in CSR but may not be the only mechanisms of DNA repair. Error-prone DNA polymerases may also play a role in the repair process and are thought to be responsible for the high frequency of mutations observed in CSR.

To summarize, $\mathcal{V(D)J}$ recombination along with hypermutation and CSR allows the use of a small number of genes to generate an open-ended repertoire. Thus, each individual inherits sketchy information — a broad game plan — which can be refined further as the need arises. The sketchy information is in the form of relatively few $\mathcal{V(D)J}$ genes from which an individual produces a comparatively large number of receptors by $\mathcal{V(D)J}$ recombination. The generated receptors recognize a range of epitopes with moderate to low affinity. If, in its lifetime, a particular B lymphocyte bearing a certain receptor does not come across its antigen, it never gets activated and never gets improved upon. However, upon antigen contact, somatic hypermutation further refines the receptor, thereby increasing its affinity for that antigen. CSR allows the same antigen to be attacked by different mechanisms, since it allows a new effector function to be endowed upon the receptor without altering its antigenic specificity. It is interesting to note that although TcR and BcR are

[10] Sterile transcripts are driven from I promoters located upstream of all S regions. They are believed not to encode proteins. Instead, they are thought to be spliced to form mature sterile transcripts that contain the C region exons and sequences upstream of the S region.

generated by similar mechanisms, TcR does not undergo somatic hypermutation. It is probable that further refinement of the T cell repertoire is likely to prove deleterious because of the high risk of self-reactivity and such mechanisms have therefore not evolved for TcR

Historical Perspective: Theories of Antibody Diversity

Two theories were proposed to explain antibody diversity. The first one was the **germline hypothesis**, which proposed that all the genes needed for generating the antibody repertoire are present in the fertilized ovum (ie, the germline) and, therefore, in every cell. These genes were postulated to arise during evolution through conventional mechanisms for gene duplication, mutation, and selection. Each antibody generating cell was thought to express only one set of V genes from the whole complement of V genes present in its germline. Thus, germline hypothesis claimed that selective gene expression determined the antibody-specificity of the lymphocyte (fig. 10.S2).

The second theory postulated that relatively few genes for the V locus were inherited. The V region of cells destined to be lymphocytes were proposed to mutate at a rate higher than the rest of the DNA (ie, the V region became a mutational hotspot) during development. It was called the **somatic mutation theory,** since non-germ cells were thought to generate the diversity. Thus, a small number of germline V genes became diversified through mutations in somatic cells, yielding a large number of clones of immunologically competent cells. It was further proposed that out of the number of clones generated by this process, only non-self reactive clones were allowed to survive, while self-reactive clones were deleted. The germline theory implies that antibody diversity was generated in a species over evolutionary time, whereas the somatic variation theory implies that antibody diversity is generated by individuals during their lifetime.

As is often the case in Science, both theories proved to be partially correct. The germline does contain a large repertoire of antibody genes. However, this repertoire is insufficient to encode for the actual repertoire of antibodies an individual is capable of producing. The antibody repertoire is increased through combinatorial and junctional diversity. It is only after antigen challenge that the antibody diversity is further increased by somatic mutations.

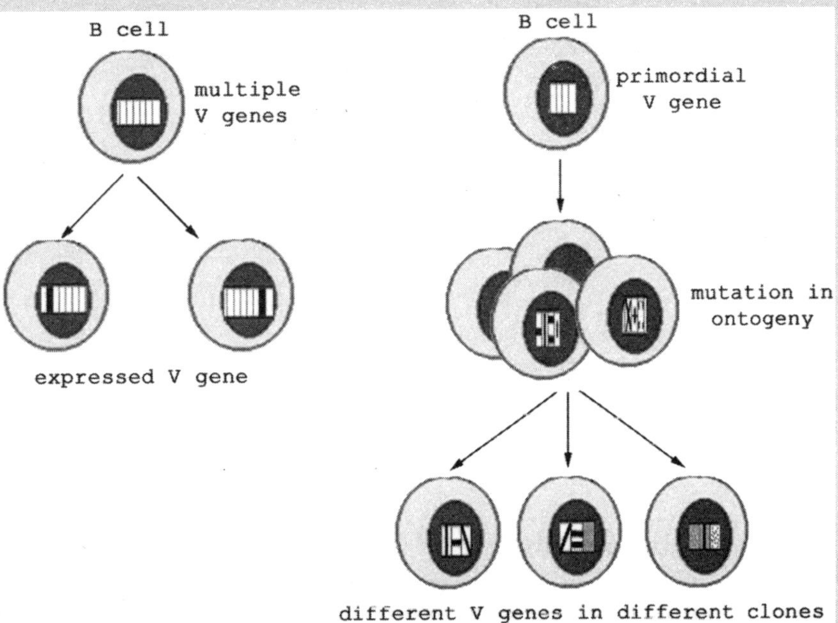

Figure 10.S2 The germline hypothesis proposed that selective expression of germline genes was responsible for antibody diversity (left panel), whereas the somatic mutation hypothesis suggested that primordial V region genes became mutational hotspots during development and resulted in each B cell having a different version of the genes, thus giving rise to a diverse antibody repertoire.

11 Cell-mediated Immunity

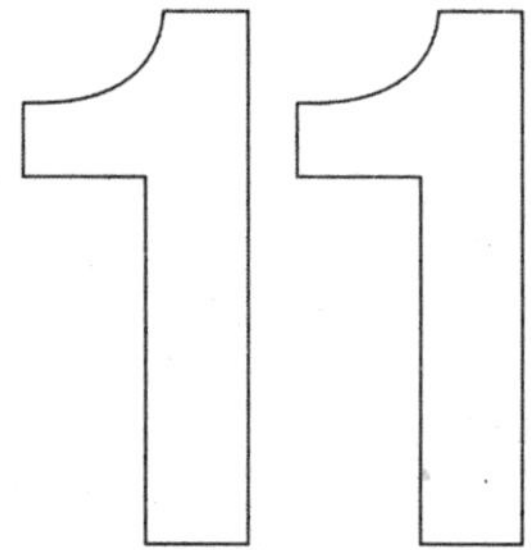

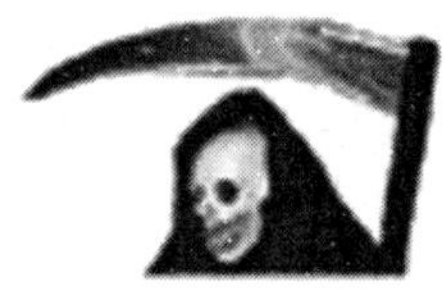

Goldeneye, I found his weakness
Goldeneye, he'll do what I please
Goldeneye, no time for sweetness
But a bitter kiss will bring him to his knees

— Tina Turner, *Golden Eye*

11.1 Introduction

The term **cell-mediated immunity (CMI) is** used for **an immune response in which cells are the 'effectors' of immunity and antibodies have only a minor role** (if at all). It is the most primitive form of immunity; CMI evolved before humoral responses. Effectors of CMI are involved in the elimination of foreign cells and infected or altered self-cells. Both, adaptive and innate arms of immunity are involved in CMI (Table 11.1) and include:

❑ CTLs and NK cells involved in the elimination of virus-infected and neoplastic cells,

❑ Macrophages and neutrophils that are important in the destruction of bacteria, viruses, and other intracellular pathogens, and

❑ Eosinophils, mast cells, and basophils engaged in the destruction of helminths.

❑ **CTLs.** As explained in section 8.3.5.2, CTLs are MHC class I restricted CD8$^+$ T cells that represent the cytotoxic arm of adaptive immunity. Like humoral responses, secondary CMI responses mediated by CTLs and aided by CD4$^+$ T cells, are more rapid and aggressive than the primary immune responses. These rapid CTL responses (in conjunction with the Ig response) help control and/or fully eliminate intracellular pathogens. As is the case with all secondary adaptive responses, the swift secondary response is partly a consequence of the clonal expansion of antigen-specific CD4$^+$ and CD8$^+$ T cells and partly due to reprogramming of the gene-expression profile that differentiating CD8$^+$ T cells undergo during the primary encounter. As a result of clonal expansion, the sheer number of CTLs capable of responding to the pathogen increases. Furthermore, genes encoding IFN-γ and cytotoxic molecules such as perforin and granzyme B, that are not expressed in naïve CD8$^+$ T cells, get constitutively expressed in effector and memory CD8$^+$ T cells. Although the synthesis of these proteins occurs only on antigen contact, elevated levels of mRNA endow memory CD8$^+$ T cells with the capacity to produce larger quantities of these proteins more rapidly than naïve T cells. Additionally, memory CD8$^+$ T cells (once again, like their CD4$^+$ counterparts) express a different pattern of surface proteins involved in cell adhesion and chemotaxis than their primary counterparts. These surface proteins allow them to extravasate into non-lymphoid tissues and mucosal sites. Lastly, the number of memory CD8$^+$ T cells is maintained for a long time because of homeostatic cell proliferation which occurs at a slow yet steady pace. IL-2, IL-7, and especially IL-15 are thought to have a role in this slow proliferation.

❑ **NK and related cells.** NK cells are large granular lymphocytes comprising between 5–15% of peripheral blood lymphocytes. They are also found in peripheral tissues such as the liver, peritoneal cavity, and even the placenta. Resting NK cells circulate in the blood. Following activation by cytokines, they are capable of extravasation and infiltration into tissues that contain malignant or pathogen-infected cells. They are a vital component of innate immunity that mediates the killing of tumour cells or virus-infected cells. They are discussed in some detail in chapter 2. IL-2 has been shown to enhance the cytotoxic activity of NK cells. IL-2-activated NK cells, called LAK cells, are used in cancer immunotherapy. The morphologically similar K cells are considered a subset of NK cells. They express FcγRIII (the low affinity receptor for IgG; CD16) and, in some instances, FcμR (receptor for IgM). These cells are effectors of ADCC.

❑ **Phagocytic cells.** Forming a link between specific and non-specific immunity, the phagocytic cells are one of the most important watchdogs of the body and have been extensively discussed in chapter 2. They have a central role in innate, humoral, and cell-mediated immunity (Table 11.2).

Macrophages and neutrophils are normally quiescent cells responsible for the removal of tissue debris and dead or dying cells. Phagocytes express a broad spectrum of receptors such as those for complement components, integrins, scavenger receptors, PRRs, etc as described in chapter 2. Contact of microbes or their products with these receptors triggers signalling processes that result in the mobilization of the phagocytic membrane and reorganization of the actin cytoskeleton. As a consequence, the microbe is internalized and eventually digested in specialized structures called phagolysosomes. Concurrent exposure to IFN-γ (produced by NK cells or T cells) and/or contact with pathogen-derived molecules leads to the activation of the phagocytic cells. Activated phagocytes have an increased number of lysosomes and secrete enzymes and cytokines that contribute to inflammation. The activated cells also show increased production of microbicidal molecules such as superoxide anion, H_2O_2, RNI, etc (Table 2.2) and are efficient effectors of CMI. They are also important in inflammatory and DTH responses. Their expression of FcRs also makes them effectors of ADCC.

Eosinophils, basophils, and mast cells produce several pharmacologically active substances that are effective in killing large parasites that cannot be phagocytosed (chapter 2). Additionally, mast cells have been shown to phagocytose microbes bound to their cell surface via complement receptors and FcγRs. All the three cell types express FcϵRs. Cross-linking of FcϵR bound IgE by a multivalent parasite leads to the degranulation of these cells. Thus, these cells can also participate in ADCC.

11.2 Mechanisms of Cell-Mediated Cytotoxicity

Cytotoxic cells employ two death-inducing strategies to bring about contact-dependent death of the target cells — Ca^{2+} dependent exocytosis of cytotoxic granules and engagement of death-receptors. The first pathway seems to be predominant in NK cells and $CD8^+$ T cells, whereas the second seems to be of special importance for T$_{H1}$ effector cells. The cytotoxic granules of CTLs and NK cells are complex organelles that combine specialized storage and secretory functions with the degradative functions of a typical lysosome. FcR expressing effector cells with a cytotoxic potential such as macrophages, neutrophils, eosinophils, mast cells, basophils, and K cells induce death by a different mechanism — by ADCC. Effectors of CMI also produce a variety of cytokines such as TNFs and IFN-γ, which, when secreted in the vicinity of target cells, have cytotoxic action but are not discussed here.

11.2.1 Perforin and Granzyme Pathway

Perforin/granzyme-mediated apoptosis is the principal pathway used by NK cells and CTLs to eliminate target cells. Granules containing these cytolytic molecules are formed during NK cell development and thus are present in mature NK cells. CTLs, by contrast, synthesize cytotoxic granules and their contents within a day of T cell activation, ie, only effector CTLs have cytotoxic vesicles. The granules reside in the cytoplasm of the cells. Signals generated by the engagement of appropriate receptors and costimulatory molecules cause the granules to migrate to the site of contact. At the cell surface, the granules fuse with the cell membrane and their contents are secreted into the tight intracellular junction (called immunological synapse[1]) formed between the two cells. Cytotoxic granules of NK cell and CTLs contain several toxic constituents.

❏ **Perforin.** Similar to complement component C9, perforin is a pore-forming, membrane-disrupting protein. It was originally thought to be the chief architect of CTL/NK cell-mediated cell death. Upon its release from granules, perforin rapidly polymerizes in the presence of Ca^{2+} to form a ring-like structure with a central pore which gets inserted into the target cell membrane. It is now recognized

[1] The immunological synapse is a distinct region formed at the contact zone between the cytotoxic lymphocyte and target cell because of the specific reorganization of cell-surface membrane proteins.

Table 11.1 Comparison of CMI and humoral responses

Characteristic	CMI	Humoral response
Effector cells	– CTLs – NK cells – Phagocytic cells such as macrophages, neutrophils, eosinophils, mast cells, etc	– B cells
Mechanism of action	– Non-specific effector molecules released in the immunological synapse bring about death of the target cell. They include cytotoxic molecules such as perforin and granzymes released by CTLs and NK cells, pharmacologically active mediators released by eosinophils and mast cells, and microbicidal products such as ROI, RNI, etc produced by macrophages and neutrophils – Induction of apoptotic pathways by CTLs and CD4$^+$ T cells	– Antibody molecules recognize and bind specifically to epitopes on antigens and result in • neutralization of viruses, enzymes, and toxins, • opsonization of the antigens, • complement activation, • ADCC, and • release of pharmacological mediators of eosinophils, mast cells, basophils, etc
Recognition system	– Innate and adaptive immune recognition molecules involved in CMI	– BcR expressed on B lymphocytes
Time of manifestation	– NK cells act within minutes of activation – CTLs usually take between 24–72 hours following secondary antigenic challenge to exert their effects – ADCC can be manifested within seconds to minutes of secondary antigenic challenge	– The response may occur within seconds to minutes of secondary antigenic challenge
Role of CD4$^+$ T cells	– They help in augmenting CD8$^+$ T cell responses – Some CD4$^+$ T cells can contribute to CMI directly via the death receptor pathway	– Cognate interaction with helper CD4$^+$ T cells is indispensable for humoral responses to TD antigens – Cytokines produced by CD4$^+$ T cells augment the humoral response to TI type 2 antigens – CD4$^+$ T cells are not required for humoral responses to TI type 1 antigens

that perforin induced cell damage by itself is not sufficient to cause apoptosis of cells, and it is suggested that it may act as a portal of entry for other cytotoxic molecules like granzymes that cause cell death. The importance of perforin in lymphocyte-mediated cytotoxicity is clear from studies in KO mice. Such mice show a deficiency in all aspects of granular killing. The exact role of perforin in causing cellular death is not clear, and its functions remain a contentious issue. Perforin is rapidly inactivated in the presence of high lipid concentrations and Ca^{2+}, and the presence of either of these factors in the immunological synapse helps cells escape from perforin-inflicted damage.

❑ **Granzymes.** These are a spectrum of serine proteases found in their active processed form in the cytotoxic granules. Out of a total of 11 reported so far, four are found in humans. The mechanism by which granzymes enter a cell is not very clear. The older model postulating that granzymes enter target cell via perforin pores is increasingly being questioned. Recent experiments seem to suggest that at least some granzymes may enter the cell via specific receptors. Perforin and granzymes are thought to act co-operatively in bringing about target cell apoptosis (fig. 11.1). Granzyme B, which cleaves target cell proteins at specific aspartate residues, is the most potent activator of apoptosis. It can cleave procaspases-3 and -8 to release the active form and thus initiate target cell death. It is also thought to activate pro-apoptotic members of the Bcl-2 family, such as Bid, which results in the leakage of pro-apoptotic mediators (eg, cytochrome c) into the cytosol.

Granzyme B is also thought to be involved in DNA fragmentation — the hallmark of apoptosis. Granzyme A, by contrast, is a tryptic protease that does not activate caspases but kills cells by the direct cleavage of nuclear proteins, facilitating the formation and accumulation of single stranded DNA breaks. The role of the other two human granzymes — Granzyme H and K — is still being elucidated. Granzyme K is reported to cause cell death in the presence of perforin, whereas granzyme H has been shown to have chemotrypsin-like activity. Since granzymes and perforin are released in the immunological synapse, the cytotoxic cells must have some protective mechanisms in place to avoid being killed by the toxins they release. CTLs and NK cells are thought to avoid suicide via granzyme B by expressing the inhibitor PI-9 (**P**rotein **I**nhibitor-**9**) in their cytoplasm and nucleus. A similar inhibitor for granzyme A has not yet been reported. Antithrombin A and α-2 macroglobulin have been shown to interact stably with granzyme A, neutralizing the enzyme. Their role in cell protection is still under investigation. Protection is also afforded by cathepsin B present in the granules (see below).

❑ **Other constituents** of cytotoxic granules include:

- **Several glycosaminoglycan complexes including a proteoglycan serglycin.** Serglycin is thought to act as a scaffold for the packaging of highly positively charged granzymes, and it may also act as a chaperone for secreted proteases. The recent discovery of macromolecular complexes of serglysin, perforin, and granzymes that bind to target cell surfaces has led to the suggestion that the toxic complexes get internalized by target cells via receptor-mediated endocytosis. The internalized perforin and granzymes then cause the death of the target cell.
- **Calreticulin** is a chaperone molecule that is a normal ER resident. It is thought to act as a regulatory molecule that dampens the effect of perforin.
- **FasL** is the ligand for CD95 or Fas. Its importance in causing apoptosis of the target cell is unclear.

Table 11.2 Macrophage cytokines and immune responses

Cytokine	*Effects*
TNF-α	– Multipotent cytokine – Increases respiratory burst and RNI production – Increases expression of adhesion molecules – Increases expression of FcRs on macrophages – Induces IFN-γ release from NK cells – Causes acute phase reaction and shock in conjunction with IL-1 and IL-6
IL-1	– Activates NK cells, macrophages, and neutrophils – Induces IL-2R expression and IL-2 synthesis in T cells – Aids in B cell differentiation
IL-6	– Causes release of acute phase proteins by hepatocytes – Aids in B cell differentiation
IL-8	– Causes chemotaxis of neutrophils and T cells
IL-10	– Promotes T$_{H2}$ responses – Suppresses macrophage function
IL-12	– Promotes T$_{H1}$ pathways – Induces IFN-γ release by NK cells
IFN-α and -β	– Have antiviral effects; important in CMI – Increase MHC class I expression on cells in vicinity
CSFs (Colony Stimulating Factors)	– Promote growth of granulocytes (G-CSF), monocytes (M-CSF), and granulocyte/monocytes precursors (GM-CSF) – GM-CSF promotes differentiation of monocytes to DCs

- **Granulysin** is synthesized by human CTLs during their activation. It has potent antimicrobial activity against many extracellular pathogens, including bacteria, fungi, and parasites. A combination of perforin and granulysin has been shown to be effective against intracellular *M. tuberculosis* as well. Granulysin can cause target cell membrane damage and induce apoptosis by causing mitochondrial polarization and release of cytochrome *c*. It also activates caspase-3, a key enzyme involved in apoptosis.
- **Cathepsin B**, unlike other constituents of the cytotoxic granules, is an enzyme involved in the protection of the effector cells. It gets sequestered on the effector cell membrane after degranulation and can inactivate perforin molecules that diffuse back to the effector cell.

11.2.2 The Death Receptor-Ligand Pathway

The induction of death in unwanted cells is essential for the normal development and functioning of a multicellular organism. As explained in chapter 8, death pathways are based on protein-protein interaction domains that lead to the activation of a cascade of proteases. These proteases, called caspases[2], have a cysteine residue in the active site and specificity for cleavage at the aspartic residues. Proteins such as FLIP (FLICE-Inhibiting Protein) or **I**nhibitors of **Ap**optosis (IAPs) can modulate the activation of caspases and protect the cell. Two different pathways can induce cell death in vertebrates.

❑ **The intrinsic pathway of cell death** is triggered by loss of tropic receptor stimulation (for example, through the withdrawal of growth factors), DNA damage (eg, because of irradiation), inappropriate loss of contact with neighbouring cells, or contact with glucocorticoids. This evolutionarily conserved pathway ensures the appropriate development of organs and the elimination of cells that have developed abnormally or with genetic errors. This pathway is also called the mitochondrial pathway of apoptosis. Bcl-2 related proteins are implicated in this pathway. These proteins have either anti-apoptotic or pro-apoptotic activities and fall in three different classes. The first class consists of anti-apoptotic proteins such as Bcl-2 and Bcl-xL, the second and third group is pro-apoptotic. Bax, Bad, and Bak belong to the second group; the third group consists of proteins like Bid and Bik. Triggering of the intrinsic pathway leads to the activation of pro-apoptotic members of the Bcl-2 family. Pro-apoptotic Bcl-2 family proteins cause the

[2] The name caspase is derived from c (for cysteine), asp (for aspartate) and ase (signifying enzymes).

CELL-MEDIATED IMMUNITY

❑ It is the immunity mediated by non-Ig secreting, cytolytic cells.

❑ CMI cannot be transferred passively by transferring serum.

❑ Effectors of CMI include CTLs, NK cells, K cells, macrophages, neutrophils, eosinophils, basophils, and mast cells.

- CTLs are MHC class I restricted CD8$^+$ T cells that kill target cells by releasing cytotoxins such as perforin, granzymes, serglycin, granulysin, etc. They can also cause cell death by inducing apoptosis in target cells.
- NK cells are a part of the innate immune mechanism that nonetheless kill by mechanisms similar to CTLs. K cells, a subset of NK cells expressing FcγRIII, can also bring about ADCC.
- Macrophages and neutrophils kill the target cell by secreting a number of microbicidal molecules such as peroxides, superoxide anions, and RNI. They are also effectors of ADCC.
- Eosinophils, basophils, and mast cells synthesize and store a large number of pharmacologically active substances that are effective in killing large, extracellular parasites. These cells can also participate in ADCC.

❑ CMI is important in defence against virally transformed cells, helminths, intracellular parasites, and tumour cells.

Table 11.3 NK cells and CTLs in CMI

Characteristic	NK cells	CTLs
Target range	Effective against tumour cells and virus-infected cells	Effective against tumour cells, virus-infected cells, and cells harbouring intra-cellular pathogens
Target recognition	Specific antigen recognition or MHC restriction is absent; a balance of activatory and inhibitory signals determines the fate of the target cell • Recognition of peptide:MHC class I complexes on target cells by KIR and NKG2 receptors on NK cells produces an inhibitory signal and allows target cell to escape death • Engagement of NCRs (or other receptors associated with adaptor molecules with ITAMs) gives an activatory signal • Recognition of antigenic epitopes by FcγRIII-bound IgG activates K cells	Specific recognition of pathogen derived peptides:MHC class I complexes occurs because of TcRs
Nature of responses	Effectors of the innate immunity Activation does not lead to proliferation; memory responses absent	Effectors of adaptive immunity Activation leads to proliferation and differentiation of cells; secondary responses are rapid and more aggressive than primary responses
Mechanism of killing	Exocytosis of granules containing perforin and granzymes Induction of apoptotic pathways Granules exist preformed during NK development, so killing can occur within minutes of activation Can take part in multiple rounds of killing; the cells re-arm themselves in response to IL-2 before engaging new targets	In addition to perforin and granzymes, cytotoxic granules also contain granulysin — a potent antimicrobial protein that can cause apoptosis of target cells Induction of apoptotic pathways Naïve CD8$^+$ T cells have no cytolytic activity; they must undergo differentiation to effector CTLs — a process that takes up to three days for maximal activity Can kill multiple cells by re-orienting their granules to another region of contact
Cytokines	IFN-γ is the major cytokine produced	Two broad types of CTLs are recognized on the basis of their cytokine profiles • Type 1 produce IFN-γ • Type 2 produce IL-4 and IL-10

mitochondria to swell, leak, and release cytochrome *c*. An apoptosome containing cytochrome *c*, procaspase-9, and other proteins is formed. Formation of the apoptosome activates procaspase-9 and yields caspase-9, which recruits other members of the caspase family, including caspase-3 (fig. 11.2). Activated caspase-3 then cleaves an inhibitor molecule tightly associated with the nuclease CAD (**C**aspase-**A**ssociated **D**NAase). Freed from the inhibitor molecule, CAD initiates DNA fragmentation and cell death. Anti-apoptotic Bcl-2 proteins bind to the mitochondrial membrane, blocking the swelling and hence the release of cytochrome *c*.

❑ **The Fas-FasL mediated death pathway** is thought to be unique to vertebrates. This pathway is initiated by the engagement of the Fas receptor (a member of the TNF family of receptors) expressed on target cells by its ligand (FasL). FasL is a

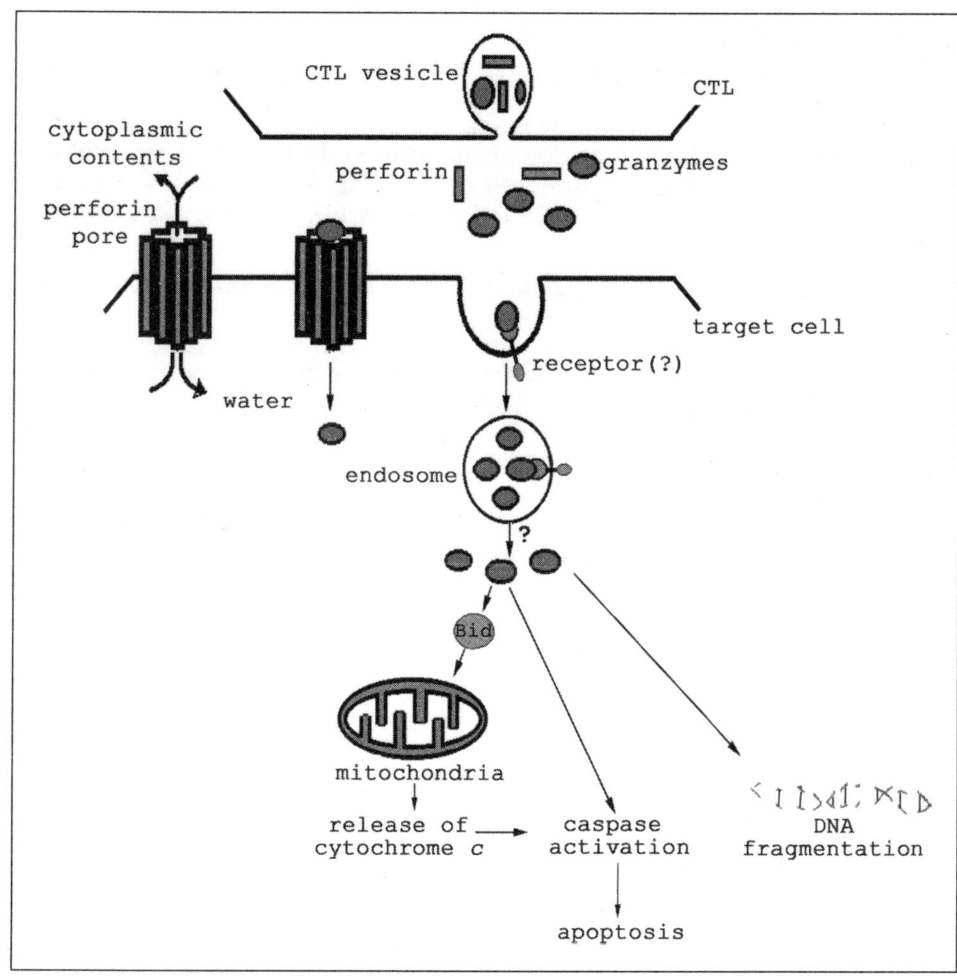

Figure 11.1 Perforin and granzymes released by CTLs and NK cells kill the target cell by activating their apoptotic pathways. Cytotoxic vesicles containing perforin and granzymes reside in the cytoplasm of the NK cells and activated CTLs, and they migrate to the site of contact upon appropriate stimulus. The vesicles eventually fuse with the cell membrane and release their contents into the tight intracellular junction formed between the two cells. The released perforin rapidly polymerizes to form a ring-like structure with a central pore and gets inserted into the target cell membrane, causing the efflux of cytoplasmic contents and an influx of water. How granzymes enter the target cell is not very clear. It has been suggested that they may enter via the perforin pore or, alternatively, undergo receptor-mediated endocytosis. The nature of the receptor and the mode of release from the endosomes are not known (denoted by question marks). Granzymes can activate the caspase pathway directly or activate the pro-apoptotic protein Bid. Activation of Bid results in the leakage of cytochrome c from the mitochondria which in turn causes caspase activation. Granzymes can also directly participate in fragmentation of nuclear proteins or DNA.

membrane-associated ligand synthesized within several hours of cytotoxic lymphocyte activation. Interaction of FasL expressed on CTL/NK surface with Fas receptors on target cells results in the aggregation of its intracellular death domain and recruitment of FADD (**F**as-**A**ssociated **D**eath **D**omain). FADD and procaspase-8 form a **D**eath-**I**nducing **S**ignalling **C**omplex — DISC. In DISC, FADD and Fas interact to activate procaspase-8. Activated caspase-8 activates additional downstream caspases, eventually leading to the activation of procaspase-3. Once caspase-3 is activated, the extrinsic and intrinsic pathways merge. Although Fas-mediated cell death is the most important pathway of inducing apoptosis by the extrinsic pathway, experimental evidence suggests that cytotoxic

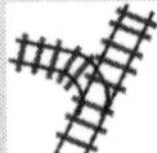

Evading the Death Penalty: Viral Evasion of Cytotoxic Lymphocyte Mediated Apoptosis

Detection and elimination of pathogen-infected cells is perhaps the most important function of CMI. One obvious strategy to avoid death by CTLs is the downregulation of MHC class I molecules of the infected cell. However, this strategy makes the infected cell susceptible to NK cell attack. Hence, viruses use other strategies to evade/survive CMI. These strategies are now being investigated for their therapeutic potential.

❑ The cowpox virus and the baculo virus encode caspase inhibitors that block caspase activity and allow survival of infected cells.
❑ A large number of viruses encode functional Bcl-2-like proteins that allow them to evade intrinsic death pathways. M1 1L from the myxoma virus and UL37 from human cytomegalovirus inhibit apoptosis by blocking the release of cytochrome *c* from the mitochondria.
❑ Adenovirus protein L4-100K directly inhibits granzyme B.

lymphocytes can also induce cell death via TRAIL (TNF-Related Apoptosis-Inducing Ligand) and TNF-R (see sidetrack 'A BAFFling, RANK-Ling TRAIL' in chapter 8). The relative roles of these different pathways in maintaining homeostasis, cancer prevention, autoimmune diseases, and transplantation immunology are still under investigation.

11.2.3 ADCC

Effector cells with cytotoxic potential and expressing FcRs can bring about ADCC. ADCC is most studied in NK cells, but several morphologically and developmentally distinctive cell types have been shown to be capable of ADCC. These include macrophages, PMNs, eosinophils, and mast cells. ADCC is dependent upon the presence of appropriate antibodies but is independent of complement and phagocytosis. The exact mechanism of the process is poorly understood.

❑ **K cells** expressing CD16 (FcγRIII) are capable of ADCC. IgG-antigen complexes bind to CD16 expressed on K cells. Ligation of multiple FcγRIIIs activates the K cell and results in target cell destruction. ADCC is thought to be the dominant component of antibody-mediated anti-tumour activity.
❑ **Eosinophils and mast cells** (and possibly basophils) use ADCC to kill parasites that are too large to be phagocytosed. When IgE antibodies combine with the epitopes on the cuticle of the worm, their Fc portions protrude from this surface and bind to FcεRI expressed by eosinophils or mast cells. Ligation of multiple FcεRI activates the cells. The activated cells flatten out along the cuticle to form a large attachment zone and spill their cytoplasmic granules into the intervening space by exocytosis. Collectively, these granules help destroy helminths and their larval forms. Recent research indicates that eosinophils express FcαR and IgA may therefore have a role in eosinphilic ADCC.
❑ **Neutrophils** have been shown to lyse tumour cells without phagocytosis *in vitro*. They appear to kill these cells via the release of cytotoxic granules, but their role in ADCC *in vivo* is still under investigation.

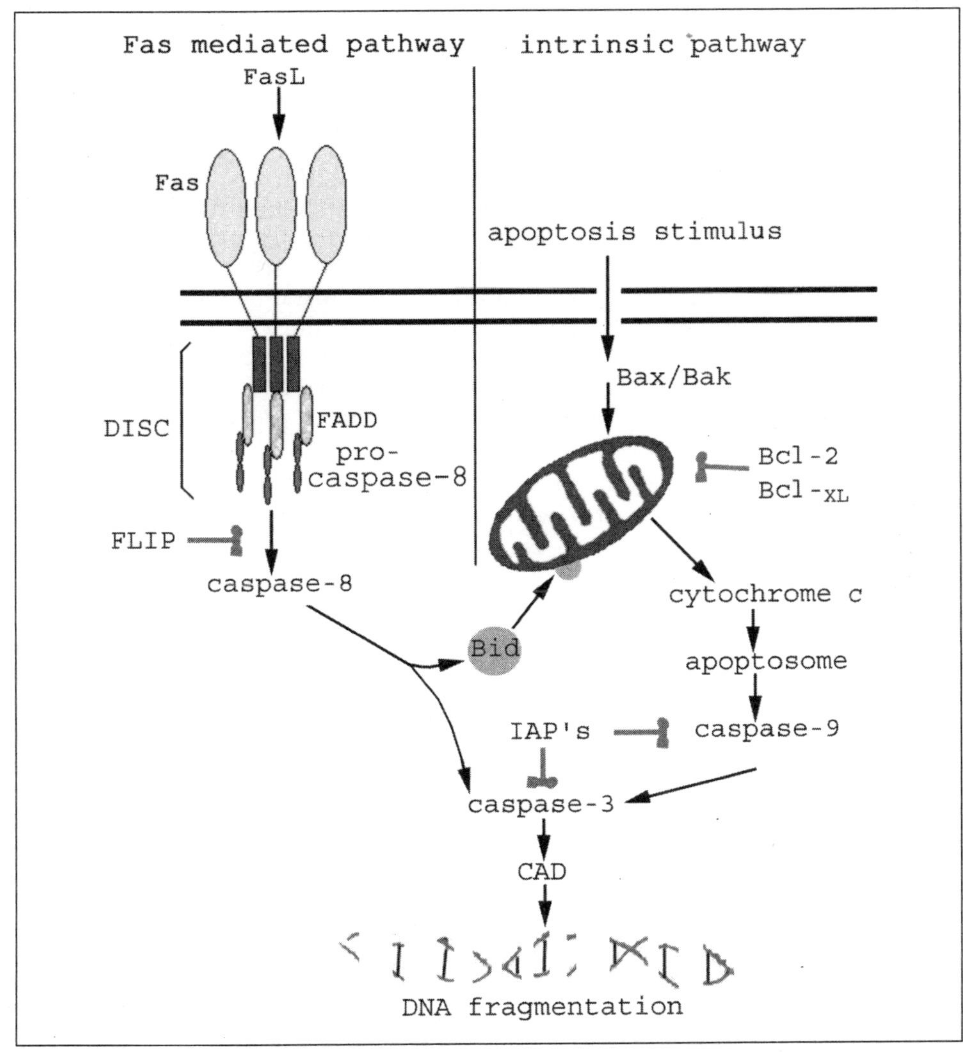

Figure 11.2 Two different pathways can induce cell death by apoptosis — the Fas-mediated or extrinsic pathway and the mitochondrial or intrinsic pathway. *The Fas-mediated pathway is triggered by the engagement of Fas via its ligand (FasL). Engagement of Fas causes the intracellular aggregation of FADD (Fas-Associated Death Domain). FADD associates with procaspase-8 to form the Death-Inducing Signalling Complex, or DISC. The interaction of FADD and Fas activates procaspase-8 and cleaves it to caspase-8. This activation is inhibited by the protein FLIP. Caspase-8 activates a cascade of downstream caspases that results in the activation of caspase-3. Activation of caspase-3 irreversibly commits the cell to undergo apoptosis. Activated caspase-3 cleaves an inhibitor molecule tightly associated with the nuclease CAD (Caspase-Associated DNAase). CAD initiates DNA fragmentation. Caspase-8 also activates the pro-apoptotic protein Bid. Bid causes the mitochondria to swell, leak, and release cytochrome c, linking the extrinsic pathway to the intrinsic death pathway. Various apoptotic stimuli such as withdrawal of growth factors, DNA damage, loss of contact with neighbouring cells, etc activate pro-apoptotic cellular proteins such as Bax and Bak, and trigger the intrinsic death pathway. Anti-apoptotic proteins like Bcl-2 and BCl-XL can inhibit this activation. Activation of Bax and Bak causes the release of cytochrome c from the mitochondria. An apoptosome containing cytochrome c and procaspase-9 is formed and results in the formation of activated caspase-9. Caspase-9 recruits other caspases in the cascade, including caspase-3. IAPs (inhibitors of apoptosis) can modulate the action of both caspase-9 and -3. Activation of caspase-3 eventually leads to DNA fragmentation and cell death.*

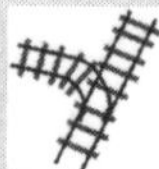

Licensing to Kill: Vaccination

Vaccination has traditionally been defined as the deliberate introduction of a pathogen or its products into the body to confer resistance to a specific infection. The term derives from the work of Edward Jenner, who showed that inoculating humans with skin lesions caused by the vaccinia (cowpox) virus protected them from small pox. The basic principle of vaccination is to actively immunize the subject and to induce a 'primed state' so that exposure to the pathogen results in a rapid secondary immune response, leading to accelerated elimination of the organism and protection from clinical disease. The first administration of the vaccine is called 'primary' vaccination, and subsequent administrations aimed at inducing a lasting secondary response are called 'booster' doses. The success of the vaccine depends upon induction of memory B and T cells and the presence of neutralizing antibodies in the serum. Traditional approaches to vaccine design are outlined below.

❑ **Introduction of live organisms into the host.** Since the organism replicates in the host, the live vaccines generate both humoral and cell-mediated responses, and immunity is long-lasting. For its success, it is essential that the organisms in the vaccine remain viable. Live vaccines are therefore especially sensitive to storage conditions. Three types of live vaccines are in common use.

- Attenuated vaccines consist of organisms whose virulence has been reduced by various means. However, since it involves introducing live organisms, the rare reversion to a virulent strain represents a potential danger. Such occurrences carry the risk of making the general populace lose faith in vaccination and then resisting its use.
- Heterologous vaccines make use of a closely related organism of lesser virulence, which shares many antigens with its virulent counterpart. These vaccines are safer than attenuated vaccines, since the danger of reversion is non-existent. Use of the cowpox virus to immunize against small pox is the most famous example of a heterologous vaccine.
- Live recombinant vaccines are the products of genetic engineering. Genes coding for the immunogenic protein of the pathogen are introduced into a harmless organism. The recombinant organism replicates and expresses the recombinant protein in the host, resulting in cell-mediated and/or humoral immunity.

❑ **Inactivated vaccines** are used when attenuation fails or when safety of the live vaccine remains an issue of concern. Inactivation can be achieved by heat or by chemical means. Instead of using the whole organism, subcellular fractions may be employed. Alternatively, the immunogenic protein is expressed in an expression vector such as *E. coli,* and the protein of interest is purified from the lysates for use in vaccines, eg, the Hepatitis B vaccine. Although they are safer than live vaccines, inactivated vaccines often have lower immunogenicity. These vaccines result in a predominantly humoral response and may fail to invoke CMI.

❑ **Toxoids** are used to confer immunity to infections like diphtheria and tetanus whose manifestations and mortality rates are due to toxins produced by the pathogens upon proliferation in host tissues. Toxoids are produced by denaturing toxins such that toxicity is lost but immunogenicity is retained.

To be effective, a vaccine must fulfil some basic criteria.

❑ **Efficacy.** Ideally, the vaccine must elicit an appropriate long-term protective response. For example, to protect against intracellular pathogens such as *M. tuberculosis*, the vaccine must elicit a cell-mediated response, whereas for respiratory pathogens like the influenza virus, a mucosal antibody response is needed. For most common bacterial and viral infections, on the other hand, a robust serum antibody response is needed to confer protection.

❑ **Safety.** This is of paramount importance. Since vaccines are to be administered to a large population, even low levels of toxicity are unacceptable. Thus, neither the constituents nor additives used for stabilization or preservation of the vaccine should be toxic or yield undesirable side effects.

❑ **Stability.** This is of particular concern in developing countries that lie in the hot equatorial belt. Ideally, vaccines should be stable (ie, retain immunogenicity) over a range of temperatures and even with fluctuations in temperatures.

❑ **Cost-effectiveness.** Vaccination is perhaps the cheapest form of large-scale health care. If vaccines are to be successfully used by the developed and developing world, it is essential that they be affordable.

❑ **Ease of administration.** This is of particular interest to infants and young children who are at the receiving end of a large number of vaccines.

DNA or gene-based vaccines have opened up a new era in vaccine technology. These vaccines introduce not the antigen, but the DNA encoding the antigen in the patient. The earliest type of DNA vaccine was an attenuated viral vector (such as vaccinia virus or adenovirus) engineered to contain DNA encoding antigenic epitopes from a pathogen. Currently, genes coding for antigenic determinant(s) of the pathogen are inserted into a plasmid, and the genetically engineered plasmid is injected into the host. The vaccines are delivered by intramuscular injection or by a device called the gene gun. The gene gun propels plasmids into the cells near the surface of the body (eg, skin or mucous membranes). The mode of vaccine introduction appears to influence the type of response — intramuscular injection seems to enhance T_{H1} responses, whereas the gene gun favours a T_{H2} type response. Once inside the cells, the recombinant plasmid enters the nucleus, and genes encoding the antigen are transcribed and translated. The protein is eventually internalized by APCs, loaded on MHC molecules, and presented to T cells, thereby eliciting an immune response. A combination approach where the immune system is primed with the DNA vaccine and boosted with recombinant viruses seems to hold the most promise, since it generates a more potent immune response than when either is used alone. The use of cytokines to further enhance the efficacy of DNA-based vaccines is also being investigated.

Autologus vaccines. DCs are the most potent APCs in the body. However, DC function is defective in many types of cancers. The generation of autologous DCs *ex vivo* is being attempted to circumvent this problem (chapter 16). Thus, monocytes (DC precursors) obtained from the patient are allowed to differentiate to DCs, matured by use of cytokines or CD154, pulsed with tumour antigens and then re-injected in the patient. Initial studies have shown that such vaccines can induce a potent antitumour response. However, since the vaccine has to be prepared individually for each patient, the procedure is expensive.

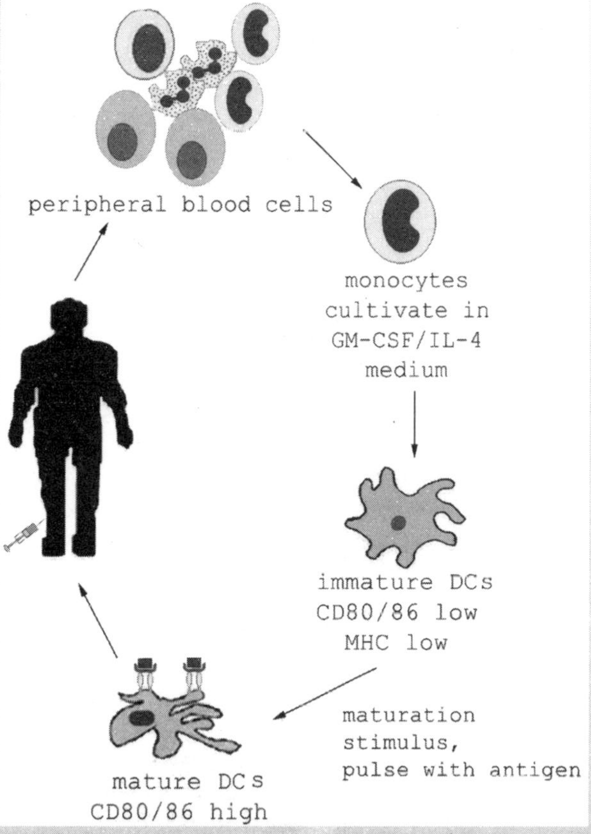

Figure 11.S1 Autologus vaccines can help overcome defective DC function observed in certain cancers and help the patient mount a potent antitumour response.

Newer approaches to vaccine design. As is clear from Table 11.S1, many infections have been successfully tackled with vaccines which mimic the natural immune response. Unfortunately, with chronic infections such as HIV and mycobacterial infections or cancers, the natural immune response is insufficient to afford protection. Therapeutic, rather than prophylactic, vaccinations are now being explored to fight these infections. The new strategies are aimed at increasing the immunogenicity, influencing the type of response, inducing local mucosal immunity, or decreasing inhibitory immune mechanisms.

❑ Epitope enhancement consists of subtly altering the T cell epitopes of a pathogen (usually a virus) to make them more immunogenic. Epitopes can be modified to achieve different goals.
  • Peptide sequences can be modified to increase their affinity for MHC molecules. Alternatively, anchor residues that bind the peptide to MHC molecules can be altered to enhance the affinity of the epitopes. This approach has been used for HIV and cancer vaccines. However, it requires detailed knowledge of the T cell epitopes of the virus or tumour that can bind multiple MHC haplotypes.
  • A second approach consists of increasing the affinity of the peptide:MHC complex for the TcR, which will allow CTLs with low affinity TcRs to be stimulated. This approach is especially useful in the case of tumour antigens, where high affinity T cells are often eliminated or rendered tolerant because of self-antigen recognition.
  • A third approach is to try to induce a broadly cross-reactive T cell response that can recognize multiple strains of the virus. This approach has been used in development of HIV vaccines — appropriate manipulation of T cell epitopes allowed the development of broadly cross-reactive CTLs that recognized multiple strains of HIV. Modified epitopes can be conjugated to a carrier protein or, alternatively, genes encoding the protein can be introduced in a viral vector for administration.
❑ Incorporation of cytokines or costimulatory molecules in a vaccine can increase its efficacy.
  • IL-2 given as a fusion protein with Fc segment of Ig was found to greatly enhance the protective immunity of a vaccine for Simian immunodeficiency virus.
  • GM-CSF has been found to be the most broadly useful cytokine. It can increase the range of T cell responses, resulting in the augmentation of both humoral and cell-mediated immunity.
  • Cytokines can skew the immune response and may be used to selectively induce CTL or humoral responses. Thus, IL-12 and IL-15 have been found to promote CTL memory and are being investigated as vaccine adjuvants.
  • Costimulatory molecules have been found to enhance vaccine efficacy and may be used synergistically with cytokines. Recently, a triple combination of CD80, ICAM-1, and LFA-3, expressed in recombinant poxvirus, has been found to be synergistic for the induction of CTL responses and anti-tumour immunity.
❑ Natural transmission of many viruses (eg, influenza and HIV) occurs at mucosal surfaces, and hence, vaccines aimed at preventing this mucosal transmission are being developed. The route of administration has been found to be important in these vaccines. The normal subcutaneous route has been found to give rise to a systemic response, leaving the mucosal sites immunologically naïve and, therefore, susceptible to infection. By contrast, mucosal immunization (either intranasally or intrarectally) has been found to give rise to CTLs in mucosal sites such as Peyer's patches as well as systemic sites like the spleen. Peptides linked to heat shock proteins have been found to be effective mucosal vaccines, whereas CpG oligonucleotides have been found to be effective mucosal adjuvants.
❑ The discovery of T$_R$ cells has stimulated research aimed at preventing their induction in diseases such as cancer. Most of the research is concentrating on the regulatory pathway involving CTLA-4. CD80/CD86 has two ligands — CD28 that gives an activating signal to the T cell and CTLA-4, which gives an 'off' signal (section 8.3.1). CTLA-4 is important in anergy induction, and preventing its interaction with CD80/86 can reverse CD8$^+$ T cell tolerance. Blocking CTLA-4 has been shown to enhance tumour immunity and is being investigated for application in tumour therapy.

Table 11.S1 Vaccines commonly in use

Infections	Vaccine preparation	Comments
Diphtheria and tetanus	Purified toxoid	Often given with pertussis as a single dose (DTP, or DTaP as it is now called)
Pertussis	Killed bacteria (P) or purified components (aP)	
Poliomyelitis	Attenuated virus — **O**ral **P**olio **V**accine (OPV; Sabin) **I**nactivated **P**olio **V**irus (IPV; Salk)	
Small pox	Attenuated virus	Use was discontinued since the world was declared small pox free; production has been resumed due to the threat of bioterrorism
Measles, mumps, rubella	Attenuated virus	Often given as a mixture (MMR)
Influenza	Haemagglutinins from type A and type B viruses	Rapid antigenic variation has caused new vaccines containing antigens derived from strains in current circulation to be produced every year
Rabies	Inactivated virus	Vaccine prepared from human diploid cell culture (HDCC) has replaced the earlier duck vaccine
Hepatitis B	Purified recombinant surface antigen (HBsAg)	
Hepatitis A	Inactivated virus	Available in a single shot with HBsAg
Typhoid, paratyphoid	Three types available — killed bacteria, oral live attenuated vaccine, and polysaccharide conjugated to a protein	
Tuberculosis	Live attenuated cells (**B**acillus of **C**almette and **G**uerin or BCG)	
Yellow fever	Attenuated virus	
Haemophilus influenzae type b (Hib)	Capsular polysaccharide conjugated to protein	Prevents ear infection in children
Menigococcal disease	Purified polysaccharides	
Anthrax	Extract of attenuated bacteria	Primarily used for veterinarians and military personnel in the developed world; for animals and farmers in some parts of India
Cholera, plague	Crude fraction of organisms	

Historical Perspective: Theories of Immunity

Cellular theory of immunity. In 1884, Metchenikoff postulated that leukocytes might play an important role in the defence of the body. His suggestion that phagocytic cells had a protective function and were the most important contributors of immunity (whether natural or acquired) resulted in a major controversy. Doubts about his theory increased after the discovery of two humoral components — complement and antibodies — involved in host defence. The death blow to the cellular theory of immunity came in 1897. In that year, Ehrlich gave convincing proof of humoral immunity. He demonstrated that a specific anti-toxin could protect an animal against a 100x lethal dose of diphtheria toxin, proving that immunity was of a humoral, not cellular, origin. It was only much later — the mid-1950s — that the concept of cellular immunity once again gained credence and led to the acceptance of the idea that both body humours and cells were involved in immunity.

Ehrlich's side chain theory. Put forward by Paul Ehrlich in 1897, this theory attempts to explain antibody formation by body cells. It postulates that body cells possess natural side chains or receptors consisting of groups or subgroups having an affinity for foreign material. Each cell was assumed to produce a variety of such receptors (fig. 11.S2, top left panel). Chemically different subgroups were presumed to combine with different antigens, ie, each cell was thought to be able to combine with more than one antigen. Ehrlich proposed that the complementarity of the receptors with analogous structures on the antigen permitted specific interaction (fig. 11.S2, top panels). It was further postulated that such combining of side chains with the antigen rendered the cell useless for normal functions. Instead, the cell was stimulated to produce and secrete more receptors (fig. 11.S2, bottom left panel), some of which were cast off into the blood stream (fig. 11.S2, botton right panel). These circulating receptors protected the body by combining with any antigen that had gained entry into blood. This hypothesis was later discarded in the 1920s when antibodies were produced against synthetic agents. It seemed inconceivable then that receptors for synthetic substances or that receptors to such a large array of substances could pre-exist in the cell. Considering that it was formulated at the beginning of the nineteenth century when not much was known about the functioning of the immune system, the theory is remarkable in its boldness and vision.

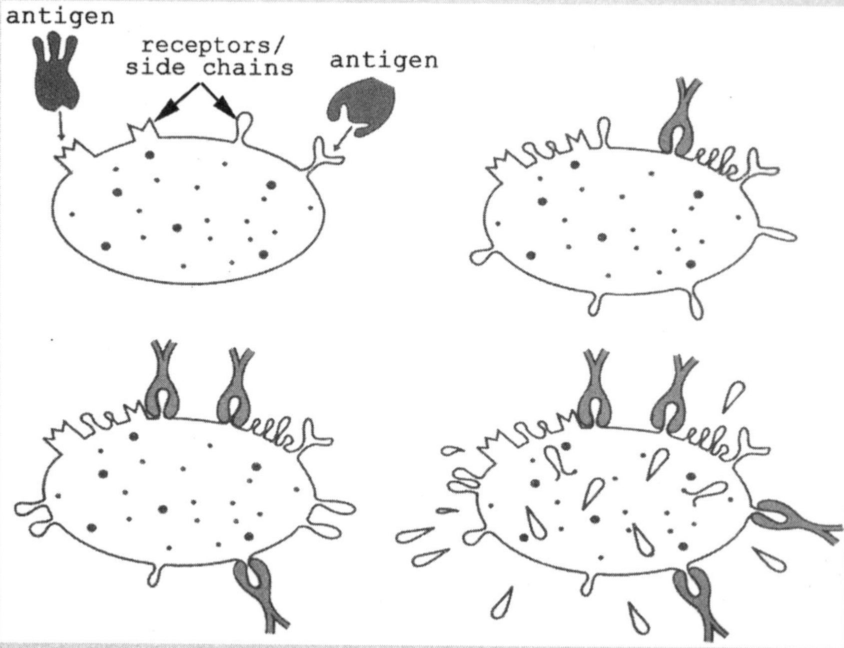

Figure 11.S2 Ehrlich's side chain theory attempted to explain antibody formation by host cells.

Immune Tolerance

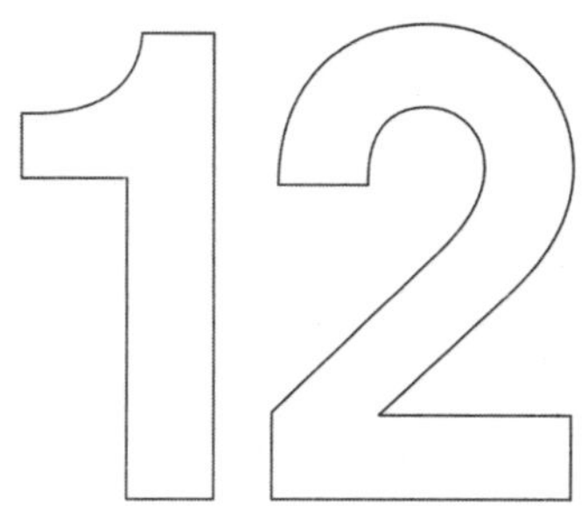

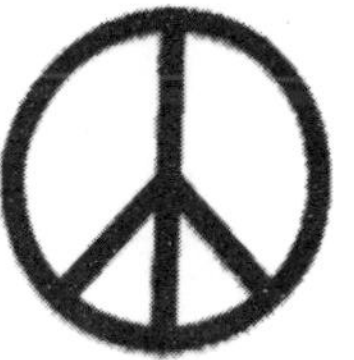

One love
One blood
One life
You've got to do what you should.
One life,
With each other,
Sisters,
Brothers.
One life,
But we're not the same.
We get to
Carry each other,
Carry each other.

— U2, *One*

12.1 Introduction

The human body produces thousands of different proteins and also comes in contact with a wide range of potential pathogens and their products. Yet, the immune system can usually distinguish between pathogens and self-tissues, attacking the former while ignoring the latter. This failure to respond to self-antigens is called self-tolerance. **Immunological unresponsiveness or tolerance can be defined as an antigen-induced block in the development, growth, or differentiation of specific lymphocytes.** It is thus an active and specific state of unresposiveness to a particular antigen that is induced by a prior exposure to that antigen. The main features of tolerance are:

- ❑ It is immunologically specific. Immune tolerance is a specific state of unresponsiveness towards a particular antigen. It is thus different from a general inability to respond to antigens that stems from immunosuppression or immunodeficiency.
- ❑ Since tolerance is specific, it can be induced only in cells expressing specific antigen receptors, ie, in B and T cells.
- ❑ It requires prior exposure to the antigen.
- ❑ It can be either natural or induced. Natural (or self-) tolerance is attained during lymphocyte development and results in absence of an immune response to self-antigens. Induced (or acquired) tolerance to external antigens is often a result of manipulation of the immune system.
- ❑ It is induced more easily in immature lymphocytes than in mature lymphocytes.

Tolerance to self-antigens is central to survival and multiple mechanisms at the central (ie, in the primary lymphoid organs viz thymus and bone marrow) and peripheral levels ensure this continued tolerance. Central tolerance mechanisms ensure that very few self-reactive clones escape to the periphery, whereas peripheral tolerance mechanisms ensure the continued silencing of the escaped self-reactive clones. The major mechanisms by which tolerance is achieved include:

- ❑ **clonal deletion** — the removal of self-reacting clones,
- ❑ **induction of clonal anergy**, ie, causing self-reactive clones to become incapable of responding to antigenic stimulus, and
- ❑ **active suppression**, wherein any surviving self-reactive clones are kept under strict regulatory controls so that they cannot respond to self antigens.

IMMUNE TOLERANCE

- ❑ Immune tolerance is an antigen-induced block in the development, growth, or differentiation of specific lymphocytes; it results in an absence of or an active suppression of an immune response to specific antigens.
- ❑ It requires prior exposure to antigen.
- ❑ Tolerance induction is dependent upon
  - the antigen — dose, nature, physical state, route of administration, and
  - the animal — its genotype, age, and immune status.
- ❑ Non-specific depression of the immune system helps in tolerance induction.

12.2 Central Tolerance

Central tolerance operates in the primary lymphoid organs and induces tolerance in T and B cells during their development. Clonal anergy, clonal deletion, and negative cell selection are important central mechanisms of induction of T and B cell tolerance. T cell tolerance is achieved by the negative selection of self-reactive clones in the thymus (chapter 8). During thymic maturation, T cells expressing TcRs having a high affinity for self-MHC molecules are induced to undergo apoptosis. Similarly, developing B cells that bind self-antigens with high affinity are pushed down the apoptosis road in the bone marrow. Clonal anergy and/or maturational arrest silence B cell clones that bind self-antigens with moderate affinity or those that encounter soluble self-antigens in the bone marrow. Since B cells require T cell help for responding to most antigens, the clonal deletion of self-reactive T cell clones further ensures the absence of B cell responses to self-antigens. As explained below, tolerance induction in the primary lymphoid organs operates under certain constraints and some self-reactive clones inevitably escape to the periphery.

❑ The success of the central deletion mechanisms depends upon the expression of all self-antigens in sufficient concentrations in primary lymphoid organs — especially the thymus. If the concentration of the relevant antigen is low, the number of MHC: peptide complexes on the thymic epithelial cells will be too low to be detected even by high affinity clones, and such clones could escape negative selection. Moreover, some proteins are expressed only after the animal attains maturity (eg, those involved in breast development or sperm development) or those expressed only during a certain phase of the life cycle (eg, during pregnancy and lactation). These proteins will not be expressed in the developing lymphoid organs in the embryo, and lymphocytes recognizing those proteins will be found in the periphery.

❑ TcR recognition is promiscuous by nature. Thus, the more stringent the negative selection, the greater the risk of dangerously narrowing the T cell repertoire and the greater the chances of allowing potential pathogens to escape. It is more cost-effective to let some thymocytes with a degree of self-reactivity to escape central deletional mechanisms and then regulate them in the periphery.

12.3 Peripheral Tolerance

Peripheral mechanisms that ensure the absence of self-reactivity are crucial for survival for multiple reasons. Firstly, mechanisms enforcing central tolerance are leaky. Secondly, since genes encoding BcR undergo mutations in the process of affinity maturation, the chance that some of the clones generated following an encounter with a foreign antigen will cross-react with self-antigens is substantial. Such clones need to be deleted or strictly regulated. Also, the body is constantly exposed to innocuous environmental antigens to which it must remain tolerant — proteins from commensals colonizing the airways and intestines of the body, food antigens, etc. Peripheral tolerance inducing mechanisms ensure the silencing of such clones and the absence of destructive immune responses. Peripheral tolerance can be induced at T cell or B cell level. Since T cells are multifunctional cells involved in humoral and cell-mediated immune responses, tolerizing T cells 'switches off' both these responses. Therefore, T cells are more strictly regulated than B cells.

❑ **T cell tolerance.** Peripheral tolerance can act at several levels in silencing T cell responses (fig. 12.1). Some mechanisms can be considered intrinsic to T cells, since they act directly at the level of T cells, whereas others exert their effect via other cells and may be considered extrinsic to T cells.
  • **Ignorance** is a term used to describe the state of self-reactive T cell clones that do not come in contact with the relevant antigen and are therefore never activated, ie, T cell ignorance[1] of self-antigens occurs when they fail to encounter the relevant self-antigens. This ignorance can be achieved by various strategies. Firstly, the trafficking of naïve T cells is restricted to blood or lymphatics so that these cells do not enter any and every tissue; it is only the memory cells that are allowed to wander. This ensures that naïve T cells encounter only antigen transported to the lymphoid organs by professional

[1] Suddenly, 'Ignorance is bliss' gets a whole new dimension ☺!

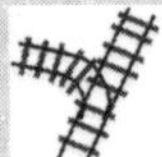

Takes Guts to Tolerate: Tolerance and Mucosal Immunity

The physiological response to food antigens and commensal flora is the induction of a state of tolerance. Conversely, inflammation or antigens associated with pathogens elicit potent immune responses in the gut. Thus, the gastrointestinal tract (specifically GALT) has a particularly difficult balancing act to conduct. It must 'tolerate' food antigens and normal gut flora, but at the same time it must mount a potent immune response to pathogens. This ability of the mucosal immune system to distinguish between the potentially harmful and harmless and focus its energies on the former is the subject of much research in immunology. A variety of strategies operative in the GALT avoid constant inflammatory responses.

❑ The epithelial layer is covered with mucus and retains most bacteria, thereby preventing their entry into the inner layers.

❑ Breach of the epithelial barrier results in an immune response consisting predominantly of IgA rather than IgG antibodies. IgA is non-inflammatory, since it does not bind complement. GALT is known to be a major source of polymeric IgA antibodies (as opposed to systemic IgA, mucosal IgA is polymeric).

❑ In the GALT, T cells are likely to receive signals via MHC in the absence of adequate costimulation, thus leading to tolerance rather than stimulation.
- APCs in the GALT express low levels of the costimulatory molecules CD80/86.
- GALT T cells express CTLA-4, which is also a ligand for CD80/86. It competes with CD28 to further reduce the available costimulatory signal.

❑ TGF-β is abundantly expressed in the GALT.
- TGF-β is thought to promote the generation of Tʀ cells involved in inducing tolerance to food antigens.
- It is vital to IgA secretion; signalling via TGF-β and its receptor is essential for isotype switching to IgA by B cells.

The phenomenon called 'oral tolerance' was described a century ago when it was observed that the oral administration of soluble proteins induces systemic tolerance. The 'default state of tolerance' of GALT and the possibility of inducing oral tolerance make success difficult with orally administered vaccines, although oral administration is the route of choice to elicit mucosal immunity. However, it is possible to actively immunize animals against orally administered antigens by combining soluble proteins with strong mucosal adjuvants such as the cholera toxin or a heat-labile derivative of *E. coli* enterotoxin. Such adjuvants can overcome oral tolerance and induce an efficient immune response, and they are now being explored in the administration of oral vaccines.

APCs. Secondly, some antigens are sequestered in sites not easily accessible to the blood/lymph-borne immune system (eg, brain, testes and eyes). In the case of reproductive organs that express new proteins post-puberty, such sequestration helps maintain ignorance of self-reactive T cell clones (see sidetrack 'The Privilege of Being and Seeing'). Lastly, the threshold of antigen required to trigger a T cell response is such that although some self-antigens may enter circulation, they will fail to elicit an immune response because their concentration does not reach the required threshold.

- **Anergy induction** causes the functional inactivation of T cells following self-antigen encounter. TcR engagement in the absence of CD28 costimulation has been shown to induce anergy in T cells *in vitro*. It is postulated that the requirement for simultaneous delivery of antigen-specific and costimulatory signals in the activation of naïve T cells ensures initiation of T cell responses by professional APCs only. By contrast, engagement of CTLA-4 and PD-1 has been reported to induce anergy. CTLA-4, a CD28 homologue with an inhibitory function, binds the same molecules (CD80/86) as CD28 but induces anergy in CTLs *in vivo*. PD-1, another member of the costimulatory molecule family, is

---

MECHANISMS OF SELF-TOLERANCE

❑ Self-tolerance inducing mechanisms are operative at the central and peripheral levels.
❑ Mechanisms important in central tolerance include clonal abortion, clonal deletion, and clonal anergy.
❑ Peripheral T cell tolerance inducing mechanisms include:
  - clonal ignorance (failure to encounter self-antigen),
  - induction of anergy in self-reactive clones,
  - phenotypic skewing,
  - induction of apoptosis in self-reactive clones,
  - skewing of the immune response by APCs, and
  - suppressive action of T_R cells.
❑ Peripheral B cell tolerance is induced by:
  - controlling T cell responses,
  - induction of anergy due to improper/incomplete activation, and
  - peripheral B cell tolerance.

---

thought to control T cell unresponsiveness by inhibiting cytokine secretion or by causing cell cycle arrest (see the sidetrack 'A Need for Stimulating Company', chapter 8).

- **Phenotypic skewing.** Regulating what self-reactive T cells make and therefore, where they go, can prevent autoimmune destruction in the periphery. Alteration in chemokine or cytokine expression patterns can avert an autoreactive T cell response in spite of activation of self-reactive cells. For example, T cells need to express CXCR5 to be able to migrate to B cell areas of secondary lymphoid tissues (section 8.3.5.1 ii). Induction of CXCR5 is dependent on CD28 ligation, and it may not be induced in the absence of an adjuvant. Thus, even if self-reactive T cells proliferate in response to a self-antigen, their migration to B cell areas of secondary lymphoid tissues is defective in the absence of CXCR5 expression, and an autoimmune response is averted.

- **Apoptosis.** Perhaps the most effective way to prevent autoimmunity is the deletion of self-reactive T cell clones by AICD. Self-antigens cannot be cleared easily and lead to repetitive T cell activation. Such repetitive activation characteristic of self-antigen-T cell encounter is thought to serve as a trigger for AICD. Recent evidence suggests that IL-2 may have a crucial role in AICD. IL-2 is thought to promote apoptosis via Stat-5 (**S**ignal **T**ransducer of **A**ctivation and **T**ranscription-**5**)-mediated induction of Fas ligand. It also downregulates the expression of the inhibitory protein FLIP. This mechanism of Fas-mediated cell death has already been discussed at some length in chapter 11.

- **Tolerance induction by APCs.** It has been accepted for many years that APCs influence the nature of the immune response (tolerance versus initiation). DCs are thought to be the key APCs in both these processes. The hypothesis in current acceptance postulates that DCs present a 'sample' of proteins in their immediate environment to T cells. Such antigen presentation by immature DCs tolerizes T cells — probably because of a lack of costimulation and/or because of the kind of chemokines expressed by immature DCs. However, the presence of products of microbial origin such as LPS, peptidoglycan, and CpG DNA causes DC maturation. Similarly, by-products of stressed or necrotic cells (possibly heat shock proteins or mitochondrial by-products) also induce DC maturation. Mature DCs are potent APCs; they express a plethora of costimulatory and adhesion molecules and produce a number of cytokines. Antigen presentation by mature DCs therefore results in an immune response. Additionally, certain types of DCs are thought to induce tolerance through their ability to generate T_R cells. Support for this idea comes from experiments where the repetitive stimulation of allogeneic naïve cord blood CD4$^+$ T cells with immature DCs was shown to result in a non-proliferating population of T$_R$ cells. It is not yet clear whether a separate subset of DCs or distinct developmental stages of DCs are responsible for T$_R$ cell generation. The idea that DCs can influence the type of immune response has enormous therapeutic potential and is being thoroughly investigated.

Induction of T$_R$ cells. T$_R$ cells have a critical role in the generation and maintenance of tolerance. However, many questions regarding their lineages, differentiation factors, antigen-specificity, and mechanisms of action remain unanswered. Many subsets of T$_R$ cells have been characterized in different experimental systems, but their relationship to each other is also not clear. *In vitro* studies have shown that instead of proliferating, T$_R$ cells suppress the proliferation of other T cells in response to an antigen. Possible mechanisms of immune suppression include signalling via cell surface markers such as CTLA-4 and production of cytokines such as TGF-b and IL-10 (chapter 8). Recent data suggests that signalling through T cell expressed CD2 in the absence of additional costimulatory signals may also be a mechanism of tolerance induction. A better understanding of their effector functions will help understand these relationships and allow the exploitation of T$_R$ cells in immunotherapy.

❑ **Peripheral B cell tolerance.** Absence of appropriate T cell help leaves B cells 'helpless' in responding to many antigens so that mechanisms effective in inducing T cell tolerance are indirectly operative at the B cell level as well. Additionally, exposure to multivalent antigens in the absence of T cell help may lead to clonal

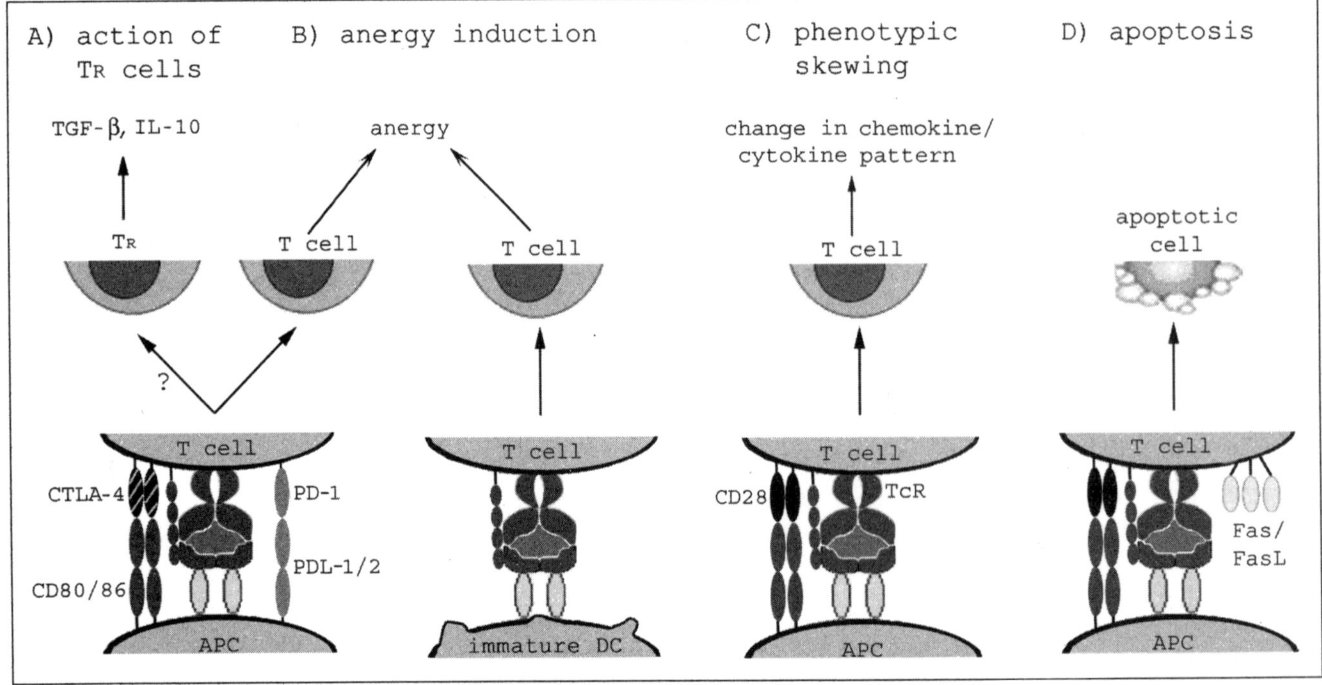

***Figure 12.1 Peripheral T cell tolerance to self-antigens is induced by multiple means.** (A) T$_R$ cells have a critical role in the generation and maintenance of tolerance. These cells are known to produce cytokines such as TGF-β and IL-10 in response to antigenic challenge, thus suppressing an immune response. The mechanism of T$_R$ cell generation is not clear (denoted by a question mark). It is proposed that engagement of CTLA-4 or PD-1 may induce naïve T cells to differentiate to T$_R$ cells. Alternatively, such engagement may render the T cell anergic and functionally ineffectual (B). Recognition on MHC:peptide complexes by TcR, in absence of costimulation may also render peripheral T cells anergic. Even if self-reactive T cells get activated, destructive autoimmune responses can be averted by phenotypic skewing (C). Thus, by altering the pattern of cytokines/chemokines secreted, the trafficking pattern or the nature of the immune response (destructive versus non-destructive) can be controlled. The most efficient way of inducing tolerance is by inducing apoptosis in self-reactive T cells (D). T cell activation causes the upregulation of FasL. It also induces Fas expression and downregulation of the inhibitory protein FLIP, causing the cells to undergo AICD.*

deletion or anergy in mature B cells. Mature mIgM⁺ mIgD⁺ cells lose IgM surface expression on exposure to high concentrations of soluble antigens (as happens with self-antigens). The critical parameter seems to be receptor occupancy; greater than 5% mIgM occupancy leads to anergy in experimental systems. Such cells are unable to enter primary lymphoid follicles, become anergic, and are eventually lost.

12.4 Tolerance Induction

Although tolerance to self-antigens is integral to survival, it sometimes breaks down, resulting in autoimmune diseases (chapter 14) and may necessitate (re-) induction of tolerance to self-antigens. Induction of tolerance to foreign antigens on the other hand happens naturally in the case of colonization of the gut with commensal flora and is done artificially to allow the survival of transplants (chapter 13). It is important to realize that tolerance is a type of immune response and hence is induced against particular epitopes. Thus, if an animal is tolerized to a particular epitope, it will show tolerance to all antigens having that particular epitope as its major antigenic determinant or immunodominant epitope, and the tolerance will be maintained so long as the antigen persists in adequate concentrations. 'Split tolerance' is observed when an animal is tolerant to some epitopes on an antigen but not to other epitopes on the same antigen. **As a rule, tolerance induction is comparatively easier, requires smaller amounts of antigen, and lasts longer in T cells than B cells**. Multiple factors affect the nature and duration of tolerance induction (outlined below). Obviously, any strategy used to induce a potent immune response (adjuvant usage, aggregating the antigen, conjugating to carrier proteins, etc) will be unsuitable for inducing tolerance.

❑ **Nature of the antigen.** Generally, monomeric or soluble antigens are tolerogenic. Monomeric antigens cannot cross-link BcR and therefore do not stimulate B cells. Also, monomeric or soluble antigens are taken up predominantly by pinocytosis and do not induce expression of costimulatory molecules. Similarly, polymers of D-amino acids are effective tolerogens, since D-amino acids can bind BcR but cannot be digested and presented to T cells. B cells therefore get tolerized in the absence of T cell help. Hapten density also seems to influence tolerogenicity. Higher densities of haptens on the carrier molecule seem to induce tolerance, whereas lower densities are immunogenic.

❑ **Dose of antigen.** Experiments to determine the relation between antigen dosage and tolerance induction in mice showed the presence of three distinct zones.
  • High concentrations of the antigen induce tolerance (called high zone tolerance). High zone tolerance is considered to be an important mechanism for maintaining tolerance to abundant ubiquitous self-proteins such as plasma proteins.
  • Medial ranges of concentrations induce an immune response.
  • Concentration ranges much below the immunizing dose induce the so-called low zone tolerance.

❑ **Route of administration.** The route of administration influences both the magnitude and type of immune response. It is possible to induce systemic tolerance by oral administration of haptens or small soluble molecules. Similarly, tolerance can also be induced to soluble proteins delivered by aerosols through airway mucosa. Administration of antigen by injection in the portal circulation has been shown to induce tolerance in animal models.

❑ **Age and immune status.** Immature lymphocytes are tolerized more easily than mature cells. Hence, neonatal or foetal exposure to the antigen induces tolerance. Thus, introduction of an exogenous antigen into the foetus renders the animal tolerant to that antigen. It is much more difficult to induce tolerance in an adult animal. Previously immunized animals are refractory to tolerance induction, since they have a much larger repertoire of memory B and T cells capable of recognizing the antigen. Moreover, memory cells are more resistant to tolerance induction than naïve cells. However, tolerance induction is possible if the mature immune system is compromised by irradiation or drugs.

❑ **Non-specific immune depression.** Generally, any treatment that depresses immune responses non-specifically facilitates the induction of tolerance. This includes immunosuppressive drugs, X-irradiation, and the use of anti-lymphocytic serum. Anti-idiotypic cytotoxic antibodies can also be used to eliminate specific clones of B cells. Drugs like cyclophosamide help in tolerance induction by delaying the regeneration of mIg receptors on the B cell surface and increasing response time.

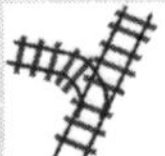

The Privilege of Being and Seeing: Immune Privileged Sites

The term 'immune privilege' is derived from the work of Medawar, who won a Nobel Prize for his pioneering work in the early 1950s. He found that grafts placed in certain areas of the eyes (cornea or anterior chamber), brain, or reproductive organs were 'privileged', in that they survived for prolonged periods of time. Immune privilege is thus the property of some sites in the body where immune responses are limited or prevented. Immune responses in these sites are 'deviant', ie, different from those in other sites. Privileged sites generally mount predominantly non-inflammatory immune responses consisting of non-complement fixing antibody isotypes, and CTL responses are limited or absent. Such deviant responses probably reflect an evolutionary adaptation to protect vital structures from the damage that normally occurs as a result of pro-inflammatory immune responses. Originally, sequestration of antigens was thought to be the major reason behind the phenomenon of immune privilege. It is now accepted that an active rather than a passive process maintains immune privilege.

The Brain. Any immune response in the brain is bad news. It is perhaps the most important and most vulnerable organ of the body ('brain-dead' is, after all, the clinical definition of death!). Multiple factors are responsible for the immunoprivileged status of the brain. A specialized **B**lood-**B**rain **B**arrier (BBB) secludes the brain parenchyma from circulating blood. BBB is the result of special characteristics of the capillary walls of the brain that prevent potentially harmful substances from moving out of the blood stream and into the brain or cerebrospinal fluid. It protects the brain from surging fluctuations in blood constituents, eg, hormones, amino acids, and K^+ ions. The endothelial cells of the cerebral blood vessels constituting BBB have tight junctions. These junctions consist of a ring of proteins that seals the epithelium and restricts the passage of molecules into and out of the brain. Most of the transport across the BBB is an active process involving specific carrier proteins; only lipophilic substances can diffuse across this barrier. BBB thus tightly regulates molecular and cellular traffic into the brain. Absence of organized lymphatic drainage further isolates the brain from immune effectors. Furthermore, normal brain cells are essentially MHC negative or low expressers; immune responses cannot occur in the absence of MHC molecules. Brain parenchyma also lacks DCs. Lack of these professional APCs significantly hampers the elicitation of an immune response. The presence of gangliosides and cytokines like TGF-β further augments the immunosuppressive environment of the brain. The downside of these multiple barriers to immune responses is acutely felt in the treatment of brain infections or tumours, since it is difficult to deliver antibiotics, chemotherapeutic agents, or vaccines to this site. It must be stressed that immunoprivileged status does not imply that the brain is devoid of any immune response. Although immune reactivity is not constitutive in the brain, CNS parenchyma can be induced to support local immune responses, usually to the detriment of the individual.

The Eyes. Much of what is known about immune privilege comes from studies of this organ. Protecting the eyes from invading pathogens is an absolute requirement for the preservation of vision. However, immune responses themselves can cause collateral tissue damage because of non-specific inflammation. Their delicate microanatomy makes the eyes particularly vulnerable to distortion from relatively trivial amounts of intraocular inflammation. Therefore, regulation of the immune response is critical to the preservation of vision. Regulatory molecules expressed by cells of the eye modulate both the induction and expression of immunity to self-antigens, resulting in the virtual elimination of immunogenic inflammation in the eyes. This regulation unfortunately also renders the eye vulnerable to those pathogens whose elimination requires participation of inflammatory molecules and cells.

The immune privileged status of the eye (specifically anterior chamber, vitreous cavity, subretinal space, and corneal stroma) is attributed to a variety of mechanisms. These mechanisms include a lack of lymphatic drainage, the presence of a physical barrier between blood and the eye (called the **B**lood-**O**cular **B**arrier), low expression of MHC class II molecules, increased expression of CD59 that inhibits complement activation, local production of immunosuppressive neuropeptides and cytokines (eg, TGF-β), and constitutive expression of FasL. Expression of FasL is known to induce death in Fas-expressing lymphoid cells. Studies have shown that FasL expression results in apoptosis of antigen-specific cells that enter the eye, preventing an immune response and promoting tolerance. Uptake of these apoptotic cells by local DCs is also thought to favour activation of T_R cells, further strengthening a tolerant response. In fact, FasL expression seems to be common in many privileged sites, including the brain, the testes, and thyroid, and it may be responsible for the immune deviation (shift from cell-mediated to humoral immune responses) observed in some of these sites.

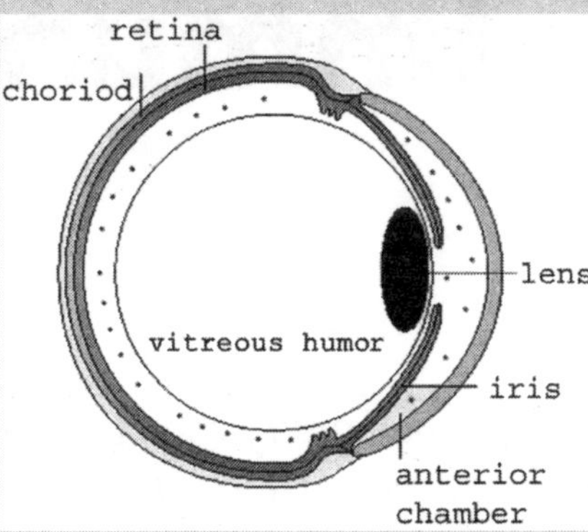

Figure 12.S1   The anterior chamber, vitreous cavity, subretinal space, and corneal stroma of the eye are immunoprivileged.

13 Transplantation and Transfusion Immunology

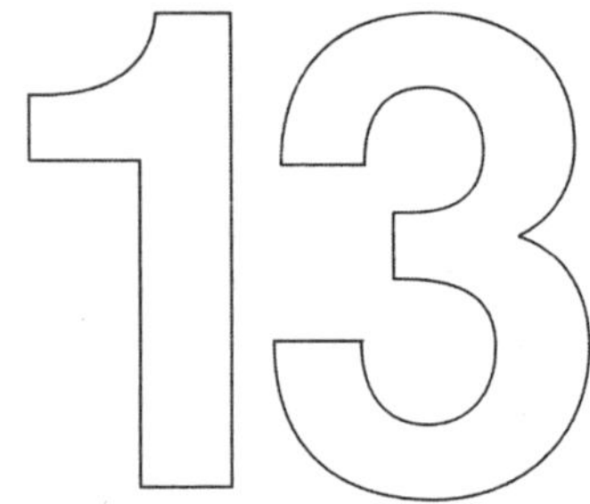

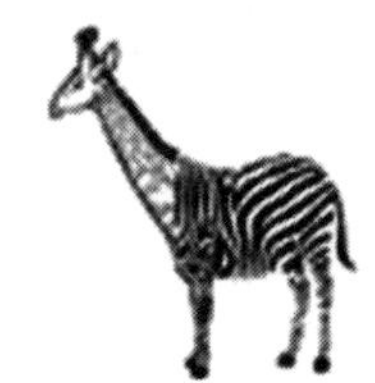

You think we look pretty good together
You think my shoes are made of leather

But I'm a substitute for another guy
I look pretty tall but my heels are high
The simple things you see are all complicated
I look pretty young, but I'm just back-dated, yeah

—The Who, *Substitute*

13.1 Introduction

The replacement of defective or damaged body parts has long been a cherished human goal. Sushruta, the ancient Indian surgeon, has been credited with using self-soft tissues in the reconstructive surgery of the nose and ears as far back as 700 BC. However, the transferring of tissues between two individuals was never successful until recent times. The problem of tissue transfer gained renewed impetus when scores of experiments in tissue and tumour transfer were undertaken in the later decades of the nineteenth century. **The transfer of cells or tissues from one individual (animal) to another was termed transplantation, and the transferred tissue was called a 'graft'.** A graft was said to be 'rejected' when the recipient's immune system mounted a vigorous response against the graft with concomitant damage to the grafted tissue. Rejection of the first graft from a particular donor is the 'first set rejection', and rejections of second or additional grafts are called 'second set rejections' (in parallel with primary and secondary immune responses). In 1912, the German scientist Georg Schöne summarized experimental work reported in the first decade of the twentieth century. He coined the term 'transplantation immunity', and formulated the rules of transplantation paraphrased below.

❑ Heterografts (xenografts), ie, the tissues transplanted from one species to another invariably fail.

❑ Allografts (homografts) consisting of transplants between genetically non-identical individuals of the same species usually fail; they may seem to survive at first but are subsequently rejected.

❑ Autografts, ie, self-tissues transplanted from one region of the body to another and isografts (syngrafts; tissues transplanted from one genetically identical individual to another) are almost always successful.

❑ Second grafts undergo accelerated rejection if the recipient has previously rejected a graft from the same donor, or if the recipient has been pre-immunized with material from the donor.

❑ Graft success is more likely when donor and recipient have a close blood relationship.

13.2 Antigens Involved in Graft Rejection

It was recognized early on that differences in the genetic make-up of the donor and the recipient were responsible for graft rejection, ie, alloantigens[1] were at the root of graft rejection.

❑ **ABO blood group antigen** incompatibility is an absolute contraindication to vascularized organ transplantation — the graft will always be rejected. After re-vascularization of the ABO incompatible graft, pre-formed anti-A or anti-B antibodies in the host circulation bind to their respective antigens, expressed on the donor vascular endothelium, and trigger complement-mediated lysis of the graft vasculature, resulting in hyperacute rejection.

❑ Experiments of Peter Gorer, George Snell, and Peter Medawar identified importance of the **major histocompatibility antigens** (ie, MHC class I and II molecules) in graft rejection. The most important MHC molecules in this respect are the classical MHC class I molecules — HLA-A, HLA-B, and HLA-C, and HLA-DR, HLA-DP, and HLA-DQ MHC class II molecules.

❑ **Minor histocompatibility antigen** mismatch can result in graft rejection, even if the donor and recipient MHC are matched. Minor histocompatibility antigens are polymorphic proteins encoded by alleles of genes on sex chromosomes, autosomes, mitochondrial DNA, etc. Minor histocompatibility alleles code for proteins that are present either in the donor (eg, H-Y antigen encoded by the sex chromosome) or are present in both the donor and the recipient, but differ from each other in a

ATG:	Antithymocyte globulin
AZT:	Azathoiprine
Crry:	Complement receptor 1 related protein y
CsA:	Cyclosporine A
FKBP:	FK506 binding protein
GPI:	glycosylphosphotidylinositol
GVHD:	Graft versus host disease
HTLV:	Human T lymphocyte virus
IDO:	Indoleamine 2,3-dioxygenase
MMF:	Mycophenolate mofetil
MNA:	Malononitrilaminde
TRALI:	Transfusion related acute lung injury
vCJD:	variant Cruzfeldt Jacob disease

[1] An antigen with the potential to elicit an immune response when transferred from one individual to another of the same species is called an alloantigen. The immunogenicity of the alloantigen is due to allelic variance of the gene encoding that antigen. The term allogeneic refers to genetic differences between individuals of the same species, whereas the term syngeneic implies genetic identity (eg, monozygotic twins or inbred laboratory animals).

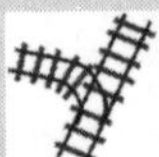

The Eyes of an Eagle and the Heart of a Lion: Xenotransplantation

Xenotransplantation is the transfer of cells, tissues, or organs between disparate species. Perceived at one time to be an experiment in biological curiosity, xenotransplantation is becoming increasingly attractive because of the severe shortage of human organs and tissues for transplantation. The advent of genetic engineering has made xenotransplants seem even more attractive. The idea of animals raised to express genes of therapeutic value or engineered expressly to reduce the risk of rejection does not seem like fantasy anymore. Nonetheless, several hurdles need to be crossed before xenotransplantation can become a reality. Not the least amongst them is the fear of unwittingly transferring infectious agents or helping in the emergence of new infectious agents.

❑ The first hurdle is physiological — whether or not the xenogeneic organ or tissue would function adequately in human patients. Porcine liver has been shown to function adequately in baboons, suggesting that physiological barriers may not be insurmountable. Such experiments with pig organs suggest that their kidneys, lungs, and hearts may function satisfactorily in humans.

❑ One of the major barriers to xenograft acceptance is non-immunological. The survivability of the xenograft will depend upon its ability to sustain angiogenesis, ie, its ability to stimulate the growth of blood vessels. The incompatibility of donor and recipient growth factors may impair the growth of new blood vessels, and the graft cells will quickly die in the absence of restoration of blood supply.

❑ If the xenograft survives this barrier, it has to face the innate immune system.

  • The complement system provides the most potent threat to xenograft acceptance. Complement can cause hyperacute rejection of the xenograft that begins within minutes of engraftment. Xenograft cells do not express complement regulatory proteins such as CD59 and DAF and are particularly susceptible to complement-mediated injury. Both classical and alternative pathways have a role in xenograft rejection. Xenoreactive natural antibodies produced by B1 B cells recognize a variety of structures on foreign cell surfaces and activate the classical pathway. Especially important are antibodies specific for Galα1,3Gal — a saccharide expressed on cells of lower mammals but not humans or apes. These anti-carbohydrate antibodies appear to be members of a class of antibodies that include anti-blood group A antibodies. They seem to arise during the first few years of life, owing to interaction of the immune system with gut bacteria. The alternative pathway, on the other hand, is activated by Factor H which inhibits association of C3b with Factor B on homologous, but not heterologous, surfaces.

  • There is some evidence to suggest that neutrophils may become activated by a direct interaction with xenogeneic cells. Macrophages, also, seem to interact directly with xenogeneic cells. Together, these cells can initiate xenograft tissue destruction without the involvement of inflammatory mediators.

  • Porcine endothelial cells seem to generate thrombin spontaneously; human platelets then get recruited to the site of thrombin generation and trigger an inflammatory response.

  • NK cells are particularly cytotoxic to xenogeneic cells. The absence of MHC class I expression by these cells, the stimulation of lectin receptors on NK cells by saccharides such as Galα1,3Gal, and ADCC mediated by xenoreactive antibodies are all thought to contribute to this susceptibility.

  • Like allografts, T cells may also be involved in xenograft rejection. Both direct and indirect pathways of MHC recognition are believed to be involved in this T cell activation.

single or a few amino acids. They were originally called 'minor' because of their weaker potential to effect rejection when compared to the HLA antigens. Subsequent studies established that multiple differences in these antigens in MHC-matched donors and recipients can elicit graft rejection with a speed comparable to MHC-mismatch. Minor H antigens are presented by the indirect pathway (section 13.3). Recipient APCs internalize, process, and present these donor proteins to recipient T cells, triggering an immune response against donor tissues expressing these antigens. Examples of mouse minor histocompatibility antigens include the autosome-encoded β_2-m, mitochondrial DNA encoded and maternally transmitted factor-α, and H-Y antigens encoded by the Y chromosome.

13.3 Allorecognition

MHC molecules are involved not only in graft rejection but also in the initiation of immune responses to antigens — whether self or foreign. As explained in chapter 8, self-MHC restriction of T cells is a consequence of selection during thymic development. These self-restricted T cells are activated because of the engagement of their TcRs by peptide:self-MHC complexes in conjunction with appropriate costimulatory signals, and this activation culminates in an immune response. Graft rejection is a consequence of a system that cannot discriminate between the deliberate introduction of a beneficial foreign immunogen and the accidental introduction of a potentially harmful one. Transplantation immunity is unique from the general model of T cell activation outlined above. It is a seeming contradiction of the imposed rule of self-restriction, since non-self MHC molecules appear to trigger T cells involved in graft rejection. Thus, although the vigorous nature of T cell responses to allogeneic MHC molecules has been known for more than half a century, the details of the mechanism by which these antigens are recognized remain controversial. Two different pathways could result in allorecognition.

❑ **Direct allorecognition.** This involves the stimulation of recipient T cells by donor APCs. This pathway is called the 'direct pathway' because the interaction occurs directly between recipient TcRs and intact MHC molecules expressed on the surface of donor APCs. It is estimated that about 1–7% of T cells show alloreactivity (ie, they recognize non-self MHC), and this seems to fly in the face of self-MHC restriction. Multiple evidence points to direct allorecognition. Firstly, matching the donor and recipient for MHC antigens improves graft survival. Secondly, depleting MHC-mismatched grafts of potential APCs (eg, DCs) improves graft survival, whereas restoring the APCs to the graft accelerates rejection. When tested *in vitro*, recipient T cells respond with vigorous proliferation in an MLR[2] with donor APCs, suggesting a similar reaction between the two cells *in vivo*. Structural analysis of alloreactive TcR indicates that recognition of allogeneic MHC occurs because of cross-reactivity. Thus, some of the TcRs specific for self-MHC cross-react with non-self MHC and proliferate in response to them. It is not clear if the alloreactive TcR recognizes the allogeneic MHC itself (ie, irrespective of the peptide bound to it) or only a particular peptide:allo-MHC complex. It is possible that these two possibilities represent two extreme scenarios, and both, MHC molecules and peptides may contribute in varying degrees to the overall binding energy between the TcR and its ligand.

❑ **Indirect pathway of allorecognition.** Originally, the direct pathway was thought to be the only major pathway of allorecognition. Recently, though, the indirect pathway has been given its due recognition. Graft rejection by the indirect pathway is triggered when peptides derived from allogeneic MHC are processed and presented in the context of self- (ie, recipient) MHC molecules. Thus, self-APCs internalize and degrade allogeneic MHC molecules, load the peptides derived from them on self-MHC molecules, and present them to self-T cells, triggering an immune response against graft tissues and cells expressing the allogeneic MHC molecules (fig. 13.1).

13.4 Graft Rejection

Clinically, allografts are usually obtained from cadavers or brain dead individuals, bone marrow transplants and some kidney transplants being notable exceptions. The organ to be transplanted is removed from the cadaver and treated before being packed in ice for transport. The process results in ischaemic/reperfusion damage[3] to the organ, characterized by complement deposition, upregulation of adhesion molecules, inflammatory cell infiltration, and cytokine release. This injury is

[2] MLR (**Mixed Leukocyte Reaction**) is used to observe a recipient T cell proliferative response to alloantigens on donor APCs *in vitro*. Donor leukocytes are irradiated to ensure that the observed proliferative response is only due to the recipient T cells.

[3] Ischaemia is the insufficient supply of blood to an organ; re-establishing the blood supply causes damage to the organ and is called ischaemia/reperfusion damage.

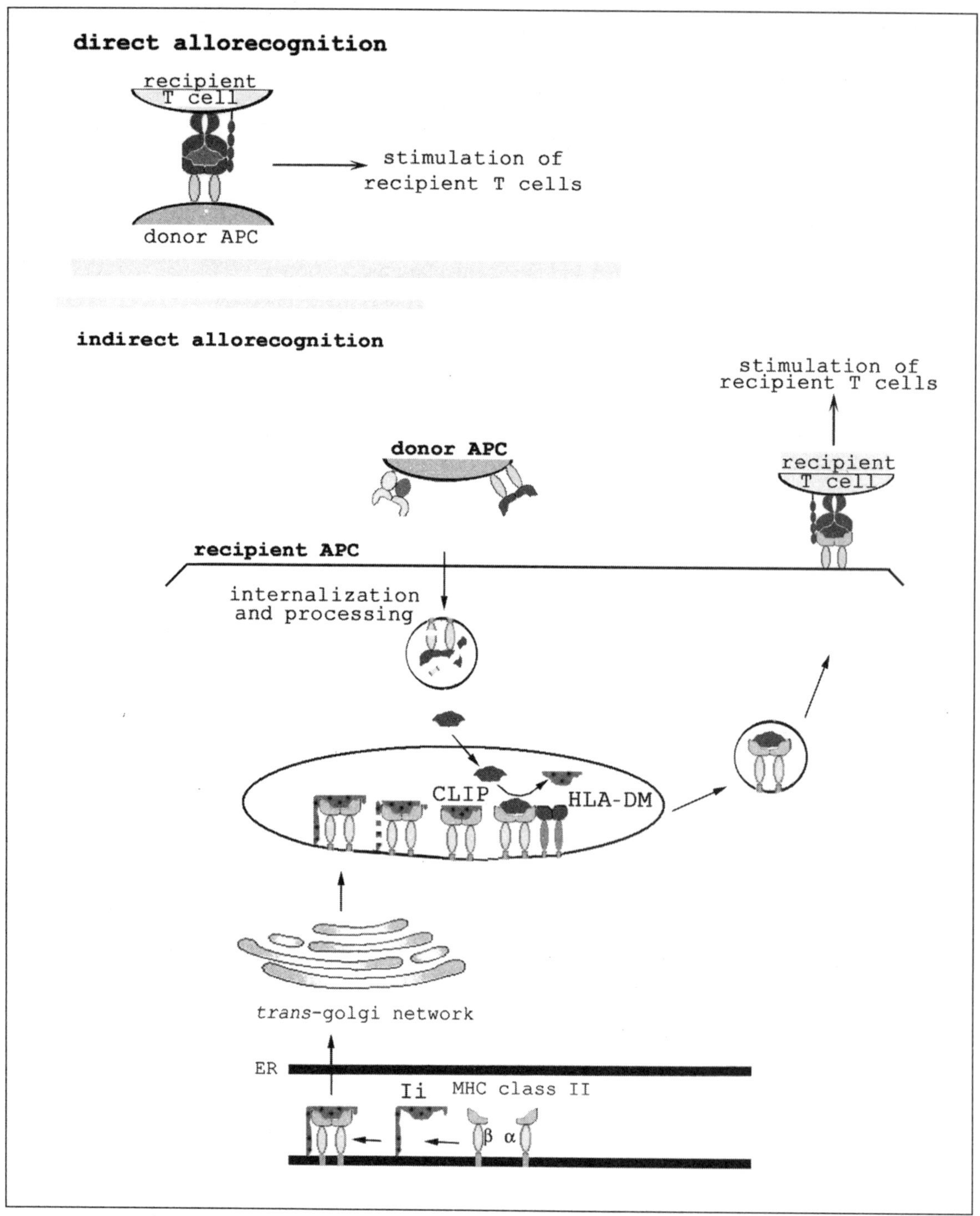

Figure 13.1 Graft antigens can activate recipient T cells through two different pathways. *Direct allorecognition occurs because of cross-reactivity between donor and recipient MHC molecules. Recipient T cells recognize and bind the non-self MHC molecules on donor APC and induce an immune response against donor antigens (top panel). In the indirect pathway, donor MHC molecules are internalized and processed by the recipient APC. Peptides derived from these molecules are loaded on recipient MHC and presented to recipient T cells resulting in their activation.*

compounded by emergency interventions that precede organ harvest. Recipients are also subjected to treatments before and during transplantation. The surgery itself also causes trauma, which worsens if the transplant site gets infected. All these factors act as immunological stimuli and play a role in graft rejection. Although the relative contributions of the direct and indirect pathways of allorecognition to graft rejection are not established, the mechanism of graft rejection and the effector pathways leading to it are becoming clearer. Three phases of graft rejection are recognized.

❑ The **hyperacute response** occurs within 48 hours of engraftment. It is induced by preformed recipient antibodies that mediate graft rejection by binding to antigens such as blood group antigens, which are expressed by the vascular endothelium of the graft. The recipient antibodies bind to antigens expressed on the graft endothelium and activate complement by the classical pathway, resulting in vasoconstriction, influx of PMNs and monocytes, formation of platelet thrombi, ischaemic damage, and infarction.

❑ **Acute rejection** typically occurs 1–2 weeks following transplantation and may be prevented or reversed using immunosuppressive regimens.

❑ **Chronic rejection** is a more insidious type of rejection and may take months or years to develop. The process is characterized by luminal narrowing, the occlusion of arteries and arterioles, and the fibrosis of the graft parenchyma, resulting in organ failure. The relation between acute and chronic rejection is not clear, but early acute rejection appears to be the most important antigen-dependent risk factor in chronic rejection.

13.4.1 Role of APCs

The immune system treats the graft as a potentially dangerous intruder, and the immunological events that follow engraftment are essentially similar to those occurring after a major infection or trauma (fig. 13.2). The pro-inflammatory signals that result from stress, ischaemia, and perfusion injury lead to the maturation of donor DCs that leave the graft and move to the draining lymph node. Here, donor APCs evoke a direct alloresponse involving both CD4$^+$ and CD8$^+$ effector T cells. This response is thought to involve cross-reactive (recipient) memory T cells primed against various environmental antigens in the context of self-MHC molecules. The activated effector T cells migrate to the graft. The ischaemic injury and resultant microvascular stress help this trafficking of leukocytes into the graft. Chemokines play a major role in this recruitment and may further increase the damage by recruiting

---

TRANSPLANTATION

❑ Transplantation is the transfer of cells, tissues, or organs from one site to another.
❑ Autografts and isografts are generally accepted; allografts and xenografts are generally rejected.
❑ Antigens involved in graft rejection include blood group antigens, and major and minor histocompatibility molecules.
❑ T cells involved in graft rejection are alloreactive, ie, they can recognize peptide:non-self-MHC complexes.
❑ Two different pathways can lead to transplant rejection.
  • Direct allorecognition, involving stimulation of recipient T cells by MHC (with or without peptides) on donor APCs.
  • Indirect allorecognition, involving the recognition of peptides derived from donor MHC in the context of self-MHC molecules.
❑ CD4$^+$ T cells have a central role in graft rejection.
❑ CMI is the major effector mechanism in rejection; eosinophils and antibodies may also play a role in the process.
❑ Graft versus host disease (GVHD) is the result of donor T cells attacking recipient tissue cells.
❑ Immunosuppressive therapies used to increase transplant acceptance include:
  • Calcineurin inhibitors such as CsA and FK506,
  • IL-2R antagonists such as Basilximab and Daclizumab,
  • Lymphocyte depleting agents such as anti-CD3 mAb and ATG,
  • Antiproliferative agents such as AZA, MMF, and MNA, and
  • Gene transcription inhibitors such as corticosteroids and sirolimus.

other effector cells such as NK cells, macrophages, and B cells to the site of the graft. The site becomes a seat of intense inflammation, resulting in necrosis and eventual graft rejection. Thus, the direct pathway is thought to be responsible for acute graft rejection. If the graft survives this phase, the direct pathway may also contribute to tolerance induction once the professional APCs in the graft die. The recipient alloreactive T cells entering the graft will recognize MHC molecules on non-professional antigen-presenting graft cells in the absence of costimulatory signals. Such non-professional antigen presentation will result in anergy, inducing tolerance to the graft.

Death of donor APCs starts in the draining lymph nodes and can set the stage for indirect pathway of allorecognition and chronic graft rejection. The dying APCs act as a source of donor MHC antigens to recipient APCs. Migrant recipient APCs trafficking through the lymph nodes can also capture alloantigens from dying donor APCs. The alloantigens are processed and presented to recipient T cells via the indirect pathway. This presentation will occur predominantly to CD4$^+$ T cells. Because of cross-presentation[4], some of the alloantigen-derived peptides will also be loaded on MHC class I molecules, resulting in the activation of CD8$^+$ T cells. Thus, both naïve CD4$^+$ and CD8$^+$ T cells are primed by recipient DCs by the indirect pathway. This pathway is thought to be important in chronic graft rejection, since the perpetual trafficking of recipient DCs through the transplanted tissue is likely to provide a continuous stimulus for the indirect alloresponse. It may therefore represent an important threat to long-term graft survival.

13.4.2 *Role of Effector Cells*

The central role of CD4$^+$ T cells in graft rejection is demonstrated by the inability of CD4-deficient mice to reject allografts. As explained in chapter 8, effector CD4$^+$ T cells can be of two types and both have a role in graft rejection. T$_{H1}$ cells produce IFN-γ and IL-2. Both these cytokines activate CD8$^+$ CTLs and NK cells, whereas IFN-γ acts on macrophages. CTLs and NK cells cause the graft cells to apoptose (chapter 11), while activated macrophages cause a DTH reaction as outlined in chapter 15. Furthermore, T$_{H1}$ cells express FasL, and hence can cause the apoptosis of Fas-expressing graft cells. Additionally, T$_{H1}$ cells promote the synthesis of complement-fixing antibody isotypes by B cells (IgG2a and IgG2b in mice, IgG1 and IgG3 in humans). Such antibodies are capable of causing lysis of graft cells. In contrast, T$_{H2}$ cells trigger eosinophil activation. Eosinophils are recruited and activated within the allograft through the combined action of IL-4, IL-5, and IL-13 produced by alloreactive T$_{H2}$ cells. Activated eosinophils have been shown to mediate graft rejection in experimental models without the participation of CTLs, macrophages, and NK cells. The importance of this pathway in clinical graft rejection is yet to be clarified. Hypereosinophilia preceding graft rejection has been reported in a number of cases, and activated eosinophils have been shown to be present within the liver, kidney, or heart allografts undergoing acute rejection.

Although not as important as T cells, B cells can also play a role in graft rejection. Antibodies are found to play a greater role in the rejection of tissues that are either directly connected to the host's blood supply, like the kidney and the heart, or in recipients sensitized to donor antigens. Patients that have undergone multiple pregnancies, blood transfusions, or previous transplantations (called hyperimmunized patients) may have B cells primed against alloantigens. These B cells can present alloantigens to recipient T cells by the indirect pathway and thus enter into cognate interaction with these T cells. Activation of B cells results in an antibody response against graft cells. Opsonized graft cells are damaged by complement-mediated lysis or ADCC. A history of transplant rejections is associated with an increase in the risk of acute humoral rejection.

---

[4] Cross-presentation is the loading of peptides derived from exogenous antigens on MHC class I molecules. Cross-presentation and the role of DCs in this process is discussed in chapter 7.

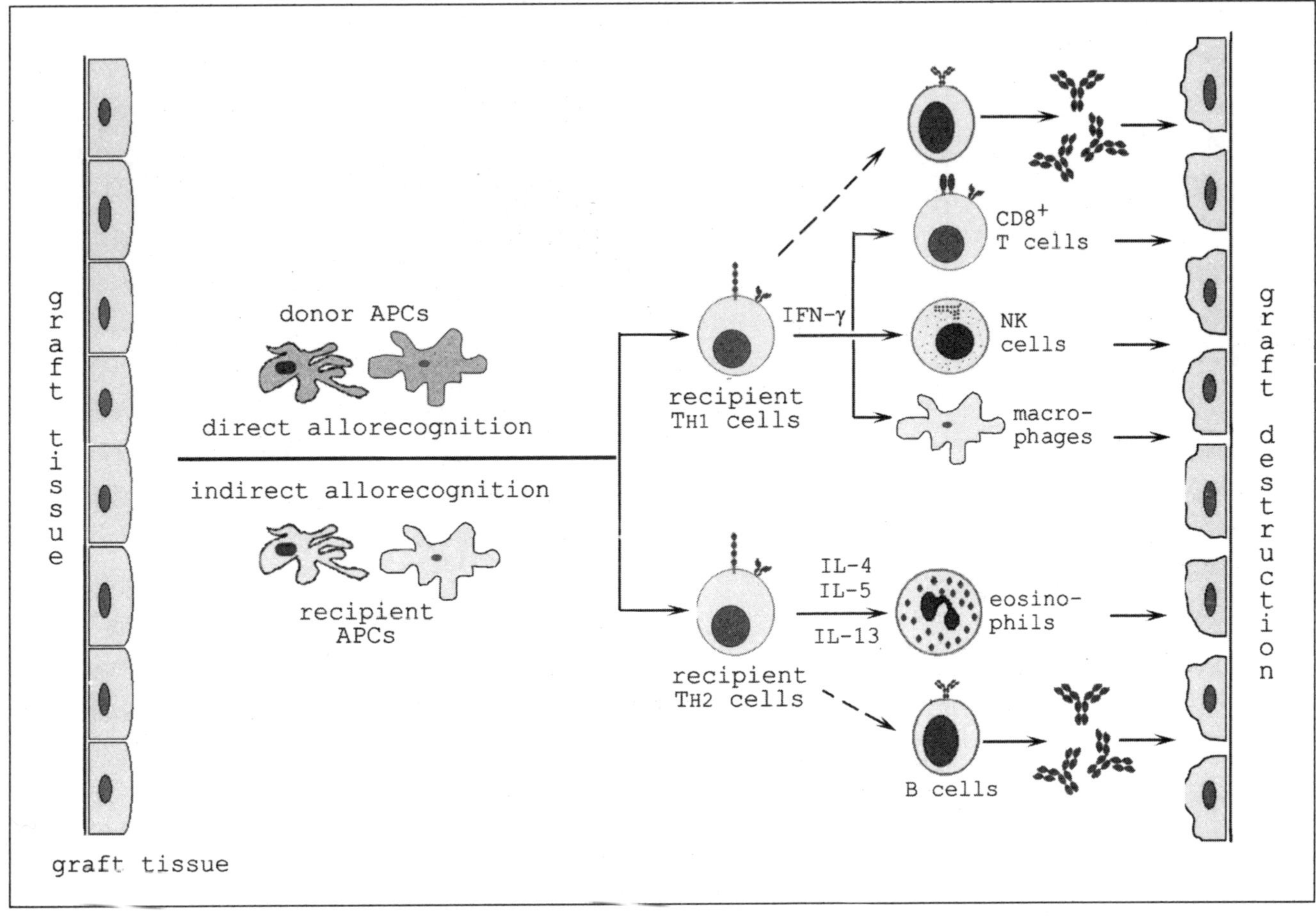

Figure 13.2 ***Both recipient TH1 and TH2 cells are involved in graft rejection.*** *Upon first exposure, graft antigens activate naïve host CD4+ T cells via both the direct and indirect pathways. The activated T cells eventually differentiate to type 1 and type 2 helper T cells. Recipient TH1 cells have a major role to play in graft rejection. Cytokines like IFN-γ secreted by the T cells help in the activation of CD8+ T cells, NK cells, and macrophages. They release cytotoxic substances that cause extensive graft tissue damage. TH1 cells also induce apoptosis in graft cells expressing Fas. Cytokines like IL-4, IL-5, and IL-13 released by TH2 cells activate host eosinophils. The activated eosinophils participate in graft destruction. Additionally, TH cells also help antigen-activated B cells to proliferate and differentiate to plasma cells. Igs secreted by the plasma cells also participate in graft rejection.*

13.5 Graft Versus Host Disease

GVHD or **G**raft **V**ersus **H**ost **D**isease is a condition that is observed after allogeneic bone marrow transplantation, and it is a significant cause of morbidity in patients. It occurs when donor immunocompetent T cells react to and attack the genetically disparate host. In stark contrast to graft rejection, the host tissue is under attack in GVHD, and the *donor T cells* are responsible for the damage. Clinical manifestations of acute GVHD include weight loss and solid organ toxicity affecting the lungs, liver, skin, and gut. GVHD is a multi-step process (fig. 13.3).

❑ **The induction phase follows a typical T cell recognition and activation cascade.** The systemic vasculature, including capillary beds, potentially represents the first extensive area of contact between donor T cells and recipient alloantigens. MHC mismatch therefore results in immediate and extensive activation of these T cells. In the event that the major MHC antigens are matched, minor MHC antigens can still activate donor T cells, resulting in GVHD. Direct allogeneic recognition (ie, recognition of recipient MHC molecules with or without peptides, expressed on recipient APCs) is thought to be responsible for activation of donor T cells. CD4+ T cells from the donors are the first to be activated, although CD8+ donor T cells do get involved later.

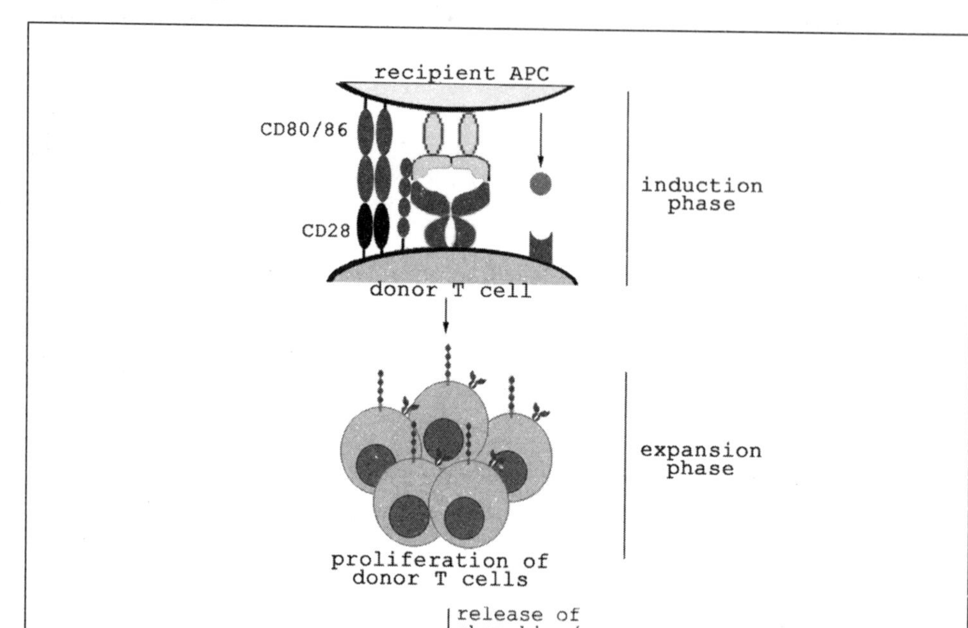

Figure 13.3 GVHD occurs in three phases. In the induction phase the donor T cells get activated by contact with recipient APCs. CD4$^+$ T cells are the first to be activated, although CD8$^+$ T cells may also get involved at a later stage (not shown). The activated T cells undergo proliferation and differentiation in the expansion phase. The cytokines and chemokines produced by these cells recruit recipient effector cells such as macrophages, PMNs, and NK cells to the graft site. Cytokines released by these cells are responsible for the extensive host tissue damage observed in GVHD.

❏ **In the expansion phase, activated donor T cells proliferate and produce cytokines and chemokines.** This release of cytokines is termed a 'cytokine storm', since the term seems to accurately describe the clinical picture. There is a suggestion that the course of GVHD may be influenced by the polarization of T cells, since some data indicates that a T$_{H1}$ type response activates CTLs and GVHD, whereas a T$_{H2}$ type response results in a humoral response and prevention of GVHD. However, other studies indicate that under certain conditions, T$_{H1}$ cytokines may also have a protective effect. It thus seems likely that the two sets of cytokines have a complex role in GVHD, and further studies are needed to clarify this.

❏ **In the effector phase, the recruited recipient cells act in tandem with donor T cells and cause damage to recipient organs.** The cytokines released by donor T cells lead to the recruitment phase, wherein other cells like NK cells, macrophages, and PMNs infiltrate the site of activation. Host tissue damage occurs by multiple pathways — release of cytotoxic molecules by NK cells and CTLs, damage due to ROI and RNI released by macrophages, induction of apoptosis by the Fas pathway, etc.

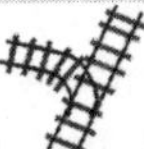

Patience of a Saint and the Tolerance of a Mother: Why the Foetus is Not Rejected

From a genetic perspective, the mother and foetus are never identical in an outbred population because the foetus inherits a set of polymorphic genes from each parent. Thus, the foetus differs from the mother in multiple tissue antigens. The mother's immune system has a difficult mandate. It must protect both, the mother and the foetus against invading pathogens or altered cells while allowing the survival and growth of the allogeneic foeto-placental unit. The chances of multiple pregnancies also mean that the mother's immune system is going to be exposed to paternal alloantigens repeatedly, allowing the formation of memory cells and the possibility of secondary responses. However, the immune system has to be subverted enough to allow these pregnancies to succeed. How the allogeneic foetus avoids immune rejection during pregnancy is one of the enduring enigmas in the field of transplantation immunology. Elucidating the mechanisms involved in the maternal tolerance of the foetus have proved difficult, since most experiments can only be carried out in animal models and then merely extrapolated to humans. Nonetheless, experiments suggest that multiple mechanisms are responsible for the acceptance of foetal allograft.

❑ **Lack of MHC expression.** Similar to other immunoprivileged sites, the cells of the trophoblastic surface that envelops the embryo and constitutes the foeto-maternal interface lack MHC class I and class II molecules and have an increased expression of FasL. The extra-villous trophoblast cells which come in direct contact with maternal blood express the classical class I MHC molecule HLA-C and the non-classical MHC class I molecules HLA-E and HLA-G, allowing them to escape both CTL and NK cell attack.

❑ **Role of NK cells.** The predominant lymphocytes at the foetal implantation site are CD56^{bright} NK cells. The infiltration of the site by NK cells is because of the influence of progesterone, endometrial IL-15, and prolactin; the cells disappear at 20 weeks of gestation. These uterine NK cells express high levels of inhibitory receptors CD94/NKG2 and are thought to influence both the cytokine milieu and innate immune responses at the foeto-maternal interface.

❑ **Cytokine milieu.** A balance of T$_{H}$1 and T$_{H}$2 cytokines is also thought to be critical to the survival of the foetus and a successful pregnancy. Local dominance of T$_{H}$2 cytokines is thought to protect the immunologically foreign foeto-placental unit against CMI and non-specific innate and inflammatory phagocytic responses. Pro-inflammatory T$_{H}$1 cytokines like IFN-γ and TNF-α have been shown to be embryotoxic. IL-1 and TNF-α have been reported to regulate trophoblastic cell apoptosis, protease production, and angiogenesis. Anti-inflammatory T$_{H}$2 cytokines such as IL-4, IL-10, and TGF-β, on the other hand, are proposed to play a role in preventing maternal rejection of the foetal allograft. They have been shown to deactivate macrophages and downregulate their cytokine production.

❑ **T$_{R}$ cells.** They are thought to have a role in the production of immunosuppressive cytokines like TGF-β and IL-10 that are responsible for the induction of tolerance.

❑ **Complement regulation.** Murine trophoblastic embryo cells express complement inhibitor Crry (**C**omplement **r**eceptor 1 **r**elated protein **y**). This protein is structurally related to DAF and MCP and inhibits the deposition of activated complement components C3 and C4 on the surface of autologous cells. It therefore prevents the inappropriate and potentially destructive effect of the activation of the complement cascade. Human placental cells and trophoblasts do not express Crry but express DAF and MCP instead. Hence, these molecules are thought to play a similar role in protecting the foetus from activated complement components.

❑ **Tryptophan starvation.** Activated T cells are sensitive to tryptophan availability; tryptophan starvation induces T cell cycle arrest and accelerated AICD. **I**ndoleamine 2,3-**dio**xygenase (IDO) is a haem-containing enzyme that catalyzes the first step in the oxidative degradation of tryptophan. Maternal cells expressing IDO are found to surround the murine embryo soon after implantation. IDO is also expressed in human placental tissue. It is therefore postulated that IDO expressing cells may help in tolerance induction or maintenance by locally decreasing the amount of available tryptophan to activated T cells. Thus, these IDO expressing cells may act as potent immunosuppressive cells.

GVHD can be divided into acute or chronic based on the time of onset, pathophysiological processes, and clinical presentations. Acute GVHD involves mostly the skin, gastrointestinal tract, and liver, and it occurs within the first 100 days of transplant. It is directed against multiple host cells, including epithelial cells and mucosa of the skin, hair follicles, bile duct, cryptic cells of the intestines, airways, mucous membranes, the bone marrow, and cells of the immune system. Between 9–50% of HLA-matched bone marrow transplants with intensive immunosuppressive therapy report clinically significant GVHD; the figure is 100% without such therapy. GVHD is said to be chronic if it appears within 100 days of engraftment. However, much remains to be elucidated on the mechanisms underlying chronic GVHD. Since donor T cells are responsible for GVHD, methods aimed at depleting them from the graft used in conjunction with immunosuppressive therapy are the only means of prophylaxis. mAbs against T cell markers like CD3, CD5, and CD2 have been used successfully in experimental models and clinical situations. Treating GVHD once it has occurred is much more difficult, and the use of steroids in conjunction with immunosuppressive therapy remains the treatment of choice.

13.6 Immunosuppressive Therapies

The ultimate aim of any transplantation procedure is the induction of tolerance to the transplant, ie, to allow the graft to survive indefinitely in the absence of immunosuppression. Although this has proven difficult to achieve, the introduction of a number of new drugs and strategies has allowed transplantation to become a standard option following organ failure. Currently, immunosuppressive drugs are used in the clinic for three purposes.

❑ **Induction therapy** is given to switch off the immune system approximately two weeks post-engraftment to reduce the likelihood of immediate rejection. Drugs used in induction therapy are broad spectrum agents that depress the entire immune response.

❑ **Maintenance therapy** is used to reduce the immune system's ability to recognize and reject foreign tissue. Often, combinations of synergistic drugs are used in maintenance. The drugs are chosen on the basis of their ability to interfere with the immune system at different sites. This allows each drug to be used at low dosages, and thus, reduce drug-related toxicity. This approach allows the immune system to remain functional at levels sufficient to protect it against infections and malignancies.

❑ **Specific treatments** are aimed at treating episodes of acute rejection.

Immunosuppression jeopardizes the well-being of transplant patients in two ways. Firstly, there is an increased risk of malignancies. Between 1–5% transplant recipients develop malignancies within a few years of receiving their allograft. This represents an almost 100% increase in risk, compared to the general population, and underscores the importance of a functional immune system in controlling neoplasms. Transplant patients are particularly prone to developing B cell lymphomas. Interestingly, there does not seem to be an increased risk of developing other types of cancers (breast, lung, colon, prostrate) that are common in the rest of the population. Secondly, the patient is at an increased risk of infections. Infections are a major cause of morbidity in solid organ transplant patients. The type of infection is often dependent upon the type of transplant — pyelonephritis and cystitis is common in renal transplants, bronchitis is common in lung transplants, etc. Administration of pre- and post-operative antibiotics is therefore necessary to combat infections. Immunosuppressive agents used in current clinical practice include the following (fig. 13.4).

❑ **Calcineurin inhibitors.** They include cyclosprine A (CsA) and tacrolimus (FK506). These are the cornerstones of successful long-term immunosuppressive regimens. Calcineurin is a phosphatase crucial for intracellular events leading to IL-2 gene transcription in T cells (chapter 6). Both FK506 and CsA are called prodrugs because they have to form complexes with cellular proteins, called

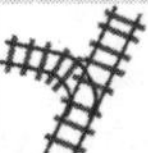

Edmonton Shows the Way: Successfully Transplanting Islet Cells

Diabetes mellitus and its associated complications affect more than 6% of people worldwide (chapter 14). Insulin administration has been the only real treatment for these patients so far. Although islet transplantation had been tried in the past, the hope that this approach would result in exogenous insulin-free life for the patient remained a dream. Less than 10% patients achieved insulin-independence for periods of a year or more. One of the major problems with this approach was that treatment used to induce immunosuppression often resulted in damage to the insulin-producing β cells or induced peripheral insulin-resistance. In 1999, researchers in the University of Alberta in Edmonton, Canada, developed a method of transplanting islet cells that allowed >80% of patients to remain insulin independent for more than a year. Called the 'Edmonton protocol', the method has since been used in international multi-centre trails in a number of patients. It involves transplanting well-characterized pancreatic islet cells into portal circulation. The protocol uses islets from two donors; for as yet unexplained reasons, the use of islets from a single donor failed to result in insulin-independence. The donor and recipients are matched for blood group antigens and cross-matched to ensure absence of lymphocytotoxic antibodies. Most importantly (and surprisingly), the protocol does not call for HLA-matching of the donor and the recipient! Islet cells are transplanted as quickly as possible to minimize cold ischaemic damage. The protocol uses a xenoprotein-free medium for preparing the islet cells. Media used in tissue culture contain between 5–10% foetal bovine serum. The researchers argued that the use of bovine serum could result in the graft cells being coated non-specifically with bovine proteins and target them for immediate destruction. Hence, they used 25% human serum albumin in place of foetal bovine serum. One of the key elements of the Edmonton protocol is the avoidance of corticosteroids. Instead, it uses a combination of sirolimus and low dose tacrolimus to achieve immunosuppression. The patients are given an inductive course of Daclizumab (anti-CD25 (IL-2R) mAb) to enhance graft survival. The combined therapy prevents the activation of T cells and therefore the triggering of an immune response.

Despite the success of the protocol, islet-transplantation remains restricted to patients with severe hyperglycaemia and is presently unsuitable for the majority of patients with type I diabetes mellitus. Most patients require two to three procedures before they can achieve complete insulin-independence. Although the risk of malignancies and life-threatening sepsis has been low in the patients treated to date, fears of these complications do limit the broader application of this technique (eg, in patients with less severe form of diabetes and in children). Also, while being less toxic than the earlier drugs, the medications used do result (amongst other things) in mouth ulcerations, weight loss, anaemia, and elevated cholesterol. Thus, though the Edmonton protocol is an important step forward in diabetes treatment, further refinements are needed to improve upon its safety and applicability.

immunophilins, to be able to exert their effects. FK506 binds FKBP (FK506 **B**inding **P**roteins) whereas CsA binds cyclophilin. Both these drugs are highly specific for T cells, and their effects are reversed upon discontinuation of the drug. They inhibit activation of mature $CD4^+$ and $CD8^+$ T cells after they have received the activation signal through an APC. Haematopoiesis and maturation of lymphoid stem cells is not affected. In clinical trials, both the drugs have been shown to prolong the survival of transplanted hearts, kidneys, livers, etc and have similar renal and hepatic toxicities.

❑ **IL-2R antagonists.** IL-2R is a complex of non-covalently linked polypeptide chains (α, β, γ). The α chain (CD25) is expressed on activated T cells. IL-2 activates T cells in an autocrine manner; the binding of IL-2 produced by activated T cells to IL-2R expressed on their cell surface results in their proliferation. Anti-IL-2R mAbs bind to IL-2R and thereby block the binding of IL-2 to the receptor. IL-2R antagonists therefore inhibit the proliferation of T cells. Two antagonists — Basilximab and Daclizumab — have been successfully used in the induction phase in clinical trials, and neither was found to increase the incidence of malignancy or opportunistic infections.

❑ **Lymphocyte depleting agents.** These can be used in the induction phase of rejection and to treat steroid-resistant rejection. They are useful in depleting T cells from donor bone marrow prior to engraftment. Being powerful immunosuppressants, they increase the risk of infections and malignancy. Consequently, use of these agents is limited to a total of less than 21 days, and they are used in conjunction with steroids to reduce adverse reactions.

- **Anti-CD3 antibody** (OKT3) is a mouse mAb against human CD3 that interferes with antigen binding and signal transduction. Its action is very rapid with peripheral T cell depletion occurring within minutes of administrating the antibody. Its effect is reversible; T cell numbers return to normal following its discontinuation. OKT3 has been used to prevent the acute rejection of heart, kidney, and liver transplants as well as to prevent GVHD. Administration of the first dose of OKT3 can cause a sudden and massive release of cytokines, resulting in manifestations ranging from mild flu-like symptoms to life-threatening shock. Other toxic side effects include encephalopathy, nephropathy, and hypotension. Repeated usage can result in the development of human anti-mouse antibodies. Although not yet in routine usage, anti-CD2 and anti-CD154 antibodies may also be used to selectively deplete T cells.
- **ATG** (Antithymocyte globulin) is a purified Ig preparation from hyperimmune serum of horses or rabbits immunized with human thymocytes. ATG administration results in the depletion of peripheral T cells. Major side effects include anaphylactic reactions, serum sickness, leucopenia, thrombocytopenia, and nephritis.

❑ **Antiproliferative agents.** These inhibit proliferation and differentiation of activated lymphocytes. Purine and pyrimidine analogues are powerful antiproliferative agents, since they interfere with DNA synthesis. Purine analogues used include azathioprine (AZT) and **M**ycophenolate **m**ofetil (MMF), whereas **M**alono**n**itril**a**minde (MNA) is the pyrimidine analogue in clinical usage.

- **AZT** is the imidazole derivative of 6-mercaptopurine. In the liver it is converted to 6-mercaptopurine which is converted to 6-mercaptopurine ribonucleotide, a structural analogue of inositol monophosphate, in the cell. It therefore causes feedback inhibition of enzymes involved in nucleic acid synthesis. It interferes

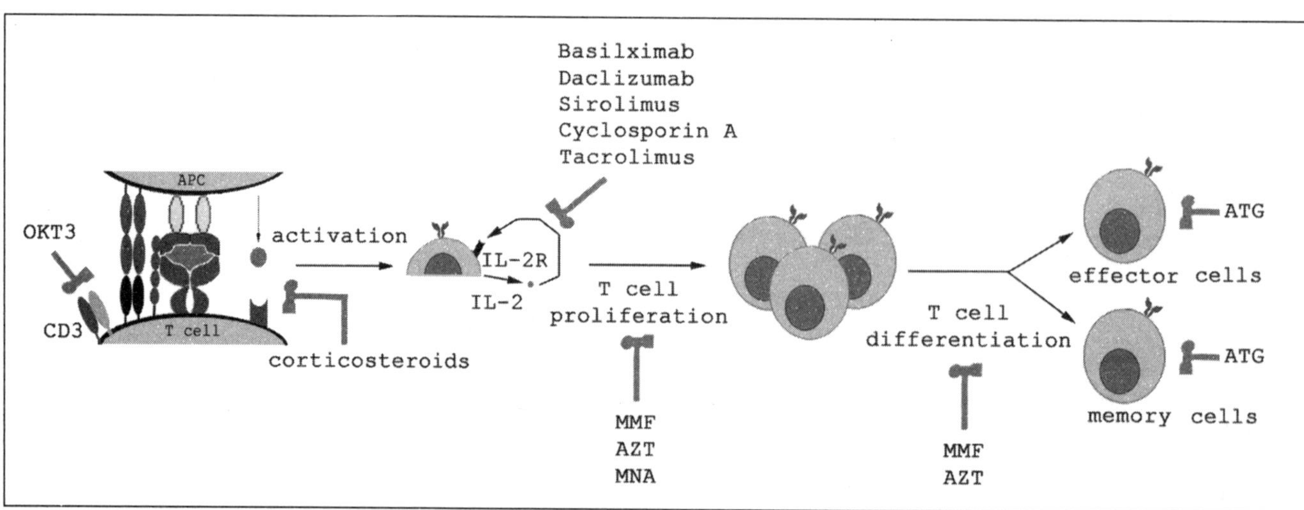

Figure 13.4 Different therapeutic agents can be used to target the various stages of a developing anti-graft immune response. *OKT3, a murine anti-human CD3 mAb, interferes with antigen binding and signal transduction. Corticosteroids inhibit gene transcription of a number of cytokines. Various agents can be used to target T cell proliferation. Basilximab, Daclizumab, and IL-2R antagonists block the binding of IL-2 to its receptor, whereas Cyclosprine A, Tacrolimus, and Sirolimus interfere with IL-2 gene expression. Sirolimus also causes the arrest of T cells in the G1 phase. Azathoiprine (AZT), mycophenolate mofetil (MMF), and malononitrilaminde (MNA) are nucleotide analogues that interfere with T cell proliferation and differentiation. ATG (antithymocyte globulin) is a purified Ig preparation. Its administration results in the depletion of peripheral T cells.*

with the proliferative cycle of B and T cells and prevents effector cell formation. It is thus a powerful inhibitor of primary but not secondary immune responses. AZT also suppresses neutrophil generation and macrophage activation. Its use is now on the decline because of potent adverse effects resulting from its ability to affect all rapidly growing cells, and its hepatotoxicity.

- **MMF** is an ester of mycophenolic acid. It inhibits the enzyme inosine monophosphate dehydrogenase involved in the 'de novo' pathway of DNA synthesis. This is the sole pathway of DNA synthesis in both B and T cells. Hence, unlike AZT, MMF is a selective inhibitor of T and B cell proliferation; other cells like bone marrow cells and parenchymal cells that can utilize the alternative 'salvage pathway' of purine synthesis are spared. MMF is therefore quickly replacing AZT in treatment of acute rejection. Preliminary results indicate that it may also be of use in the treatment of chronic rejection and may promote tolerance to donor antigens. Adverse effects are less severe than those of AZT and include diarrhoea and gastritis.

- **MNA** inhibits both B and T cell proliferation by interfering with pyrimidine biosynthesis. It is also thought to interfere with T cell tyrosine kinases. It is now undergoing clinical trials for use in the treatment of acute rejection.

❑ **Agents interfering with cytokine gene expression.** Two main types of agents fall in this category — those that interfere with the expression of a number of cytokine genes and those that interfere with downstream IL-2 signalling.

- **Corticosteroids** are the most commonly used immunosuppressive and anti-inflammatory agents in clinical practice, although due to their adverse side-effects, most regimens try to minimize their use. Predinisone, the prototypic agent, is analogous to the major endogenous corticosteroid cortisol (hydro-cortisone) except that it is four times more potent than cortisol. Corticosteroids inhibit gene transcription of a number of cytokines such as IL-1, IL-2, IL-6, IFN-γ, and TNF-α by cells of the immune system. They also induce lympho-cytopenia by causing redistribution of lymphocytes from the intravascular space to the lymphoid space, although the reason for this redistribution is not clear. Low doses of corticosteroids are used in combination with other drugs such as CsA and MMF for maintenance therapy whereas high doses may be used for short terms to treat acute rejections. They may also be used to minimize hypersensitivity reactions to ATG or mAbs. High doses of the drug can cause severe side effects, including hypertension, diabetes, weight gain, osteoporosis, gastrointestinal bleeding, opportunistic infections, cataracts, and the poor healing of wounds.

- **Sirolimus** (rapamycin) is a macrolide antibiotic structurally similar to FK506. It binds to FKBP but causes the arrest of T cells in G1 phase by binding to a unique cellular target, called mammalian target of rapamycin. Binding of sirolimus to this protein inhibits activation of p70^{s6} kinase and thus arrests synthesis of proteins required for cell cycle progression. In addition, it also blocks signals delivered by IL-2, IL-4, and IL-6 to T cells. It thus interferes with late events in the signalling cascade. Although they bind to the same protein, FK506 and sirolimus are found to be synergistic *in vivo*. Use of sirolimus in combination therapy with FK506 and CsA has allowed a reduction in dosages of all the drugs involved. It also has relatively fewer side effects, though it can cause hypercholesterolaemia and hence increase the risk of heart disease. It is often used in maintenance regimens as well as in treating chronic rejection.

13.7 Blood Transfusion

Although Jean-Baptiste Denis in France and Richard Lower in England separately reported the transfusion of blood from lambs to humans in 1667, it was Karl Landsteiner who opened the door to routine transfusions with his discovery of antigens on human erythrocytes. He described the presence of the A and B blood groups and called the third O (ie, lacking both A and B). His colleagues Descatello and Sterli reported the fourth (AB) blood group. To date, the international society of blood transfusion recognizes 270 blood group determinants ascribed to 26 blood group systems. Most erythrocytic surface antigens are located on the integral membrane polypeptides and glycoproteins or, in some cases, membrane glycolipids. Most blood group antigens are proteinic in nature, with the blood group specificity determined primarily by the amino acid sequence. The membrane proteins are divided into four types, based on their integration in the lipid layer. The first two categories consist of antigens that pass the membrane once and are anchored in it by either their NH_2– or COOH– terminus (the Indian and Kell group antigens respectively). A third group consists of antigens that span the membrane several times (eg, Rh and Duffy group antigens). The last type consists of glycoproteins that are anchored in the membrane by a **glycosylphosphatidylinositol** (GPI) anchor. This is a fatty acid anchor that is inserted into the membrane and is attached to the protein through a carbohydrate (fig. 13.5).

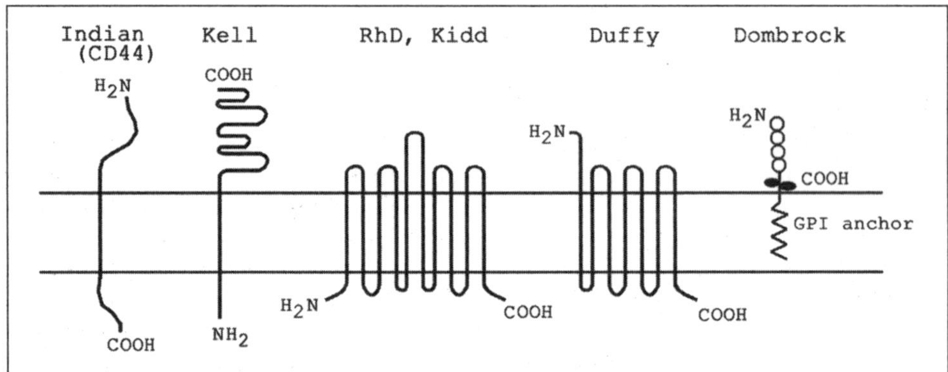

Figure 13.5 Different types of integral cell membrane proteins confer antigenicity to erythrocytes. The proteins are anchored either at their Amino– or Carboxy– termini or via a GPI anchor (Adapted from Weiner Klinische Wochenschrift (2001) 113:781).

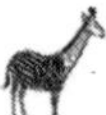
O Bombay, No *Kidd*ing: Blood groups in the Indian Subcontinent

While the blood group O is the most common in the world, the incidence of type B is unusually high in Asia; the concentration of type B reaches a whopping 21% in Northern India. Interestingly, the recognition that the O group has the H antigen and is due to Hh alleles was a result of a report by Bhende et al., in 1952. They reported the first three individuals who completely lacked A and B antigens, but did not belong to the O group. This null phenotype was named 'Bombay' after the city it was first reported in. Although this phenotype is extremely rare in most populations, it is relatively easier to find in India. The reported frequency of the Bombay phenotype is 1:7600. The Bombay phenotype is due to a recessive gene at the H locus (labelled h). Persons with the Bombay phenotype do not have the H gene and hence cannot produce α(1,2) fucosyl transferase. Without the basic H structure, the A and B enzymes cannot function since they use UDP-N-acetylgalactose or UDP-galactose to convert the H antigen to A and B antigens respectively. Individuals with the Bombay phenotype have severe transfusion reactions if transfused with the 'normal' O blood group, because of the presence of anti-H antibodies in their serum.

The first example of the Kidd antibody was reported in 1951, and it is named after Mrs. Kidd, who had antibodies that caused haemolytic disease in her newborn son. Many individuals of Asian or Polynesian backgrounds, including Indians and Japanese, completely lack the Kidd antigen. The Kidd antigen is on the urea transporter found not only on erythrocytes but also on kidney cells. RBCs from the Kidd⁻ phenotype (called Jkᵃ⁻ᵇ⁻) have been shown to be resistant to lysis in high concentrations of urea as opposed to normal cells that lyse within a minute of urea exposure.

Despite the cloning and sequencing of most of the genes involved in the antigenicity of erythrocytes, relatively little is known about their functions and/or the biological significance of their polymorphisms.

❑ Some blood group antigens are membrane transporters involved in the transport of molecules across the erythrocyte membrane.
- The Diego blood antigen is an anion transporter.
- The Kidd glycoprotein is an urea transporter.
- The Colton glycoprotein is a water channel.
- The Rh proteins and Rh associated glycoproteins have a structure characteristic of a transporter. They belong to a family of proteins that facilitate ammonium transport in lower organisms, leading to the suggestion that Rh proteins could be involved in ammonium transport and that erythrocytes may protect against ammonium toxicity to the brain by transporting ammonium ions to the liver or kidney for metabolism or excretion.

❑ The Duffy glycoprotein is a member of G protein coupled superfamily of chemokine receptors.

❑ The Kell glycoprotein is an endopeptidase and may be involved in the formation of endothelin, a vasoconstrictor.

❑ The Cromer antigen is the complement regulatory protein DAF (CD55).

13.7.1 ABO and Rh Blood Groups

Out of the myriad blood groups recognized, only the ABO and Rh groups are matched for routine transfusions, and only those will be considered here.

❑ The **ABO** (and the related Lewis or Le) blood group antigens are different from other groups described above in that these are not proteinic but carbohydrate antigens, ie, the epitopes are the result of oligosaccharides attached to glycoproteins or glycolipids. The genes that govern their polymorphisms do not encode the antigen directly but encode glycosyl transferases that catalyse the addition of the defining monosaccharide to an oligosaccharide substrate. The ABO antigens are attached to a variety of glycoproteins on erythrocyte surfaces. Most are attached to antigens such as Diego, glycophorin A, and MN, or to glucose transporters, though they may also be present on any of the other glycoproteins and glycolipids. These carbohydrates at the erythrocyte surface comprise the glycocalyx (or cell coat), and this extracellular matrix of carbohydrates protects the cell from mechanical damage and microbial attack. It may also prevent cellular aggregation.

Many of the original assumptions about these antigens have now proven erroneous. Originally, four groups had been recognized based on the presence or absence of two epitopes, A and B. It is now established that the A group consists of two subgroups A_1 and A_2. A_2, being less prevalent than A_1, was missed in earlier investigations[5]. The group O was originally thought to lack any antigen but is now known to possess the H antigen. The Bombay group lacks this H antigen and is thus truly O (see sidetrack '*O* Bombay, No *Kidd*ing'). Structures similar to ABO antigens are found on some plants and micro-organisms. Consequently, individuals who do not express these antigens produce anti-A, anti-B, or anti-O antibodies upon encountering them via food or infections. Transfusion of ABO incompatible blood to a recipient therefore results in severe reactions.

The structure and synthesis of ABO antigens is well established. A core polysaccharide consisting of N-acetylgalactose-galactose-N-acetylglucose-galactose attached to proteins or lipids anchored in the erythrocyte cell membrane forms the backbone of the ABH and Le antigens. H^6 antigen is the result of the addition of a fucose to this core polysaccharide by a fucosyl transferase enzyme (FUT1, H glycosyl transferase, or H enzyme). Hexoses attached to the branched

[5] Type A_1 appears to exist to the exclusion of type A_2 among Australian aborigines and Eskimos, and amongst the inhabitants of parts of Indonesia, Pacific islands, Canada, India, and northern USA. The highest incidence is amongst the Blackfoot and Blood Indians in Canada and USA. Its highest frequency is 50% among the Lapps.

[6] Why H? Because it is a **H**eterophile antigen shared with many plants and microbes.

polysaccharide H antigen give the A, B, or Le epitopes (Table 13.1). The A allele of the ABH gene codes for the A enzyme and the B allele codes for the B enzyme. Being codominant, when present together, both A and B epitopes are added to yield the AB blood group. Lack of both the enzymes results in an inability to modify the H antigen and generates the O blood group (Table 13.1). The structurally related Lewis groups are also coded by allelic genes that result in four groups (Le^a, Le^b, Le$^-$, and Le^{a+b+}). Interestingly, synthesis of these glycolipids does not occur in erythroid tissue, but the epitopes are acquired by erythrocyte membranes from other tissues through the circulating soluble forms bound to lipoproteins.

Table 13.1 ABO blood group system

Group	Genotype	Enzyme(s) present	Structure of minimal epitope		Serum antibodies
A	AA, AH	A (N-acetyl galactosaminyl transferase) H (α(1,2) fucosyl transferase)	A H	GalNAc–α1–3 ╲ Gal–β1–l ╱ Fuc–α1–2	anti-B
B	BB, BH	B (galactosyl transferase) H (α(1,2) fucosyl transferase)	B H	Gal–α1–3 ╲ Gal–β1–R ╱ Fuc–α1–2	anti-A
AB	AB	A (N-acetyl galactosaminyl transferase) H (α(1,2) fucosyl transferase) B (galactosyl transferase)	A H B H	GalNAc–α1–3 ╲ Gal–β1–R ╱ Fuc–α1–2 Gal–α1–3 ╲ Gal–β1–R ╱ Fuc–α1–2	none
O	HH, Hh	H (α(1,2) fucosyl transferase)	H	Fuc–α1–2–Gal–β1–R	anti-A, anti-B
Bombay	hh	α(1,2) fucosyl transferase absent	–	Gal–β1–R	anti-A, anti-B, anti-H

❑ **The Rh system.** Discovered by Landsteiner and Weiner, this antigen was called Rh because it is also found in the Rhesus monkey. Those who had the antigen were called Rh$^+$ whereas those who lacked it were termed Rh$^-$. It was later realized that the **Rh antigen is not a single antigen but a group of alloantigens**. It is one of the most complex of blood group systems with 45 determinants. The D antigen is the most immunogenic of all the protein blood groups. D$^-$ individuals lack the whole RhD protein and therefore mount an immune response to a variety of epitopes on the extracellular domains of the RhD protein. Rh incompatibility is found to cause Erythroblastosis foetalis, a severe haemolytic disease in new borns. The disease is a result of Rh incompatibility between the foetus and the mother, ie, when the mother is Rh$^-$ and the foetus Rh$^+$ (due to an Rh$^+$ father). If the mother has been previously exposed to Rh antigens (eg, during previous pregnancies), IgG antibodies from the sensitized mother cross the placenta and coat foetal erythrocytes. Such coated erythrocytes are destroyed by the phagocytic cells in the liver, causing haemolytic anaemia in the foetus and newborn infant (chapter 15).

13.7.2 Potential Transfusion Hazards

Two major hazards have to be considered while transfusing blood or blood products.

❑ **Transfusion reactions.** The identification of alloantigens on the surface of erythrocytes is called blood typing or blood grouping (Appendix III). The matching of donor and recipient blood groups for ABO and Rh antigens is essential for the

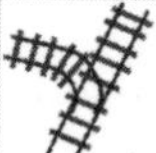

Sweet Disposition Sweet Advantages: Secretors and Non-secretors

ABH and Le alloantigens are present not only on the erythrocytes but also on other tissue cells such as cells of the kidneys, liver, and even sperm. About 80% of the human population also produces blood group alloantigens in a soluble form, and these are found in saliva, sweat, gastric juices, etc. People belonging to this majority are called secretors. The remaining 20% do not produce soluble blood group antigens and constitute the non-secretors. Alleles of a single gene (Se/se) control this trait. It is thought that the presence of these secreted blood group mucins may influence the type of bacteria that take up residence in gut—some gut bacteria produce enzymes that allow them to degrade the terminal sugar of the ABH blood type antigens and use it as a source of energy. The secreted antigens may also bind and neutralize dietary lectins. Such lectins that can bind ABH antigens could otherwise have a disruptive effect on cells expressing these antigens. Secretors are found to have less dental cavities than non-secretors, giving rise to the suggestion that salivary ABH antigens may aggregate some oral bacteria, preventing them from colonizing dental surfaces. Overall, non-secretors seem to be at a higher risk of infections including those caused by *Helicobacter pylori*, *Neisseria* spp., and *Candida* spp., and to bacterial urinary tract infections. It is thought that the ABH non-secretor state is associated with the strategy of allowing the invader in and then attempting to destroy it internally (defence in depth strategy), whereas the secretor state does not allow the invader to enter in the first place (preclusive strategy).

success of solid organ transplants and for blood transfusion. Transfusion of improperly matched blood can result in severe immunological reactions that may prove fatal (Table 13.2). Although transfusion reactions are often due to the activation of the recipient's humoral response against antigens on donor erythrocytes, it is possible that antibodies in the donor blood may cause lysis of recipient erythrocytes. This reaction is akin to GVHD and results in acute respiratory distress and lung injury or TRALI (**T**ransfusion **R**elated **A**cute **L**ung **I**njury). Cross-matching of the donor and recipient blood ensures absence of a high titre of anti-recipient antibodies in the donor's blood and helps in avoiding TRALI.

❑ **Infections.** Asymptomatic blood donors suffering from infections such as AIDS, Hepatitis, and malaria can transmit the infection to unsuspecting recipients. Transfusion-related AIDS cases have been reported in many countries in the early 1980s. A number of tests developed since then have dramatically reduced the risks of transfusion-related infections. Blood may also get contaminated with skin contaminants during venupuncture and/or collection, which multiply during storage. Proper collection and storage procedures are therefore essential.

Donor procedures that help protect blood supplies from infectious agents include:

- The collection of blood only from volunteers who have nothing to gain from the procedure.
- Extensive screening to ensure that donating blood is not going to harm the donor and the recipient; donor health history is interpreted strictly to assure highest recipient safety.
- A donor's physical examination to ensure good health.
- Examination of donor's arms to confirm that he or she is not a drug user.
- Extensive laboratory testing of each unit of blood to eliminate potentially infectious units — blood group and antibody titre is established; blood is also tested for its haemoglobin content, presence of hepatitis B antigen, and antibodies to infections such as hepatitis C, HIV-1 and -2, syphilis, and HTLV-I and -II (**Human T L**ymphocyte **V**irus). Nonetheless, blood cannot be tested for all possible infectious agents, including ones that can prove fatal (eg, Bovine Spongiform Encephalitis). There is thus a certain inherent risk in any transfusion.

Table 13.2 Transfusion Reactions

Type of reaction	Signs and symptoms	Comments
Febrile (non-haemolytic)	Rise in temperature, rigours, headache, malaise, vomiting	Usually occurs in patients with a history of previous transfusions or pregnancies and is caused by HLA-mismatch
Acute haemolytic reaction (immediate)	Symptoms occur within 15 minutes of transfusion and include fever, chills, haemoglobinuria, renal failure, hypotension, oozing from IV site, back pain, and pain along infusion vein	Caused by the administration of ABO or Rh incompatible blood. Bacterial contamination of the blood can also result in similar symptoms; treatment is aimed primarily at prevention of renal failure
Delayed haemolytic reaction	Weakness, unexplained fall in post-transfusion haemoglobin, elevated serum bilirubin	Usually caused by a previous sensitization to red cell antigens; antibody titre usually too low to be detected in the initial screening
Anaphylactic shock	Urticaria, erythema, respiratory distress, hypotension, laryngeal or pharyngeal oedema, bronchospasm	Caused by antibodies to donor plasma proteins or ingested substances (eg, drugs, foods, chemicals) in donor plasma; treatment consists of administrations of antihistamines and epinephrine
Allergic reaction	Rash, urticaria, flushing	Caused by antibodies to plasma proteins or ingested substances and treated with antihistamines
TRALI	Shortness of breath, hypoxaemia, chills, fever, cyanosis, hypotension, pulmonary oedema	Caused by *donor* antibodies to recipient HLA antigens; treatment is aimed at reducing respiratory distress

13.7.3 Transfusion Alternatives

The advent of the AIDS epidemic led to the emergence of alternatives to blood transfusions. Emergence of vCJD (**variant C**ruzfeldt **J**acob **D**isease, the human variant of the so-called mad cow disease) has given a further impetus to their development. One approach is to stimulate RBC production by the administration of recombinant human erythropoietin or altered erythropoietin. A second approach is the development of artificial oxygen carriers. Such carriers have multiple advantages. They are non-antigenic, sterilizable, and have an extended shelf-life and unlimited availability. However, many carriers in clinical trials seem to have a short intravascular life (about 1–2 hours) and have shown renal toxicity. Additionally, they have also been shown to cause pulmonary and systemic hypertension and immune suppression. Perfluorocarbon emulsions that can dissolve any gas (including O_2 and CO_2), raffinose cross-linked and polymerized human haemoglobin, and recombinant human haemoglobin are being tested in clinical trials. The two principal applications for these artificial oxygen carriers are in patients with trauma and those undergoing surgery, not to forget individuals belonging to religious sects or groups (eg, Jehovah's witnesses) that object to blood transfusions.

Autoimmunity

14

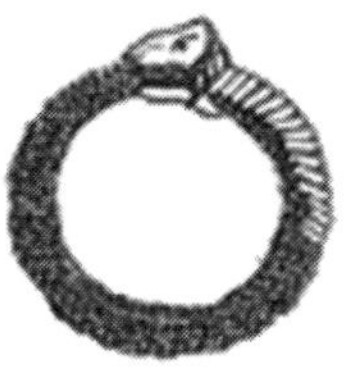

I am the hate you try to hide and I control you
I take you where you want to go
I give you all you need to know
I drag you down, I use you up
Mr. Self Destruct

    —Nine Inch Nails, *Self-Destruction (Final)*

ACh: Actylcholine
ALPS: Autoimmune lymphoproliferative syndrome
EAE: Experimental autoimmune encephalomyelitis
HPA: Hypothalamus-pituitary-adrenal
IDDM: Insulin-dependent diabetes mellitus
MBP: Myelin basic protein
RA: Rheumatoid arthritis
SLE: Systemic Lupus Erythematosus
SNS: Sympathetic nervous system
TNFR: TNF receptor
VLA-4: Very late antigen-4

14.1 Introduction

Armies or arms are considered means of protection. Yet, a bullet shot by a soldier can kill an ally or an enemy; it is where the bullet is targeted that will determine who dies. This harsh reality of weapons possession applies equally to the immune system, the body's private army. The famous immunologist Ehrlich used the term 'horror autotoxicus' to describe what he considered the unwillingness of the organism to endanger itself by the formation of toxic autoantibodies. He thought that an organism would never imperil itself by allowing autoimmune reactions. As it turns out, that was to be one of the few times when this great immunologist was wrong.

In chapter 8, we have explained how T cells bearing high-avidity receptors for self-antigens are negatively selected during development. This process seems to be incomplete, however, and autoreactive T cells[1] and autoreactive antibodies can be found in the peripheral blood of healthy animals. A number of tolerance mechanisms are operational in the periphery to keep potentially dangerous self-reactive cells in check (section 12.3). Most autoreactive antibodies found in healthy individuals are directed against ubiquitous proteins such as albumin, transferrin, cytochrome c, and nucleic proteins, or cytoplasmic filaments such as actin. These are low-affinity antibodies of the IgM isotype that are often cross-reactive with exoantigens such as bacterial cell walls. They are usually produced by $CD5^+$ B cells, do not undergo affinity maturation, and therefore, do not pose a threat to the host. Thus, some physiological autoimmune reactivity against self-antigens is normal. It is suggested that autoantibodies may in fact serve as physiological regulators of the immune system and may be found at normal physiological levels as components of the body's homeostatic mechanisms. Autoantibodies are also thought to act as 'biological taxis', transporting cellular breakdown products for their ultimate disposal. For example, after myocardial infarction, apparently harmless autoantibodies to heart tissue are found in the patient's blood and are thought to help clear away damaged tissue. Thus, transient autoimmune responses are common and require no medical intervention.

Autoimmunity can be defined as the specific breakdown of mechanisms responsible for tolerance to self-antigens, and autoimmune diseases result when a specific adaptive immune response against self-antigens is serious enough to cause tissue damage. A large spectrum of diseases with varying symptoms falls under this umbrella. Both, humoral immunity and CMI are involved in autoimmunity. A breakdown in the peripheral tolerance mechanisms allows the formation of T_{H1} cells and CTLs, and is accompanied with an inappropriate activation of macrophages. This results in perturbation of normal immunoregulatory mechanisms. The autoreactive T cells can help self-reactive B cell clones produce autoantibodies. These are usually complement-fixing IgG antibodies that can undergo affinity maturation. Together, the autoreactive CTLs and antibodies are responsible for the extensive and indiscriminate damage observed in some autoimmune disorders.

14.2 Interplaying Factors

Immune diversity generating mechanisms are active throughout life, and both B and T cell repertoires are open-ended, since they have to respond to a world of forever evolving pathogens. Put simply, this implies that cells capable of recognizing self-antigens can exist or be formed throughout the individual's life. Strict regulatory control mechanisms at the central and peripheral level ensure that this self-reactivity does not translate into a threat to the organism. In the foregoing chapters, we have already discussed the processes that ensure the absence of autoimmune disorders in healthy individuals, and they are summarized below.

❑ During maturation in the primary lymphoid organs, most self-reactive clones — both B and T — are deleted rendering the immune system tolerant to self-antigens.

[1] One could argue that autoreactivity is a built-in feature of the immune system. The T cell receptor repertoire is positively selected on MHC:self-peptide complexes in the thymus, and naïve T cells require contact with self-MHC molecules in the periphery for their survival and effector function. This means that all T cells in the periphery are, by definition, autoreactive! It is when T cells that recognize self-peptide:self-MHC complexes with moderate to high affinity, are allowed to proliferate that autoimmune diseases develop.

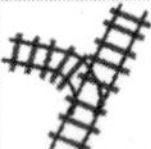

Too Much of a Good Thing:
Type 1 and Type 2 Diabetes Mellitus

Diabetes mellitus is a chronic disorder of carbohydrate, fat, and protein metabolism, characterized by hyperglycaemia resulting from defects in insulin secretion or signalling. Insulin, a hormone produced by the β cells of the pancreatic islets of Langerhans, is indispensable for glucose metabolism. Entry of glucose in the β cells triggers the secretion of insulin. The secreted insulin is then carried in the blood to peripheral tissues. Binding of insulin to its receptors starts a cascade of events that allows the uptake of glucose by cells. Defects in the β cell-peripheral tissue pathway can result in hyperglycaemia — that is too much glucose in the blood and not enough in the cells. Diabetes is a case of biology imitating a depressing reality — starvation in the midst of plenty. Two forms of diabetes are recognized clinically. Type 1 (**I**nsulin-**D**ependent **D**iabetes **M**ellitus (IDDM) or juvenile onset) diabetes is caused by the deficiency in the production of insulin due to the immune-mediated destruction of β cells. By contrast, type 2 (non-insulin dependent or adult onset) diabetes is caused by inappropriate or inadequate insulin secretion coupled to insulin resistance.

IDDM has a major autoimmune component, showing the presence of inflammatory infiltrate in pancreatic islets, antibodies to islet cell autoantigens, and a strong MHC allele linkage (Table 14.1). IDDM patients show the presence of at least three different autoantibodies. Antibodies to an isoform of **G**lutamic **A**cid **D**ecarboxylase (GAD65) are commonly observed in most patients. Also observed are antibodies to IA-2, a member of the transmembrane protein tyrosine phosphatase family, that is thought to play a role in insulin secretion. Anti-insulin antibodies are especially common in young children developing IDDM. Frequency of anti-insulin antibodies is much less in those who develop the disease at an older age. These antibodies appear in the patients months or years before the development of clinical disease. The number rather than the titre of the antibodies seems to be of predictive value.

In spite of their predictive value, antibodies are thought to play a minor role in the pathogenesis of disease. Two different processes result in cell-mediated destruction of β cells. Antigen-specific destruction occurs because of the recognition of autoantigens in the context of MHC class I molecules on β cells by CD8$^+$ CTLs and culminates in the death of β cells. β cells do not express MHC class II molecules and therefore are not susceptible to antigen-specific CD4$^+$ T cell destruction. However, APCs in the islets internalize dead or dying cells, degrade the autoantigens, load them on MHC class II molecules, and eventually export them to the cell surface. Engagement of these petide:class II complexes by T$_{H1}$ cells recruited to the site of insulitis (inflammation of the pancreas) results in the release of cytotoxins by these cells. These cytotoxins cause the death of not only the APCs but also bystander β cells in the vicinity. The nature of the autoantigens is not clear, but GAD and insulin are believed to be strong candidates. Childhood viral infections that cause pancreatic inflammation are thought to be responsible for breaking tolerance to these antigens.

Type 2 diabetes begins as a syndrome of insulin resistance — ie, the target tissues fail to respond to insulin appropriately. Typically, the disease manifests itself in adulthood, usually around age 40 or above. It is the most common type of diabetes; 85–90% of diagnosed diabetes cases are of this type. The exact cause of the disease is not clear. In some instances, type 2 diabetes can be of autoimmune origin, although it is not the major cause. For example, antibodies to insulin receptor can prevent binding of insulin to the receptor and cause perturbation of glucose metabolism. It is often called a self-induced disease, since life-style choices (lack of adequate exercise and obesity) seem to be the major pre-disposing factors, although genes do play a role. People of Native American, Asian, and Hispanic origin show an increased susceptibility to the disease. India has earned the dubious distinction of being the diabetes capital of the world, with the number of people suffering from diabetes approaching 10% of the population.

❑ Most tissue antigens are expressed at levels that are too low to initiate a T cell response; if they are present at higher concentrations, the corresponding T cells are deleted in the thymus because of the negative selection of clones that recognize self-antigens with a high affinity.

❑ Presentation of tissue-specific antigens by non-professional APCs (ie, in the absence of costimulation) induces tolerance to self-antigens through clonal anergy. These surviving self-reactive clones that exist in the body, but cannot be activated, are said to be in a state of immunological ignorance.

❑ T$_R$ cells have a major role in keeping self-reactive T cell clones in check. Since B cells cannot respond to TD antigens in the absence of T cell help, controlling self-reactive T cell clones automatically controls B cell responses to most antigens.

- Innate immune mechanisms also have a role in preventing autoimmunity by promoting self-tolerance.
- Self-reactive low affinity IgM antibodies are thought to be important in the negative selection of autoreactive B cell clones formed in the bone marrow. It is postulated that cross-linking of BcR by these IgM-self-antigen complexes triggers negative selection.
- Components of the complement cascade are involved in the opsonization and clearance of apoptotic cells and immune complexes. This prompt clearance of cell debris helps reduce the incidence of autoimmunity. Interference with these clearance mechanisms leads to chronic inflammation and is found to increase susceptibility to autoimmune diseases in animal models.

The relatively low incidence of autoimmune diseases points to the success of these controls. Currently, no general unifying theory can explain the start of an autoimmune disease in healthy individuals. The induction and perpetuation of autoimmune diseases seems to depend upon the interplay of three parameters — genetic predisposition, environmental factors, and immune regulation. The importance of each single component in the appearance of these diseases may vary for different individuals and diseases; however, the appearance of an autoimmune disease requires the convergence of all three components as shown in fig. 14.1.

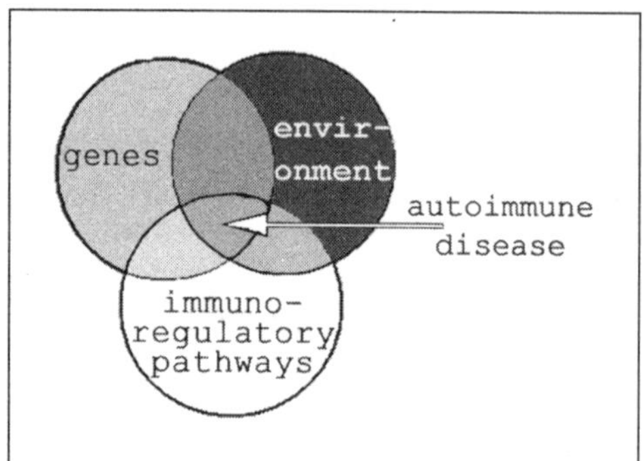

Figure 14.1 An interplay of three factors leads to the development of autoimmune diseases. The relative importance of the individual factors may vary in individuals and diseases, but convergence of all three is required for the manifestation of the disease (Adapted from Nature Immunology (2001) 2: 759).

❑ **Genetic predisposition.** Autoimmune diseases run in families, which suggests a genetic component in their incidence. Only a few genes involved in the pathogenic mechanisms that underlie autoimmune diseases are actually known. One of the most important ones implicated is the gene cluster that codes for MHC molecules. Certain MHC alleles are found to be associated with specific autoimmune disorders with much greater frequency (Table 14.1). However, autoimmune diseases can develop in the absence of the 'disease-associated' MHC haplotype, and not everyone who has the disease-haplotype develops autoimmunity, which argues for the involvement of other genes as well. The manner in which MHC molecules affect predisposition to autoimmune diseases is not understood. MHC molecules serve as 'thymic selection elements' to create the repertoire of naïve T cells, and then, in the periphery, present antigenic determinants to the same T cells. Amino acids lining the peptide-binding groove of an MHC molecule dictate the peptides that can be loaded on that molecule. Consequently, during thymic development, the predisposing MHC gene products could lead to positive selection of a repertoire of T cells that are specific for certain autoantigens (ie, a failure of negative selection). Alternatively, it is also possible that some MHC alleles are better at presenting foreign peptides resembling self-peptides in the periphery. The possibility that certain haplotypes tend to bind and present autoantigenic peptides to T cells in the periphery also cannot be ruled out. Thus, it is not clear whether the role of predisposing MHC gene products is in the selection process in the thymus, in the presentation of (auto) antigenic peptides in the periphery, or both. Interestingly, the presence of a T cell receptor with a particular $V\alpha$ or $V\beta$ region has also been linked to some autoimmune pathologies, including **E**xperimental **A**utoimmune **E**ncephalomyelitis (EAE) in mice and its human counterpart — Multiple Sclerosis, and Myasthenia gravis.

Table 14.1 Association between MHC alleles and autoimmune diseases

Allele	Disease
B8 and DR3	Myasthenia gravis Sjogren's syndrome
B27	Ankylosing spondylitis Reiter's syndrome Enteropathic arthropathy
B38	Psoriatic arthritis
DR2	Goodpasture's syndrome Multiple Sclerosis
DR3	Grave's disease SLE IDDM
DR4	IDDM Pemphigus vulgaris RA
DR5	Autoimmune pernicious anemia Hashimoto's autoimmune thyroiditis

Genes other than the MHC cluster are also important in the development of autoimmune diseases. Thus, in humans, inherited deficiency of the early proteins of the complement pathway (C1, C2, and C4) is very strongly associated with SLE (**S**ystemic **L**upus **E**rythematosus). Similarly, a point mutation in the Fas-FasL system (CD95-CD95L) is known to induce SLE-like disease in a number of mouse models. A similar defect results in ALPS (**A**utoimmune **L**ympho**p**roliferative **S**yndrome) in children, though once again, all children who develop this disorder do not have the defect. An inherited variation in the levels of expression of certain cytokines (eg, TNF-α) is also thought to increase susceptibility to autoimmune disorders.

❑ **Environmental factors**. Although autoimmune diseases run in families, both siblings of an identical pair of twins do not necessarily suffer from them. This clearly points to the importance of factors other than genetic makeup in autoimmune disease development. This low concordance rate within identical twin pairs can only be explained if an environmental factor is required to trigger disease in a genetically predisposed individual. Infectious agents are proposed to be one such trigger. Thus, for SLE, an infection with Epstein-Barr virus has been established as a trigger. Recent work suggests that autoimmunity may also be triggered by an immune response to the highly conserved stress proteins (eg, heat shock proteins) of human and bacterial cells. Smoking has been shown a predisposing factor for psoriasis. In some autoimmune pathologies, smoking is shown to be linked to certain manifestations of that disease. For example, in Goodpasture's syndrome, pulmonary haemorrhage is almost exclusively found in smokers. Similarly, smoking is a major factor in opthalmopathy associated with Grave's disease.

❑ **Disruption of immunoregulatory pathways.** In spite of having the necessary predisposition and exposure to predisposing environmental factors, some individuals develop only a low titre of autoreactive antibodies and do not suffer from full blown autoimmune diseases. This suggests the importance of a third factor — the disruption of immunoregulatory pathways. Though such disruptions are difficult to prove in humans, they have been clearly shown to occur in mouse models.

- **Disruption of apoptotic pathways.** Fas-FasL signalling is involved in cell apoptosis. MRL *lpr/lpr*[2] mice harbour a disruption of the gene that encodes Fas. These mice spontaneously develop a multi-organ autoimmune disease with symptoms that are similar to SLE. The same phenotype is found in *gld/gld* mice in whom the gene that encodes FasL is disrupted, establishing the importance of apoptotic pathways in autoimmune diseases.

- **Interference with development of T$_R$ cells.** Studies in a number of experimental models of organ-specific autoimmune disease provide convincing evidence that specialized T$_R$ cells capable of controlling autoimmunity are an integral part of the T cell repertoire in normal animals, and interference with their development leads to autoimmune disorders. For example, IL-2 signalling pathways are known to be important in development of T$_R$ cells. Mice with targeted mutations of IL-2 or CD25 also develop a fatal disease characterized by lymphoproliferation, lymphocytic organ infiltration, colitis, autoantibody formation, and anaemia. Similarly, CTLA-4$^{-/-}$ mice deficient in CTLA-4, a key molecule in the development of T$_R$ cells, succumb to a severe lymphoproliferative syndrome with organ infiltration within the first 3–4 weeks of life[3].

- **Dysregulation of cytokine and neuroendocrine networks.** The integrated immunoregulatory circuit consisting of immune-derived cytokines, the **H**ypothalamus-**P**ituitary-**A**drenal (HPA) axis, and the **S**ympathetic **N**ervous **S**ystem (SNS) is thought to be essential in maintaining homeostasis. The disruption of this circuit can predispose to autoimmunity in animal models of spontaneous autoimmune thyroiditis, lupus-like disease, and experimental arthritis. Cells of the immune system are responsive to neurotransmitters like norepinephrine. Both norepinephrine and epinephrine can inhibit the production of pro-inflammatory cytokines such as TNF-α by cells of the immune system. They also stimulate the production of anti-inflammatory cytokines such as IL-10 and TGF-β. Several autoimmune diseases are characterized by alterations of the balance of T$_{H1}$, T$_{H2}$, or T$_R$ cells (fig. 14.2). Both **r**heumatoid **a**rthritis (RA) and Multiple Sclerosis show a skew towards T$_{H1}$ cytokines with overproduction of TNF-α and IL-12 and a deficiency of IL-10. These cytokines appear to be the critical factors that determine the proliferation of autoreactive T cells in these diseases. SLE on the other hand shows a shift towards T$_{H2}$ cells (fig. 14.2). Restoration of this balance through intervention has been shown to prevent or moderate the severity of the disease. Similarly, in experimental models of EAE, animal recovery has been shown to be dependent on an increase in endogenous glucocorticoid levels. It has recently been shown that this endocrine response is, at least in part, triggered by the immune response to the encephalitogenic antigen and mediated by endogenous IL-1 produced during the disease.

---

[2] Animal mutations are denoted by simple three letter codes meant to aid recall, though it may not always help people not in the field! The *'lpr'*, in this case, stands for 'lymphoproliferative', and *'gld'* for 'generalized lymphoproliferative disease'.

[3] CTLA-4 has been mapped as a susceptibility gene in both human autoimmune thyroid disease and IDDM, whereas IL-2 and CTLA-4 are found in genetic regions linked to disease susceptibility in NOD (Non-Obese Diabetic) mice.

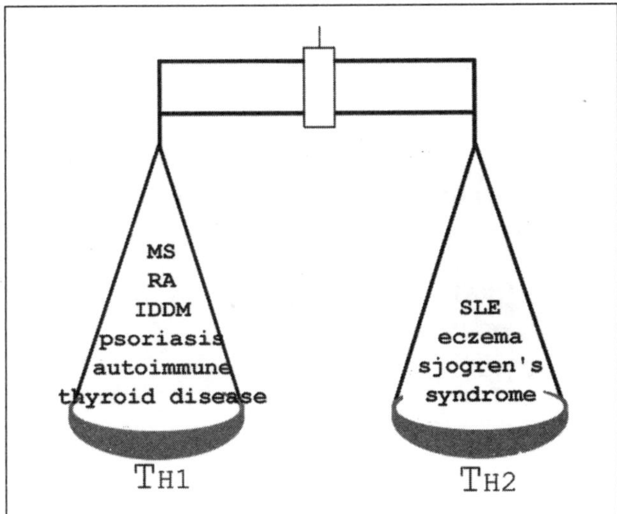

Figure 14.2 An alteration in the balance of T_{H1}:T_{H2} cytokines may result in autoimmune diseases and restoring this balance can prevent or reduce the severity of the disease.

14.3 Triggering Factors

Autoimmune responses are a direct consequence of a breakdown of normal tolerance mechanisms. Factors that can act as triggers in this breakdown are discussed below.

❏ **Infections.** There is a strong association between infection and the onset of autoimmunity. Multiple mechanisms could be involved in infection-associated breakdown of tolerance (fig. 14.3).

- **Antigen-specific mechanisms** of breakdown of tolerance include the following.
  - ◆ **Release of hidden/sequestered antigens due to infection.** Such release of normally sequestered antigens could lead to a reversal of anergy, triggering an autoimmune response against these antigens. For example, sperm formed in later stages of development is sequestered from the immune system. Male infertility results when cells of the immune system gain access to sperm-forming tissues in infections like mumps. Similarly, an autoimmune reaction against eye lens protein is observed after a trauma makes this normally sequestered antigen accessible to cells of the immune system.
  - ◆ **Cross-reactivity between a foreign and self-antigen** may lead to induction of an immune response to self-antigens. This phenomenon is called molecular mimicry and implies that an antigenic determinant on some microbial protein is structurally similar to a determinant on a host protein. In the case of T cells, this would imply a linear peptide of about 8–15 amino acids in length that would be recognized in the context of a particular MHC haplotype. Most post-infection autoimmune diseases are therefore linked to a particular MHC allele. An initial T cell response to one epitope can lead to B cell autoimmune responses to other closely related, diverse determinants, and is called epitope spreading. Some examples of infection precipitated autoimmune damage are listed below.
    - Cross-reactivity between *S. pyogenes* and myosin present in cardiac muscles is thought to be responsible for the cardiac damage observed in acute rheumatic fever that follows a streptococcal infection.
    - Coxsackie B virus apparently shares an antigen with myocardium, and infection with this virus can trigger lethal myocarditis.
    - The outer surface protein of the spirochete *Borrellia burgdorferi* induces the formation of T cells that recognize a peptide derived from LFA-1 (CD11a or CD18) in the context of HLA-DR4. Lyme arthritis that does not resolve after antibiotic treatment is thus thought to be a result of this

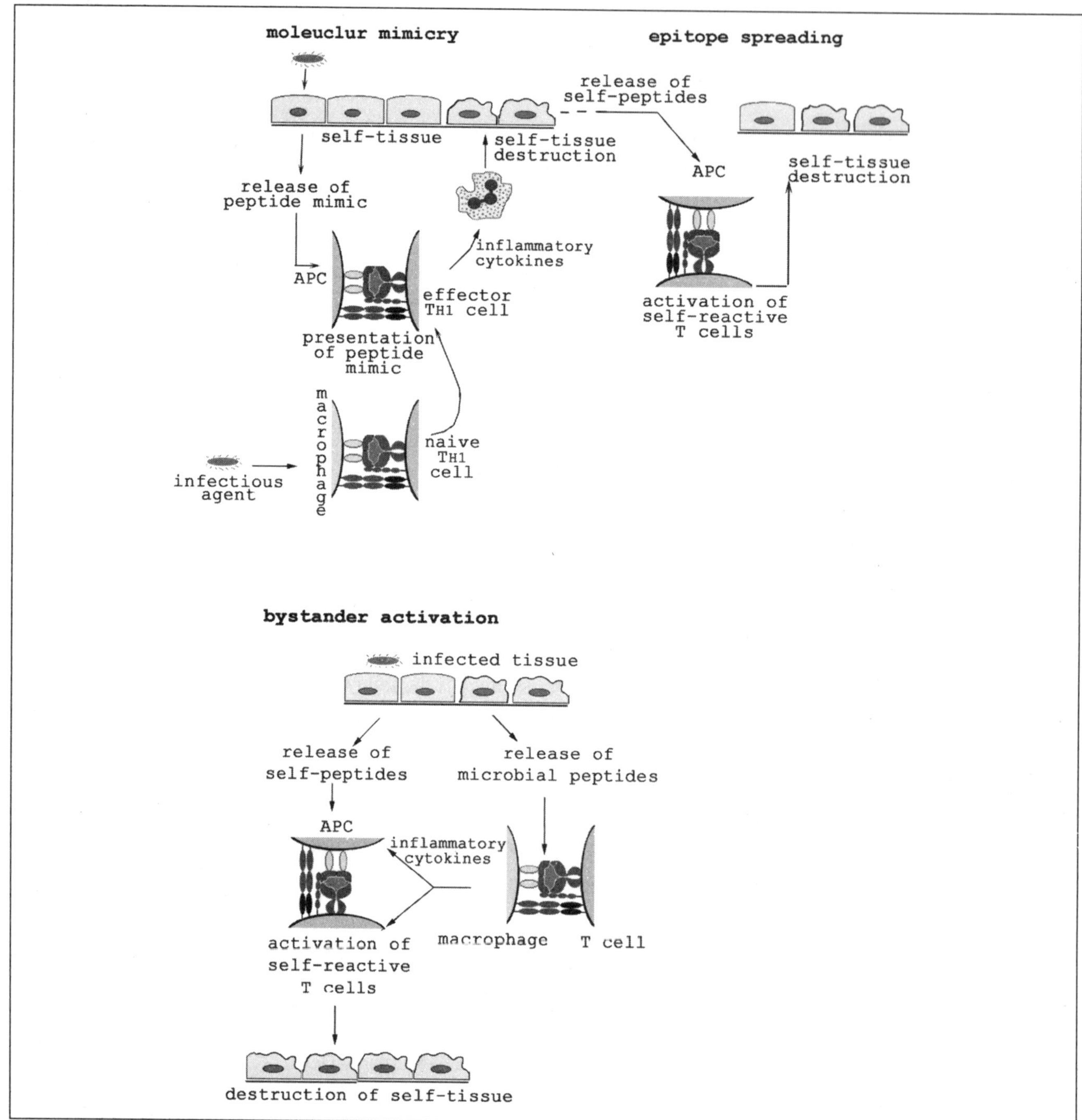

Figure 14.3 Infections can induce autoimmunity by multiple mechanisms. *Following infection, macrophages and DCs internalize and process the infecting agent and its products, load fragments derived from these proteins on MHC molecules, and display them at the cell surface. Recognition of these MHC:peptide complexes along with appropriate costimulatory signals results in the activation of naïve T cells. The activated T cells proliferate and differentiate to effector T cells. Stimulation of effector T cells by MHC:peptide complexes causes them to release pro-inflammatory cytokines that activate the macrophages and switch on their destructive potential. If an antigenic determinant on a microbial protein is structurally similar to a host epitope, the process results in activation of cross-reactive T cells and destruction of self-tissues (molecular mimicry, upper left panel). The subsequent release of self-tissue antigens and their uptake by APCs perpetuates the disease. In epitope spreading (upper right panel), self-tissue damage caused by a persistent microbial infection causes the release of multiple self-peptides. The pro-inflammatory environment caused by the infection results in the upregulation of MHC and costimulatory molecule expression by APCs. Internalization and presentation of self-peptides by APC under these conditions causes the spreading of the autoimmune response to multiple self-epitopes. Bystander activation is the non-specific activation of self-reactive cells caused by the pro-inflammatory environment in persistent infection (bottom panel). Activation of T cells specific for microbial antigens results in the influx of more T cells to the site of infection. Some of these T cells are likely to be self-reactive and get activated. These activated T cells cause self-tissue damage and perpetuate the autoimmune response.*

cross-reactivity. Nerve toxicity observed in this disease is attributed to cross-reactivity between flagellin of *B. burgdorferi* and axon protein.

- A recent study has established a link between *Klebsiella* infection and ankylosing spondylitis in HLA-B27 individuals.
- Herpes simplex virus-1infection of the eye can provoke chronic inflammation of the corneal stroma called herpetic stromal keratitis, a leading cause of human blindness. Recently, it has been shown that the blindness is the result of inflammation caused by T_{H1} cells against a viral peptide (UL6) cross-reacting with a peptide in the corneal antigen.
- Reiter's syndrome is a crippling arthritis linked to infection with *Chlamydia trachomatis* and is associated with HLA-B27. Similarly, infection with *Proteus mirabilis* is linked to reactive arthritis in HLA-DR1 and DR4 alleles.

- For **antigen non-specific mechanisms**, no particular microbial determinant has been implicated. Possible causes of tolerance breakdown include:
  - Induction of costimulatory molecules on tissue cells because of a local inflammatory response; such induction would allow non-professional APCs to present self-antigens to T cells, triggering a deleterious autoimmune response,
  - Binding of infectious agents or their products to self-proteins may result in the proteins acting as haptens conjugated to the pathogenic carrier, resulting in an autoimmune response,
  - Dysregulation of cytokine networks due to the induction of pro-inflammatory cytokines such as TNF-α and IL-1 by an infection can lead to autoimmune disorders in predisposed individuals, and
  - Polyclonal lymphocyte activation via a mitogen or a superantigen may result in autoimmunity. B cell stimulation by polyclonal activators or infectious agents like the Epstein-Barr virus or T cell activation by bacterial superantigens could lead to polyclonal activation of autoreactive T cells and precipitate an autoimmune response.

❏ **Inappropriate expression of MHC class II molecules** may result in the stimulation of autoreactive clones. Normal tissue cells do not express MHC class II molecules. However, during viral infections they secrete IFN-γ, a potent inducer of both MHC class II and costimulatory molecules. Mitogens such as phyto-haemagglutinin can also induce MHC class II expression. It is suggested that this inappropriate expression of MHC class II molecules could allow cells to present self-antigens, leading to a breakdown of self-tolerance.

AUTOIMMUNE DISEASES

❏ They are the result of a breakdown in self-tolerance.
❏ The interplay of three independent factors (genetics, environment, and breakdown of immunoregulatory pathways) results in autoimmunity.
❏ Triggering factors include:
  - infections resulting in the breakdown of tolerance,
  - inappropriate expression of MHC class II molecules, and
  - hormones.
❏ Mechanisms of autoimmune damage include:
  - cytolysis due to complement fixation,
  - failure to clear immune complexes,
  - autoantibody caused compromised cellular function, and
  - inappropriate CTL activation.
❏ Treatment includes alleviation of symptoms by metabolic correction and the administration of anti-inflammatory and/or immunosuppressive agents.

❑ **Sex hormones,** in addition to their effects on sexual differentiation and reproduction, also influence the immune system. This results in a gender dimorphism in the immune function with females having higher Ig levels and mounting stronger immune responses following immunization or infection than males. Thus, women tend to have a T_{H2} pattern of immune responses, and this state is further heightened during pregnancy. This greater immune responsiveness in females is also evident in their increased susceptibility to autoimmune diseases. Autoimmune diseases show a clear gender bias with women suffering from them at a much higher frequency than men (Table 14.2). Studies in normal mice show that estrogen treatment induces polyclonal B cell activation with increased expression of autoantibodies that is characteristic of autoimmune diseases. Several mechanisms appear to contribute to this breakdown in tolerance, including a reduction of bone marrow mass and altered susceptibility of B cells to death. In addition, recent data indicates that sex hormones influence both apoptosis and cytokine profile of T cells. Thus, patients suffering from SLE improve with androgen treatment. In animal studies, androgens change the cytokine profile from predominantly IL-4, IL-5, IL-6, and IL-10 (ie, T_{H2} type) to TNF-α and IFN-γ (ie, T_{H1} type). Conversely, patients with RA (characterized as a T_{H1} disease) improve with estrogens (oral contraceptives).

Table 14.2 Gender bias in autoimmune diseases

Disorder	Female:Male ratio
Hashimoto's thyroiditis	50:1
Sjorgen's syndrome	9:1
SLE	9:1
RA	4:1
Multiple Sclerosis	2:1
Myasthenia gravis	2:1
IDDM	2:1
Chronic idiopathic thrombocytopaenic purpurea	2:1
Ankylosing spondylitis	1:3
Acute anterior uveitis	1:2

14.4 Mechanisms of Damage

The pathology of an autoimmune disease is determined by both, the specific antigen or group of antigens against which the autoimmune response is directed and the mechanism of damage of the antigen-bearing tissue. These mechanisms are essentially similar to those operative in protective immunity except that they cause damage since they are directed against self-tissues instead of infectious agents or tumours. Furthermore, since the offending antigen is an integral part of the body, there is a constant supply of the antigen, amplifying rather than diminishing the response.

❑ **Damage caused by complement-fixing autoantibodies.** Complement-fixing autoantibodies can cause tissue damage by two different mechanisms.
  • **Cytolysis.** Autoantibodies against cell surface antigens cause extensive damage because of complement-associated cytolysis, especially in non-nucleated cells. For example, in autoimmune haemolytic anaemia, IgG autoantibodies bind to blood group antigens and cause the destruction of erythrocytes. Likewise, autoantibodies against the fibrinogen receptor on platelets lead to the depletion of platelets and cause haemorrhage in autoimmune thrombocytic purpurea. Similarly, antibodies against the basement membrane[4] collagen are responsible for the acute vasculitis and renal failure observed in Goodpasture's syndrome.

[4] A basement membrane is a specialized form of extracellular matrix that consists of laminins, collagen type IV and a variety of glycoproteins that separates the epithelium from the underlying supporting tissue. Basement membranes of different organs have different compositions.

- **Immune complex formation.** Binding of autoantibodies to soluble antigens leads to the deposition of immune complexes in tissues, blood vessels, etc. The immune system fails to clear the large quantities of complexes formed, resulting in the chronic activation of the complement cascade. The resultant release of C3a and C5a initiates an inflammatory response with phagocytic cell recruitment that is destructive to tissues. NK cells recruited to the site cause further tissue injury through ADCC. This is the underlying mechanism of tissue damage in systemic autoimmune diseases such as SLE. Weakening of muscles observed in Myasthenia gravis is also partially attributed to complement mediated degradation of **A**cetyl**ch**oline (Ach) receptors. In some individuals with RA, formation of autoreactive IgM antibodies against the Fc region of IgG leads to deposition of IgM-IgG complexes in the joints and chronic complement activation that results in joint inflammation.

- ❑ **Compromised cellular function because of the binding of autoantibodies to cell surface receptors.** The binding of autoantibodies to cell surface receptors can either mimic the normal function of the receptor, block binding of the ligand to the receptor, or even lead to degradation of the receptor. Thus, in Myasthenia gravis, antibodies to myocyte acetycholine receptors, located at the neuromuscular junction, interfere with proper neurotransmission. Binding of these antibodies to receptors is also believed to promote their internalization and degradation, leading to diminished contractility and progressive weakness of muscles. By contrast, in Graves' disease, binding of autoantibodies to the receptor of the thyroid-stimulating hormone mimics the action of the normal hormone, resulting in over-stimulation of the thyroid gland.

- ❑ **Damage due to CTL activation.** If the autoimmune response is a predominantly cellular one, extensive damage to specific organs or tissue is observed because of the destruction of cells expressing specific MHC class I:self-antigen complexes by CTLs. An example of this type of damage is seen in autoimmune thyroiditis where accumulation of phagocytic and cytolytic cells can be found in thyroid lesions. Similarly, in IDDM, infiltrating CTLs destroy β cells located in the islets of Langerhans in the pancreas. Autoreactive T cells have a role in Multiple Sclerosis and EAE as well. In Multiple Sclerosis, T cells cause the destruction of the myelin sheath of nerve fibres, resulting in neurologic dysfunction. EAE is a classic T cell-related autoimmune disease where autoreactive cells to **M**yelin **B**asic **P**rotein (MBP) cause damage to brain cells.

14.5   Diagnosis and Treatment

Laboratory diagnosis of most autoimmune diseases entails the detection of autoreactive antibodies in tissue or serum of the patient. Presence of autoreactive antibodies in tissue can be determined by immunofluorescence, whereas RIA or ELISA/EIA remain techniques of choice for detection of antibodies in serum. The Coomb's test is used to detect autoantibodies in haemolytic anaemias (Appendix III). With diseases like IDDM, treatment is symptomatic, and diagnosis of the nature of the disease is secondary. Autoimmune disorders can be divided into two categories.

- ❑ **Organ specific** autoimmune diseases have localized lesions such as Hashimoto's disease and pernicious anaemia.
- ❑ **Non-organ specific** diseases, which do not have localized lesions but lesions distributed in the body. Examples include RA, Multiple sclerosis, and SLE (Table 14.3).

Alleviation of symptoms of organ specific diseases can be achieved by metabolic correction, eg, administration of thyroid hormones in thyrotoxicosis or vitamin B$_{12}$ in pernicious anaemia. However, these treatments do not address the underlying

Table 14.3 Common autoimmune disorders

Disorder	Autoantigen	Description
Organ-specific diseases		
Hashimoto's disease (Chronic thyroiditis)	Thyroglobulin, thyroid peroxidase	Binding of antibodies to the autoantigen causes malfunctioning of the thyroid and interferes with iodine uptake resulting in hypothyroidism.
		Infiltration of lymphocytes and phagocytes in thyroid causes inflammation, enlargement (goitre) and destruction of thyroid gland
		Common in middle aged women
Thyrotoxicosis (Graves' disease)	Thyroid hormone receptor	Uncontrolled stimulation of thyroid caused by the binding of autoantibodies to the receptor, leads to hyperthyroidism
Autoimmune gastritis and pernicious anaemia	α, β subunits of gastric proton pump (H^+/K^+-ATPase)	Perturbation of the gastric proton pump causes loss of acid, gastritis (inflammation of gastric mucosa) and atrophy of the gastric mucosa
	Membrane protein on gastric parietal cells called intrinsic factor involved in transport of vitamin B_{12} across small intestine	Binding of autoantibodies to gastric parietal cells causes their destruction and results intrinsic factor deficiency; these antibodies also interfere with binding of vitamin B_{12} to intrinsic factor
		Deficiency of the vitamin affects haematopoiesis and results in a change in the size, shape, and number of mature erythrocytes in the blood
Autoimmune haemolytic anaemia	Rh or Ii blood group antigens	Binding of antibodies to antigen on surface of erythrocytes results in complement-mediated lysis of erythrocytes and severe anaemia
		Anti-Ii antibodies are cold agglutinins that bind RBC associated Ii antigen; result in severe necrosis of body extremities, especially in winter
	Drugs like penicillin or methyldopa (used to treat hypertension) that attach to erythrocytes and act as haptens	Drug-induced anaemias caused by an autolytic reaction against the drug-coated erythrocytes
Goodpasture's syndrome	$\alpha 3$ chain of Type IV collagen found in the basement membrane of kidney glomeruli and/or lung alveoli	Binding of autoantibodies to the collagen causes progressive kidney damage and/or pulmonary haemorrhage
Male infertility	Antigens on spermatozoa	Antibodies cause agglutination of spermatozoa and prevent fertilization
Thrombocytopenic purpurea	Glycoprotein antigens on cell surface; most common is platelet integrin GpIIb/IIIa	Anti-platelet antibodies cause agglutination and destruction of platelets, resulting in uncontrolled haemorrhage
Myasthenia gravis	Nicotinic acetylcholine (ACh) receptor, especially peptides derived from the α subunit involved in muscle contraction; signal generated by the binding of ACh (a neurotransmitter released by somatic motor neurons into the neuromuscular junction) to its receptor results in the contraction of skeletal muscle cells	Binding of autoantibody to ACh receptors causes endocytosis of ACh receptors or destruction of the cell by ADCC
		The resultant loss of receptors interferes with muscle contraction and causes progressive muscle weakness
IDDM (type I diabetes)	Antigen on β cells in the islets of Langerhans of the pancreas; β cells produce insulin, a hormone, needed for the transport of glucose into cells	Hyperglycaemia caused by insufficient insulin production due to CTL-mediated destruction of insulin-producing pancreatic β cells
		Autoantibodies have only a minor role in the destruction

Systemic diseases

SLE[5]	Three main antigens nucleosome, the spliceosome and a ribonuleoprotein complex containing Ro and La proteins[6]	Chronic inflammatory multi-organ disorder
		Deposition of immune complexes in renal glomerulii, joints, and other organs results in widespread damage with a spectrum of symptoms
	Other ubiquitous self-antigens (DNA, histones, ribosomes, etc) also involved	Damage to kidneys and brain may prove fatal
RA	Antigen unknown	Autoantibodies against the Fc domain of IgG/IgM found in the synovial fluid of affected joints; whether cause or effect of disease unclear
		Deposition of immune complexes causes joint inflammation and destruction
Multiple Sclerosis (EAE in mice)	Myelin basic protein (MBP), proteolipid protein and myelin oligodendrocyte glyco-protein; components of myelin	$CD4^+$ T cell-mediated attack on the myelin sheath of neuronal cells causes paralysis in affected individuals
Pemphigous vulgaris	Desmoglein, the skin glue that attaches adjacent cells	Attack of autoantibodies causes virtual ungluing of skin, causing burn-like lesions or blisters that do not heal.

cause of the disease. The ideal treatment for autoimmune diseases (whether organ-specific or non-organ specific) is to induce long-lasting, antigen-specific tolerance. Commonly used immunosuppressive and anti-inflammatory drugs have clinical benefits but are associated with significant side-effects. The use of conventional immunosuppressive therapy is now being reduced or replaced with new biological agents.

❑ **Neutralization of cytokines.** TNF-α is a pro-inflammatory cytokine acting directly on multiple target tissues and inducing other pro-inflammatory cytokines such as IL-1, IL-6, and IL-8. Moreover, it potentiates lymphocyte activation and facilitates recruitment of leukocytes to sites of inflammation by inducing expression of adhesion molecules and chemokines. Increased levels of TNF-α are found in several autoimmune diseases such as Crohn's disease, Multiple Sclerosis, and RA. Therapies aimed at neutralizing TNF-α include:
  - Administration of chimeric mouse-human anti-TNF-α mAbs has met with encouraging success in clinical trials of RA patients and was found to be especially beneficial with low doses of methotrexate.
  - Instead of targeting the cytokine, neutralization can also be achieved by the use of modified cytokine receptors that bind the cytokine, inhibiting it from activating cellular responses. Engineered **TNF R**eceptor (**TNFR**) has been successfully used in the treatment of RA. Etanerecept, a dimeric molecule comprising two extracellular domains of TNFR attached to the Fc portion of human IgG1 antibody, has been given FDA approval in the USA.

❑ **mAbs against T cell surface molecules** such as CD3, CD4, CD52, and CD25 have been used successfully in the treatment of autoimmune diseases.

❑ **Targeting T cell trafficking pathways** with mAbs against LFA-1, LFA-3 and VLA-4 (**V**ery **L**ate **A**ntigen-**4**) has shown promise in clinical trials. These mAbs have the advantage of interfering with lymphocyte trafficking without decreasing T cell numbers.

❑ **Administration of antigens by oral or mucosal routes** has been found to induce antigen-specific tolerance in animal models. The reasons behind tolerance induction are not clear. It is generally believed that oral or mucosal administration of the antigens leads to the formation of TR cells. Generation of TR cells may also cause immune deviation — a shift from a pathogenic (TH1 or IFN-γ driven) to a protective (TH2 or IL-4/TGF-β) T cell response. Though antigen-specific therapy is logically appealing and demonstrably effective in animal models, the approach has not met with appreciable success in clinical trials, and much remains to be done before antigen-specific tolerance becomes a reality.

[5] 'Systemic' refers to the multi-organ involvement observed in this disease, *Lupus* (Latin for wolf) describes the characteristic butterfly facial rash, resembling the colouring of a (European) wolf and 'Erythematosus' refers to the redness of the skin rash.

[6] The spliceosome are located in the nucleus and splice out intronic nucleotides from pre-mRNA to yield mRNA that is then translated into proteins on ribosomes. Ro and La stand for the first two letters of the surnames of patients in whom these autoantibodies were first discovered.

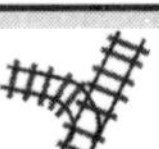

Jamming the Joints: Rheumatoid Arthritis

RA, an autoimmune disease, is a chronic destructive disease of the joints, characterized by inflammation, synovial hyperplasia, and abnormal cellular and humoral responses. It is the most common form of inflammatory arthritis that affects primarily the synovium[7], although integrity, resilience, and water content of the cartilage are also impaired. RA can be distinguished from other forms of arthritis by the location and number of joints involved — neck, shoulders, elbows, wrists and hands, especially the joints at the base and middle of the finger as well as hips, knees, ankles, and the joints at the base of the toes. Interestingly, the affected joints tend to be involved in a symmetrical pattern. About one-fifth people with RA also develop rheumatoid nodules, which are lumps of tissue that form under the skin, often over bony areas. The disease shows a sex bias; it is three times more common in women than men. The synovium of inflamed rheumatoid arthritic joint shows the presence of CD4$^+$ T cells, B cells (especially plasma cells), monocytes, and macrophages. Neutrophils, in contrast, are found almost exclusively in the synovial cavity (fluid) and only rarely in the synovial tissue. Also found in the synovial cavity are 'rheumatoid factors', autoantibodies against IgG and collagen type IV. Though characteristic of RA, it is not clear whether these autoantibodies are the cause or the result of the disease.

RA was originally believed to be a T cell driven disease. It was thought that activation of CD4$^+$ T cells by as yet unidentified antigen triggered and maintained the inflammatory process in the rheumatoid joint. The large number of CD4$^+$ T cells in the joint, skewed TcR gene usage, and the association of RA with MHC class II haplotypes (eg, HLA-DR4) lent support to this idea. However, T cells appear to be inactive in the chronic phase of the disease and secretion cytokines such as IL-2, IL-4, or IFN-γ that are associated with an activated T cell state are also very low. By contrast, cytokines such as IL-1, IL-6, IL-8, TNF-α, and GM-CSF known to be produced primarily by macrophages and connective tissue cells are expressed in abundance in RA synovium and synovial fluid, and this has led to the suggestion RA is an inflammatory immune complex disease. Thus, while T cells are thought to be important in initiating the disease, chronic inflammation perpetuated by macrophages and fibroblasts in a T cell independent manner is thought to be the cause of RA. According to this hypothesis, T cell dependent B cell activation to viral or bacterial antigens results in the formation of autoantibodies and leads to immune complex deposition. Inflammatory mediators released by this deposition cause the migration of monocytes into the synovium and start a self-perpetuating cycle of inflammation and tissue destruction. Thus, secretion of IL-1 and TNF-α by chronically activated macrophages maintains the synovial fibroblasts in an activated state, while cytokines such as IL-6, IL-8, and GM-CSF, secreted by the activated fibroblasts, contribute to further recruitment and maturation of monocytes and activation of PMNs. Prostaglandins and proteases, secreted by the fibroblasts, erode and destroy nearby connective tissues such as bone and cartilage resulting in the characteristic painful joints of RA.

There is no cure for RA at present. The goals of current treatment methods therefore are to relieve pain, reduce inflammation, stop or slow down joint damage, and improve function and patient well-being.

---

[7] Synovium is the membrane that lines and lubricates a joint. Cartilage is normally a very resilient tissue that absorbs considerable impact and stress and is composed primarily of type II collagen and proteoglycans.

Hypersensitivity

15

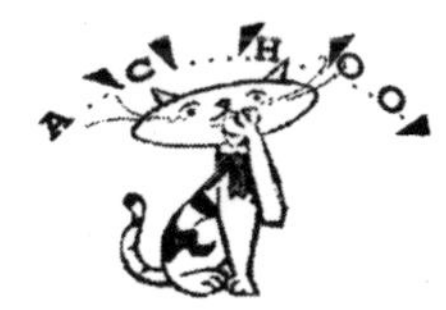

I know, I get cold
'Cos I can't leave things well alone
Understand I'm accident prone

—Natalie Imbruglia, *Wishing I Was There*

DTH:	Delayed-type of hypersensitivity
MCP-1:	Macrophage chemoattractant protein-1
MIP-1α:	Macrophage inflammatory protein-1α
NCA:	Neutrophil chemotactic factor-A
PCA:	Passive cutaneous anaphylaxis
PDGF:	Platelet-derived growth factor
PG:	Prostaglandins
VEGF:	Vascular endothelial growth factor

15.1 Introduction

The term hypersensitivity or allergy is used to describe any adaptive immune response to innocuous antigens in a presensitized (or immune) host that is exaggerated or inappropriate, which causes tissue damage, and is detrimental to the health of the individual. The term anaphylaxis (from the Greek *ana* — against, *phylaxis* — protection) was introduced to describe the detrimental effect of a second encounter with a foreign substance. Von Pirquet introduced the term allergy (once again, Greek *allos* — altered, *ergon* — action) to suggest any alteration in the immune status of an individual after exposure to the antigen. He suggested that the term 'immunity' be used to describe increased resistance, whereas 'hypersensitivity' be used to describe the deleterious effect of allergy. However, allergy and hypersensitivity (especially type I) are now used synonymously, and the antigen triggering the hypersensitivity reaction is termed the allergen.

The current classification of hypersensitivity reactions is based on the classification used by Coombs and Gell. They described four types of hypersensitivity reactions (type I to IV); type I, II, and III are antibody-mediated, whereas type IV is T cell-driven cell-mediated response (Table 15.1).

Table 15.1 Types of Hypersensitivities

Characteristic	Type I (anaphylactic)	Type II (cytotoxic)	Type III (immune complex)	Type IV (delayed-type)
Effectors	IgE	IgG, IgM	IgG, IgM	T cells
Antigen	Exogenous	Cell surface	Soluble	Tissues and organs
Response time	Immediate (15–30 minutes)	Minutes to hours	Hours to days	48–72 hours
Manifestations	Wheal and flare reaction, smooth muscle contraction, bronchoconstriction, mucus production	Lysis and necrosis of tissue; erythrocyte damage very common	Erythema, oedema, and necrosis; kidney damage very common	Erythema and induration
Pathophysiology	Accumulation of basophils, neutrophils, and eosinophils	Complement-mediated destruction of tissue/cells	Immune complexes, complement, neutrophils, and macrophages at site of tissue damage	Infiltration of monocytes/macrophages and lymphocytes, granuloma formation
Mediators of injury	Bioactive products of mast cells/basophils	Complement components, perforin/granzymes	Complement components, neutrophil exocytosis	Cytokines and chemokines
Examples	Asthma, hay fever, atopic dermatitis, urticaria	Erythroblastosis foetalis, autoimmune haemolytic anaemias, transfusion reactions	Glomerulonephritis, SLE, rheumatoid arthritis, pigeon fanciers' disease, serum sickness,	Granulomatous diseases such as tuberculosis and leprosy, contact dermatitis

15.2 Hypersensitivity Type I

Also referred to as immediate, or anaphylactic hypersensitivity, **hypersensitivity type I is characterized by an *immediate* inappropriate response to a secondary exposure to allergens.** The main players in type I hypersensitivity are basophils/mast cells and IgE. The primary exposure to the allergen that causes IgE production is called sensitization, and the secondary exposure that results in manifestations of type I hypersensitivity is termed allergenic challenge. Since anti-allergen IgE

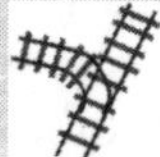

Taking Your Breath Away: Asthma

Asthma is a pulmonary disorder characterized by a generalized reversible obstruction of airflow that results in wheezing, shortness of breath, chest tightness, reversible airway inflammation, etc. Airway hyper-responsiveness (an exaggerated bronchospastic response to non-specific agents such as cold air or specific antigens) is a cardinal feature of asthma. It is thought to result from complex interactions between genes and the environment. The pathology of asthma is characterized by various changes in the airways, including mucus plugging, shedding of epithelial cells, thickening of the basement membrane, engorgement of vessels, angiogenesis, inflammatory cell infiltration, and smooth muscle hypertrophy and hyperplasia.

Increased IgE levels are a major feature of allergic asthma. DCs seem to be the key APCs that cause a $T_{H}2$ type response with the concomitant production of IgE upon initial exposure to antigen. Cross-linking of FcεRI on mast cells by IgE-allergen complexes activate and degranulate these cells. Bioactive mediators liberated by them are responsible for the acute bronchospasm that occurs within 15–30 minutes of exposure. The toxic mediators are also responsible for an inflammatory response in the airways. Chemokines released by mast cells result in neutrophil recruitment (due to IL-8) and eosinophil recruitment (due to RANTES, eotaxin, IL-5, etc), and a late-phase response that peaks 4–6 hours after exposure and causes prolonged symptoms. The presence of activated eosinophils is a defining feature of asthma. Perhaps because of their cytotoxic potential, eosinophils are under tight regulatory controls. Few eosinophils are normally present in circulation, and these do not express FcεRI. Only activated eosinophils express FcεRI. Chemokines like eotaxin cause their activation, and $T_{H}2$ cytokines like IL-5 increase the production of eosinophils from the bone marrow. Once activated, however, eosinophils can contribute to airway epithelial damage by the release of products like MBP. A type IV hypersensitivity that is caused by $T_{H}2$-dependent IL-4 and IL-13 may also contribute to the pathology of asthma. Both these cytokines, but especially IL-13, are thought to contribute to airway hyper-responsives and goblet cell metaplasia[1].

Epithelial damage and the loss of its protective barrier function caused by repeated asthmatic episodes may be responsible for smooth muscle proliferation in the airway, thickening of basement membranes, and fibrosis. These changes lead to a reduction of airway diameter and increase in bronchial responsiveness. Thus, chronic asthma is thought to be the result of a disturbance in repair and remodelling. Although allergens and endotoxins have long been identified as modifiers of asthma, the genes involved have proven hard to identify. Recent research indicates that the *ADAM-33* gene, located on the short arm of chromosome 20, is significantly associated with asthma. It is expressed by lung fibroblasts and bronchial smooth muscles and is a member of a subfamily of metalloproteinases. Although the exact role of ADAM-33 is not clear, it is suggested that ADAM-33 may be involved in small airway remodelling or cytokine shedding and may thus be responsible for turning an allergic runny nose into an asthmatic wheezy response.

Factors that commonly provoke asthma include allergens, upper respiratory tract infections, exercise, perfumes, fumes, changes in temperature and humidity, drugs (eg, aspirin and other non-steroidal anti-inflammatory drugs), food additives (metabisulphite or tartrazine), and food and drink (peanuts, alcohol, cola). Chemicals in the workplace such as ink, paints, adhesives, Pt salts, or epoxy resin hardening agents can also cause asthma. Conventional asthma treatment includes inhaled corticosteroids, β-agonists, and agents that interfere with Ca^{2+} influx or increase cytoplasmic cAMP levels. New therapies involving humanized mAb to IgE, IL-4 and IL-5, soluble IL-4R, etc are currently under investigation.

antibodies must develop to cause type I hypersensitivity, at least 14 days must elapse between sensitization and challenge for the hypersensitivity to manifest itself. Both mast cells and basophils, the major cell types responsible for type I reactions, are derived from $CD34^{+}$ haematopoietic stem cells, and express FcεRI, the high affinity receptor for IgE but differ in a number of characteristics.

❑ **Mast cells** do not circulate in blood. They are a heterogeneous population of cells that vary in patterns of expression of cell surface proteins and granule constituents. They express FcεRI and can bind and retain IgE for prolonged periods. Their maturation occurs in vascularized peripheral tissues and is tightly

[1] Goblet cells are found in the epithelium of the intestines and respiratory tracts. They secrete mucus, a viscous fluid composed primarily of highly glycosylated proteins called mucins.

regulated by various cytokines. Although traditionally mast cells were classified into 'mucosal' and 'connective tissue', it is now established that their phenotypic features can change markedly in response to a change in the cytokine milieu. Mature mast cells proliferate in response to $T_{H}2$ cytokines; their numbers increase dramatically during $T_{H}2$-type responses but later return to 'baseline' level after the resolution of the process. **Stem Cell Factor (SCF)** regulates many aspects of mast cell development and survival, although other cytokines such as IL-3 can also promote their survival. Mast cells produce an impressive array of mediators and signalling molecules (Table 15.2). Many of these mediators (eg, histamine, serotonin, proteases like tryptase, chimase, and kininogenase, TNF-α, NCF-A (**N**eutrophil **C**hemotactic **F**actor-A), and ECF-A) are preformed and stored in intracellular granules. Upon activation, mast cells rapidly synthesize bioactive metabolites of the archidonic acid pathway, including leukotrienes (LTC4, LTD4, LTE4), prostaglandins (PGD2) and PAF, cytokines (GM-CSF, IL-1 through IL-8, IL-10, IL-13 through IL-16, neuronal growth factor), chemokines (MIP-1α (**M**acrophage **I**nflammatory **P**rotein-1α) and **M**acrophage **C**hemoattractant **P**rotein-1 or MCP-1), and angiogenesis factors (eg, **V**ascular **E**ndothelial **G**rowth **F**actor (VEGF) and **P**latelet-**D**erived **G**rowth **F**actor or PDGF). This second wave of response occurs after the first immediate hypersensitivity reaction and helps amplify it. Together, these molecules are responsible for the recruitment and activation of inflammatory cells (because of increased vascular permeability, increased adhesion of vascular endothelium, and chemoattraction) as well as the smooth muscle contraction, bronchoconstriction, mucus production by goblet cells, and increased gastrointestinal motility observed in anaphylactic shock.

Table 15.2   Pharmacological mediators of basophils and mast cells

Mediator	*Biological effects*
	Preformed mediators
Histamine	Vasodilation, increased capillary permeability, chemokinesis, mucus secretion, bronchoconstriction, cytotoxicity to parasites
Serotonin*	Smooth muscle contraction, increased vascular permeability
Heparin	Anticoagulant; cytotoxicity to parasites
Proteases (tryptase, kiniogenase)	Activation of complement cascade, hydrolysis of plasma kininogen to release bradykinin, connective tissue degradation
NCF-A, ECF-A	Recruitment of neutrophils and eosinophils
TNF-α	Pro-inflammatory; activation of vascular endothelium
	Synthesized mediators
PAF	Aggregation and lysis of platelets resulting in the release of vasoactive amines, heparin, histamine, etc that cause smooth muscle contraction, neutrophil chemotaxis, bronchoconstriction
Leukotrienes** (LTB4, LTC4, LTD4, LTE4)	Prolonged bronchoconstriction and mucus secretion — leukotrienes are a thousand times more potent bronchoconstrictors than histamine; vasoactive, cause pain and oedema; LTB4 causes chemotaxis of basophils
Prostaglandins (PGD2)	Bronchoconstriction, platelet aggregation, vasodilation
Thromboxanes	Bronchoconstriction
Bradykinin	Bronchoconstriction, vasodilation
Cytokines (GM-CSF, IL-1 to IL-8, IL-10, IL-13 to IL-16, neuronal growth factor, MIP-1α, MCP-1, TNF-α, VEGF, PDGF, etc)	Activation of vascular endothelium, recruitment and activation of neutrophils and macrophages, angiogenesis, etc

* Only in mouse; platelet-derived in humans

** Originally called SRS-A (**S**low **R**eacting **S**ubstance of **A**naphylaxis), since they were released in the later phase of the anaphylactic reaction

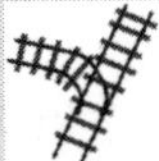

One Man's Food, Another's Poison: Food Allergy

Food allergy is defined as an adverse immunological (hypersensitivity) response to food. Manifestation of the disease is almost as varied as the foods that cause it. Thus, the same food (eg, wheat) can cause in an individual atopic dermatitis, urticaria, anaphylaxis, asthma induced by inhalation of wheat antigens, or coeliac disease caused by gluten. Food allergic disorders mediated by IgE have an acute onset of symptoms after ingestion and affect one or more target organs — skin (urticaira or angioedema), respiratory tract (rhinitis or asthma), gastrointestinal tract (pain, emesis, diarrhoea), and cardiovascular system (anaphylactic shock). Reactions can be triggered by direct exposure of the involved organ to the food or by systemic distribution of proteins after digestion. Food allergic disorders mediated by T cells are subacute or chronic and of delayed onset (occurring after a few hours of ingestion). They typically affect the gastrointestinal tract or skin, with a propensity to affect infants and children. Sensitized T cells can home to different organs or tissues (eg, skin) and result in food-responsive atopic dermatitits. Coeliac disease and the related skin disorder dermatitis herpetiformis are rather serious manifestations of T cell-mediated food allergies to gluten.

Food hypersensitivity is caused by malfunction of the normal immune responses to dietary antigens. In healthy non-allergic individuals, oral tolerance ensures that the gastrointestinal immune system does not react to dietary antigens or commensal bacteria colonizing the gut. Furthermore, humoral immune responses in the gut are of the non-complement fixing, non-inflammatory IgA type. The exact cause of the breakdown of tolerance and a switch from IgA to IgE response is not clear. An alteration in intestinal permeability is often observed in patients with allergies; however, it is not clear if it is a cause or effect of the disease. Cytokines such as IL-4, superantigens, and dietary lectins are all known to affect mucosal membrane permeability. In both animals and humans with food allergy, increases in the number of IELs, mucosal mast cells, and eosinophils are observed in intestinal biopsies. It is therefore proposed that alterations in TH1/TH2 balance may result in food hypersensitivity.

Potent food allergens are usually water-soluble glycoproteins of about 10–60 KD that are stable at low pH. Cooking can affect allergenicity variably; it can reduce allergenicity because of the destruction of allergenic epitopes (as is the case with eggs and fish), but increase the allergenicity of other foods because of covalent modifications that lead to formation of new epitopes or improved stability (eg, roasting of peanuts results in greater resistance to digestion and heightened allergenicity). IgE-mediated food allergies can be diagnosed with the skin-prick test or by detection of antigen-specific IgE. An improvement with dietary elimination of suspected foods is often a presumptive evidence of the disease. Antihistamines can be used for symptomatic treatment. However epinephrine injections remain the mainstay of treatment for anaphylaxis. Currently at least, avoidance of the culprit foodstuff is the only way of preventing allergic episodes.

❑ **Basophils,** like other granulocytes, mature in the bone marrow and then circulate in peripheral blood. In contrast to the long-lived mast cells, basophils have a short life span of a few days. Production and survival of human basophils is dependent upon IL-3. They also require IL-5 and GM-CSF. Like mast cells, basophils have granules with preformed mediators such as histamine, chondroitin sulphate, and neutral proteases. However, they synthesize a rather limited array of mediators following degranulation. These include LTC4, PGD2, IL-4, and IL-13. Although basophils also express FcεRI, being circulating cells, they are recruited to the site of allergenic challenge by the mediators released by mast cells.

The first step in an immediate hypersensitivity reaction is the preferential production and secretion of IgE in response to innocuous substances. Most common allergens are small, readily soluble molecules of low MW. Inhalation or contact with minute doses of the allergen results in a TH2-driven response. B cells undergo an isotype switch from IgM to IgE when exposed to TH2-derived cytokines IL-4 and IL-13 (chapter 8). Once the B cells switch to IgE, subsequent exposures also result in an IgE response. The type of antigen, dose and route of administration, as well as the cytokine milieu are important in this response (chapter 4).

Since both mast cells and basophils express FcεRI, they get coated with any IgE present in their vicinity. Cross-linking of FcεRI-bound IgE by a multivalent antigen results in degranulation of the cells and release of bioactive mediators responsible for manifestations and symptoms of type I hypersensitivity[2]. The primary dose of the allergen that results in the IgE response is called the 'sensitizing dose', and the later dose that precipitates the reaction is the 'shocking dose'. Ligation of FcεRI-bound IgE by the antigen induces the activation of protein tyrosine kinases associated with the receptor and results in phosphorylation of ITAMs present on the receptor subunits. The ensuing activation of downstream signalling pathways leads to the degranulation of cells and the synthesis and release of lipid mediators, cytokines, chemokines, and growth factors that are responsible for symptoms of anaphylaxis.

Mast cell degranulation is preceded by the massive influx of Ca^{2+} ions into cells. This is a crucial step in the process, since ionophores that cause an increase in cytoplasmic Ca^{2+} can cause degranulation even in the absence of IgE ligation, and agents that deplete cytoplasmic Ca^{2+} suppress degranulation[3]. **The immediate result of IgE-mediated degranulation is an inflammatory response that starts within seconds and is followed by a late phase response that takes six to twelve hours to develop.** The immediate inflammation is due to the release of preformed pharmacological mediators such as histamine and the rapid synthesis and release of prostaglandins and other toxic metabolites following degranulation.

The pharmacological mediators cause a rapid increase in vascular permeability and smooth muscle contraction. ECF-A, IL-4, IL-5, LTC4, and histamine cause an influx of eosinophils, whereas MIP-1α, MCP-1, NCF-A, and IL-8 are responsible for recruitment of phagocytic monocytes and neutrophils. PAF, released in the later phase of the response, causes platelet aggregation and further release of histamine, heparin, and vasoactive amines. The combined effect of these mediators is an influx of leukocytes to the site of allergenic challenge and results in a sustained late-phase reaction (fig. 15.1). Thus, even though the initial cells involved in anaphylactic reactions are mast cells and basophils, platelets, neutrophils, and eosinophils also get involved in the later phases. Although most of these responses to allergen challenge are transient and reversible, repeated challenges can lead to chronic inflammation with progressively increasing severity of symptoms, and it may even prove fatal.

Binding of IgE to FcεRI has biologically important consequences beyond sensitization and eventual degranulation of mast cells and basophils. IgE also upregulates surface expression of FcεRI by mast cells and basophils. In addition, IgE-bound cells have an enhanced ability to secrete histamine, MIP-1α, and lipid mediators following FcεRI aggregation. MIP-1α (like IL-4 and IL-13 also produced by mast cells) has been reported to increase IgE production by B cells, suggesting a potential positive feedback mechanism — increase in IgE leads to increased FcεRI expression, which in turn increases the probability of degranulation, increasing release of IL-4, IL-13, and MIP-1α themselves responsible for increased IgE production. Monomeric IgE has also been shown to increase mast cell survival by an unknown mechanism *in vitro*, raising the possibility that it may affect mast cell survival *in vivo* as well. Monocytes and DCs are known to express a trimeric version of FcεRI. Cross-linking of the receptor prevents apoptosis and triggers IL-10 production. In individuals with high levels of FcεRI, ligation of the receptors on monocytes and DCs was found to activate the pro-inflammatory transcription factor NFκB. Together, these data suggest that IgE may contribute directly and indirectly to chronic allergic inflammation and the persistence of symptoms associated with it.

Manifestations of type I hypersensitivity vary according to the site of the response (Table 15.3).

❑ The local reaction is limited to the target organ or tissue. It is often observed when the allergen comes in contact with epithelial surfaces or respiratory mucus membranes. Thus, involvement of skin results in urticaria or eczema, the eyes in

---

[2] IgE can also bind other FcRs other than FcεRs (FcγRII, FcγRIII) expressed by some mast cell populations. However, ligation of these FcRs does not result in degranulation.

[3] Degranulation can also be triggered by other stimuli such as exercise, emotional stress, chemicals, anaphylatoxins such as C3a, C5a, as well as MBP released by eosinophils. Although the resulting symptoms are similar to anaphylaxis, these are not hypersensitivity reactions, since IgE is not involved.

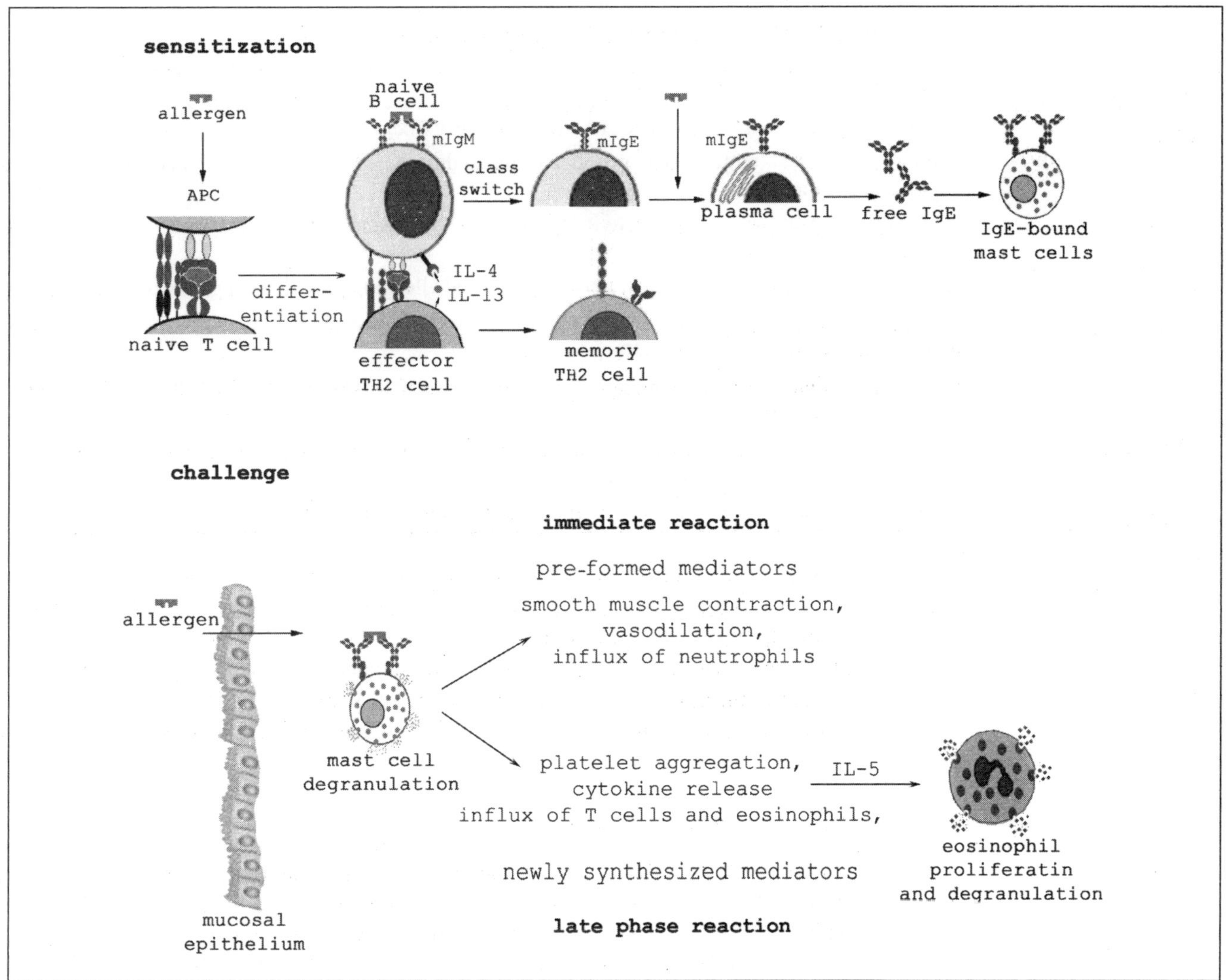

Figure 15.1 Allergen-mediated cross-linking of FcεR-bound IgE causes degranulation of mast cells, basophils, and eosinophils and results in manifestations of hypersensitivity type I reactions. Hypersensitivity type I responses can be divided into two phases. In the sensitization phase (top panel), naïve T cells differentiate to TH2 effector and memory cells. The effector TH2 cells help antigen-activated B cells to switch their isotype to IgE by producing cytokines like IL-4 and IL-13. Sensitization leads to the establishment of allergen-specific memory TH2 cells and memory B cells that produce IgE on further antigenic challenge. IgE produced by the B cells binds to FcεRs expressed by mast cells and basophils. Upon subsequent challenge (lower panel), the allergen will bind to FcεR-bound IgE on mast cells present in the mucosal epithelia and trigger their degranulation. The release of preformed mediators present in the granules is responsible for the immediate effects of type I hypersensitivity. Degranulation also causes the synthesis and release of new mediators that result in platelet aggregation and influx of T cells and eosinophils. Cytokines like IL-5 produced by the T cells induce proliferation and degranulation of eosinophils, resulting in the late phase reaction.

conjunctivitis, a reaction in the nasopharynx results in rhinitis, bronchopulmonary tissue involvement results in hay fever and/or asthma, whereas gastritis is caused by a reaction in the gastrointestinal tract.

❑ The systemic form of hypersensitivity is often fatal and develops when the allergen is given parenterally. Called anaphylactic shock, it occurs within minutes of allergen administration. Disseminated mast cell activation causes widespread increase in vascular permeability (causing disastrous capillary leakage and a precipitous fall in blood pressure), constriction of airways (causing difficulty in breathing), laryngeal oedema, etc. The syndrome can be controlled by the immediate injection of epinephrine. A wide range of substances can trigger systemic anaphylactic shock including insect venom, anti-toxins, seafoods, and

Table 15.3 Classical anaphylactic reactions

Type of reaction	Characteristics
Hay fever (allergic rhinoconjunctivitis)	Is characterized by catarrh of conjunctiva and respiratory tract
	Occurs when inhaled allergens such as pollen, (house) dust, or mold spores come in contact with exposed mucous membranes
Asthma	Is characterized by airway hyper-reactivity and obstruction of small bronchioles, resulting in difficulty in breathing
	Is caused mainly by inhaled allergens, although ingested allergens may also trigger an asthmatic attack
Urticaria	Is characterized by the appearance of skin rashes — crops of intensely itching wheals with raised white centres surrounded by erythema
	Is caused by contact with or inhalation of a wide variety of sensitizers — sea food, egg whites, wheat, tomatoes, chocolates, etc
Angioedema	Is characterized by skin rashes similar to urticaria, but with larger wheals restricted mainly to the face and neck
	Is caused by contact with or inhalation of the sensitizing substance

peanuts. Administration of drugs like penicillin, vitamin B$_6$, or insulin, or exposure to anaesthetics such as benzocaine and lidocaine can also result in anaphylactic shock in sensitized individuals[4].

❑ A mixed reaction may develop if the allergen enters the body via the mucus membranes of the gut. It is characterized by gastrointestinal symptoms (vomiting, diarrhoea, etc caused by the activation of intestinal mast cells), as well as skin rashes, asthma, etc.

15.2.1 Interplaying Factors

Although allergic diseases have been described since ancient times and countless studies have been undertaken to determine the underlying causes, the factors responsible for the onset and maintenance of type I hypersensitivities are not clear. The determination of these factors has become all the more urgent, since it is now well established that the incidence of allergies has increased dramatically in the last 50 years. Like autoimmune diseases, a number of interplaying factors are thought to contribute to the occurrence of allergic disorders.

❑ **Genetic factors.** It has been recognized since the 1920s that allergic parents tend to have a higher proportion of allergic children, ie, type I hypersensitivity tends to run in families. The word 'atopy' is used to describe this propensity to develop allergies which is strongly linked to T$_{H2}$ type responses and raised IgE levels. Three atopic diseases in particular are inherently connected within families — asthma, atopic eczema, and rhinoconjunctivits. There is almost a 50% chance of children suffering from these if both their parents are allergic. The figure reduces to 30% if one of the parents is allergic. Several loci for specific atopy-associated genes have been determined on various chromosomes (Table 15.4). Not surprisingly, these include genes for cytokines, TcR, and MHC class II molecules. Interestingly, a particular HLA-DR locus seems to increase the risk of allergy to a specific allergen. Thus, the HLA-DR2 allele is found to be associated with ragweed pollen allergy whereas the HLA-DR3 allele is associated with allergy to grasses. However, genetic background alone cannot explain the incidence of allergies, particularly the increase observed over the last few decades.

❑ **Environmental factors.** The environment clearly influences the incidence of allergies. Allergies are more prevalent in urban rather than rural areas, whether in Ethiopia or Germany. This has led to the suggestion that the traditional lifestyles of indigenous peoples in tropical environments tend to reduce the occurrence of

[4] Although drug induced, this reaction is different from type II hypersensitivity, since the damage is caused by IgE-mediated degranulation of mast cells and it is not the result of complement activation by anti-drug IgG antibodies.

Table 15.4 Genetic loci associated with allergic diseases

Chromosome	Gene product
5q31-35	T_{H2} cytokines: IL-3, IL-4, IL-5, IL-9, IL-13
	CD14
	β-adrenergic receptor
	Glucocorticoid receptor
6p21	MHC class II molecules
	MHC class III molecules (TNF-α)
7	TcR α chain
11q13	β chain of FcεRI

allergic disease, and their progressive westernization places them at a greater risk of developing these conditions. This hypothesis is supported by studies that compared the incidence of asthma in immigrant groups in industrialized countries with that of the populations in the native developing country; the prevalence of asthma in the immigrant groups was significantly greater than in their compatriots in the native country. The observed increase of allergies in urban areas has given credence to the idea that increased environmental pollution results in increased type I hypersensitivity. However, different pollutants seem to affect humans differently. Type I pollutants are characterized by SO_2, large particles, and dust emitted from predominantly outdoor sources and have adverse health effects such as upper respiratory tract inflammation and infection. Type II air pollutants are emitted from outdoor and indoor sources and include volatile organic acids, ozone, NO_x, and cigarette smoke. These have been found to lead to allergic sensitization of the airways and are considered risk factors for atopic disease.

Exposure to allergens is a pre-requisite for allergies. The increased use of indoor furnishings such as carpets and curtains, tends to concentrate house-dust mites (*Dermatophagoides pteryonyssinus*) in the immediate environment of an individual, and this has been recorded to increase the incidence of adult asthma in case studies. House dust mites and especially their faecal pellets are a major allergen in the house environment and removal of fixtures that house these allergens has often shown to decrease the severity of asthma attacks in patients. Pollen grains are a common outdoor allergen whose counts seem to have increased because of increased pollution. Also, the release of allergens from pollen grains seems to have altered in urban areas. Interaction of pollen grains with type II air pollutants has been shown to lead to agglomeration and changes in surface structure, with a concomitant increase in allergen release.

❑ **Lifestyle choices.** Lifestyles seem to influence the incidence of allergies. Recent studies have indicated that children raised in big families and on farms tend to have a lower incidence of allergies then those raised in nuclear families. This has given rise to the hygiene hypothesis (see sidetrack 'Too Clean For Comfort'). Cigarette smoking and exposure to cigarette smoke is also known to predispose an individual to allergies. Other lifestyle choices such as increased psychological stress, lack of exercise — linked to increased TV viewing and therefore greater exposure to indoor allergens — changed food habits with early introduction to exotic foods, etc have all been implicated in increased allergies. However, in the absence of clear experimental data, it is difficult to draw firm conclusions about the effects of these factors on the incidence of allergies.

15.2.2 Diagnosis

The passive transfer of allergy via serum was first demonstrated by the famous experiment of Prausnitz and Kustener. Kustener was allergic to fish, but Prausnitz was not. Prausnitz injected Kustener's serum intracutaneously in his own forearm

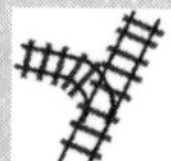

Too Clean For Comfort: Hygiene Hypothesis

There has been a remarkable increase in allergy-linked diseases such as asthma, atopic dermatitis, and hay fever in developed (read 'westernized') countries. Even after accounting for factors such as better diagnosis and a hereditary component, there is little doubt that this increase in the incidence of allergies is real. The best documented has been asthma — the prevalence of asthma has increased 75%, in the USA alone, from 1980 to 1994. By contrast, the low baseline prevalence of allergic disease has not changed appreciably over the same period in the developing world. The rapidity of the epidemiological shift suggests a change in environment as a possible culprit. Interestingly, a similar trend has been observed for the incidence of autoimmune diseases as well. While the incidence of childhood infections has shown a continuous downward trend since the 1950s in Western Europe and USA, there is an almost parallel upward trend in the incidence of autoimmune diseases. The 'hygiene hypothesis', put forward to explain this phenomenon, is increasingly gaining acceptance in the scientific community. It is derived from a number of studies across the developed world. These studies noted an inverse relation between the risk of allergy and family size (bigger the family, less the chances of developing allergies), exposure to animals (allergies are less frequent in children growing on farms), and a direct correlation between parental economic status (the higher income group, the more prone to allergies), educational background (more educated the parents, greater the chances of allergy), and even birth order (only or first-born children seem to be more likely to develop allergies). Thus, childhood infections show an overwhelming and consistent negative association with allergic disorders.

The hygiene hypothesis postulates that infectious stressors guide the development of the immune system. Children with a western lifestyle who are protected from childhood infections and/or exposure to a variety of infectious agents fail to get this 'education' and have an increased risk of developing allergic and/or autoimmune diseases. Thus, exposure to food and orofecal pathogens such as the hepatitis A virus, *Toxoplasma gondii*, or *Helicobacter pylori*, reduces the risk of atopy by >60%. Studies have also revealed a difference in the rate and quality of bacterial colonization in children with and without a predisposition to allergy. An early colonization with enterobacteria or lactobacilli has a protective effect against allergy, whereas early exposure to antibiotics changes the bacterial flora and is a risk factor. It was initially thought that a shift in the balance from T_H1 to T_H2 might be responsible for allergy development. However, worldwide, helminth infections and allergic diseases do not overlap, despite both conditions being accompanied by strong T_H2 type responses. Recent work on DCs and induction of T_R cells has resulted in a plausible explanation for this phenomenon and provided an immunological framework for the hygiene hypothesis. Chronic parasitic infections are known to cause T cell hyporesponsiveness in humans. Downregulatory molecules such as IL-10, TGF-β, and NO are implicated in this suppression, and they seem to be effective against both T_H1 and T_H2 type responses. It is therefore proposed that a high overall infection turnover (such as observed in developing countries) may be instrumental in the development of an immunoregulatory network. When uncontrolled, strong T_H1 or T_H2 responses can lead to autoimmunity and allergy. High pathogen burden is thought to endow DCs with the ability to induce T_R cells. These T_R cells produce immunosuppressive cytokines such as IL-10 and TGF-β and thus ensure that inflammatory responses (either of the T_H1 or T_H2 type) with their negative health repercussions are kept under control. It is rather ironic that just as we were about to breathe a sigh of relief for winning the war against childhood infections, we have to find a way to increase our exposure to them in order to avoid increasing our chances of contracting allergies.

(life, or for that matter science, was definitely easier in pre-AIDS days). An injection of fish extract in the area elicited a wheal and flare (oedema and erythema) reaction characterized by inflammation and reddening, indicating the successful passive transfer of hypersensitivity. The reaction is called the P-K reaction in their honour. The **PCA** (**P**assive **C**utaneous **A**naphylaxis) test developed by Ovary is essentially similar to the P-K test and is used to demonstrate the presence of sensitizing IgE antibodies in serum. The test is performed by injecting antiserum or purified antibodies intradermally in the test animal (guinea pig) and challenging it with a subcutaneous injection of antigen a few hours later. A dye such as Evan's Blue is injected along with the antigen to facilitate observation. An irregular circular stained area appears at the site of challenge; the size of the area is an indication of the concentration of antibodies in the preparation.

The allergic status of an individual can be determined using a patch test. It can be used to determine hypersensitivity to drugs, cosmetics, surfactants, botanicals, etc. The test is performed by placing antigen extract in contact with the skin of the arm and occluding the area for up to 48 hours. A negative control (without the antigen extract) is placed on the other arm to eliminate false positive reactions. A positive test is characterized by a typical wheal and flare reaction at the site of contact with the allergen. Hypersensitivity may also be determined by demonstrating allergen-specific IgE in the patient's serum by ELISA or RIA (see Appendix III).

15.2.3 Treatment

The best treatment for allergy is to avoid the allergen, although this may not always be feasible. In case of contact with the allergen, immediate treatment is needed to alleviate symptoms.

❑ Administration of anti-histamines such as diphenylhydramine is used to relieve the early phase symptoms or to prevent mast cell degranulation.

❑ Sodium chromoglycate inhibits mast cell degranulation, probably by inhibiting Ca^{2+} influx.

❑ Cyclic nucleotides appear to play a significant role in the modulation of immediate hypersensitivity reactions. Substances that increase intracellular cAMP seem to relieve allergic symptoms (especially bronchopulmonary symptoms) and are used therapeutically.

- Isoproterenol derivatives such as isoprenaline or salbutamol stimulate β-adrenergic receptors and prevent release of pharmacological mediators from mast cells; they are used in bronchodilators for short term relief.

- Epinephrine (also known as adrenaline) has a similar mode of action as isoproterenol and is a mainstay of anaphylactic shock treatment. People who have experienced anaphylactic shock or who have scored very high on skin-prick allergy tests are advised to carry a single dose of epinephrine in the form of an autoinjector at all times to avoid life-threatening episodes of anaphylactic shock.

- Theophylline increases intracytoplasmic cAMP levels by inhibiting cAMP-phosphodiesterase. It also inhibits intracellular Ca^{2+} release and is used to relieve bronchopulmonary symptoms in asthma.

- Phenoxybenzamine elevates cAMP by blocking β-adrenergic receptors and is used for therapeutic relief of symptoms.

❑ Late onset symptoms such as bronchoconstriction that are mediated by leukotrienes can be treated with leukotriene receptor blockers or inhibitors of cyclooxeganase pathways or corticosteroids.

Immunotherapy (desensitization or hyposensitization) aimed at the elicitation of a non-IgE response to the allergens can be successful, especially for insect venom and pollen allergy. It consists of repeated injections of small, but increasing amounts of the adjuvant bound antigen extracts. Although the mechanism of desensitization is not clear, the treatment results in an increase in allergen-specific serum IgG levels and a decrease in IgE levels. Owing to their ability to inhibit immediate skin reactions to allergen provocation, these IgG antibodies are called 'blocking antibodies'. However, immunotherapeutic administration of allergens is itself likely to cause local or systemic side effects such as urticaria or even anaphylactic shock. The allergen is therefore chemically modified or adsorbed to an adjuvant to delay systemic release. Since most extracts are not chemically pure, there is also the risk that the therapy itself may induce new IgE reactivities towards extract components.

15.3 Hypersensitivity Type II

Multiple factors are brought into play when IgG or IgM antibodies recognize and bind to antigens expressed on cell surface of pathogens or transformed cells. Briefly, the process is as follows.

❑ Complement is activated, MAC is formed and results in the lysis of the target cell (chapter 3).

❑ C3a and C5a released during complement activation cause vasodilation and chemotaxis of PMNs to the site of the reaction. Additionally, the released anaphylatoxins cause the degranulation of mast cells so that the cytotoxic and pro-inflammatory arsenal of these cells is also available for the destruction of target cells.

❑ Neutrophils recruited to the site of interaction phagocytose dead and dying cells. They also liberate an array of microbicidal agents.

❑ K cells may also be recruited to the site of infection and are responsible for complement-independent ADCC.

❑ Antigen-antibody complexes bind to platelets via their FcRs and result in platelet aggregation and microthrombus formation; aggregation leads to the release of vasoactive amines, further increasing PMN influx.

❑ If the antigen-antibody complex is embedded in tissue or is too large for engulfment, phagocytosis fails; neutrophils release their lysosomal contents in the external milieu by exocytosis, thereby releasing a corrosive cocktail of enzymes/acids in surrounding tissue.

❑ The end result of these events is an inflammatory response that helps get rid of intruders. However, other cells in the vicinity (called bystanders) may also be killed in the process, ie, the protective process is not without collateral damage. Healing and tissue remodelling begins immediately, and the system returns to normal.

This protective response can become destructive if the antibodies are against cell surface or tissue antigens, and the reaction is then called cytotoxic or type II hypersensitivity. The antigen could be endogenous (molecules expressed by cells) or exogenous (eg, hapten adsorbed to tissue cells). The kind of tissue or organ affected and the intensity of the reaction depends upon the location and concentration of the antigen. Manifestations of type II hypersensitivities include:

❑ **Autoimmune diseases.** A variety of autoimmune diseases are a result of type II hypersensitivity and include Myasthenia gravies, Goodpasture's syndrome, autoimmune gastritis, autoimmune haemolytic anaemia, and Pemphigous vulgaris.

❑ **Transfusion reactions.** In chapter 13, we explained that erythrocytes express multiple membrane antigens and that the transfer of incompatible blood results in severe transfusion reactions (Table 13.2). Other components of blood, including leukocytes and platelets, may also give rise to transfusion reactions though they are often of less severity. The transfusion reaction is acute and immediate if the recipient has been previously exposed to donor antigens. If considerable amount of antibodies are present in the blood at the time of transfusion, a rapid intravascular (ABO incompatibility) or extravascular (Rh incompatibility) lysis of the donor red blood cells is observed. Symptoms include fever, chills, nausea, and vomiting. Circulatory shock as well as acute necrosis of the kidneys is a complication associated with intravascular lysis. A previously unsensitized transfusion recipient may develop antibodies to antigens on donor erythrocytes over a period of time, and this may give rise to delayed jaundice and anaemia.

❑ **Haemolytic disease of the newborn (Erythroblastosis foetalis).** This may be observed when blood groups of the foetus and the mother are mismatched and maternal IgG antibodies to foetal erythrocytic antigens cross the placenta. The antibodies cause the destruction of foetal erythrocytes resulting in the development

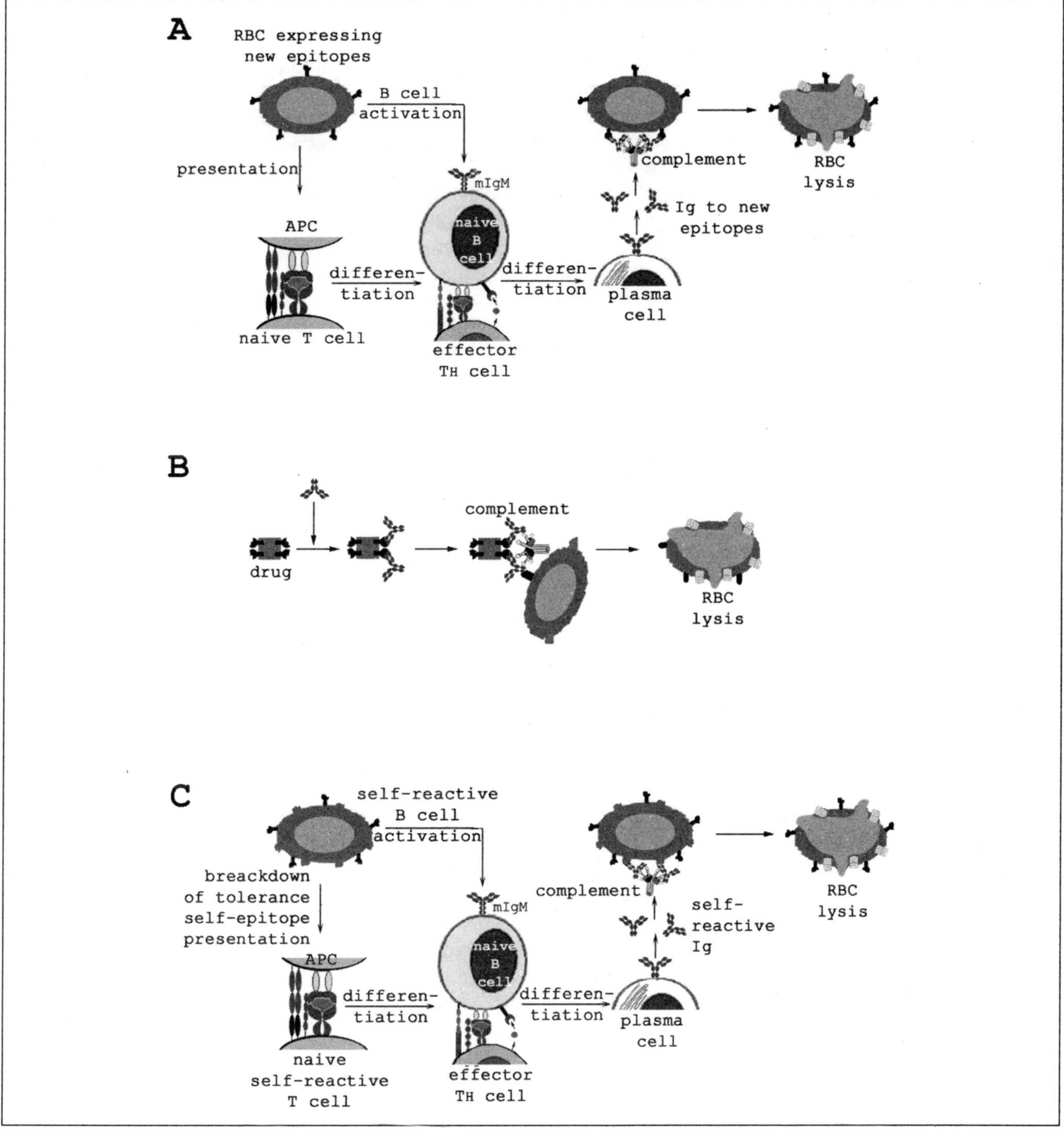

Figure 15.2 Adsorption of drugs to erythrocytes can trigger an immune response that results in complement-mediated lysis of RBCs. *Multiple mechanisms can result in drug-induced anaemias. The primary event common to all of them is the induction of an immune response to the drug. Drugs that get adsorbed to erythrocytes or tissue cells appear as new epitopes to the immune system. Processing and presentation of such drug-adsorbed cells by professional APCs results in activation and differentiation of helper T cells. Cross-linking of BcRs on naïve B cells by the drug-erythrocyte complex causes B cell activation. On receiving appropriate T cell help, these B cells differentiate to plasma cells that secrete anti-drug antibodies. Recognition of the drug epitopes on RBCs by the antibodies results in complement-mediated lysis of the erythrocytes (top panel; A). Lysis of incompatible donor RBCs observed in transfusion reactions also occurs by a similar mechanism. Complement-mediated erythrocyte lysis can also occur if drug-Ig complexes bind to RBCs via FcRs or complement receptors (central panel; B). The lowermost panel (C) depicts the third mechanism of drug-induced anaemia. The presence of the drug on the erythrocyte may result in altered processing and presentation by the APCs (eg, expression of new proteases or alteration in the epitopes being presented). This altered presentation can cause a breakdown of self-tolerance and the formation of autoantibodies, and it may result in extensive lysis of RBCs.*

of anaemia and jaundice within the first 24 hours of life. Rh incompatibility —
Rh^- mother and Rh^+ foetus — is one of the most common causes of this
disease. Since the mother has to be sensitized to the antigen, the disease is not
manifested during the birth of the first Rh^+ child. Sensitization may occur during
this first childbirth, when foetal cord blood can enter the mother's circulation,
and the risk of the disease increases exponentially with each new Rh^+ foetus.
Sensitization can be avoided by the administration of anti-RhD serum within 72
hours of delivery of the first Rh^+ child. As explained in chapter 8, memory B cells
suppress naïve B cell activation. The administration of anti-Rh antibodies
exploits this phenomenon. The anti-RhD antibodies will also opsonize any foetal
erythrocytes that may have entered the mother's circulation and facilitate their
removal before they can activate the mother's immune system. The administration
of anti-RhD antibodies must occur before the sensitization of the mother since
activation of memory B cells is not inhibited by the presence of antibodies. Severe
haemolytic disease during pregnancy can be treated with intrauterine blood-
exchange, wherein foetal Rh^+ blood is replaced with Rh^- blood[5]. Haemolytic
disease can also be caused by ABO incompatibility; however, the disease is rarely
severe enough to entail any treatment.

❑ **Drug induced anaemias**. A variety of drugs (eg, quinines, sulphonamides, and
penicillins) can get adsorbed to erythrocytes, platelets, etc and provoke
hypersensitivity type II reactions (fig. 15.2). Autoimmune anaemias (whether drug
induced or otherwise) can also be a result of phagocytosis of autoantibody
coated erythrocytes.

15.4 Hypersensitivity Type III

**Type III hypersensitivity (also called 'immune complex disease') is caused by
the persistence of immune complexes in circulation.** Although both type II and
type III reactions are at least partly the result of complement activation, unlike the
type II reaction, **the antigen in type III reaction is soluble and not attached to the
tissue.** As seen in chapter 3, complement is activated as a consequence of antigen-
IgG (or IgM) interaction and results in cytolysis, PMN and mast cell recruitment,
etc. Scavenger cells such as macrophages and monocytes remove these immune
complexes by FcR-mediated endocytosis. However, moderate antigen excess can
result in the formation of small complexes (Ag.Ab2 or Ag3.Ab2) that are not easily
removed by the scavengers. Consequently, they tend to remain in circulation and
become deposited on tissues, initiating complement-mediated and neutrophil
exocytosis-mediated tissue injury and inflammation (fig. 15.3). Kidneys are often
the site of this immune-complex damage and nephrotoxicity is an identifying feature
of type III hypersensitivity. Experiments in KO mice suggest that mast cells may
have a major role in the pathology of immune complex disease. On the basis of these
experiments, it is being postulated that mast cell degranulation caused by binding of
IgG-antigen complexes to FcγRIII may contribute significantly to the type III reaction.

**Many human diseases are associated with circulating immune complexes
and the spectrum of symptoms depends upon the site of immune complex
deposition.** Chronic immune complex formation is often observed in chronic and
persistent infections that elicit a weak antibody response (eg, malaria and viral
hepatitis). Since small antigen-antibody complexes are barely soluble and are often
filtered out in capillary beds or may be driven into vessel walls at places of especially
turbulent flow, the kidneys and lungs are often the site of tissue damage in immune
complex disease. Complex deposition may occur in the small blood vessels, kidneys,
joints, and skin, resulting in vasculitis, glomerulonephritis, scar tissue formation,
and urticaria respectively. In contrast, repeated inhalation of an antigen (spores of
fungi, actinomycetes, tissue (or hair) of animals or plants) may result in the deposition
of complexes in the lungs, eg, Farmer's lung, and Pigeon Fancier's disease. Immune

---

[5] Detection of Erythroblastosis foetalis is
done by Coombs' test described in
Appendix III.

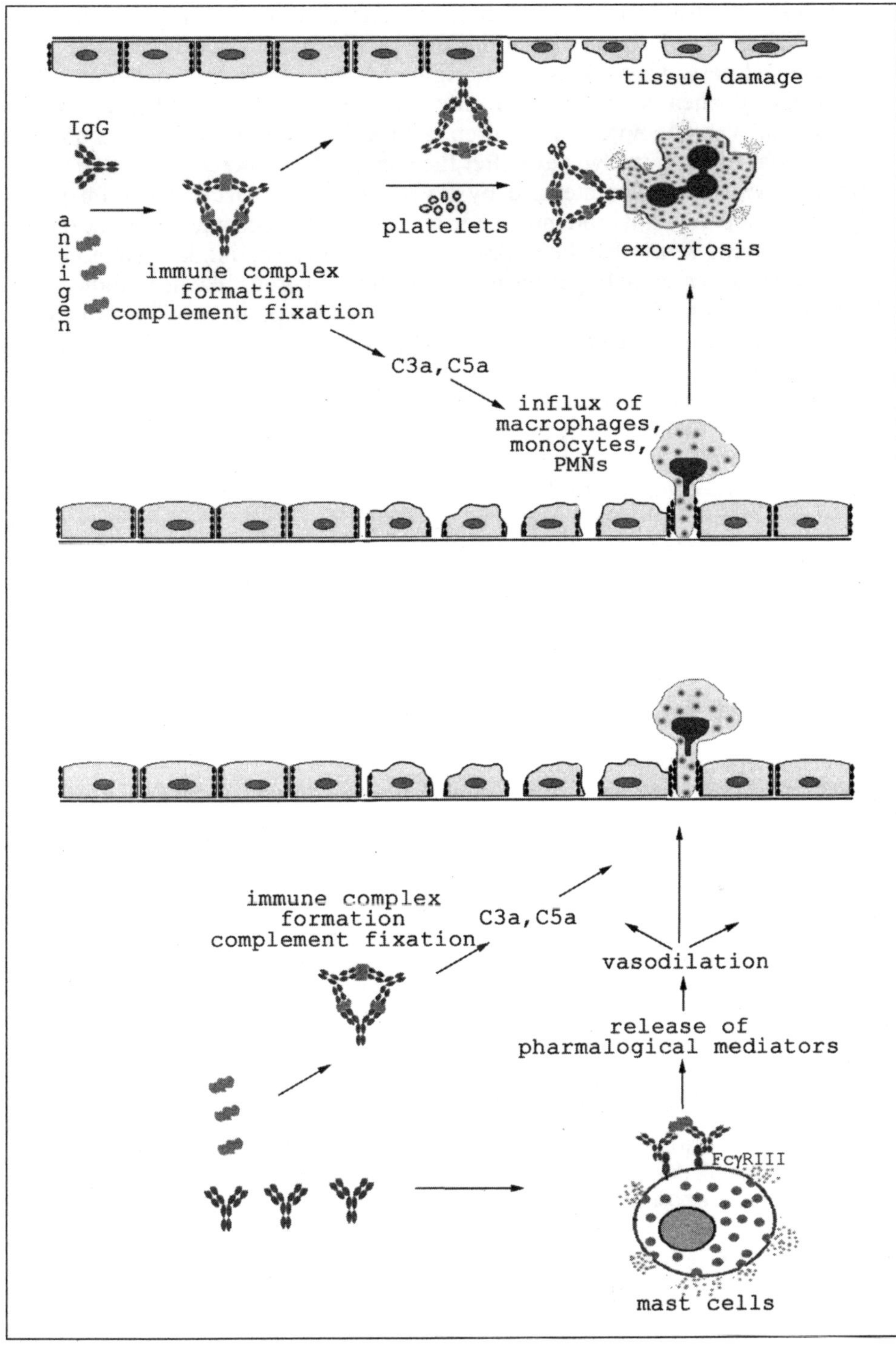

Figure 15.3 Type III hypersensitivity is caused by the persistence of large quantities of small, soluble immune complexes in circulation. *Small antigen-antibody complexes are barely soluble and are often filtered out in capillary beds or may be driven into vessel walls at places of turbulent flow such as the kidneys. The immune complexes also adhere to platelets via FcRs and result in microthrombus formation. C3a and C5a released as a result of immune complex formation, and chemokines released by the platelets attract PMNs and monocytes to the site. Unable to endocytose the complexes, the scavengers release their intracellular contents by exocytosis, causing tissue injury and inflammation. Mast cells have a major role in localized reactions (lower panel). Cross-linking of FcγRIII expressed on tissue mast cells by the immune complexes causes their degranulation. The pharmacological mediators and chemoattractants released result in the influx of inflammatory cells to the site and subsequently cause tissue damage.*

complexes may also be formed by autoantibodies and may result in autoimmune diseases like SLE or RA. Manifestations of type III hypersensitivity include:

- ❑ **Serum sickness.** This disease was originally observed in the beginning of the 20th century when passive immunization with massive doses of horse or rabbit antiserum was attempted in children with acute bacterial infections such as diphtheria. Eight to twelve days after the therapy, the children developed a self-limited syndrome characterized by fever, urticaria, muscle and joint pains, lymphadenopathy, and proteinuria. Serum sickness has become rare since the use of heterologus serum has been discontinued. However, similar symptoms are sometimes observed in hypersensitivity reactions to drugs like penicillin.
- ❑ **Arthus reaction.** This is the name given to a local type III reaction that can be demonstrated experimentally by a subcutaneous injection of a soluble antigen in pre-immunized animals having a high titre of IgG antibodies. Oedema and haemorrhage develop at the site of the injection within four to ten hours and subside within 48 hours. The reaction is slower than the type I reaction, since the $Fc\gamma RIII$ receptor is a low affinity receptor, and the threshold of activation of mast cells via this receptor is considerably higher than for the $Fc\varepsilon RI$ receptor. A passive cutaneous form of the Arthus reaction can be demonstrated by injecting a high titre antiserum intravenously in a non-sensitized animal and challenging it later with an intradermal injection of the antigen.
- ❑ **Generalized type III reactions.** Persistent soluble complexes are found in post-infection complications and result in glomerulonephritis, arthritis, etc. Type

---

HYPERSENSITIVITY TYPE I

- ❑ IgE antibodies play a central role in this type of hypersensitivity.
- ❑ It is triggered by the degranulation of mast cells, basophils, or eosinophils by cross-linking of IgE-bound $Fc\varepsilon RI$.
- ❑ The early phase reaction begins seconds to minutes after allergenic challenge and is caused by the release of preformed mediators.
- ❑ The late phase reaction sets in 6–12 hours later, and is caused by leukotrienes and cytokines released by mast cells.
- ❑ Its manifestations include uticaria, hay fever, rhinitis, asthma, and anaphylactic shock.
- ❑ Treatment:
  - Medications to alleviate symptoms such as antihistamines, sodium chromoglycate, epinephrine, isoprenaline, salbutamol, theophylline, phenoxybenzamine, and corticosteroids.
  - Immunotherapy aimed at the elicitation of a non-IgE response.

HYPERSENSITIVITY TYPE II

- ❑ Type II hypersensitivity is a cytolytic reaction caused by antibodies to cell surface antigens.
- ❑ Complement-mediated cytolysis is responsible for some of the damage observed.
- ❑ Manifestations are seen in blood transfusion reactions, Erythroblastosis foetalis, and drug-induced anaemias.

HYPERSENSITIVITY TYPE III

- ❑ Persistence of small complexes consisting of a soluble antigen and low affinity antibodies are responsible for type III hypersensitivity.
- ❑ Tissue damage is often seen in areas of turbulence and high blood pressure such as the kidneys, alveoli, joints, etc.
- ❑ Examples of type III hypersensitivity include Farmer's lung, Pigeon Fancier's disease, Serum sickness, and autoimmune disorders such as RA and SLE.

HYPERSENSITIVITY TYPE IV

- ❑ Type IV reaction is of the delayed-type with symptoms observed a minimum 24 hours after antigenic challenge.
- ❑ It is observed in a number of diseases where the pathogen tends to persist intracellularly.
- ❑ Manifestations of the type IV reaction are observed in leprosy, tuberculosis, leishmaniasis, blastomycosis, histoplasmosis, schistosomiasis, etc.

III reactions are also observed in a variety of autoimmune diseases such as RA, SLE, and Sjogren's syndrome.

15.5 Hypersensitivity Type IV

Although first described by Koch in 1882, it was not until the 1940s that Landsteiner and Chase proved that type IV hypersensitivity was caused by cellular and not humoral components of immunity. For the first time, they experimentally demonstrated that this type of immunity can be transferred solely by transferring cells. Unlike the antibody-mediated type I, type II, and type III responses that are manifested within minutes or hours after antigen exposure, type IV hypersensitivity takes between 24 and 72 hours to develop and is therefore called DTH (**D**elayed-**T**ype of **H**ypersensitivity). **DTH is mediated by CD4$^+$ T cells in conjunction with CD8$^+$ CTLs.** The lag between antigenic challenge and manifestation of DTH thus reflects the slower nature of cellular responses which require induction of cytokines/ chemokines and an influx of cells. Thus, if type I, II, and III hypersensitivity responses are humoral responses gone awry, DTH can be argued to be CMI gone awry. Unfortunately, the exact relation between the protective and destructive functions of

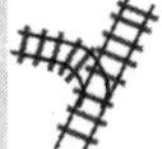

Cellular Ghettos: Granulomas

A granuloma can be described as localized inflammatory reaction; immune granulomas contain T cells and represent a form of DTH. The central feature in granuloma formation is the persistence of antigen that cannot be easily cleared by phagocytic cells. In infection-induced granulomas, the lesions represent a localized interface between infectious agents and the immune system. Persistence of pathogens in macrophages causes their chronic activation. Such activated macrophages fuse to form characteristic epitheloid and multi-nuclear giant cells around the source of irritation, ie, the pathogen. An extracellular matrix shields this cellular conglomerate from healthy tissue.

Macrophages are the prominent cell types in all granulomas. γδ T cells and NKT cells are also found in granulomatous lesions, although their role in these lesions is unclear. T cells and myeloid inflammatory effector cells are recruited to the complex. T cells provide TNF-α that is crucial for the initiation and maintenance of granulomas. In addition, they are also the source of chemokines required for macrophage recruitment. T cells are also involved in complex regulatory circuits that determine every aspect of these localized inflammatory lesions. Such granuloma formation is protective for the host, since the inflammatory reaction gets isolated and insulated while adjacent tissue remains healthy. Moreover, the expansion and spread of infectious agents is also inhibited. This idea is supported by the fact that compromised granuloma formation results in disseminated infection and host death. Granulomas are now believed to represent a mutually advantageous compromise between some infectious agents (such as *M. tuberculosis*) and their hosts. They ensure a longer life for the host while the infectious agent is allowed to survive in the granuloma but is subjected to a restrictive and harsh environment. However, under certain conditions, granulomas can contribute to disease pathology. Granuloma formation and the fibrotic scarring that follows can cause progressive organ damage and are a significant part of the pathology of granulamatous diseases such as schistosomiasis. Schistosome egg-induced granulomas induce fibrosis and result in increased portal blood pressure. It was previously thought that the pathogen remained dormant in the granuloma and bided its time until the individual was immunocompromised so that the pathogen could establish a focus of infection. However, new evidence shows that *M. tuberculosis* does not exist in a dormant state in the granuloma; instead it expresses an array of granuloma-specific genes that are actively induced by this specific microenvironment. It was initially suggested that DTH responses and granuloma formation is a TH1 response. It is now known that both TH1 and TH2 cells are involved in granuloma formation. TH1 cells are involved in granulomas caused by bacterial, viral, and fungal pathogens (eg, tuberculosis, leprosy, listeriosis, Q fever, blastomycosis, histoplasmosis, and infectious mononucleosis), while TH2 cells are involved in granulomas caused by helminths such as schistosomiasis and ascariasis.

CMI is not clear. DTH responses are characterized by erythema and induration[6] with a large influx of macrophages/monocytes and lymphocytes at the site of antigen challenge.

Like other hypersensitivity reactions, type IV hypersensitivity also requires sensitization, ie, it is a secondary response to the sensitizing antigen. The sequence of events in the development of DTH responses is similar to that of CMI responses. Upon primary exposure to the antigen, APCs such as Langerhans[7] cells and macrophages internalize the antigen, transport it to the draining lymph node, and present it to $CD4^+$ T cells. The resulting activation and differentiation gives rise to T_H cells and CTLs capable of responding to epitopes on that antigen. A subsequent exposure to antigen induces the effector phase of the response. It is a result of a complex interaction between cells of innate and adaptive arms of the immune system. The secondary antigenic challenge results in the release of pro-inflammatory cytokines such as TNF-α and IFN-γ by DCs. Antigen-specific T_{H1} cells that recognize the MHC class II:peptide complexes on the DCs also secrete chemokines and cytokines. The result is increased vascular permeability and influx of monocytes to the site of injection; monocytes and neutrophils begin to infiltrate the site of antigenic challenge within hours of antigen challenge. The infiltrating monocytes differentiate to activated macrophages during this process. IL-3 and GM-CSF produced by the activated T_{H1} cells stimulate monocyte production by bone marrow stem cells, further enhancing their influx into the site of inflammation. Each of these events can take several hours to develop. As explained in chapter 2, activated macrophages have a potent arsenal of antimicrobial substances that are crucial in host defence against intracellular parasites or pathogens that are not accessible to circulating antibodies. The cocktail of enzymes and microbicidal factors released by the macrophages can damage cells in the immediate vicinity and is a small price to pay for rapid pathogen clearance.

Unfortunately, prolonged macrophage activation becomes destructive to the host. Persistence of antigen/pathogen results in an intense inflammatory response and chronic macrophage activation. High concentrations of lytic enzymes liberated by these cells cause the destruction of surrounding tissues and may even lead to tissue

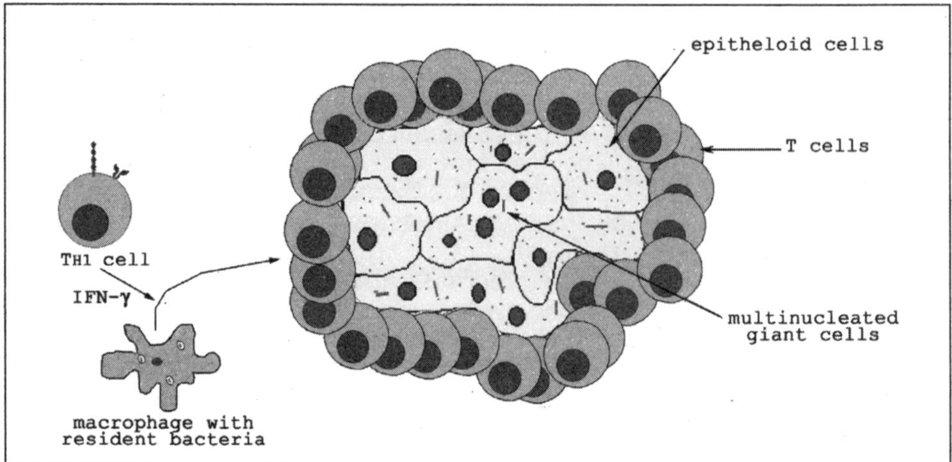

Figure 15.4 A granuloma is a characteristic localized inflammatory response that is the result of persistent macrophage activation coupled with a failure to eliminate intracellular pathogens or their constituents. Failure to get rid of the intracellular pathogen causes the macrophages to remain in a continuously activated state. The macrophages assume an epitheloid shape and closely adhere to each other. Some of them fuse to form multi-nucleated giant cells. This central macrophage-derived core is surrounded by T cells. T cells provide TNF-α which is crucial for the initiation and maintenance of granulomas. An extracellular matrix shields this cellular conglomerate from healthy tissue. The pathogen may survive in the granuloma, but its proliferation and spread are inhibited.

[6] Dervied from Latin (*indurare* — hard), induration is a hardening or lumpiness observed at the site of physical trauma or antigen challenge.

[7] Langerhans cells are a kind of DC; see chapter 5.

necrosis. Continuous activation causes the macrophages to adhere closely and assume an epitheloid shape (fig. 15.4). They may even fuse together to form multi-nucleated giant cells that displace normal tissue cells. Deposition of fibrous scar tissue around these cells results in the formation of palpable nodules called granulomas. Such granulomatous immune responses are observed both in protective immune responses and disease pathology. Only 5% of the participating cells are antigen-specific T cells in a fully developed DTH reaction. A variety of intracellular pathogens (eg, *Schistosoma* spp., *Leishmania* spp., herpes simplex virus, mumps virus, blastomycosis, and histoplasmosis) or their products can give rise to deleterious DTH responses.

The prototypical type IV response is the tuberculin test used to determine the immune status of an individual to *Mycobacterium tuberculosis*. Other substances that can induce DTH responses include insect venom, poison ivy, and chemicals like Ni or chromium salts. Some of these give rise to painful cutaneous (or contact) hypersensitivity responses. Substances like picryl chloride or the lipid soluble pentadecacatechol present in the leaves of poison ivy interact and modify cellular proteins upon contact with the skin, and elicit a deleterious T cell response to the modified proteins. Although originally DTH was proposed to be an exclusively T_{H1} phenomenon, later experiments have proven that both T_{H1} and T_{H2} cells can participate in DTH reactions. IL-4 seems to be crucial for systemic DTH responses, although IFN-γ and TNF-α appear to be key cytokines in the initial phase of the response. In support of this idea is the fact that IL-4 KO mice cannot mount contact hypersensitivity responses. Paradoxically, T_{H2} cytokines such as IL-4 and IL-10 may also be important in DTH suppression and lesion healing. Different types of DTH responses are listed in Table 15.5.

Table 15.5 Type IV hypersensitivity or DTH reactions

Type	Time (days)	Features
Jones-Mote reaction	1	Characterized by infiltration of basophils in the epidermis; basophils constitute 50% of cellular exudate Induced by soluble antigens
Contact hypersensitivity	2–3	Characterized by a local epidermal reaction (eczema) at site of contact Induced by small haptens conjugated to tissue antigens; caused by contact with poison ivy, salts of nickel, chromates, etc
Tuberculin type	1–2	Characterized by fever, generalized sickness, induration, and swelling at site of injection Caused by injection of soluble antigens of *M. tuberculosis*, *M. leprae*, etc; certain non-microbial antigens may also induce a similar reaction
Granulomatous type	Minimum 14	Characterized by a nodular mass consisting of a core of multi-nucleated giant cells and epitheloid cells surrounded by fibrotic scar tissue; T cells are instrumental in the formation and maintenance of granulomas Caused by the persistence of antigen that cannot be cleared by phagocytes

16 Cancer and the Immune System

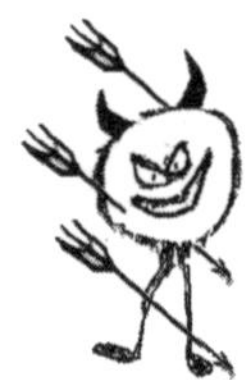

I think I'll find another way
There's so much more to know
I guess I'll die another day
It's not my time to go

For every sin, I'll have to pay
I've come to work, I've come to play
I think I'll find another way
It's not my time to go

I'm gonna avoid the cliche
I'm gonna suspend my senses
I'm gonna delay my pleasure
I'm gonna close my body now

I guess, die another day

—Madonna, *Die Another Day*

16.1 Introduction

Mature cells of multicellular organisms have a fixed life span and die a natural death. Death may also be caused by other factors such as trauma or infections. These dying cells must be replaced by the proliferation and differentiation of appropriate stem cells. However, this process of proliferation must be strictly regulated so that the number of any given cell type remains more or less constant, ie, cell renewal and cell death must be properly balanced to maintain the status quo, ie, homeostasis. These growth control mechanisms ensure that most cells grow in a density dependent manner and cease proliferation after a certain number of cell divisions or after reaching a certain density. The occasional formation of cells that do not respond to growth control mechanisms and hence refuse to die is the bane of all multicellular organisms. **The term 'neoplasm[1]' is used for such an abnormal mass of tissue, the growth of which exceeds and is uncoordinated with that of normal tissues and persists in the same excessive manner after cessation of the stimuli that evoked changes.** The process that converts the cell from a normal to a malignant form is called transformation.

To understand what causes a cell to become malignant, you could think of the cell as a car and cancer the car accident. There is an appropriate speed at which a car should travel (or a cell should divide). Any increase in speed is an accident waiting to happen. Just as the accelerator and the brake determine the speed of the car, two sets of genes determine the rate of cell proliferation. Genes that function to speed up growth are the accelerators; those that control the rate of cell division are the brakes. Unrestricted multiplication occurs when the brakes fail. Fortunately, a cell has two copies of every gene, so even if one mutates (ie, if one brake fails), the other copy will still control the rate of proliferation. It is only when both the brakes fail that unrestricted multiplication (and cancer) result. It is more difficult to understand how accelerator failure can result in increased growth. Consider what will happen if the accelerator gets jammed to the floor. The car will hurtle at breakneck speed, and trying to brake the car will prove futile. Unlike with the brakes, having two copies of

ALL:	Acute lymphocytic leukaemia
BRCA-1:	Breast cancer-1
BRCA-2:	Breast cancer-2
CALLA:	Common acute lymphocytic leukaemia antigen
CML:	Chronic myelogenous leukaemia
IAP:	Inhibitors of apoptosis
MAGE:	Melanoma antigens
MIF:	Migration inhibitory factor
RNI:	Reactive nitrogen intermediates
ROI:	Reactive oxygen intermediates
TAAs:	Tumour associated antigens
TILs:	Tumour infiltrating lymphocytes
TRAIL:	TNF-related apoptosis inducing ligand
TRAs:	Tumour rejection antigens
TSAs:	Tumour specific antigens
TSTAs:	Tumour specific transplantation antigens
VEGF:	Vascular endothelial growth factor

[1] The term derives from 'neo' meaning 'new', and 'plasia' meaning 'growth'.

Understanding Terminology

A tumour is a swelling caused by a mass of cells. Benign tumours are normally slow-growing, circumscribed, and encapsulated, with well-defined edges. They do not invade surrounding tissue. Malignant tumours are often rapidly growing, aggressive, invasive masses of cells that can spread through the blood or lymph, ie, metastasize. The term 'cancer' refers specifically to malignant tumours. **Oncology** is the study of malignant tumours, ie, cancers.

Metastasis is the transfer of pain, function, or disease from one organ to another through contact, blood vessels, or lymphatics. It is usually used in reference to the transfer of tumour cells. The original tumour is the primary tumour, and tumours caused by metastasis are secondary tumours.

Malignant tumours are classified according to the embryonic origin of the tissue from which they are derived.

❑ A **carcinoma is a malignant tumour arising from ectodermal or endodermal tissues** such as the skin or epithelial lining of internal organs or glands. More than 80% of all tumours are carcinomas; a majority of breast, lung, prostrate, or colon tumours are carcinomas, eg, mammary adenocarcinoma, hepatocarcinoma, and colon carcinoma.

❑ A **sarcoma arises from mesodermal** tissues such as bone, fat, and cartilage. Examples include fibrosarcoma, osteosarcoma, and liposarcoma.

❑ **Lymphomas and leukaemias are tumours of the haematopoietic cells of the bone marrow**. Lymphomas tend to grow as solid masses. Examples of lymphomas include Hodgkin's disease and Multiple myelomas. Carcinomas, sarcomas, and lymphomas are called solid tumours. By contrast, leukaemias are circulating cancerous cells that proliferate as single cells, eg, ALL (**A**cute **L**ymphocytic **L**eukaemia) and CML (**C**hronic **M**yelogenous **L**eukaemia).

genes that speed up growth is a disadvantage. Increase in growth rate caused by a single copy is enough to cause malignancy.

Tumour suppressor genes are recessive genes that 'brake' cell division and cycling at various points during the cell cycle. Being recessive, the loss of both copies of the normal genes is required before cancer becomes likely. p53 and the related p63 and p73 proteins belong to this family. Both p63 and p73 have functions in normal development, whereas p53 seems to have evolved in higher animals exclusively to prevent tumour development. p53 is the most commonly transformed gene, being found in about 50% of human tumours. The p53 protein is induced in response to stress signals encountered during tumour development and malignant progression (such as DNA damage, hypoxia, telomere erosion, and loss of survival signals; also called oncogenic stress). It acts in the nucleus to stop the replication of damaged cells. In most cases, induction of p53 results in irreversible inhibition of cell growth, sometimes by the induction of apoptosis. So long as one allele of p53 is active, tumour suppression continues. Loss of both alleles of p53 causes the cell cycle to continue despite oncogenic stress or mistakes in DNA transcription. The proto-oncogenes are dominant genes that regulate cell growth, division, and differentiation (the accelerators). If a proto-oncogene undergoes mutation that makes it work better, it can cause cancer. Proto-oncogenes that have undergone such changes are called oncogenes, ie, oncogenes are derived from proto-oncogenes by mutation, retroviral transduction, etc. Primary candidates for oncogenes include genes that normally regulate expression of growth factors and their receptors, signal transducing proteins, nuclear transcription factors, and cyclins that are involved in the progression of the cell cycle.

Mutations or transformations in two other sets of genes can also result in cancer. The first set is genes involved in DNA repair. To carry the car analogy further, if mutations can be looked upon as damage to the car, DNA repair machinery is the team of mechanics that keeps it in good shape. If you lose your mechanic, you lose your car. The second set of genes that can result in malignancy is those involved in apoptosis regulation. Apoptosis regulating genes involved in the regulation of cell-death are the highway patrolmen. These traffic police keep the roads safe by pulling off speeding cars. Major accidents will result if these cops fail to do their job. Mammalian cells use two main pathways to undergo apoptosis. The extrinsic pathway is initiated by the ligation of cell surface death receptors such as TNF-α and Fas (CD95). The intrinsic pathway is centred on dysregulation of mitochondrial function and release of cytochrome c. Two gene families of apoptosis regulators have been identified (chapter 11), and mutations in either of them can result in cancer.

❑ The **Bcl-2 family** comprises molecules with pro- and anti-apoptotic functions. Anti-apoptotic proteins include Bcl-2 and Bcl-$_{XL}$, whereas the pro-apoptotic ones are Bax, Bad, Bak, and Bid. Bcl-2 proteins affect apoptosis by decreasing (anti-apoptotic) or increasing (pro-apoptotic) mitochondrial permeability, thereby affecting the release of cytochrome c.

❑ **IAP** (Inhibitors of **AP**optosis) **proteins** are the other family of apoptosis regulators. They inhibit caspases, the enzymes involved in apoptosis.

The process by which a malignant neoplasm is produced is called carcinogenesis. A random or single mutation cannot cause the cell to become malignant. Apart from a non-lethal mutation that imparts the ability to grow indefinitely (ie, immortality) and resist apoptotic signals, cancerous cells often show a diminished requirement for growth factors and altered biochemical activities that allow them to survive and multiply (fig. 16.1). Malignant neoplasms grow by progressive infiltration, invasion, destruction, and penetration of surrounding tissues. For a tumour to grow, it must have an adequate supply of nutrients. Most solid tumours often secrete angiogenesis factors that result in the formation of new blood vessels. To invade, a cancerous cell must detach from the tumour, adhere to the

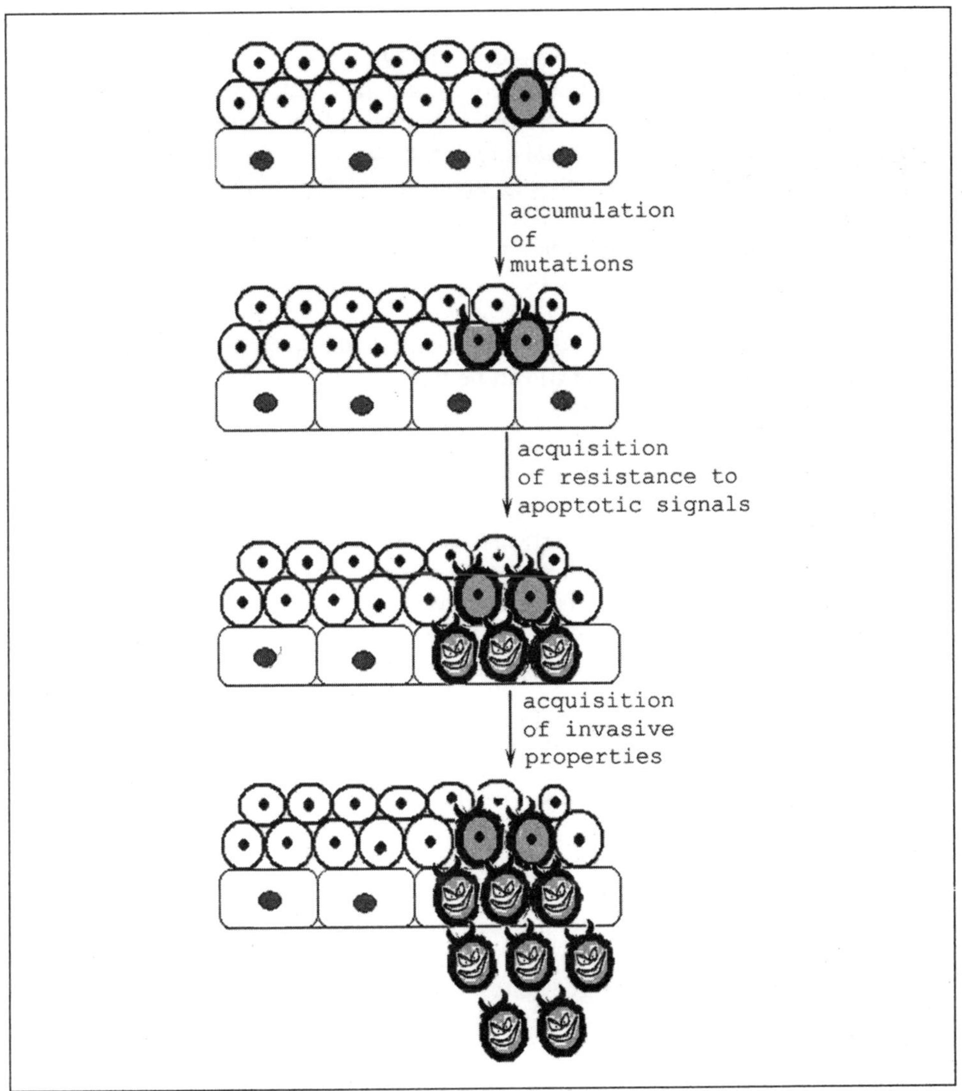

Figure 16.1 Tumour transformation involves the progressive accumulation of multiple mutations that allow the tumour cells to survive, proliferate, and resist apoptotic signals.

extracellular matrix, proteolytically degrade the matrix, and then find its way out of the basement membrane that allows it to migrate to other tissues or organs. A single mutation cannot endow all these characters on the malignant cell. Thus, **tumour formation is a multi-step process requiring the accumulation of numerous mutations in the cells.** This is called tumour progression.

Both environmental and genetic factors can be involved in the induction of malignant transformation in normal cells.

❑ **Environmental factors** that lead to genetic changes increase the chances of malignancies. These include:

- **Viruses.** Some viral infections can result in increased cellular proliferation and hence lead to cancer. Examples include infection by the human papilloma virus (causes cervical cancer), hepatitis B virus (causes hepatocellular carcinoma), Epstein-Barr virus (linked to Burkitt's lymphoma and Hodgkin's lymphoma), Human T cell Leukaemia Virus type 1, Mouse Mammary Tumour Virus, and Rous sarcoma virus[2].
- **Chemicals.** A variety of chemicals, called carcinogens, can cause malignant transformations — arsenic, asbestos, benzene, benzo(a)pyerenes in cigarette smoke, vinyl chloride, and aflatoxins just to name a few.

[2] Studies on v-src encoded by the virus helped prove that oncogenes alone could induce malignant transformation; a group of tyrosine kinases is named after this gene; see sidetrack 'Arch SAARC' in chapter 6.

- **Radiations.** Radiations such as UV rays and ionizing radiations can cause cancers through their ability to induce mutations.
- ❑ **Genetic factors.** Until the 1980s, environmental factors were thought to be predominantly responsible for cancer. However, in the last decade of the 20th century, the role of genetics in causing cancer came to be better understood and appreciated. The first predisposing gene to be identified was the *RB1* gene associated with retinoblastoma. **Mutations in genes involved in apoptosis or signalling or genes encoding enzymes involved in angiogenesis, DNA repair, and genome stability have since been identified as being responsible for cancer.** Notable examples include:
  - Mutations in genes encoding key molecules such as p53 or Ras involved in signal transduction (chapter 6) can be inherited in the germline, and they can predispose a person to cancer.
  - Majority of inherited breast cancers are due to a mutation in *BRCA-1* and *BRCA-2* (**Br**east **Ca**ncer-1 and -2) genes; a mutation in tyrosine receptor kinase gene *ERBB2* can also result in breast cancer.
  - Mutations in the phosphatase PTEN increases the risk of Cowden's syndrome (resulting in gastrointestinal, breast, or thyroid cancers).
  - Xeroderma pigmentosum is caused by a defect in the gene that encodes UV-specific endonuclease (a DNA repair enzyme) and the resultant inability to repair UV-induced mutations results in multiple types of skin cancers.

16.2 Effectors of Anti-tumour Immunity

Although the role of the immune system in protecting against tumours was conceptualized by Ehrlich in the early 1900s, the notion was formalized by Burnet and Thompson in 1967 when they outlined the 'immunosurveillance concept'. They suggested that the lymphocytes acted as sentinels in recognizing and eliminating continuously arising nascent transformed cells. Experimental evidence for this concept emerged after the advent of KO mice; mice deficient in certain key features of the immune system (eg, *RAG* genes, perforin, or IFN-γ) showed increased susceptibility to tumours. A similar trend emerged from data on transplant and immunocompromised patients. Thus, data obtained from both murine and human studies provide strong support for the existence of, and physiologic relevance of cancer immunosurveillance.

Tumours represent a unique problem to the immune system. The immune system is 'educated' to discriminate between self and non-self and to focus its destructive powers on the latter. Thus, the presence of non-self molecules or 'danger signals' are required to 'switch on' the defensive powers of the immune system. Tumours develop

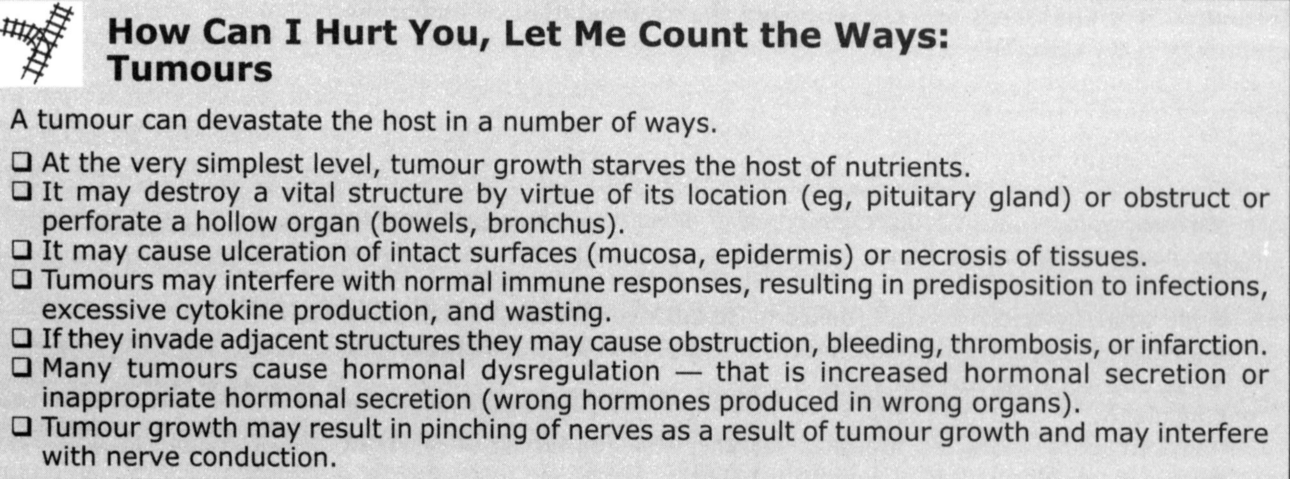

How Can I Hurt You, Let Me Count the Ways: Tumours

A tumour can devastate the host in a number of ways.

- ❑ At the very simplest level, tumour growth starves the host of nutrients.
- ❑ It may destroy a vital structure by virtue of its location (eg, pituitary gland) or obstruct or perforate a hollow organ (bowels, bronchus).
- ❑ It may cause ulceration of intact surfaces (mucosa, epidermis) or necrosis of tissues.
- ❑ Tumours may interfere with normal immune responses, resulting in predisposition to infections, excessive cytokine production, and wasting.
- ❑ If they invade adjacent structures they may cause obstruction, bleeding, thrombosis, or infarction.
- ❑ Many tumours cause hormonal dysregulation — that is increased hormonal secretion or inappropriate hormonal secretion (wrong hormones produced in wrong organs).
- ❑ Tumour growth may result in pinching of nerves as a result of tumour growth and may interfere with nerve conduction.

from self-cells, and at least in the initial stages, do not send out distress 'danger signals'. They may therefore remain invisible to the immune system and are likely to escape immunosurveillance during the initial phases of development. Once solid tumours reach a certain size, they begin to grow invasively and require enhanced blood supply. This blood supply occurs as a consequence of the production of angiogenic proteins by the tumour. Such invasive growth causes disruption in surrounding tissue and starts the immune response. The sequence of events that results in an anti-tumour response is outlined below (fig. 16.2).

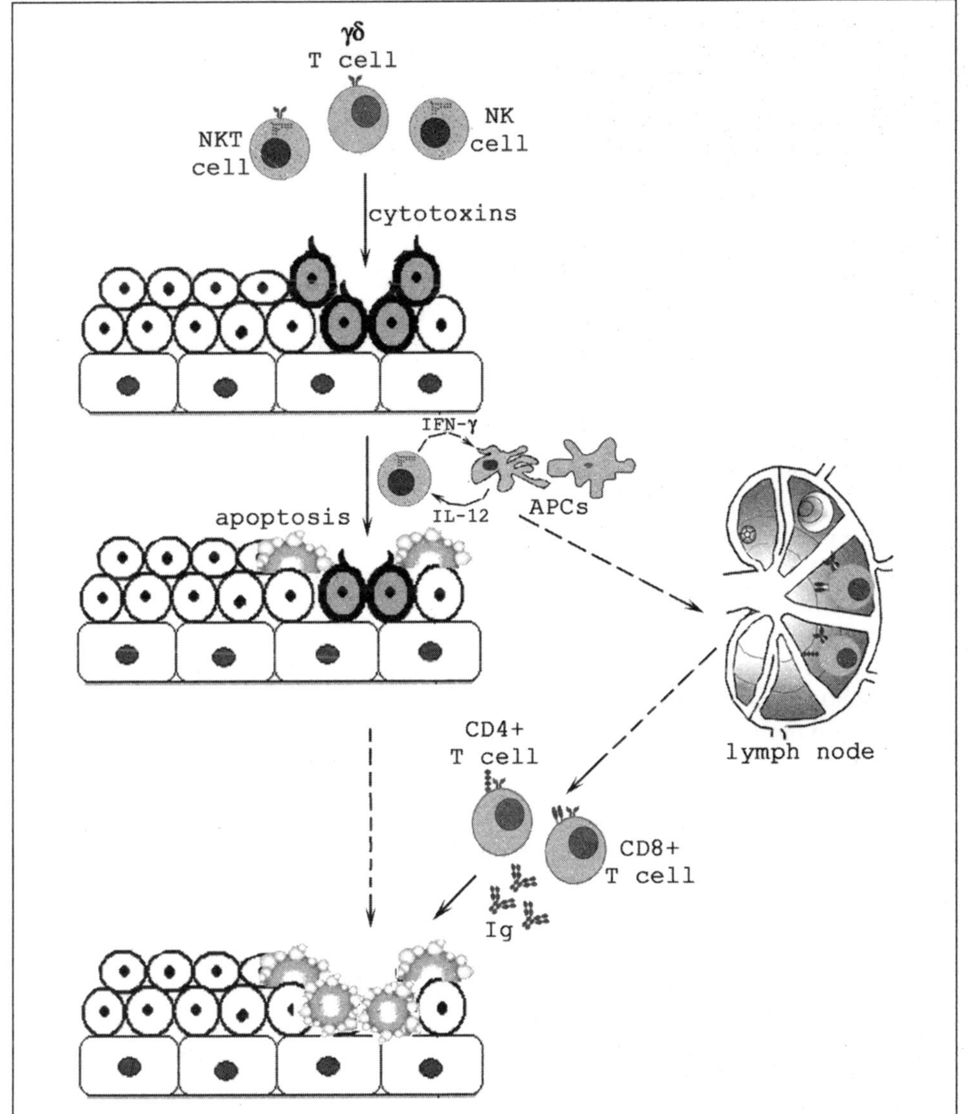

Figure 16.2 Cells of the innate and adaptive immune system work in tandem to eliminate tumours. Pro-inflammatory signals released by tumour cells result in the recruitment of cells of the innate immune system such as γδ T cells, NKT cells, and NK cells. These cytotoxic cells bring about the death of the tumour cells by inducing apoptosis and secreting pro-inflammatory cytokines like IFN-γ. Chemokines and cytokines released as a result of the inflammatory response recruit APCs such as DCs and macrophages to the site. The NK cells and macrophages activate one another by reciprocal production of IFN-γ and IL-12. Activated macrophages help in further eliminating tumour cells. IFN-γ and tissue debris from the dead and dying cells causes maturation of the DCs. The APCs transport tumour antigens to the regional lymph node where they induce the development of tumour specific CD4+ Th1 cells and CD8+ CTLs. These effector T cells home to the tumour site and destroy tumour cells. The CD4+ T cells also help the B cells in mounting a humoral response.

❑ Invasive growth induces inflammatory signals such as stress-induced proteins, leading to the recruitment of cells of the innate immune system (NK, NKT, γδ T cells, macrophages, and DCs).

❑ NK and NKT cells have been shown to act against tumour initiation, growth, and metastasis. These cells are cytotoxic cells that can induce cell death by the perforin-granzyme pathway as well as by the induction of apoptosis in cells (chapters 2 and 11). Additionally, NK cells secrete a number of effector cytokines such as IFN-γ, TNF-α, and GM-CSF.

❑ Structures on the transformed cells are recognized by the infiltrating cells, and this results in the production of IFN-γ.

❑ IFN-γ production in particular aids antitumour immunity in multiple ways.

- Induction of limited amount of tumour cell death occurs because of its anti-proliferative and apoptotic mechanisms.
- Induction of chemokines having angiostatic capacities such as CXCL19, CXCL10, and CXCL11 block the formation of new blood vessels within the tumour. The lack of blood supply and effect of IFN-γ accelerates tumour cell death.
- Stimulation of NO production by phagocytes.
- Increased leukocyte-endothelium interaction results in a further influx of leukocytes, ie, apart from the influx induced by invasive growth.
- Upregulation of MHC class I and class II molecules on many cell types — including tumour cells.

❑ Chemokines produced during the escalating inflammatory responses recruit more NK cells and macrophages to the site; the tumour infiltrating NK cells and macrophages activate one another by reciprocal production of IFN-γ and IL-12. Cytotoxic granules, TRAIL (**T**NF-**R**elated **A**poptosis **I**nducing **L**igand), ROI, and RNI are all responsible for further death of tumour cells.

❑ It is thought that NK cells may regulate DC activation in non-microbial scenarios such as tumourogenesis; the IFN-γ produced by NK cells and the tissue debris resulting from the lysis of tumour cells by NK cells are central to DC activation. The debris from tumour cell death is internalized by DCs which home to the local draining lymph node.

❑ DCs in the draining lymph node induce tumour specific CD4+ TH1 cells that in turn facilitate the development of CD8+ CTLs. These CD4+ and CD8+ T cells home to the tumour site where the CTLs destroy tumour cells.

❑ Memory CD4+ and CD8+ T cells formed as a result of CD4+ and CD8+ T cell differentiation are critical in maintaining protective immunity.

❑ Humoral responses to tumour antigens are triggered when B lymphocytes internalize tumour antigens and enter into a cognate interaction with activated CD4+ T cells. Antibodies against tumour cells or their constituents have been observed in the sera of patients with Burkitt's lymphoma, malignant melanoma, osteosarcoma, and lung and breast cancers. However, antibodies often have difficulties in reaching peripheral tumours and may have a limited role in their elimination. Paradoxically, some antibodies may even promote tumour survival. Such antibodies, called enhancing antibodies, are non-cytotoxic antibodies whose mechanism of action is unclear. They are thought to promote tumour survival by binding the cell surface molecules critical for tumour lysis and inducing their downregulation.

16.3 Tumour Immune Evasion

As explained, tumour formation is a multi-step process in which transformed cells undergo a series of changes that allow their survival and proliferation. Although it originates from self-cells, the tumour is a parasite, and this host-parasite relationship is as dynamic as the more conventional host-parasite/pathogen relationship. A newly forming tumour will inevitably express self-antigens. It is also likely to express new or altered proteins because of mutations or viral transformation. These new/altered proteins are the ones that trigger the immune response and eventually result in the tumour becoming a target of immune effector mechanisms. Tumours that survive or flourish through this immune attack are often the ones that can withstand the tumour suppressing actions of the immune system. Thus, the immune system exerts selective pressure on the tumours — highly immunogenic tumours are unlikely to survive the defensive mechanisms of the immune system and will be eliminated, whereas weakly immunogenic tumours will survive. Aggressive tumours that replace cells faster than those destroyed by the immune attack are also more likely to survive even if they are immunogenic. Multiple pathways lead to tumour survival.

❑ **Downregulation of MHC class I antigen processing and presentation pathways.** Decreased or absent HLA class I expression is associated with invasive and metastatic tumours, and total loss of MHC class I expression is not uncommon in many tumours including melanomas, colorectal carcinomas, prostate adenocarcinomas, and breast cancers. Some of the mechanisms reported in cancer patients that result in the loss or downregulation of MHC class I expression include:
- Loss of or defective β_2-m gene.
- Downregulation of the proteasome multi-catalytic complex units LMP-2 and LMP-7.
- Downregulation of peptide transporters TAP-1 and TAP-2.
- Selective loss of MHC class I haplotype because of loss of transcription factors.

❑ **Loss/downregulation of the MIC-A and MIC-B molecules.** Loss of MHC class I molecules should make tumours more susceptible to NK cell lysis. However, such tumours also lose or downregulate the MIC-A and MIC-B molecules required to engage NKG2D activatory receptors on NK cells. In the absence of these activating signals, NK cells do not attack tumour cells.

CANCER AND THE IMMUNE SYSTEM

❑ Tumour formation is a multi-step process requiring the accumulation of numerous mutations in the cells that allows them to survive, proliferate, and obtain nutrients from surrounding tissues.

❑ Genes often involved in malignant transformation include:
- Proto-oncogenes involved in the regulation of cell growth, division, and differentiation,
- Tumour suppressor genes involved in breaking cell division and cycling at various points during the cell cycle,
- Apoptosis genes involved in the regulation of cell-death, and
- Genes involved in DNA repair.

❑ CD4+ TH1 cells and CD8+ CTLs are especially important in destroying tumour cells; Igs play a relatively smaller role in antitumour immunity.

❑ Strategies that allow tumours to evade host immune responses include:
- Downregulation of MHC class I antigen processing and presentation pathways,
- Downregulation of MHC class I-like MIC-A and MIC-B molecules,
- Absence of costimulatory molecule expression,
- Overexpression of MIF, which contributes to angiogenesis,
- Downregulation of tumour antigen expression,
- Defective apoptosis-inducing pathways or overexpression of FasL,
- Expression of cytokines and chemokines that can negatively affect maturation and function of immune cells,
- Interference with IFN-γ signalling pathways, and
- Overexpression of PI-9.

❑ Immunotherapeutic strategies for selective targeting of tumour cells include:
- Injecting irradiated tumour cells with adjuvants to stimulate host immune system,
- Administration of cytokines,
- Enhancing the expression of costimulatory molecules, and
- Using engineered mAbs that deliver the drug/radionucleotide/cytokine directly to the tumour cells.

❑ **Lack of costimulatory molecule expression.** This can allow tumours to escape NK cell and CTL attack. Engagement of MHC class I:peptide complexes in the absence of costimulation will result in CTL anergy and suboptimal NK cell activation, allowing tumour escape.

❑ **Overexpression of MIF (Migration Inhibitory Factor).** Macrophage MIF is an immunomodulator associated with tumour progression and is found to be overexpressed by many tumour cells. It contributes to neoangiogenesis and epithelial cell proliferation. Furthermore, it may contribute to genetic instability in tumours as it suppresses p53 function.

❑ **Loss or decreased surface antigen expression** often correlates with disease progression. The exact mechanisms of the downregulation of tumour antigens are not known. However, a decreased expression of T cell epitopes such as MAGE or gp100 (see next section) is associated with disease progression. Such decreased expression has also been observed with residual tumours following peptide vaccination.

❑ **Defective apoptosis-inducing pathways.** FasL and TRAIL are important in the induction of apoptosis (chapter 11). Engagement of Fas on tumour cells by FasL expressing cells (eg, CTLs or NK cells) results in the activation of death receptors and induces cell death. Multiple sites in the death receptor pathways can favour tumour escape.

- Defective death receptor signalling may contribute to tumour survival and proliferation.
- Downregulation of Fas expression itself may also contribute to resistance to apoptosis. Mutation and loss of the gene encoding Fas has been identified in multiple myelomas, non-Hodgkin's lymphomas, and melanomas.
- Many tumours show an increase in FLIP, an inhibitor of caspase-8, and are therefore resistant to apoptosis.
- Tumour cells may also show a defect in downstream signalling pathways in apoptosis following engagement of the death receptor, eg, low expression of death receptors, and loss or mutation in caspase-8 or caspase-3.

❑ **Expression of FasL.** This is also suggested to be another mode of tumour escape. Engagement of Fas on T cells by FasL on tumour cells will cause the death of Fas expressing T cells. However, this mode of tumour escape is controversial, and clear proof of FasL expression on tumour cells is still lacking.

❑ **Overexpression of PI-9.** PI-9 is a protease inhibitor that inactivates granzyme B and allows tumours to block CTL- or NK cell-mediated cytotoxicity via the perforin pathway (chapter 11).

❑ **Expression of a variety of cytokines and chemokines** can negatively affect maturation and function of immune cells and create an immunosuppressive environment.

- Most tumour cells secrete VEGF (**Vascular Endothelial Growth Factor**). *In vitro*, VEGF has been shown to inhibit DC differentiation and maturation through suppression of the transcription factor NFκB in haematopoietic stem cells. In patients with lung, head, neck, and breast cancers, a decrease in the function and number of mature DCs was found to be associated with increased plasma concentrations of VEGF.
- Increased concentration of serum IL-10 is also frequently detected in patients with cancer. IL-10 inhibits DC differentiation, antigen presentation, IL-12 production, and induction of TH1 responses. It also enhances spontaneous DC apoptosis. It may also protect tumour cells from CTLs by downregulation of MHC class I, MHC class II, TAP-1, TAP-2, and ICAM-1 expression.
- PGE2 is also found to be expressed in many tumours. This is often the result of enhanced expression of cycloxeganse 2, the rate-limiting enzyme in PGE2 synthesis. PGE2 increases the production of IL-10 by lymphocytes and macrophages while inhibiting IL-12 production by macrophages.

- High concentrations of TGF-β are frequently found in cancer patients and are associated with disease progression and poor response to immunotherapy. TGF-β is an immunosuppressive cytokine that directly inhibits NK cell activation. It also inhibits the activation and proliferation of B and T lymphocytes. Both IL-10 and TGF-β may also result in the formation of T_R cells. These cells suppress the activation and proliferation of CD4+ and CD8+ T cells and therefore aid in tumour escape.

❑ **Interference with IFN-γ signalling pathways,** a cytokine crucial to antitumour immunity helps tumour survival. Many tumour cells have been found to have defective IFN-γ signalling pathways which render them resistant to its actions.

16.4 Treatment

Tumours have a greater population of dividing cells than normal tissue which makes them relatively more susceptible to chemotherapeutic drugs than normal tissue. γ-radiation and chemotherapeutic agents interfere with cell division and hence are more toxic to dividing than non-dividing cells. However, the drugs (and radiation) cause severe side-effects since they also kill healthy cells undergoing cell division, such as cells in the bone marrow, gastrointestinal tract, and hair follicles. These side effects limit the dosage of anticancer drugs, and they often have to be given in suboptimal doses, resulting in eventual failure of therapy and/or development of drug resistance and metastatic disease. Newer approaches to cancer treatment include the development of immunotherapeutic strategies that allow the selective targeting of cancer cells. As explained, tumours may escape immunosurveillance by

---

Have Chemistry, Will Kill: Chemotherapy

Antitumour chemotherapeutic agents in common use kill target cells primarily by causing cellular stress and induction of death by apoptosis. Four broad classes of chemotherapeutic agents are recognized.

❑ **Alkylating agents** generally interact non-specifically with DNA and tend to cross-link it. Alkylation of nucleic acids involves a substitution reaction in which a nucleophilic atom on the nucleic acid is replaced by an alkyl group from the alkylating agent. Alkylating agents in clinical use include Cyclophosphamide, Melphalan, Mitomycin C, and Chlorambucil. Platinum compounds such as Cisplatin and Carboplatin are also considered to be alkylating agents.

❑ **Antitumour antibiotics** tend to target DNA or other structures such as tubulin that are common constituents of all eukaryotic cells. They tend to be more selective for cancerous cells than the non-specific alkylating agents. Most antibiotics in use introduce protein-associated strand breaks by stabilizing DNA-topoisomerase I or II complexes, eg, Doxorubicin, Etoposide, Mitoxantrone, and SN-38. Other modes of action include inhibition of translation (Actinomycin D), introduction of double stranded DNA breaks (Bleomycin), and DNA-DNA cross-linking (Mitomycin C).

❑ **Tubulin binding agents** prevent microtubule assembly so that the cell is arrested in the G2 phase of growth — examples include Vinblastine, Vincristine, Toxotere, and Paclitaxel.

❑ **Antimetabolites** disrupt or inhibit essential metabolic processes by getting incorporated in nuclear material or combining irreversibly with vital cellular enzymes. Many anticancer antimetabolites exploit the dividing cells' need for a constant supply of nucleic acid bases that are required for DNA synthesis.

- **Methotrexate** inhibits the enzyme dihyrofolate reductase essential for the synthesis of purines and pyrimidines.
- **5-fluorouracil** inhibits thymidylate synthase.
- **Folic acid analogs** such as tomudex also act by interfering with thymidylate synthase.
- **Purine analogs** in clinical use include mercaptopurine and thioguanine, whereas floxuridine and fludarabine are the **pyrimidine analogues.**

promoting immunosuppressive pathways. Non-specific immunostimulatory therapies are aimed at activating macrophages and NK cells and promoting pro-inflammatory pathways. Such antigen non-specific approaches have the advantage of not requiring extensive knowledge of the immunogenicity of the tumours being treated.

❑ **Injecting irradiated[3] tumour cells or tumour extracts mixed with bacterial products** such as BCG or suspension *Corynebacterium parvum*. It was thought that the injection of adjuvant would result in an inflammatory response, stimulate DCs to internalize and present tumour cell debris to T cells, and generate a tumour-specific antigen response. BCG, whether given intralesionally or locally, has resulted in tumour regression in a number of melanoma cases. However, the treatment has failed to live up to its promise when it comes to other kinds of tumours.

❑ **Administration of cytokines.** Although a number of cytokines qualify for immunotherapy, the complexity and redundancy of cytokine functions makes their clinical use difficult. Severe side effects are another factor limiting their usage.

  - Pro-inflammatory cytokines such as IFN-γ and TNF-α have yielded some promising results in clinical trials. Apart from activating innate effector cells such as NK cells and macrophages, these cytokines also upregulate the expression of MHC molecules on tumour cells. As explained, many tumour cells escape immunosurveillance by downregulating expression of MHC molecules. IFN-γ and TNF-α therapy may help in restoring MHC expression and allow the development of CTL responses. Moreover, IFN-γ may also act directly because of its anti-proliferative effect on tumour cells.

  - IL-2 is a potent activator of lymphocytes. It also induces their proliferation. NK cells obtained from cancer patients can be activated with IL-2 *in vitro*. When re-injected in the patient, these activated cells, called LAK cells, have potent antitumour activity. **Tumour Infiltrating Lymphocytes (TILs)** can be similarly isolated and activated *in vitro* with IL-2. When administered to the patient, such activated TILs have been shown to have specific cytolytic activity against the tumour.

❑ **Increasing the expression of costimulatory signals.** In animal models, tumour immunity can be enhanced by providing costimulatory signals. Thus, the injection of tumour cells transfected with genes encoding costimulatory molecules CD80/86 in tumour-bearing mice has been shown to result in tumour regression. A similar approach can be used in the treatment of melanomas, since melanoma antigens are shared by a number of different tumours.

Successful development of tumour-specific immunotherapies requires the knowledge of tumour antigens. The past two decades have resulted in the identification of many such antigens that can be used as targets in antitumour therapy. Tumour antigens may be expressed as cytoplasmic constituents, membrane proteins, or secreted in fluids. Membrane expressed tissue antigens can be used as a target for antibody-based immunotherapies. The role of secreted tumour antigens (also called neoantigens) in such therapies is questionable. However, they find a use in the diagnosis and monitoring of tumour progression, and in gauging the response of the tumour to treatment. Tumour antigens are divided into two broad classes.

❑ **Tumour Specific Antigens (TSAs) are expressed exclusively by tumour cells and are not found on normal body cells.** TSAs are the obvious choice as targets for immunotherapy. They could be of two types—those encoded by genes exclusively expressed by tumours such as antigens expressed as a result of viral transformation or antigens expressed by variant (mutated) forms of normal genes. Most tumours induced by physical, chemical, or viral agents express neoantigens. By contrast, spontaneously occurring tumours are often non- or weakly immunogenic. TSAs induced by physical or chemical agents are specific for each tumour, since the mutations induced by such agents are likely to be unique to

---

[3] Irradiation ensures that the injected tumour cell is incapable of multiplying in the patient.

each cell. Thus, multiple tumours induced by these agents in the same animal will have different TSAs. TSAs induced by viral transformation are characteristic of the tumour-inducing virus and are shared by all tumours induced by that virus. Since TSAs contribute to tumour rejections, they are also referred to as **Tumour Specific Transplantation Antigens (TSTAs)** or **Tumour Rejection Antigens (TRAs)**. Some examples of TSA are:

- Mutated proteins found in melanomas such as the cyclin-dependent kinase-4 involved in cell cycle regulation, and β-catenin involved in signal transduction,
- Mutated caspase-8 found in squamous cell carcinoma, and
- Viral gene products E6 and E7 of human papilloma virus found in cervical cancer.

❑ **Tumour Associated Antigens (TAAs) are found on both normal and cancerous cells.** Some TAAs are antigens expressed at only certain stages of differentiation or only by certain differentiation lineages in normal cells whereas others are antigens overexpressed on cancer cells. Examples include the following.

- Oncofoetal antigens that are normally expressed only in foetal cells such as α-foetoprotein that is secreted in patients with hepatomas and testicular cancers, and carcinoembryonic antigen expressed on cell membranes and secreted in fluids of patients with colorectal tumours. Since these antigens are normally expressed before the immune system gains competence, they are recognized as foreign and can elicit an antitumour response.
- CALLA (**C**ommon **A**cute **L**ymphocytic **L**eukaemia **A**ntigen) has now been identified as CD10 normally expressed at low levels on B cells.
- Differentiation antigens are overexpressed in tumours and are found in only certain types of normal tissue such as prostate-specific membrane antigen found in prostate cancer, Mucin-1 and ERBB2 (also called HER2/neu; receptor tyrosine kinase) found in breast and ovarian cancers, cancer-testis antigens such as **M**elanoma **A**ntigens (MAGE), etc. MAGE are a family of proteins expressed only in the testes or tumour cells, especially in skin cancer. MAGE-1 was the first tumour-specific T cell epitope to be defined. The group also includes a number of differentiation antigens expressed by melanocytes but overexpressed by melanoma cells, eg, tyrosinase (involved in melanin synthesis), gp75, gp100, MART-1, and Melan-A. Since some of these proteins are expressed only in trace amounts in normal cells (eg, ERBB2, MART-1), mAbs against these antigens can be used to selectively target the tumour cells.
- Telomerase and Survivin (an IAP) are TAAs that are expressed by most tumour-bearing individuals.

Active antigen-specific immunotherapy is often referred to as antitumour vaccination. In contrast to anti-infection vaccines, however, antitumour vaccines are therapeutic (ie, curative) rather than prophylactic (ie, preventive). Tumour vaccines make use of tumour antigens usually derived from proteins produced by the tumour. The aim of the vaccination is to trigger a CTL response to that tumour. Peptides derived from TSA and TAAs can be good candidates for vaccine preparation. The major hurdle in successful vaccination is the individual differences between patients — both in types of HLA molecules and in the epitopes that are presented and recognized. Thus, identifying T cell epitopes that are most likely to trigger the immune response requires extensive knowledge of tumour antigens and patient MHC haplotype. Antitumour vaccines are therefore tailored for the individual and cannot be mass-produced. Needless to say, they are therefore expensive. Pre-clinical and clinical trials of antitumour vaccines show that they are well tolerated and thus demonstrate the safety of this approach. Although tumour regression has been reported in some patients, the clinical outcome has not been as successful as was hoped. However, with an increasing knowledge of T cell epitopes, coupled with a better understanding of tumour immunoevasion, it is hoped that the antitumour vaccinations will bring some real benefits to cancer patients in the near future.

Although inducing antitumour immunity using autologous DCs is a complicated and expensive process, it is one of the most promising new approaches in cancer therapy. Administration of peptide-adjuvant mixtures has also been attempted but has met with less success than peptide-pulsed DCs. DCs are the most potent APCs of the body and can be used to induce tumour specific CTLs and T$_H$ cells in the patient (see sidetrack 'Licensing to Kill', chapter 11). Briefly, pre-DC cells such as monocytes isolated from the patient are allowed to proliferate and differentiate *in vivo* by exposure to GM-CSF and IL-4. They are then pulsed with tumour antigens. Originally, DCs were pulsed with tumour extracts, but now tumour-derived peptides are used to ensure safety and standardization. The DCs are also exposed to maturation stimulus such as IFN-γ or TNF-α. The peptide-loaded mature DCs are then injected into patients. DC vaccination has resulted in efficient CTL responses and tumour regression in a number of clinical trials against a variety of cancers including melanoma, renal carinoma, breast cancer, ovarian cancer, and prostate cancer. Moreover, it appears to be safe, with minimal side effects (transient fever, local reactions, and autoimmune vitiligo in melanoma patients).

The general principle and application of antibody-based therapy has already been discussed in chapter 9. Here, clinical strategies for increasing the efficacy of anti-cancer therapies will be discussed briefly (fig. 16.3).

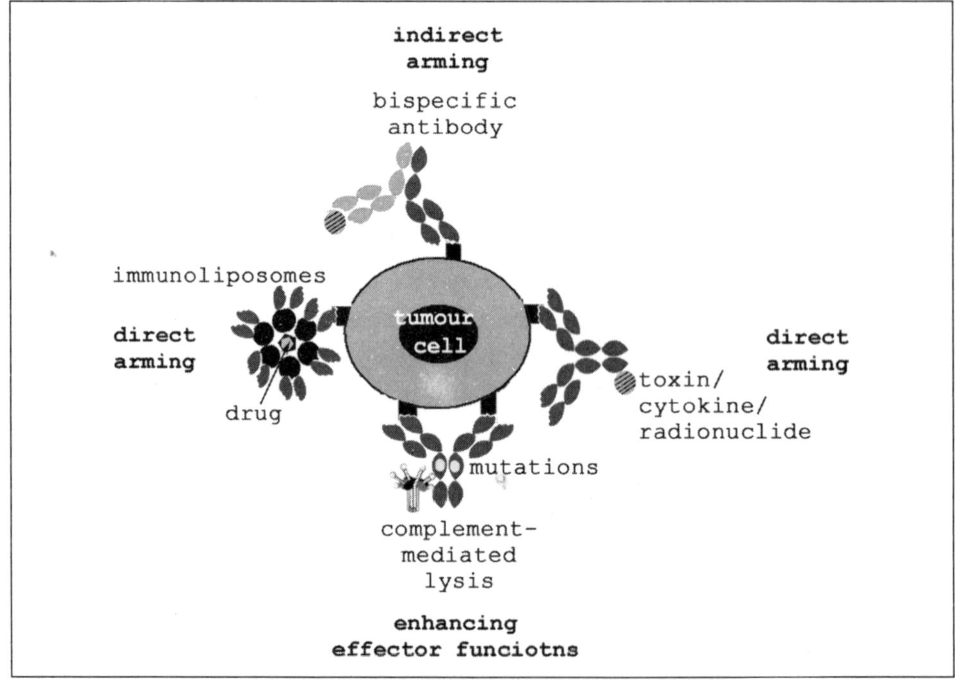

Figure 16.3 Several strategies can be used to increase the efficiency of anticancer immunotherapies. The simplest strategy is to enhance the cytotoxic potential of antibodies by site-directed mutatgenesis. Alternatively, mAbs can be linked to toxins or radionucleotides to enhance their killing potential (direct arming). This strategy has the advantage of requiring lower doses of the toxic substance, since the antibodies deliver the toxic cargo directly to the tumour cell. The mAbs can also be armed with toxic cytokines like IFN-γ or TNF-α. Indirect arming can be achieved in two ways. Engineering of bispecific antibodies capable of binding to different antigens allows the targeting of the cytotoxic substance directly to the tumour. Immunoliposomes containing an immunotherapeutic agent can be linked to engineered antibody fragments, allowing selective tumour targeting (Adapted from Nature Reviews in Cancer (2001) 1:118).

❑ **Combination therapy.** Use of mAbs in conjunction with cytotoxic drugs has been found to increase the success of treatment. For example, Herceptin (humanized anti-ERBB2 mAb) has been found to be synergistic with

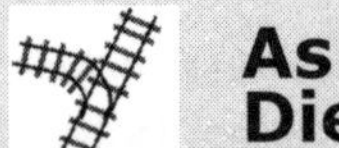

As You Sow So Shall You Reap: Diet and Cancer

The importance of nutrition in cancer development is an area of active study and continued controversy. Diet is estimated to contribute to about one-third of preventable cancers. Several studies have examined the association between diet and specific cancers. The most convincing epidemiological evidence for the role of dietary factors in cancer risk is the inverse relationship between the consumption of fruits and vegetables and many types of cancers, including lung, oral, oesophageal, gastric, pancreatic, ovarian, and breast cancers. Similarly, consumption of whole grains has been associated with a decreased risk of developing stomach and colorectal cancers. However, it must be emphasized that a causal link between foods and cancer has not been established. It is also not clear which of the particular constituents of fruits, vegetables, and grains are responsible for this protective effect. Neither are the cellular or molecular processes that are responsible for the protection understood. Some of the vitamins and micronutrients with a protective effect against cancer are listed below.

❑ Reduced folate intake has been associated with a higher risk of colon cancer, breast cancer, gastric and oesophagal cancer, and pancreatic cancer in smokers. *In vitro* studies have shown that folic acid deficiency causes a dose-dependent increase in uracil incorporation into human lymphocyte DNA and results in an increased number of chromosome breaks.

❑ Vitamin B_6 and B_{12} deficiencies can cause increased chromosome breaks by a uracil-misincorporation mechanism similar to folate deficiency. Epidemiological studies indicate an association between B_6 deficiency and increased lung and prostate cancer.

❑ Reduced intake of antioxidants such as vitamins C, D, and E are all associated with an increased risk of cancer. Although both experimental and epidemiological data indicate that vitamin C protects against stomach cancer, especially when consumed in the form of fruits and vegetables, studies on vitamin C diet supplements have proved largely inconclusive. Increased vitamin C intake is found to reduce DNA strand breaks. Vitamin C intake is especially important in smokers; smoking depletes vitamin C, which is required to protect sperm DNA from oxidative damage. A smoker needs to consume 40% more vitamin C than a non-smoker to maintain a comparable blood plasma level. Several studies have examined the association between paternal smoking, vitamin C intake, oxidative damage, and childhood cancer in the offspring. Available evidence indicates that the risk of cancer is likely to be increased in the offspring of male smokers, especially when dietary antioxidant intake is low.

❑ Deficiencies in minerals such as Fe, Se, and Zn have also been associated with increased cancer risk.

chemotherapeutic agents like the Pt salt cisplatin. It was also found to work well when administered with a number of other drugs such as doxorubicin, methrezate, taxol, and cyclophosphamide. Similarly, anti-CD20 antibody is found to increase the efficacy of these drugs. On the down side, combination therapies often show increased cytotoxicity.

❑ **Use of immunoliposomes.** Liposomes are self-assembled lipid bilayers that encapsulate some of the surrounding medium during their formation. Liposomal formulations of chemotherapeutic agents such as doxorubicin have been approved for clinical use. Engineered antibody fragments can be attached to these liposomes for selective tumour targeting of drugs or toxins or even DNA for gene therapy. Results from studies in animal models are highly encouraging. One major difficulty is the size of the immunoliposomes (usually ~100 nm in diameter). This large size makes extravasation into the tumour difficult. This drawback could be used to an advantage by targeting the immunoliposomes to tumour vasculature rather than the tumour itself, and this approach is now being investigated.

❑ **Targeting tumour vasculature.** Angiogenesis is a process by which tumours become vascularized by the proliferation of new blood vessels. Beyond a certain size, tumours cannot survive in the absence of angiogenesis. mAbs that neutralize VEGF or its receptor have potent antitumour activity and are now being tested in clinical trials.

❑ **Targeting minimal residual disease**[4]. Since the difficulties associated with penetration of mAb in solid tumours are reduced in minimal residual disease, mAbs could be used in their treatment. The anti-epithelial adhesion molecule mAb Panorex has recently been approved for treatment of colorectal cancer minimal residual disease and Herceptin is being tested in clinical trials for breast cancer minimal residual disease treatment.

[4] Minimal residual disease is the tumour remaining in the patient following surgery/chemotherapy/radiotherapy.

AIDS

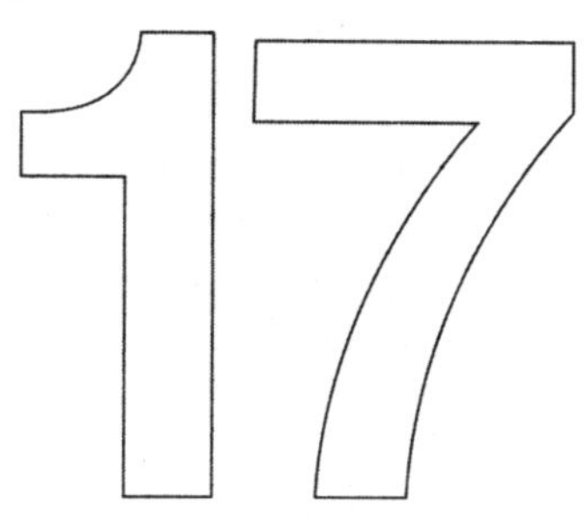

I ain't got a fever got a permanent disease
It'll take more than a doctor to prescribe a remedy
I got lots of money but it isn't what I need
Gonna take more than a shot to get this poison out of me
I got all the symptoms count 'em 1, 2, 3

—Jon Bon Jovi, *Bad Medicine*

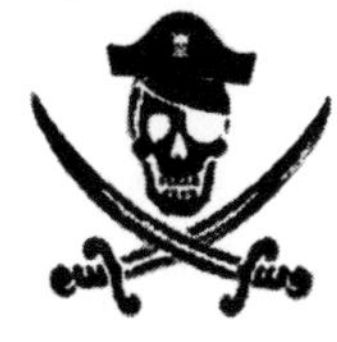

AIDS:	Acquired immunodeficiency syndrome
gag genes:	group-specific antigen genes
HAART:	Highly active antiretroviral therapy
HIV:	Human immunodeficiency virus
LTRs:	Long terminal repeats
Nef:	Negative effector
NNRTI:	Non-nucleoside reverse transcriptase inhibitors
NRTI:	Nucleoside/nucleotide reverse transcriptase inhibitors
PI:	Protease inhibitors
pol genes:	polymerase genes
Rev:	Regulator of virion expression
Tat:	Transcriptional transactivator
vif:	viral infectivity factor
vpr, vpu or vpx:	Viral proteins r, u or x

17.1 Introduction

AIDS (**A**cquired **I**mmuno**d**eficiency **S**yndrome) was recognized as a new disease in 1981, and its aetiological agent, HIV (**H**uman **I**mmunodeficiency **V**irus), was identified in 1983. AIDS is a fatal immunodeficiency that, unlike SCID, is acquired, not inherited. It leads to a progressive decrease in the efficiency of the victim's immune system and leaves the patient susceptible to opportunistic infections and neoplasms. HIV infection is called a syndrome because of the wide spectrum of signs and symptoms that characterize it. HIV is present in the secretions of infected persons — blood, semen, breast milk, saliva, urine, and tears; the concentration of HIV in saliva, urine, tears, and sweat is too low to be of clinical importance. AIDS is primarily a sexually transmissible disease, although contaminated blood or blood products, infected needles, or breast milk can also transmit it. The current AIDS epidemic surfaced predominantly among intravenous drug abusers and homosexual males in the USA. Nevertheless, heterosexual contact (unprotected sex involving exchange of body fluids) remains the major mode of transmission around the world. There has been a shift in the sex of the victims as well. More women than men are now infected, with a concomitant rise in vertical transmission (from mother to child) occurring during childbirth or via the placenta or breast milk.

In the 20 odd years since its recognition, HIV has infected more than 70 million people worldwide, and the epidemic shows no sign of receeding. AIDS has affected many areas of human life. It has laid waste a whole continent (Africa), altered the practice of medicine, made us take a closer look at the choices we make, and changed the way we live. It is in recognition of its impact on human life in general, and the field of immunology in particular, that a separate chapter has been devoted to AIDS. Preliminary knowledge of principles of virology will make reading this chapter easier.

17.2 The Virus

HIV is a human retrovirus closely related to animal lentiviruses (Latin *lentus* — slow acting). Two strains of the virus are recognized — HIV-1 and HIV-2. Both are similar in gross structure. Most infections are due to HIV-1; HIV-2 has limited distribution, being relatively more common in Portugal and parts of the world that have ties with it (eg, West Africa or parts of Southern India). The mature virus is about 90–100 nm in diameter. It consists of a bar-shaped electron dense core containing the viral genome and enzymes (reverse transcriptase, protease, ribonuclease, and integrase) enclosed in an outer lipid envelope having 72 surface projections. The genome of the virus consists of two strands of RNA about 9 kilobases in length encoding 16 distinct proteins (fig. 17.1).

❑ **Long Terminal Repeats** (LTRs), present at either end of the genome, contain regions that bind host transcription factors such as NFκB and NFAT. LTRs are required for initiating transcription.

❑ *gag* (group-specific **antigen**) **genes** encoded protein precursors are processed by a viral protease into matrix and capsid proteins.

❑ *pol* (**pol**ymerase) **genes** encoded precursors are also processed by the viral protease into a variety of viral enzymes, including a protease, a reverse transcriptase (needed to synthesize DNA from the viral RNA), RNAse, and an integrase (needed to integrate viral DNA into host DNA).

❑ *env* **genes** encode the precursor glycoproteins 160 (gp160) and gp140[1]. gp160 is cleaved by host protease into gp120 or gp125 surface glycoproteins (HIV-1 and HIV-2 respectively). By contrast, gp140 is cleaved to gp41 (HIV-1) or gp36 (HIV-2) transmembrane glycoproteins. These surface glycoproteins are important for gaining entry into target cells.

[1] The number signifies the MW of the molecules.

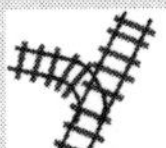

The Relentless March: AIDS in 2004

Within 10 years of being recognized as a disease, 173 out of 193 countries reporting to World Health Organisation had registered AIDS cases. In its third decade, more than 40 million people are now estimated to be infected with HIV. The AIDS epidemic seems to be on the decline in developed countries. Unfortunately, its spread continues unabated in much of the rest of the world.

The global HIV/AIDS epidemic killed more than 3 million people in 2003, and an estimated 5 million more humans became infected with HIV, bringing the total number of people living with the virus to around 42 million. Of those newly infected worldwide, 50% were women. In 2003, the infection was transmitted to 800,000 children by their mothers; with the increase in women suffering from the infection, this number too, is slated to increase in the coming years. Fifty percent of all new infections occurred among young individuals between 15 and 24 years of age, pointing to the dismal failure of educative measures. Current projections suggest that as many as 45 million people will be infected by 2010, and more than 40% of these infections will occur in Asia and the Pacific regions.

Currently, sub-Saharan Africa is by far the worst affected. Around 35% adults in countries such as Botswana, Zimbabwe, and Lesotho are thought to harbour the virus. Although India, China, and Indonesia have less than 1% infected individuals, thanks to them being heavily populated, this translates to between 6–7 million infected people. While injected drug use still remains the major mode of transmission in the Asia-Pacific region, recent evidence suggests a major shift to heterosexual transmission, particularly amongst wives and sex partners of previously infected males. Eastern Europe and Central Asia have the dubious distinction of having the world's fastest growing HIV epidemic. The majority of this spread is because of the abuse of injected drugs. In the first six months of 2002, some countries in the region reported as many new HIV infections as had been reported in the whole previous decade. In Latin America and the Caribbean, homosexual and heterosexual transmissions continue to be major modes of transmission, although abuse of injected drugs is also on the rise. In the developed countries, the epidemic seems to be shifting to the marginalized and poorer sections of society. In the USA, AIDS remains the leading cause of death amongst African-American men and the third leading cause of death amongst Hispanic men. Unfortunately, unsafe sex practices seem to be on the increase, especially in the homosexual population of countries like Australia, USA, Great Britain, and Canada, raising the spectre of resurgence of the epidemic in these countries. With its propensity to strike the young, its long periods of latency, and the lack of a cure, HIV may turn out to be by far the biggest challenge humanity will ever face.

❑ Apart from the above listed proteins that are common to other retroviruses, HIV genome also encodes for HIV-unique proteins.

  ● **Regulatory proteins. T**ranscriptional **T**ransactivator (Tat) along with Nef listed below is crucial for high levels of HIV replication and viral immune evasion, whereas **R**egulator of **V**irion expression (Rev) regulates the transport of viral mRNA from nucleus to cytoplasm.

  ● **Accessory proteins.** These include **v**iral **i**nfectivity **f**actor (vif), **V**iral **p**roteins **r** (Vpr), **u** (Vpu; HIV-1 only), or **x** (Vpx; HIV-2 only), and **N**egative **ef**fector (Nef). Nef is an ironical misnomer, since it enhances virion infectivity and seems to promote the progression of disease.

HIV enters the body through the exchange of bodily fluids and infects mainly T_H cells, macrophages, microglial cells, and DCs. This selectivity in infection is due to specific receptors and coreceptors used by the virus to gain entry into the cell. The probability of infection is a function of the number of infective virions in the body fluid which contact the host, as well as the number of cells available at the site of contact that have appropriate receptors. The major steps in HIV infection of host cells and its replicative cycle are outlined below.

❑ HIV infection occurs predominantly through mucosal surfaces of the genital tract. DCs and Langerhans cells in mucosal tracts express the chemokine receptor CCR5

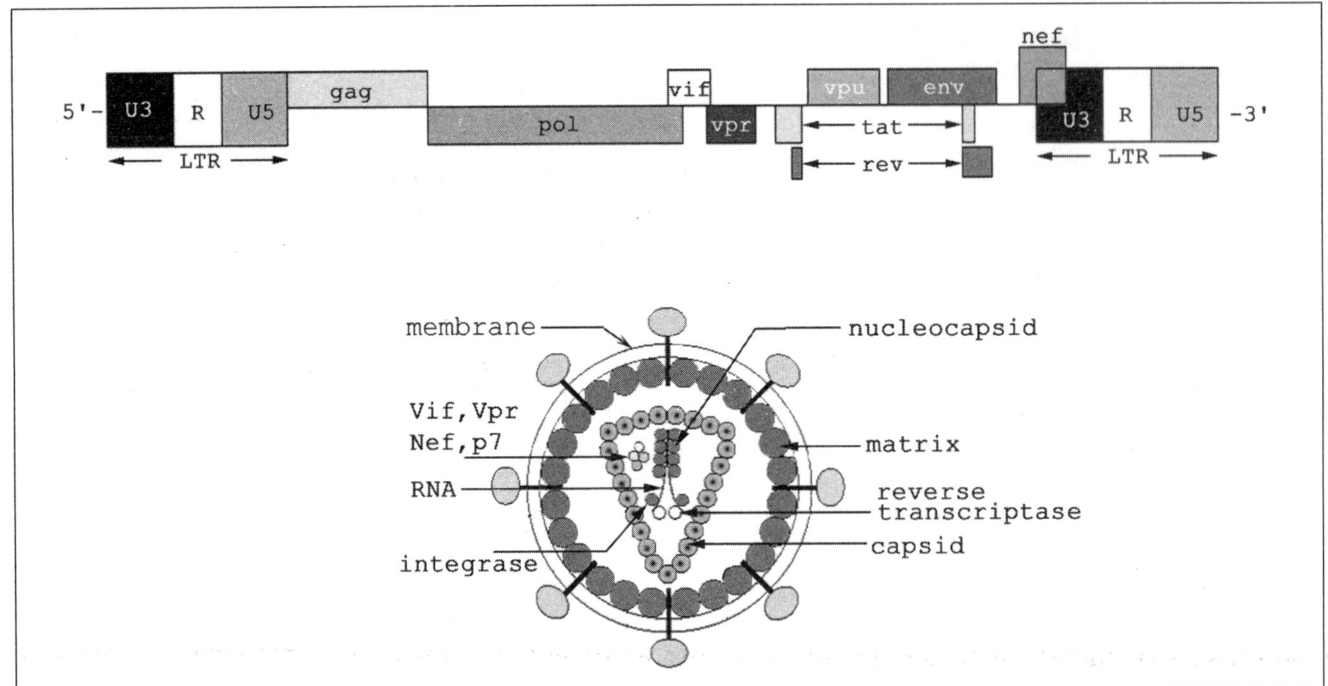

Figure 17.1 *The genome of the HIV provirus encodes 16 proteins that yield the mature enveloped virus. A schematic organization of the 9 kilobase genome is given in the top panel and does not reflect actual distances. The different genes and the proteins they encode are explained in the text. The bottom panel is a schematic organization of the virion particle. The mature virus is about 90 – 100 nm in diameter and consists of a bar-shaped electron dense core containing the viral genome and enzymes (reverse transcriptase, protease, ribonuclease, and integrase), and regulatory and accessory proteins (Vif, Vpu, Nef, etc) enclosed in an outer envelope of matrix proteins. gp120 molecules, important for gaining entry into the cell, protrude from surface of this envelope as projections. The virus is enveloped in a membrane derived from host cell membrane.*

that is needed for the entry of the virus (see below). These cells act as both vectors and reservoirs of infection. Submucosal DCs express DC-SIGN, a C-type lectin that binds HIV gp120 with high affinity. However, this interaction does not trigger the conformational changes necessary for viral fusion with the DC membrane. Instead, the virus is internalized and subsequently displayed on the DC surface, following DC migration and maturation. Transit of the virus through the acidic DC compartments is thought to enhance its ability to fuse with T cells, and it can easily infect any T cell to which the DC is presenting antigen. Thus, DCs expressing DC-SIGN act as 'Trojan horses', facilitating spread of the infection from the mucosal surfaces to lymphatic organs.

❑ Productive infection occurs when HIV enters the cell by engagement of gp120 on the virus surface with CD4 on host cells. gp120 binds CD4 and undergoes conformational changes to express additional sites for chemokine receptors (fig. 17.2). Although several chemokine receptors have been reported to function as coreceptors for viral entry *in vitro*, only two receptors, CCR5 and CXCR4, seem to be important for cell entry *in vivo*. These chemokine receptors are preferentially found in lipid rafts and are similar to the lipid bilayer envelope of the virus; removing cholesterol from the virions or target cells greatly reduces their infectivity.

● CCR5 is expressed on macrophages, DCs, and T cells, and isolates that bind this receptor are called R5 (the earlier M tropic) isolates[2]. R5 viruses mediate both mucosal and intravenous transmission of HIV infection.

● CXCR4 is expressed mainly on T cells, and isolates that preferentially bind it are called X4. Early in the infection, only R5 isolates are found in the infected individual, but X4 dominate in the later phase of infection.

[2] HIV is prone to mutation and several mutants can co-exist in a single host. Historically, variants that replicated slowly, did not form multinucleated giant fusion cells (syncitia) in infected T cells, had a propensity to infect macrophages, and predominated in the early phases of infection were called M tropic or slow/low viruses; preferentially T cell-infecting mutants that formed syncitium, replicated rapidly, and predominated the later phases of the infection were called T tropic or rapid/high viruses.

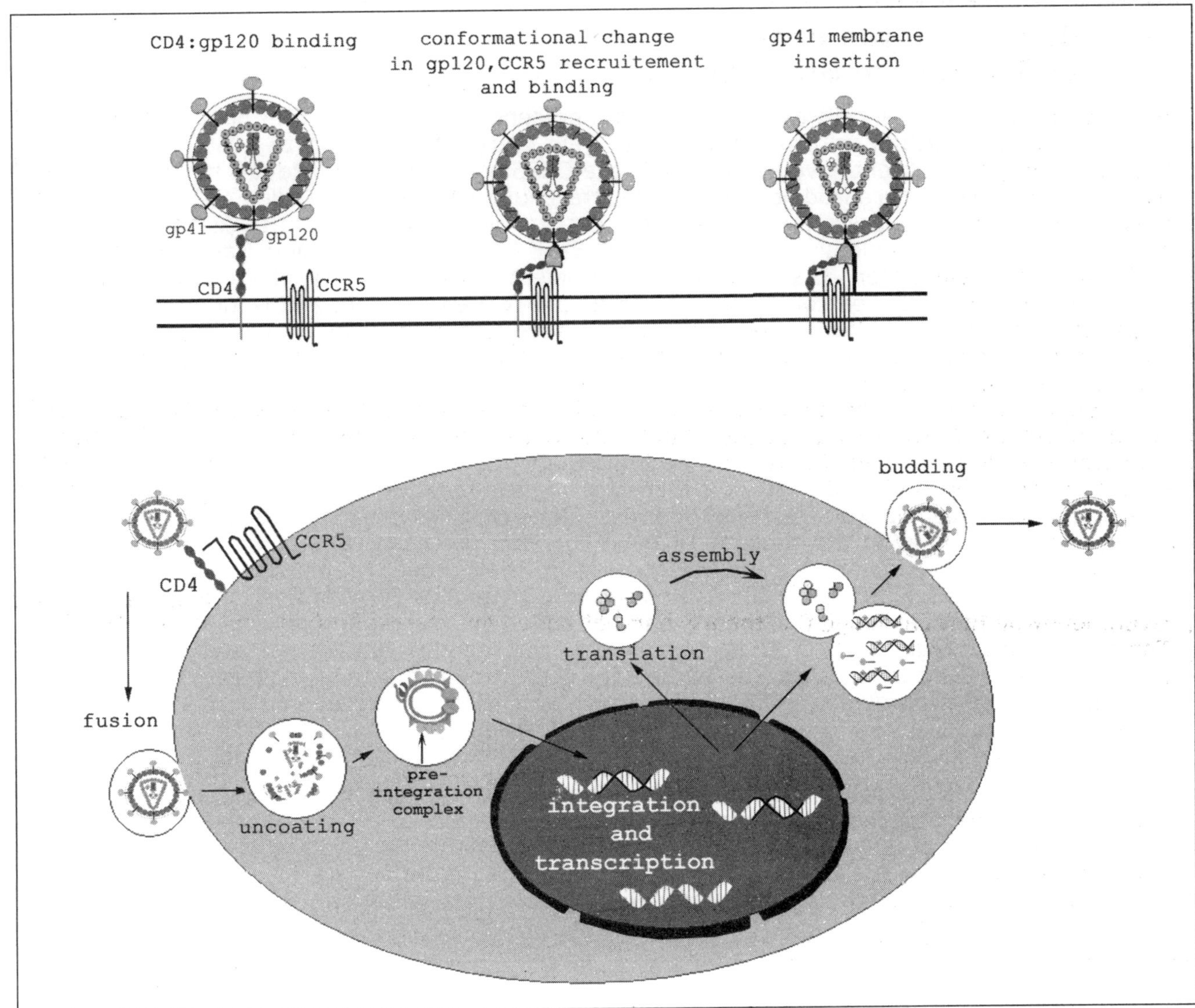

Figuer 17.2 The replicative cycle of HIV begins when the virus gains entry into the cell by binding to CD4 and CCR5 receptors. *The top panel depicts the major events that allow the virus to enter the target cell. Conformational change in gp41 allows the fusion of viral membrane to target cell membrane and the release of the viral core into its interior. After gaining entry, the virus rapidly uncoats. Completion of reverse transcription yields a pre-integration complex comprising double stranded viral cDNA, enzymes (IN, RT), Vpr, matrix protein, and some host proteins. Upon reaching the nucleus, the viral cDNA is transcribed, and the transcripts are rapidly transported to the cytoplasm where they are translated to structural and enzymatic proteins. The final phase of the assembly takes place at the cell surface. Accessory glycoproteins such as Nef and Vpr as well as some host proteins are incorporated into the virions. The assembled virion buds through lipid rafts, yielding virions with cholesterol-rich envelopes (Adapted from Nature Reviews in Immunology (2003) 3:97).*

❑ The sequential engagement of gp120, CD4, and chemokine coreceptors prompts a conformational change in gp41. This conformational change promotes the fusion of the virion and target cell membrane, leading to the release of the HIV viral core into the cell interior.

❑ Viral uncoating occurs once the virion gains entry into the cell and generates the viral reverse transcriptase complex, comprising the diploid viral RNA genome, tRNA primer, enzymes such as reverse transcriptase and integrase, Vpr, matrix protein, nucleocapsid protein, and various host proteins. Vif stabilizes the complex which docks with actin microfilaments in the host cell.

❑ The completion of reverse transcription yields the HIV pre-integration complex,

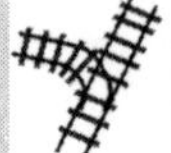

Blast from the Past: CCR5 and the Black Plague

HIV-1 entry into mucosal cells depends upon the presence of CD4 and CCR5 on the cells. Many other viruses use such chemokine receptors to gain entry into cells. Up to 10% individuals of Northern European descent have a mutation in the *CCR5* gene. These individuals have a 32 base-pair deletion in the region encoding the second extracellular loop of CCR5. Called Δ32, this deletion prevents cell surface expression of CCR5. By contrast, less than 2% central Asians carry this mutation, and it is completely absent amongst East Asians, Africans, and Native Americans. Individuals homozygous for Δ32 show an almost complete resistance to HIV infection, underscoring the importance of CCR5 in person-to-person spread of HIV. Heterozygous Δ32 is found in 10 – 15% of Caucasians, and cell surface expression of CCR5 is reduced in these individuals. Entry of the R5 strain of HIV-1 is reduced but not prevented, the viral load is decreased, and progression to AIDS is delayed in such individuals.

Although the origin of the mutation is obscure, it appears to have suddenly become relatively common among Northern Europeans about 700 years ago — coinciding with the biological catastrophe called the 'Black Death' that decimated about a quarter to one-third of the European population between 1347 and 1350. It is therefore suggested that the mutation arose during this infection, and in keeping with Darwin's theories, conferred a selective survival advantage. Thus, people with this mutation are thought to have survived the Black Death, or bubonic plague, caused by *Yersinia pestis* and passed the gene on to their progeny. This sidetrack would have ended here, if two scientists—Susan Cameron and Christopher Duncan from the University of Liverpool—who now challenge this theory, had not added an interesting (yet controversial) twist. The survival advantage of Δ32 CCR5 is not what they question but rather the assumption that the Black Death was the bubonic plague. After having sifted through historical evidence, they suggest that the infection was probably an Ebola-like virus that spread through person-to-person contact. If indeed the history books have it wrong, the theory raises the scary possibility of other severe outbreaks of viral infections. In support of their theory, they point to the following facts:

❑ Quarantine measures used to contain the infection would not have been successful if rat-borne fleas spread the infection; rats have no respect for quarantines.

❑ Large scale death of rats was not reported before the outbreak; in any case, black rats were not introduced to Europe until 50 years later than the Black Death.

❑ The symptoms described included black splotches that are typical of Ebola-like haemorrhagic fever and not of bubonic plague.

composed of double stranded viral cDNA, enzymes (reverse transcriptase and integrase), Vpr, matrix protein, and some host proteins.

❑ The process by which the pre-integration complex reaches the cell nucleus is an area of intense research. The matrix protein contains the nuclear localization signal. Vpr and integrase also contain nuclear targeting signals. The role of these proteins and the nature of their co-operation (if any) in nuclear localization is not yet established. It is thought that the viral genome passes through nuclear pores. In resting cells, reverse transcription is inefficient, and energy levels are too low for effective nuclear import; ds viral genomes can accumulate in these cells without integrating.

❑ Integrase plays a central role in the integration of the viral cDNA into host DNA. The HIV provirus can integrate at many different chromosomal locations, although it has a preference for active genes. Integration can lead to either latent or transcriptionally active forms of the virus. Most infected cells contain more than one provirus, and the possibility that at least one of them will be transcriptionally active is high. The formation of the latent provirus helps HIV escape from the vigorous immune response mounted in the initial phases of infection. It also allows the re-emergence of the virus when the host defence gets weaker. This ability to establish transcriptionally latent forms helps HIV escape potent antiviral therapies as well.

❑ Once integrated, the provirus behaves like any human gene — transcription is initiated at the 5' end and terminated at the 3' end.
  - The 5' LTR acts as a promoter and has binding sites for host transcription factors such as NFκB and NFAT that are formed in activated cells. Activation of T cells therefore results in increased viral protein synthesis.
  - The 3' LTR behaves as a polyadenylation and termination site.
  - Tat shifts viral gene expression to higher gear by recruiting multiple host factors that promote transcription.
❑ The HIV transcripts are rapidly transported to the cytoplasm. Transport is dependent upon the production of adequate amounts of Rev; Rev has nuclear export signals and ensures that the viral transcripts reach the cytoplasm.
❑ Structural and enzymatic viral proteins are synthesized and transported to the plasma membrane.
❑ The final phase of virion assembly occurs at the cell membrane. Molecular chaperones from host cells are thought to be involved in the process. These chaperones allow the conformational changes in gag that are needed for assembly of capsids. gag associates preferentially with cholesterol- and glycosphingolipid-enriched membrane microdomains called lipid rafts (chapter 6) and recruits multivesicular bodies to the site of budding. The assembled virion buds through these specialized regions in the lipid bilayer, yielding virions with cholesterol-rich envelopes (fig. 17.2).

17.3   HIV and the Immune System

The success of HIV as a pathogen is evident from the fact that in less than a quarter of a century since it was first recognized, it has managed to reach almost all parts of the globe. What started as an infection of chiefly marginalized sections of society (gay men and intravenous drug abusers) in the USA has now become a mainstream epidemic spread predominantly through heterosexual contact. The special features that make HIV such a formidable pathogen include:

❑ Its persistence in the host, owing to an ability to integrate irreversibly in the host genome and remain latent for extended periods of time; the host remains asymptomatic for years, ensuring the spread of the virus.
❑ Its ability not to kill host cells indiscriminately; HIV seems to strike the host in a target- and time-specific manner, allowing the host to survive for a long time; death is due to opportunistic infections and neoplasm, not the virus.
❑ Its propensity to hijack the immune system for its own proliferation and spread.
❑ Its capacity to evade and destroy the immune system.

17.3.1   Dynamics of HIV Infection

The primary target of the HIV is the immune system itself, which gets slowly destroyed as the disease progresses. HIV infects cells expressing CD4 and chemokine receptors such as CCR5 or CXCR4. Although CD4$^+$ T cells are the main targets of the virus, various accessory cells are also infected and have a role in disease progression.

❑ DCs play a primary role in the establishment of HIV infection. Their ability to migrate to secondary lymphoid tissues and their close association with T cells make them important in the initial seeding of secondary lymphoid tissues with the virus.
❑ FDCs appear to play a role in pathogenesis after initial infection and seeding has occurred. FDCs have the ability to trap antigen-antibody complexes for prolonged periods with the antigen maintained in its native form (chapter 10). In HIV infection, this ability converts the FDC network into a reservoir of infectious

virions. Although FDCs trap HIV in the form of virion-antibody complexes, experimental evidence suggests that HIV remains infectious in such complexes. Furthermore, FDCs appear to provide signals that increase HIV infection and replication, although the precise nature of these signals is unclear. The continued presence of the virus in the lymph nodes results in destruction of its architecture, unfortunately the exact mechanism of destruction is not known.

❑ Even though monocytes and macrophages harbour large quantities of the virus, they appear to be relatively resistant to HIV killing. Since these cells travel throughout the body, they disseminate the infection to various organs such as the lungs and brain.

❑ Microglial cells are thought to be the major reservoir of the virus in the brain. Patients with clinical AIDS often show CNS and peripheral nervous system abnormalities. The brain is heavily infected, and histological evidence points to extensive viral replication. It is not clear if AIDS related dementia is a consequence of virus replication or a result of an immune response to this replication.

The precise course of HIV infection and disease onset varies considerably from patient to patient[3]. Three major phases of infection are recognized (Table 17.1).

❑ **Primary HIV infection** is followed by a burst of viraemia in which the virus is easily detected in peripheral blood PMNs and plasma. The number of $CD4^+$ T cells decreases by 20–40%. Two to four weeks after infection, 70% people suffer from flu-like symptoms related to the acute infection. It is often associated with fever, lymphadenopathy (swollen lymph glands), and a rash. These symptoms quickly subside, and the patient enters a chronic asymptomatic phase. After initial entry, the virus establishes an infection in macrophages, Langerhans cells, and submucosal DCs at the site of infection or within peripheral blood mononuclear cells. R5 isolates predominate in this phase of the infection. Infected DCs migrate to regional lymph nodes and form clusters with T cells that initiate explosive viral replication in these cells. The major site of replication quickly shifts to the lymphoid tissues of the body, including the lymph nodes, spleen, liver, and bone marrow. Dissemination of the virus to the lymphoid system results in a strong CTL response. Seroconversion, with detectable antibodies to the virus, is observed at this stage. This immune response keeps viral replication in check so that after an initial burst of viraemia, the viral levels in circulation achieve a steady state.

[3] HIV disease is not uniformly expressed in all individuals. Most infected individuals develop full-blown AIDS within 10 years of primary infection. A small proportion of infected individuals develop AIDS and die within months of primary infection, whereas about 5% of infected individuals exhibit no signs of disease even after 12 years or more — they are called long term non-progressors.

Table 17.1 Major phases in HIV infection

Stage of infection	Time	$CD4^+$ T cells (cells/μl)	Characteristics
Acute infection	4–8 weeks	Transient decrease	Transient viraemia Seroconversion; neutralizing antibody found in serum Mild symptoms — fever, headache, lymphadenopathy, malaise, rash
Latent phase	Early — upto 5 years	> 500	Mostly asymptomatic, though patients may report frequent bouts of diarrhoea and night sweats Viral replication continues at low rate
	Intermediate — 5–10 years	500–200	Opportunistic infections and malignancies set in — dermatitis, oral candidiasis, hairy leukoplakia, Herpes zoster infection, Kaposi's sarcoma, etc CNS abnormalities observed
Clinical AIDS	10 years and beyond; 50% patients die within 9 years of infection	< 200	Neutralizing antibody levels start falling Viral load increases dramatically Infections with cytomegalovirus, atypical mycobacteria, cryptopneumocystis, and severe encephalopathy and/or dementia observed

The CD4$^+$ T cell numbers rebound to 80–90% of pre-infection levels (fig. 17.3). Once the virus has reached the lymph nodes, at any given moment there are three major forms of HIV in the body.

- Cell-associated virus is a major source of the virus. About 98–99% of total virus production occurs in activated memory CD4$^+$ T cells, whereas monocytes, macrophages, and microglial cells account for about 1–2% of the total virus produced. It is estimated that 10^9 virions are released daily by the infected cells. Additionally, a minor proportion of CD4$^+$ T cells are latently infected by the virus.
- Free HIV, present in plasma and interstitial fluids, represents only about 1% of the total virus.
- FDC-associated virus may represent >95% of the total HIV present in the body. It is estimated that the lymphoid tissue represents a major reservoir of HIV, and majority of the trapped virus (estimated at 1.5 × 10^8 copies of viral RNA/ gm of lymphoid tissue) exist on the surface of FDCs.

❑ In **the asymptomatic phase**, the patient remains largely free of symptoms despite smouldering low-level viral replication in the lymphoid organs and ongoing immune system destruction. During this latency period, enough of the immune system remains sufficiently intact to provide immune surveillance and to prevent most infections. The provirus latency ensures that cells remain infectious even though antiviral antibodies are found in the serum, and there is an absence of detectable virus in the plasma. The lymph nodes and GALT tissue act as reservoirs of HIV. The virus continues to replicate and infect CD4$^+$ T cells. As more and more CD4$^+$ T cells get infected, their numbers in the peripheral blood falls below 500/μl, with a concomitant increase in opportunistic infections. Almost all facets of the immune system show abnormalities. The structure of

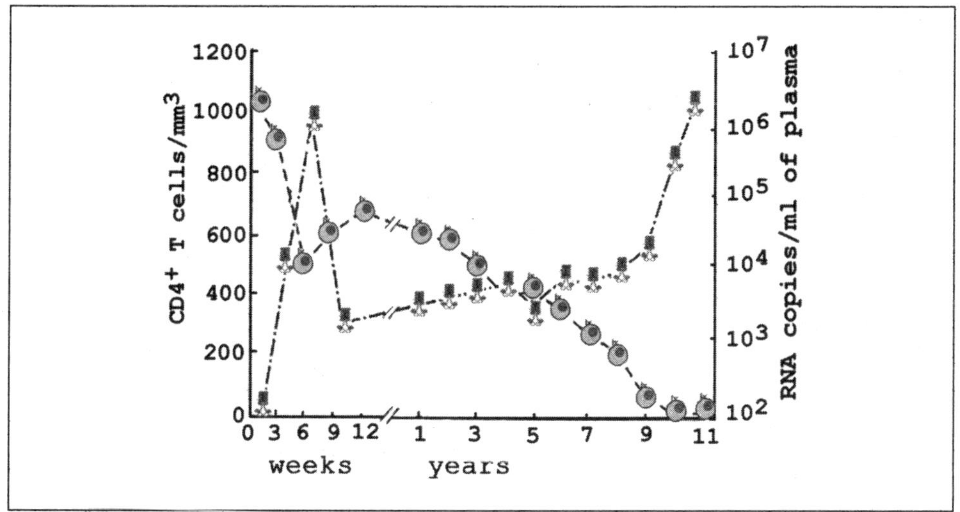

Fgiure 17.3 HIV infection is characterized by a rapid decline in CD4$^+$ T cells, followed by a brief rebound before resuming their downward trend. *Primary HIV infection is followed by a burst of viraemia, when the virus disseminates widely throughout the body, with a concomitant and rapid decline in the number of CD4$^+$ T cells. As an immune response ensues, the numbers of CD4$^+$ T cells recover but never reach the pre-infection level. Although culturable virus is absent from the plasma at this point (not shown), viral mRNA (shown as the central viral core) can be detected easily in the plasma. The number of T cells declines slowly but steadily with an attendant increase in plasma viral mRNA. The patient is largely asymptomatic in this phase and can remain so for years. When the CD4$^+$ T cell numbers fall below a critical threshold (~ 200/μl), patients enter the clinical phase of the infection with a rapid increase in the number of copies of viral mRNA and detectable viraemia. The patient becomes susceptible to opportunistic infections and continues to deteriorate from this point onwards (Adapted from New England Journal of Medicine (1993) 328:327).*

the lymph nodes gets completely destroyed. Cellular parameters of immune functions such as proliferation in response to mitogens, antigens, or alloantigens, decrease and are eventually lost. Chronic activation also results in massive stimulation of B cells, impairing their ability to mount humoral responses.

❑ **The final phase** of infection occurs when the number of CD4$^+$ T lymphocytes declines to a stage where the production of new cells cannot match the numbers of those destroyed. Patients exhibit fatigue, persistent fever, and weight loss. Clinical AIDS is defined by a CD4$^+$ T cell count of <200/μl of blood and the appearance of one or more opportunistic infections or malignancies such as Kaposi's sarcoma, *Pneumocystis carnii* pneumonia, atypical mycobacterial infections, and severe HIV encephalopathy.

17.3.2 HIV Immune Evasion

How HIV evades and survives effectors of the immune system has been a matter of intense scientific interest. The immune system has evolved a two-pronged system for detecting and destroying intracellular pathogens — one antigen-specific (by virtue of CTLs) and other antigen non-specific (via NK cells; chapter 11). Recognition of pathogen-derived peptides loaded on MHC class I molecules results in antigen-specific activation of CD8$^+$ T cells. Downregulation of MHC class I expression can allow a pathogen to escape CTL recognition. However, such downregulation makes the infected cells susceptible to NK cell attack. Nevertheless, HIV encoded proteins reshape the cellular environment of the virus and allow it to evade the immune system.

❑ **HIV reverse transcriptase is error-prone.** The low fidelity of the enzyme allows the virus to mutate at extremely high rates; it is estimated that the enzyme introduces a mutation once per 2000 nucleotides incorporated. Due to epitope imprinting, this high variability allows newly developing strains to escape effectors of adaptive immunity (see sidetrack 'Trying to Fit In' in chapter 9).

❑ **HIV encoded Nef help make virus-infected cells invisible to CTLs and NK cells.**
  - Nef ensures that MHC class I molecules do not reach the cell surface. In the presence of Nef, MHC class I molecules (HLA-A and HLA-B) are diverted from the cell surface to the endosomes and eventually to the *trans*-golgi network, where they get trapped.
  - Nef does not decrease the expression of HLA-C and HLA-E which bind inhibitory effectors on NK cells.

❑ **Tat interferes with MHC class II transcription** in infected monocytes and macrophages, thus interfering with their ability to present antigen via MHC class II molecules and the generation of an adaptive immune response.

❑ **HIV induces the death of uninfected immune effectors.** Cross-linking of CD4 by the HIV envelope in the presence of soluble Tat can induce FasL expression and apoptosis of uninfected cells. Similarly, interaction of the HIV envelope with CXCR4 on macrophages leads to the death of bystander CD8$^+$ T cells through the induction of TNF expression.

17.3.3 HIV Immune Destruction

Much like a pirate taking over a ship and using it till it is destroyed, HIV commandeers the immune system to ensure its own spread, and in the bargain, destroys it. Nef has a major role in this destruction.

❑ Nef triggers accelerated endocytosis and subsequent lysosomal degradation of CD4 in infected cells. It thus ensures that the released virions do not rebind CD4 on infected cells but remain free to bind CD4 and chemokine receptors on fresh cells.

❑ Nef induces upregulation of FasL expression on the surface of infected cells. This FasL interacts with neighbouring cells expressing Fas (such as virus-specific CTLs), and triggers their apoptosis.

❑ Nef ensures the survival of infected cells by blocking mitochondrial apoptotic pathways. It thus prevents the premature death of infected cells and facilitates the completion of the viral replicative cycle.

17.4 Treatment

Virtually all compounds currently in use or in advanced clinical trials for treatment of HIV infections belong to one of four classes.

❑ **Nucleoside/nucleotide Reverse Transcriptase Inhibitors** (NRTIs). These nucleotide analogues need to be metabolically activated before they can interfere with viral DNA (vDNA). They are converted by cellular kinases to 5-triphosphates, which then get selectively incorporated by reverse transcriptase into vDNA, resulting in the termination of vDNA synthesis. Examples include thymidine analogues such AZT and Stavudine (d4T), cytidine analogues such as Zalcitabine (ddC) and Lamivudine (3TC), the inosine analogue Didanosine (dd), and guanine analogue Abacavir. NRTIs can cause myriad side effects, including myelotoxicity, gastrointestinal problems, neurological symptoms, and pancreatitis.

❑ **Non-Nucleoside Reverse Transcriptase Inhibitors** (NNRTIs). These are structurally diverse, non-competitive inhibitors of reverse transcriptase. They do not require metabolic activation. They are extremely effective in halting virus replication, especially when used in combination with NRTIs. The most commonly used NNRTIs include Nevirapine and Efavirenz. Cytochrome P450 enzymes metabolize both these drugs. Resistance development is a major problem, since a single point mutation can result in resistance to the entire class of drug.

❑ **Protease Inhibitors** (PIs). These lipophilic compounds function by inhibiting the HIV protease that cleaves gag-pol protein into its functional subunits. It thus interferes with HIV maturation and replication. PIs, when used in combination

---

THE HUMAN IMMUNODEFICIENCY VIRUS

❑ HIV is a human retrovirus about 90 – 100 nm in diameter, consisting of a bar-shaped core containing the viral genome and enzymes, enclosed in an outer lipid envelope.

❑ The primary target of the HIV is the immune system itself, which gets slowly destroyed as the disease progresses.

❑ HIV enters the body through the exchange of bodily fluids and infects cells expressing CD4 and CCR5 but spreads by hijacking the cells of the immune system.
  - CD4$^+$ T cells are the primary target of infection.
  - DCs are important in the initial seeding of secondary lymphoid tissues with the virus.
  - FDCs are a reservoir of infectious virions.
  - Although macrophages and monocytes are relatively resistant to HIV killing, their migratory properties cause them to disseminate the infection to various organs.
  - Microglial cells are thought to be the major reservoir of the virus in the brain.

❑ Primary HIV infection is followed by a burst of viraemia; following this burst, the immune system keeps the virus in control until the CD4$^+$ T cells decline to a critical level (200 cells/µl), after which the patient suffers from full blown clinical AIDS.

❑ The virus uses a multi-pronged strategy to evade the immune system.
  - The low fidelity reverse transcriptase allows the virus to mutate at extremely high rates; the mutants co-exist in the individual.
  - HIV encoded Nef interferes with MHC class I expression while allowing non-classical MHC class I expression.
  - Tat interferes with MHC class II transcription in infected monocytes and macrophages.
  - HIV induces the death of uninfected immune effector cells by inducing apoptosis.

❑ The best way to treat the infection is to hit early and hit hard by using a combination of drugs. The classes of drugs used include reverse transcriptase inhibitors, protease inhibitors, and fusion inhibitors.

with RTIs, have been shown to reduce plasma HIV RNA levels by 99–99.9%. PIs in current use include Saquinavir, Indinavir, and Ritonavir. Common side effects include gastrointestinal disturbances and lipid abnormalities (lipodystrophy and dyslipidaemia), insulin resistance, and premature artherosclerosis.

❑ **Fusion inhibitors.** T-20, a 36 amino acid peptide corresponding to 127–162 residues of gp41, inhibits viral fusion and had been recently approved for clinical use.

All antiretroviral drugs in current use have severe side effects. The high turnover and mutation rate of the virus results in rapid development of resistance to any drug used singly. The paramount therapeutic aim is to reduce viral load in the infected individual as rapidly as possible and at as early a stage of infection as possible. To put it succinctly, the motto is — hit hard and hit early. A combination therapy consisting of a cocktail of two or more drugs has been found to be effective in bringing down and maintaining the viral load to undetectable levels and is often referred to as HAART (**H**ighly **A**ctive **A**nti**r**etroviral **T**herapy). Nevertheless, therapy does not eradicate infection. Hence, newer approaches are being developed to activate and eradicate the latent virus, eg, treatment with cytokines like IL-2 and GM-CSF. However, these therapies are as yet in investigative stages.

Although HIV-1 was successfully grown in tissue culture and completely sequenced within four years of recognition of AIDS, a successful therapeutic vaccine against HIV still eludes us. The same reasons that make HIV a difficult target for the immune system also make it a uniquely difficult problem for vaccine development. Firstly, HIV-1 and HIV-2 are so divergent in their genetic sequence that their envelope glycoproteins are often not cross-reactive. Hence, separate vaccines need to be developed for them. Other problems such as the co-existence of several antigenically disparate mutants in an individual, formation of latent proviral DNA with a long half-life in early stages of infection, and heavy glycosylation of exposed epitopes has led to the failure of traditional approaches to vaccine development. The most promising approach to fighting HIV appears to be the induction of CMI by DNA vaccines (see sidetrack 'Licensing to Kill' in chapter 11). However, the inefficient expression of HIV-1 mRNA remains a major problem in the development of these vaccines. A new adjuvant consisting of IL-2 fused to Ig H chain has been shown to augment T cell immunity in mouse models and is being studied. Another approach is the use of live viral vectors. Use of recombinant modified vaccinia Ankara virus (rMVA) or recombinant human Adenovirus (Ad5) to deliver the DNA vaccine has met with moderate success in animal trials. Despite all efforts, effective chemo- and immunotherapy for AIDS remains a distant dream. The only way to prevent infection is to take adequate preventive measures (using double gloves when handling human blood and body fluids, using disposable needles and ensuring their proper disposal, avoiding multiple sex partners, using condoms, etc).

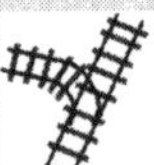

The Pandora's Box:
Moral and Ethical Issues Related to the HIV Epidemic

HIV/AIDS is scary not only because it starkly exposes and manipulates our vulnerabilities — both biological and socio-cultural — but also forces us to face up to the realities of the society we live in. HIV/AIDS is biologically potent, but its potency is magnified tenfold by the brilliance with which it manipulates our illusions of invincibility, our prejudices, and our societal denial mechanisms.

The current HIV/AIDS pandemic surfaced amongst gay men and drug abusers in North America. It became associated in the public mind with homosexuality and drug abuse — issues normally swept under the carpet. In Africa and Asia, the epidemic has spread through heterosexual contact — mainly through prostitutes or people with multiple partners. It is for this reason that HIV/AIDS came to be conveniently viewed as a disease of the depraved. Early in the pandemic's history (and arguably even now), most countries adopted a 'holier than thou' attitude; HIV/AIDS was a problem faced by 'other' societies and cultures. The fact is, we cannot rely on moral solutions to solve biological problems. The rapid spread of HIV/AIDS amongst heterosexual populations shatters our illusions of 'civilized' societies. It makes us take a long hard look at grey areas in our morality. It throws up evidence of promiscuity, prostitution, the closeted double lives people lead, and rampant drug abuse. Even more scarily, it shows us conclusive evidence of the magnitude and frequency of their prevalence. But it does not stop there.

Many of its victims innocently contract the disease, and this is not counting the blood transfusion recipients. Amongst heterosexuals, women are more likely to catch the infection than men. What makes it worse is the fact that the vast majority of the women in the developing world have very little say in sexual matters. Whether prostitutes or housewives, most women cannot insist on condom usage by their partners. In countries like India, women in monogamous relationships are found to have contracted the infection from promiscuous partners. Even sadder — they often pass it on to their children during childbirth and whole families are laid waste by the disease.

The only way the epidemic can be controlled is through education. Forewarned is forearmed. Education can dispel the many myths surrounding the infection, myths that run the gamut from bizarre ideas that HIV does not cause AIDS to claims that having sex with a virgin cures the infection[4]! The resistance to open discussion about sexual practices is one of the major barriers to stemming the spread of the epidemic. Sex, needless to mention, has always been a touchy issue, something that we as a society are more comfortable not talking about. The resistance of the religious right (of whichever religious denomination/country) to sex education and/or condom usage plays right into the hands of the virus. The fact remains that except for abstinence, no method of protection can guarantee an HIV/AIDS free life. Even abstinence does not guarantee freedom from receiving infected blood during transfusions or accidentally acquiring the disease eg, by getting pricked with a tainted needle. If we could better control our impulses, STDs would not have survived for more than 2000 years. At least condoms reduce the risks of catching the disease by offering 90% protection — which is much better than no protection at all!

HIV/AIDS has in a matter of decades become mainstream. The stigma attached to the infection, however, remains. A lack of awareness about the disease has resulted in HIV-infected people facing varying degrees of discrimination. Fear of contagion has sometimes even led to discrimination against the HIV infected by medical personnel, and legal struggles to rectify this situation continue. At the family level, an adult with HIV infection translates into a severe crunch on resources because the person's capacity to work reduces while the cost of treatment multiplies. The high cost and long-term nature of the treatment makes AIDS a death sentence for the poorer sections of the society. The result is families abandoning the infected — be it babies or adults.

Discrimination is only one of the ethical issues that HIV has raised. It also throws up the issue of personal choice *vis à vis* risk to the society. The high rate of mutation in the virus makes it necessary to use a combination of three or more drugs, and this may cost up to USD10,000 or more annually. To make matters worse, multiple drug therapy involves taking a minimum of eight HIV fighting pills (and frequently many more) a day on an often complex schedule, in addition to any other medicines the individual might need. Trying to adhere to this schedule while trying to find and hold down a job is a daunting task. Patients who fail to follow the directions risk encouraging the proliferation of drug-resistant virus in the body, making subsequent treatment more difficult and increasing the risk of infecting others with a resistant strain of the virus.

The current HIV/AIDS pandemic seems to successfully emphasize the weaknesses of our societies — in terms of moral issues, notions of sexuality and sexual repression, gender inequalities, class inequalities, egocentrism, ignorance, discrimination, and denial. HIV has an advantage over the human population not only biologically, but also psychologically. Unless we face up to the realities exposed by the disease, we may never be able to win this biological battle. The costs of this disease are not limited to infected individuals or even their families. Ultimately, they will be borne by whole sections of the societies and economies that it has spread to. Although the current pandemic originated in the USA, the global burden of HIV/AIDS will be overwhelmingly borne by people in the developing world, and inequalities of gender, race, class, and wealth will dictate the future course of this pandemic.

---

[4] If that does not make you sick to your stomach, nothing else will!

Appendix I

List of CDs Mentioned in the Book

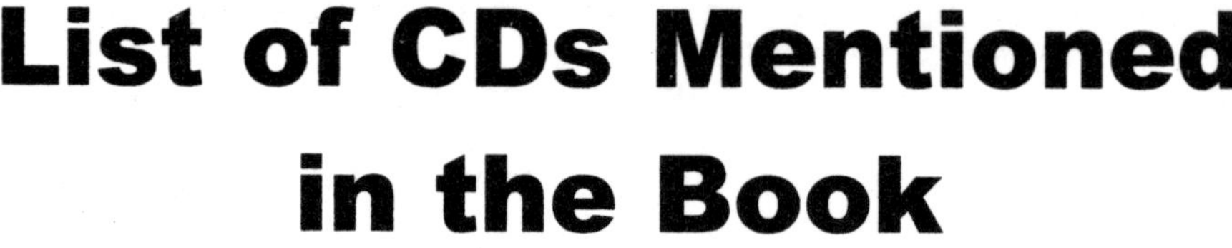

CD (alternate name)	Cellular expression	Known functions
CD1	Cortical thymocytes, Langerhans cells, DCs, B cells, cells in the intestinal epithelium, smooth muscles, blood vessels	• MHC class I-like molecule associated with β_2-microglobulin • Presents lipid antigens
CD2	T cells, thymocytes, NK cells	• Adhesion molecule, binds CD58 (LFA-3) • Binds Lck intracellularly and activates T cells
CD3	Thymocytes, T cells	• Associated with TcR • Required for cell surface expression of and signal transduction by the TcR
CD4	Thymocyte subsets, T_{H1} and T_{H2} cells, monocytes, macrophages	• Coreceptor for MHC class II molecules • Binds Lck • Receptor for HIV-1 and HIV-2 gp120
CD5	Thymocytes, T cells, subset of B cells	• Modulates signalling through the antigen-specific receptor complex (TcR and BcR) • Is a phenotypic marker for a subset of B cells (the B1 subset) • Is a phenotypic marker for some B cell lymphoproliferative disorders (B cell lymphocytic leukaemia, mantle zone lymphoma, Hairy cell leukaemia, etc)
CD7	Pleuripotent haematopoietic stem cells, thymocytes, T cells	• Function not known • Marker for T cell acute lymphatic leukaemia and pleuripotential stem cell leukaemias
CD8	Thymocyte subsets, CTLs	• Coreceptor for MHC class I molecules • Binds Lck
CD9	Pre-B cells and a subset of B1 cells, eosinophils, basophils, platelets, activated T cells, cells in the brain and peripheral nerves, vascular smooth muscles	• Mediates platelet aggregation and activation via FcγRIIa • May play a role in cell migration
CD10	B and T cell precursors, bone marrow stromal cells	• Zinc metalloproteinase • Marker for pre-B acute lymphatic leukaemia

CD11a	Lymphocytes, granulocytes, monocytes and macrophages	• Subunit of integrin LFA-1 (associated with CD18) • Binds to CD54 (ICAM-1), CD102 (ICAM-2), and CD50 (ICAM-3) • Intercellular adhesion and costimulation
CD11b (Mac-1)	Myeloid cells and NK cells	• Subunit of integrin associated with CD18 to form complement receptor 3 • Binds CD54, complement component iC3b, and extracellular matrix proteins • Promotes phagocytosis of iC3b or IgG coated particles
CD11c	Myeloid cells	• Subunit of integrin associated with CD18 to form complement receptor 4 • Binds fibrinogen • Similar in function to CD11b/CD18 with which it co-operates
CD14	Myelomonocytic cells	• Receptor for complex of LPS and LBP
CD16	Neutrophils, NK cells, macrophages	• Component of low affinity Fc receptor — FcγRIII • Mediates phagocytosis and ADCC
CD18	Leukocytes	• Integrin β-2 subunit, associates with CD11a, b, c, and d
CD19	B cells	• Forms a complex with CD21 (CR2) and CD81 (TAPA-1) • Coreceptor for B cells • Cytoplasmic domain binds tyrosine kinases and PI 3-kinase
CD20	B cells	• Oligomers of CD20 may form a Ca^{2+} channel • May have a role in regulating B cell activation
CD21	Mature B cells, FDCs	• Complement receptor 2; binds C3d • Receptor for Epstein-Barr virus • Forms a part of the BcR complex along with CD19 and CD81
CD22	Mature B cells	• Binds sialoconjugates
CD23	Mature B cells, activated macrophages, eosinophils, FDCs, platelets	• Low affinity receptor for IgE • Regulates IgE synthesis • Ligand for CD19:CD21:CD81 coreceptor complex
CD25	Activated T cells, B cells, monocytes	• IL-2 receptor α chain
CD28	T cell subsets, activated B cells	• Activation of naïve T cells, • Binds CD80 (B7.1) and CD86 (B7.2) and delivers a costimulatory signal
CD31 (PECAM-1)	Monocytes, platelets, granulocytes, T cell subsets, endothelial cells	• Adhesion molecule • Mediates both leukocyte-endothelial and endothelial-endothelial interactions
CD32	Monocytes, granulocytes, B cells, eosinophils	• FcγRII, a low affinity IgG receptor
CD33	Myeloid progenitor cells, monocytes	• Binds sialoconjugates
CD34	Haematopoietic precursors, capillary endothelium	• Ligand for CD62L (L-selectin)
CD35	Erythrocytes, B cells, monocytes, neutrophils, eosinophils, FDCs	• Complement receptor 1 • Binds C3b and C4b • Mediates phagocytosis
CD40	B cells, macrophages, DCs, basal epithelial cells	• Binds CD154 (CD40L) • Receptor for costimulatory signal for B cells • Promotes growth, differentiation, and isotype switching of B cells, and cytokine production by macrophages and DCs
CD44	Leukocytes, erythrocytes	• Binds hyaluronic acid • Mediates adhesion of leukocytes
CD45	All haematopoietic cells	• Tyrosine phosphatase • Augments signalling through BcR and TcR

CD46	Haematopoietic and non-haematopoietic nucleated cells	• Membrane cofactor protein • Binds C3b and C4b and allows their degradation by Factor I
CD50 (ICAM-3)	Thymocytes, T cells, B cells, monocytes, granulocytes	• Binds integrin CD11a/CD18
CD54 (ICAM-1)	Haematopoietic and non-haematopoietic cells	• Binds CD11a/CD18 integrin (LFA-1) and CD11b/CD18 integrin (Mac-1) • Receptor for rhinovirus or RBC infected with the malarial parasite
CD55 (DAF)	Haematopoietic and non-haematopoietic cells	• Binds C3b • Inhibits formation of C3 convertase • Disassembles C3/C5 convertase
CD56	NK cells	• Isoform of neural cell adhesion molecule (NCAM)
CD58 (LFA-3)	Multiple cell types of haematopoietic and non-haematopoietic origin	• Adhesion molecule, Ligand for CD2
CD59	Haematopoietic and non-haematopoietic cells	• Binds C8 and C9, and blocks assembly of MAC
CD62L	B cells, T cells, monocytes, NK cells	• Leukocyte adhesion molecule (LAM) • Binds CD34 • Mediates rolling interactions with endothelium
CD69	Activated T and B cells, activated macrophages, and NK cells	• Function unknown, early activation antigen
CD72	B cells (except plasma cells)	• Function unknown
CD79a and CD79b (Igα and Igβ)	B cells	• Components of BcR • Required for cell surface expression and signal transduction
CD80	B cells	• Costimulatory molecule • Ligand for CD28 and CTLA-4
CD81 (TAPA-1)	Lymphocytes	• Associates with CD19, CD21 to form BcR
CD86	Monocytes, activated B cells, dendritic cells	• Ligand for CD28 and CTLA-4
CDw90 (CD90.1, thy-1)	Haematopoietic stem cells, neurons, murine thymocytes and peripheral T cells, may be found on a subset of monocytes	• Function not clear, may contribute to inhibition of proliferation and differentiation of haematopoietic stem cells
CD91	Monocytes, many non-haematopoietic cells	• α2-macroglobulin receptor
CD94	T cell subsets, NK cells	• A C-type lectin • CD94-NKG2A complex inhibits NK cell function
CD95 (Fas)	Wide variety of cell lines, *in vivo* distribution uncertain, but expressed by activated T and B cells	• Binds FasL; induces apoptosis • One of the molecules involved in lysis of target cells by CTLs
CD100	Haematopoietic cells, upregulated on activated T cells, expressed on germinal centre but not MZ B cells	• Function largely unknown • Increases CD3 and CD2 induced T cell proliferation

CD102 (ICAM-2)	Resting lymphocytes, monocytes, vascular endothelium cells (strongest)	• Binds CD11a/CD18 (LFA-1) but not CD11b/CD18 (Mac-1)
CD117 (c-kit)	Developmental marker for most haematopoietic cells	• Stem Cell Factor receptor
CD122	T cells, B cells, NK cells, monocytes/macrophages	• IL-2 receptor β chain • A critical subunit of IL-2R and IL-15R
CD127	Bone marrow lymphoid precursors, pro-B cells, mature T cells, monocytes	• IL-7 receptor
CD134 (OX40)	Activated T cells	• May act as adhesion molecule • Costimulatory molecule • Promotes T cell survival
CD134L (OX40L)	Activated B cells, DCs, vascular endothelial cells	• T cell costimulatory molecule • Enhances Ig production in B cells
CD152 (CTLA-4)	Activated T cells	• Receptor for B7.1 (CD80), and B7.2 (CD86) • Negative regulator of T cell activation
CD154 (CD40L)	Activated CD4+ T cells	• Induces B cell proliferation and activation
CD161	NK cells, T cells	• Regulates NK cytotoxicity
CD178 (CD95L)	Most T cells, NK cells, neutrophils, breast epithelial cells, microglia, a subset of DCs	• Activates apoptotic pathways • Key effector of cytotoxicity • Expression upregulated upon cell activation

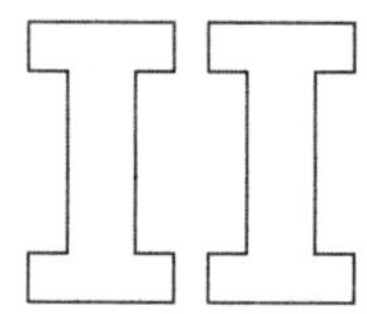

'Nobel' Immunologists

Year	Recipient(s)	*Citation* and the Prize-winning Discovery
1996	Peter C. Doherty and Rolf M. Zinkernagel	*'For their discoveries concerning the specificity of cell-mediated immune defence'*
		They established that CTLs' co-ordinate-recognition of self-H-2:viral antigen defined the basis of MHC restriction of immune responses in 1974.
1987	Susumu Tonegawa	*'For his discovery of genetic principle for generation of antibody diversity'*
		He established that single immunoglobulin proteins were encoded by separate rearranging genes in 1976.
1984	Niels K. Jerne, Georges J.F. Kohler, and Cesar Milstein	*'For theories concerning the specificity in development and control of the immune system and the discovery of the principle of production of monoclonal antibodies'*
		Jerne was cited for the influence of his theories concerning the development and control of the immune system.
		Kohler and Milstein were awarded the prize for their 1975 discovery of the principle for production of monoclonal antibodies.
1980	Baruj Benacerraf, Jean Dausset, and George D. Snell	*'For their discoveries concerning genetically determined structures on the cell surface that regulate immunological reactions'*
		They were recognized for their separate work over three decades to define genetically the H-2 and HLA molecules that regulate immunological reactions.
1977	Rosalyn Yallow	*'For the development of radio-immunoassays of peptide hormones'*
		She shared the prize with R. Guillemin and A.V. Schally who were awarded the prize for their work concerning peptide hormone production in the brain.
1972	Gerald M. Edelman and Rodney R. Porter	*'For their discoveries concerning the chemical structure of antibodies'*
		Their work done during the late 1950s and early 1960s showed that immunoglobulins were composed of covalently bonded two heavy and two light chains.
1960	Sir Frank MacFarlane Burnet and Peter Brian Medawar	*'For discovery of acquired immunological tolerance'* MacFarlane Burnet was cited for developing the theories of clonal selection of antibody production and for applying this to the concept of acquired immunological tolerance.
		Medawar was awarded the prize for experimentally confirming Burnet's theory, showing that graft rejection is due to an immunological reaction and that tolerance can be built up by injections into embryos.

| 1951 | Max Theiler | *'For his discoveries concerning yellow fever and how to combat it'* |

He was awarded the prize for his contribution to the 1938 development of the universally successful vaccine for yellow fever.

| 1930 | Karl Landsteiner | *'For his discovery of human blood groups'* |

He was cited for serologically defining the ABO blood group system.

| 1919 | Jules Bordet | *'For his discoveries relating to immunity'* |

He was awarded the prize for developing the basis of immune haemolysis of foreign erythrocytes including the involvement of separate heat labile (complement) and heat stable (antibody) components.

| 1913 | Charles Robert Richet | *'In recognition of his work on anaphylaxis'* |

He showed that injection of dead or attenuated microbes not only led to specific immunity but that subsequent re-exposure could provoke severe illness or death due to anaphylactic shock.

| 1908 | Ilya Ilyich Metchnikov and Paul Ehrlich | *'In recognition of their work in immunity'* |

Metchnikov was cited for developing the cellular theory of immunity, emphasizing a key role for phagocytes.

Ehrlich was awarded the prize for developing the first general theories of specific immunity and natural self-tolerance. His side chain receptor theory anticipated Burnet's clonal selection theory by half a century.

| 1901 | Emil Adolf von Behring | *'For his work in serum therapy, especially its application against diphtheria'* |

He was awarded the prize for defining the concept of serum therapy by showing that diphtheria and tetanus exotoxins could be used to raise antitoxins that could be passively transferred to protect against disease.

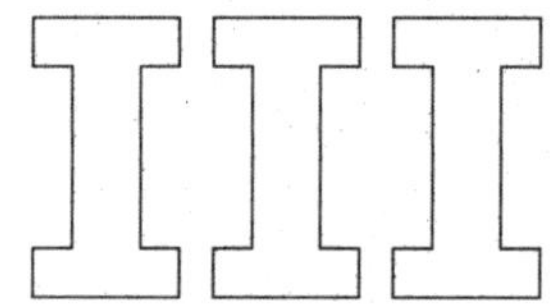

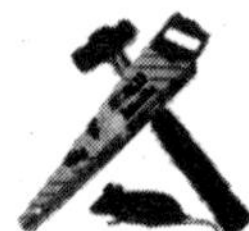

Tools of the Trade

Science is all about asking questions and designing experiments to answer them. The foregoing chapters are intended to help in identifying the questions that need to be asked. To be able to design experiments for answering those questions, a basic understanding of the available techniques is necessary. This appendix is meant to be a general aid to understanding common techniques used in immunology — the tools you will need to practice the trade. Igs, with their high specificity and their ability to specifically recognize and bind antigens in the presence of high concentrations of other molecules, are excellent tools for detection and/or measurement of virtually any biological molecule. They are almost indispensable to immunological techniques. We therefore start this appendix with a brief introduction to the physicochemical principles of antigen-antibody interactions.

Kinetics of Antigen-antibody Interaction

The basic thermodynamic principles of monovalent antigen-antibody reaction are the same as those for any reversible bimolecular chemical binding. The reaction between an antigen and its homologous antibody is essentially a reaction between the antigenic epitope and the paratope (or antigen-binding site) of the antibody. The antigen-antibody binding involves multiple non-covalent bonds such as hydrogen bonds, electrostatic bonds, hydrophobic bonds, Van der Waal's bonds, and salt bridges (Table 4.1). Although each single bond is weak, the sheer numbers of bonds formed add up to a considerable binding energy[1]. However, the interacting groups must be closely associated to allow the formation of these bonds, since the forces of attraction that form these bonds rapidly decline with increasing distance.

Consider the reaction between epitopes at concentration $[E]$ and paratopes at concentration $[P]$. Both the reactants will be in thermal motion and will be colliding with each other. The rate of complex formation will be governed by the Law of Mass Action.

Epitope-paratope complexes $[x]$ will be formed at a rate proportional to
— the concentrations of the free reagents, ie, $[P - x]$ and $[E - x]$, and
— the rate of effective collisions, k_1
The rate of complex formation with respect to time can be given by the equation:

$$\frac{d[x]}{dt} = k_1[E - x][P - x] \tag{1}$$

The formed complexes will dissociate at a rate — k_1, proportional to the concentration of the complex, and this decrease in its concentration with respect to time can be defined by the equation —

[1] This is similar to the Liliputians immobilizing Gulliver with a large number of ropes nailed to the ground. Although he could have easily broken any one of them, the sheer number of these ropes prevented his getting free.

$$-\frac{dx}{[dt]} = k_2[x] \tag{2}$$

The rate of change of concentration of the complex with respect to time will be obtained by combining equations (1) and (2)

$$\frac{dx}{[dt]} = k_1[E-x][P-x] - k_2[x] \tag{3}$$

When the reaction reaches equilibrium, the rate of the forward reaction (complex formation) will be equal to the rate of backward reaction (complex dissociation) and therefore $dx/[dt] = 0$, ie,

$$k_1[E-x][P-x] = k_2[x] \text{ or,}$$

$$\frac{[E-x][P-x]}{[x]} = \frac{k_1}{k_2} = \frac{[\text{free epitopes}]\,[\text{free paratopes}]}{[\text{complexes}]} \tag{4}$$

This ratio of k_1/k_2 is called the equilibrium constant and is denoted by K_D. It has the dimensions of concentration, and is conventionally expressed in terms of molarity (M). The equilibrium constant may also be expressed in terms of K_A which is the inverse of K_D, and has the peculiar dimension of M^{-1} (or litres/Mole). The equilibrium constant (whether K_D or K_A) is a measure of the affinity of the antibody for the antigen (*affinity*—liking or attraction). Smaller the K_D, greater the forward reaction, stronger the bonds between the antigen and the antibody, and more stable the complex. Like any chemical reaction, the antigen-antibody binding is affected by temperature, pH, ionic strength, etc.

Equation (3) describes an interaction of monovalent reactants (eg, haptens and Fab fragments). K_D is thus a summation of all the attractive and repulsive forces of a reaction of monovalent reactants. In practice, however, the situation is much more complicated since a multivalent antigen reacts with a bivalent or multivalent antibody. When a multivalent antigen combines with more than one of the antibody's combining sites, the strength of the binding is considerably more than just the sum of the binding energies of the individual site. This is because all the antigen-antibody bonds must be simultaneously broken before the reactants can dissociate. The strength with which a multivalent antibody binds to a multivalent antigen is termed avidity.

Determination of K_D

Information regarding the antigen-antibody reaction is contained in its equilibrium constant K_D, the ratio of backward and forward reaction constants at equilibrium. To estimate the equilibrium constant, one needs to be able to separate at least one of the three entities from the equilibrium mixture (free epitopes, free paratopes, and epitope-paratope complexes), without disturbing the equilibrium in any way. Equation (4) above can be transformed to a linear form ($y = mx + C$) and used to estimate the K_D.

Thus,

$$\frac{[x]}{[E-x]} = \frac{[P-x]}{K_D} = \frac{[P]}{K_D} - \frac{[x]}{K_D} \tag{5}$$

Use of this equation requires the determination of the amount of bound $[x]$ and free fraction $[E-x]$ of one of the reactants at equilibrium, over a range of concentrations, keeping the concentration of the other reactant $[P]$ in large excess. The values can then be fitted in a graph of $[x]$ vs $[x]/[E-x]$; the inverse of the slope of this graph is K_D.

❑ **Equilibrium dialysis** is one of the most unequivocal methods of K_D determination. It is particularly suited for determining the K_D of antibodies to small dialyzable haptens. In this technique, antibodies are retained on one side of a semi-permeable membrane whereas the antigen (hapten) can freely pass through it. K_D is computed by fitting the initial and the bound concentrations of the hapten in equation (5).

❑ **Labelled reactant techniques.** The major drawback of equilibrium dialysis is that the method is only applicable to small haptens (MW<3000 daltons). To determine the reaction between large antigens and antibodies one of the reactants (usually the antigen) is labelled and the complexes formed at equilibrium separated by a variety of methods (eg, centrifugation, filtration, precipitation, and adsorption to a solid surface), to obtain the data needed for equation (5). These techniques presume that both the labelling and the separation of one of the reactants at equilibrium do not alter binding kinetics.

❑ **Optical biosensors.** These instruments allow the measurement of biomolecular interactions with minimal distortions, since they enable interaction monitoring in real-time (ie, as they are occurring). To measure K_D by this method one of the reactants is immobilized to a non-reactive gel. The kinetics of the interaction at the gel surface is subsequently measured by adding the second reactant. The measurements are done as the reaction proceeds, ie, before it reaches equilibrium, and allows the application of equations (1), (2), and (3).

A. Antibodies as Diagnostic Tools

Binding of the antibody to its homologous antigen can alter the physical state of the antigen and this property is used in a variety of ways in immunodiagnosis.

IMMUNODIAGNOSTIC ASSAY PARAMETERS

❑ The specificity of an assay is the ability to give a positive reaction with only the ligand, and is dependent on the quality of the detecting reagents.
❑ The detection limit of a test is defined as the lowest concentration of the ligand that gives a response that differs significantly from zero concentration response (ie, the negative control).
❑ Sensitivity of an assay is the change in response per unit amount of reactant.
❑ Precision and reproducibility of an assay are defined by the **S**tandard **D**eviation (SD) obtained with multiple readings of the same concentration of reactants; smaller the SD, greater is the precision and reproducibility.
❑ Practicability of the assay refers to speed and ease of performance, possibility of automation, etc.

A.1 The Precipitin Reaction

Complexing of Igs with soluble antigen results in the formation of insoluble aggregates that precipitate out of the liquid. The quantitative precipitin assay was described by Heidelberger in 1897 and has been used as a qualitative and semi-quantitative procedure for serum antibody detection and measurement. The highest dilution of the serum that gives a positive reaction is called its titre. When fixed aliquots of antiserum are added to increasing concentrations of the homologous soluble antigen, the amount of precipitate obtained increases until a maximum is reached after which the quantity of precipitate decreases. The curve obtained by plotting the concentration of antigen added against the amount of precipitate formed is called the precipitin curve (fig. A.1). If the presence of the unused reactant in the supernatant is correlated with the precipitate formed, three distinct zones are observed.

❑ The initial antibody excess zone in the ascending limb of the precipitin curve,
❑ a zone of equivalence at the plateau (when neither excess antigen nor antibody is left in the supernatant; the concentrations of reactants that yield maximum precipitate are termed 'equivalent concentrations'), and
❑ a zone of antigen excess in the descending limb of the curve.

The Lattice hypothesis explains the nature of the precipitin curve. It assumes that precipitation is a consequence of growth of aggregates wherein each antigen/antibody molecule is linked to other molecules through multiple linkages. As the aggregate size reaches a critical volume the complex becomes too large to remain suspended, and precipitates spontaneously. Such large linear aggregates are formed in the zone of equivalence (fig. A.1). By contrast, small complexes that fail to precipitate are formed in the antigen or antibody excess zones. *In vivo* formation of such small antigen-antibody aggregates (termed immune complexes) may cause significant pathology (chapters 14 and 15). With the advent of accurate and easy techniques such as RIA and ELISA, precipitin reaction based assays are more of historical interest than practical use and are summarized in Table A.1.

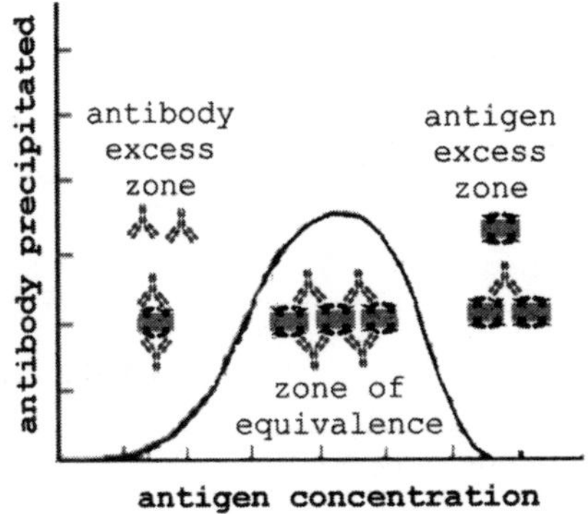

Figure A.1 *The precipitin curve*

Table A.1 Precipitin tests

Test	Application	Comments
Interfacial ring test	Antigen identification	• The antigen and antibody are allowed to react in a capillary tube • A ring of precipitate is formed at the zone of equivalence
Precipitation in gels	Determination of homogeneity and identity of the reactants	• The reactants are added to wells bored in gel • A band of precipitate is formed at the zone of equivalence • The position of the bands is dependent upon rate of diffusion and concentrations of the reactants
Immunoelectrophoresis	Identification of antigen components	• Components of a complex antigen are separated electrophoretically • Precipitin bands formed upon antiserum addition give information about the different components
Flocculation tests	Diagnosis of syphilis	• A colloidal suspension of an alcoholic extract of beef-heart is used as the antigen • An autoimmune reaction caused by the infection elicits an anti-cardiolipin response which is detected in the test eg, VDRL and Kahn tests

A.2 Agglutination

When a particulate antigen reacts with its homologous antibodies, the antigen is clumped or agglutinated because it gets cross-linked by antibody molecules. Agglutination tests have multiple applications.

❑ **Diagnosis.** Antibodies against the infecting organisms generally appear in the peripheral blood a week after the onset of the infection and can be demonstrated by using the agglutination reaction. It is therefore used for presumptive diagnosis of the infection. Agglutination is normally carried out in a physiological salt solution (0.8% or 0.15M NaCl, pH 7.4). Although easy to perform, the interpretation of agglutination tests are complicated by a number of factors.
  - Low or moderate titres can be observed in healthy individuals in the case of endemic or widely prevalent infections (eg, cholera or typhoid/paratyphoid in parts of India),
  - Anamnestic responses can result in false positive reactions with moderate titres (section 9.3).
  - Vaccinated individuals may have a high titre of antibodies. To avoid a false positive diagnosis, two consecutive tests are performed a week apart — an active infection gives a rising titre.

- Some antibiotics are immunosuppressive; early antibiotic therapy can lead to false negative results.
- An anomalous phenomenon called the prozone phenomenon is sometimes observed in certain infections, eg, brucellosis; lower dilutions of the antiserum fail to agglutinate the antigen, but higher dilutions do. What causes the prozone, however, is not clear.

Table A.2 Diagnostic applications of agglutination

Infection (sample)	Antigen	Diagnostic titre
Typhoid (serum)	*S. typhi* H/O	1:80/1:80 active infection 1:80/<1:80 carriers, previous infection <1:80/1:80 usually infection with related organism A four-fold increase in paired sera taken 10 days apart is confirmatory
	S. typhi Vi	>10 suggestive of carrier state
Paratyphoid (serum)	*S. paratyphi A, S. paratyphi B* H/O *S. paratyphi A, S. paratyphi B* Vi	As above As above
Undulating fever (serum, milk)	*B. abortus* strain 456 O	>1:80 of diagnostic value
Typhus (serum)	*Proteus* spp OXK/OX2/OX19	1:80 diagnostic
Atypical pneumonia (serum)	Human O RBCs	>40 diagnostic High titre may also be found in other diseases
Infectious Mononucleosis (serum)	Sheep RBCs	1:10 or more; differential adsorption of antibody by bovine RBCs but not guinea pig kidney extract confirmatory

- ❑ **Serotyping.** Classification of strains on the basis of their antigenic make up is called serotyping. Identification and typing of bacteria is a major application of the agglutination reaction.
- ❑ **Haemagglutination** is used to determine blood groups (chapter 13). For typing, a drop of the patient's blood is mixed with standard high titre sera and observed for the pattern of agglutination (Table A.3). Serum or plasma of the donor is also tested to ensure the absence of antibodies to recipient erythrocytes and avoid TRALI. If a 1:10 dilution of the donor serum agglutinates recipient erythrocytes, the donor blood is deemed unsuitable for transfusion to that recipient. For anti-D antibodies the acceptable titre of donor serum is 0.5 IU/ml or lower.
- ❑ **The Coombs' test**, developed by Robin Coombs, is used for the detection of anti-Rh antibodies. Rh incompatibility (Rh⁻ mother carrying a Rh⁺ foetus) can cause Erythroblastosis foetalis, a potentially fatal complication (chapter 13). Detecting these anti-Rh antibodies is difficult. For unexplained reasons, anti-Rh antibodies do not agglutinate erythrocytes and standard agglutination tests cannot be used for their detection in maternal serum. The presence of these antibodies can also not be detected on foetal RBCs, since Rh antigens are widely spaced on the erythrocytic surface. Consequently, they cannot form the doublet of antigen-bound IgG molecules necessary for C1q activation (chapter 3). As a result, even if the foetal erythrocytes are coated with maternal anti-Rh IgG, the presence of these antibodies cannot be demonstrated by complement-mediated lysis. To circumvent these problems, Coombs suggested the use of anti-IgG antibodies. Two types of tests are used. The direct Coombs' test allows the detection of sensitized foetal erythrocytes, ie, *after* the foetus is endangered, whereas the indirect Coombs' test allows the detection of the antibodies *before* they can harm the foetus. In the direct Coombs' test, anti-IgG antibodies are added to washed foetal RBCs. Anti-IgG antibodies cross-link any maternal antibody coating the

foetal erythrocytes, causing the RBCs to agglutinate (fig. A.2a). The indirect Coombs' test is used to detect non-agglutinating anti-Rh antibodies in maternal serum. In this test, the maternal serum is incubated with Rh$^+$ RBCs. After thoroughly washing the cells, anti-IgG antibodies are added to the erythrocytes and checked for agglutination (fig. A.2b). The principle of Coombs' test is used in the diagnosis of autoimmune haemolytic anaemia.

Table A.3 ABO blood typing

Blood type	Antiserum A	Antiserum B
A	agglutination	–
B	–	agglutination
AB	agglutination	agglutination
O	–	–

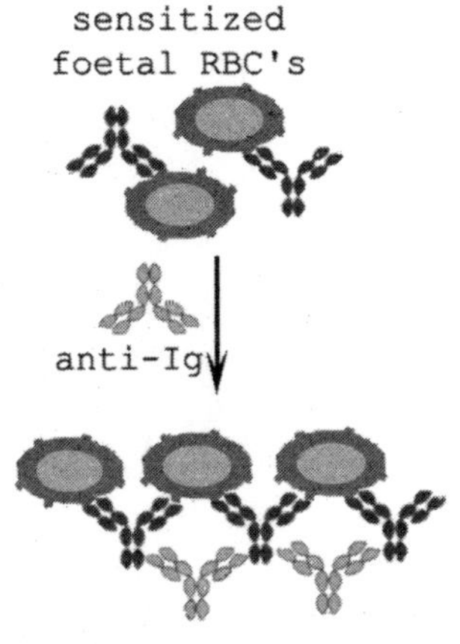

Figure A.2a *The direct Coombs' test*

❑ **Haemagglutination inhibition test** is an interesting variation of the haemagglutination test used in the diagnosis of some viral infections. Many viruses — from picorna to pox — can bind to receptors on human RBCs and agglutinate them. Antibodies to the virus inhibit this agglutination. In the test, dilutions of patient's sera are mixed with aliquots of viral suspension. The mixture is then added to washed test erythrocytes. The highest dilution of the serum that can inhibit haemagglutination is the antibody titre of the serum.

❑ **Passive agglutination**. One of the most versatile applications of the agglutination test is to passively adsorb or conjugate the antigen to latex or sepharose beads and use these in immunodiagnosis. For example, in the agglutination test for rheumatoid arthritis, IgG-coated latex beads are used to detect anti-IgG antibodies in patient's serum. Similarly, the latex pregnancy test utilizes latex beads coated with the antibodies to human choriogonadotropin. This hormone is found in the urine of pregnant women and hence agglutination of the beads confirms pregnancy.

A.3 Complement Fixation Test

Although not in common use now, this test was routinely used in the diagnosis of many viral infections (such as those caused by Enteroviruses, Myxoviruses, Varicella virus, Rubella virus, and Variola virus) and mycoplasmal infections. The complement cascade is activated when IgG or IgM antibodies react with their homologous antigens (chapter 3). The amount of complement used up in an antigen-antibody reaction is a function of the amount of the two reactants and hence activation (or 'fixation') of complement can be used as a measure of the reaction. The quantity of complement left over from the primary interaction is detected using a mixture of Sheep RBC (SRBC) and Rabbit serum containing anti-sheep RBC (aSRBC); the sensitized SRBC are lysed in the presence of complement. The test was used to diagnose any infection that elicited an IgM or IgG response. Since IgE or IgA antibodies cannot fix complement the test could not be used to demonstrate their presence.

In the test, dilutions of the patient's serum are added to aliquots of the antigen in the presence of complement. The patient's serum is decomplemented by heating to 56°C for 30 minutes and standardized guinea pig serum is used as the source of complement. The indicator system (SRBC-aSRBC) is next added to the tubes. Absence of SRBC lysis indicates the absence of free complement in the system, and implies the utilization of all the complement in the primary reaction. In contrast, SRBC lysis implies the presence of free complement in the system and indicates that the primary reaction was negative. The highest dilution of the patient's serum that fails to give a predetermined degree of lysis is its titre.

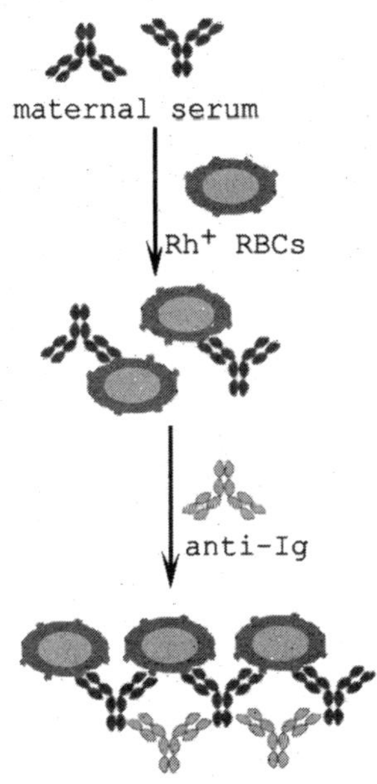

Figure A.2b *The indirect Coombs' test*

A.4 Labelled Antibody Techniques

Most of the earlier immunodiagnostic techniques described so far use polyclonal antisera raised by repeatedly injecting whole cell extracts or crude antigen preparations along with an adjuvant in animals (eg, rabbits or mice). Since the antisera contained a mixture of antibodies with different specificities and affinities, the preparations had limited applications. Most of these techniques also had low sensitivities (Table A.4).

Table A.4 Relative sensitivities of serodiagnostic assays

Assay	Sensitivity
Precipitation	1 – 20 mg/ml
Double diffusion in agar	1 – 5 mg/ml
Radial immunodiffusion	0.5 – 0.05 mg/ml
Immunoelectrophoresis	20 – 50 mg/ml
Agglutination	0.1 – 0.01 mg/ml
Complement fixation	0.5 – 1 mg/ml
Haemagglucination inhibition	0.001 – 0.005 mg/ml
RIA	picogram/ml achievable
ELISA	picogram/ml achievable

The development of mAb technology by Kohler and Milstein changed this. It allowed large scale production of antibodies with a defined specificity and increased the number of applications manifold. mAb production is now routinely done in a number of laboratories. In this technique the animal (usually a mouse) is injected with an antigen repeatedly so as to elicit a strong immune response and ensure a large population of plasma cells specific to the antigen. The animal is sacrificed and the harvested splenocytes fused with a myeloma cell line that lacks the enzyme **Hypoxanthine Guanine Phosphoribosyl Transferase** (ie, **HGPRT⁻**). Myeloma cells lacking this enzyme cannot use exogenous hypoxanthine to synthesize purines and die when placed in purine deficient medium. The fused cells are grown in a medium containing **Hypoxanthine Aminopterin Thymidine** (HAT) for a few weeks. Plasma cells, being short-lived end cells, die within a few days. Unfused myeloma cells die because they cannot utilize HAT as a source of purines. Hybridoma cells that have the unlimited capacity for growth of the myeloma cell and the capability of utilizing HAT of the plasma cell, survive. The survivors are tested for Ig secretion and Ig-secreting hybridomas are further cultured and expanded for use (fig. A.3). It is possible to obtain T cell hybridomas in a similar manner. For this, it is necessary to establish a clone of T cells from splenocytes of immunized animals. The T cell clone is fused with a malignant T cell lymphoma line. Such T cell hybridomas recognize a particular peptide loaded on a particular MHC class I, class II, or CD1 molecule.

Labelled mAbs are used as probes in detection of particular molecules in or on cells, tissues, or biological fluids. Antibodies are usually labelled at their Fc region or the C_{H1} domain of the Fab region. Two types of assays are in common use. In the direct assays, labelled antibody is allowed to react with unlabelled ligand and the residue examined after removing the excess of the labelled antibody by washing. In the indirect assays both the antigen and the antibody are unlabelled and the bound antibody is detected by the use of labelled anti-Ig antibodies. The advantage of the indirect technique is that the same labelled reagent can be used to detect a variety of antigens.

❑ **Immunofluorescence.** Use of antibodies labelled with fluorescent dyes is one of the most popular methods of detecting antigens in tissues or cells. The dyes chosen for immunofluorescence are usually excited by light of one wavelength (usually blue or green) and emit a light of a different wavelength in the visible spectrum. The use of appropriate filters allows the detection of the light emitted only from the dye. The most commonly used dyes include green light emitting fluorescein, and red light emitting phycoerythrin and Texas Red. In immunofluorescent microscopy, tagged antibodies are used in diagnosis (eg, to detect viruses or rickettsiae) or research (eg, to detect expression of molecules) in tissue sections or cells. The confocal microscope takes this one step further. It uses computer-aided techniques to produce ultrathin optical sections of a cell or tissue allowing the study of localization of molecules in different organelles of the cell without the need for elaborate sample preparation.

One major application of fluorescent labelled antibodies is in flow cytometry and FACS (**F**luorescent **A**ssisted **C**ells **S**orter) analysis. These instruments allow the study of subsets of cells in a mixed population. In flow cytometry, individual cells in the population are tagged by treating with fluorescent labelled antibodies. The tagging can be done either directly or indirectly. The mixture of labelled and unlabelled cells is mixed with a large volume of saline (called sheath fluid) and forced through a nozzle to create a fine stream of liquid containing cells spaced singly. The stream of cells passes through a laser beam. As each cell passes through the laser beam it scatters the laser light. Fluorescent antibody tagged cells fluoresce and emit a light in the visible range. A sensitive photo-multiplier tube detects the intensity and polarization of scattered light as well as the fluorescence emission. Both the forward light scatter (generally over a range of 2° to 15°) and side light scatter (at 90°) is detected separately and gives information about the size as well as granularity of the cell respectively. By contrast, the fluorescence emission gives information of the extent of binding of the tagged antibody and hence the extent of expression of molecule of interest. The data from the flow cytometer is usually displayed as histogram of fluorescence intensity versus cell numbers in case the cells are labelled with a single dye. If two dyes are used for labelling, the data is usually in the form of a scatter plot where fluorescence from one dye label is plotted against the other (fig. A.4). Each

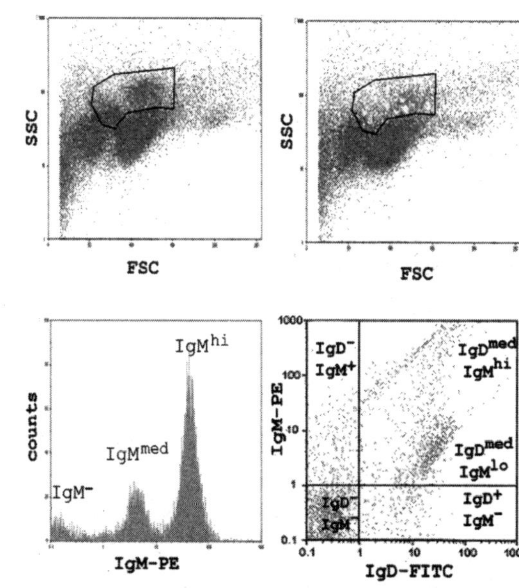

Figure A.3 *Major steps in mAb production*

Figure A.4 Flowcytometric analysis. *Each dot in the plot represents a cell. Cell types can be separated on the basis of their size and granularity by a FSC vs SSC plot. Macrophages, being larger and more granular than lymphocytes, fall in a separate region than the less granular and smaller lymphocytes (indicated by the marked region). The top panels are dot plots of splenocytes before (left panel) and after (right panel) macrophage depletion. The lower left panel is a histogram of IgM$^+$ cells in the sample. The sample contains three subsets — IgM$^-$ cells, cells expressing moderate IgM (middle peak) and those expressing high levels of IgM (right peak). The lower right panel is a dot plot of cells stained for IgM and IgD. The sample shows the presence of four distinct subsets. Cells that express neither of the molecules fall in the lower left quadrant. Cells expressing either one of the markers fall in the upper left and lower right quadrant. Cells expressing both the molecules fall in the top right quadrant. Thus, by double staining it is possible to differentiate the populations based on the extent of expression of IgM and IgD. The IgD^{med}IgM^{hi} population represents the B1 B cell compartment, whereas the IgD^{med}IgM^{lo} cells are the conventional (B2) B cells.*

dot in the plot represents a single cell and FACS analysis allows the separation and purification of sub-population of cells based on the degree of binding of the labelled antibodies. These instruments are the staple of every immunological research laboratory.

❑ **Radioimmunoassay (RIA).** This highly sensitive method was introduced by Barsson and Yallow for measuring insulin concentrations in serum. Although it has multiple applications, the most common one is the measurement of peptide hormones in blood and tissue fluids (fig. A.5). RIA is based on radioactive isotope labelling and both direct and indirect assays are in use. Iodine isotopes are most commonly employed for labelling. A variety of methods are used to separate the labelled complexes from the mixture. The most common method is to conjugate or adsorb the unlabelled antigen to a solid support — plastic tubes, cellulose beads, etc. The excess labelled ligand can therefore be easily separated from the complexes by simple washing or centrifugation. The amount of radioactivity on the solid support is a direct measure of the labelled complexes formed.

❑ **Enzyme-Linked ImmunoSorbent Assay (ELISA):** Since its introduction by Engvall and Perlmann in 1971, the ELISA test has become the most widely used of all immunological tests. It is a quick, sensitive, and specific assay that allows the detection/quantification of antigens (or antibodies) in the picogram range even in the presence of a large quantity of background proteins (fig. A.5). One of the reactants (usually the antigen) is adsorbed to a solid support. PVC (**polyvinylc**hloride) or polystyrene trays (microtitre plates) are most commonly used, although beads or tubes can also be employed. Direct ELISAs are very simple to perform but may be limited in their sensitivity. Sandwich ELISAs (indirect ELISA) are much more sensitive. A high affinity antigen-specific antibody (called the catching antibody) is adsorbed to the solid support. The solid-bound antibodies bind any antigen present in the solution and concentrate it on the surface of the plate. This technique thus allows antigen detection even when it is present at very low concentrations, eg, cytokines or hormones in secretions. A secondary antibody that recognizes a separate epitope on the antigen is linked to an enzyme and used as the detecting reagent. The two most commonly used enzymes are Alkaline Phosphatase and Horseradish Peroxidase. The amount of the soluble coloured product formed is a direct readout of the amount of antigen present.

❑ **Immunohistochemistry.** This technique is essentially similar to ELISA in that it too utilizes enzyme-linked Ig antibodies. The difference is that the reaction occurs in tissues instead of plates, and the localized deposition of the insoluble coloured product is observed under a light microscope. Since the antibodies usually recognize only the native structure of the proteins, tissue

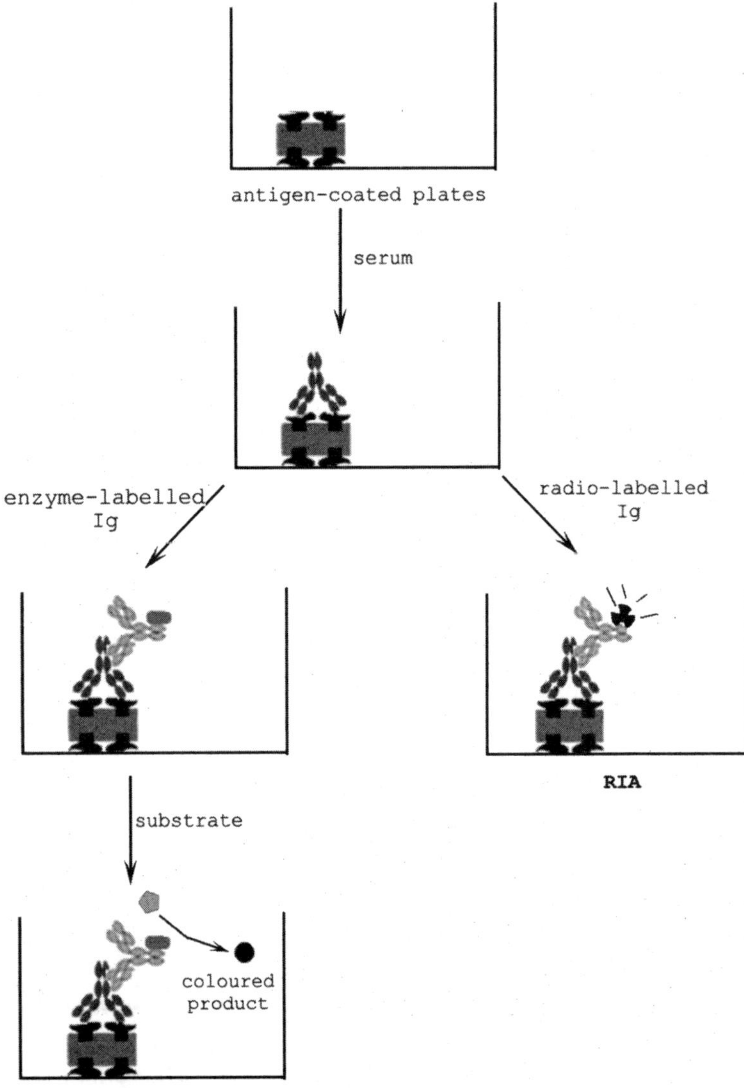

Figure A.5 *Schematic representation of Direct ELISA and RIA*

fixation techniques need to be very gentle. Alternatively, the reaction is allowed to be completed on frozen tissues before fixing it.

☐ **Use of magnetic beads.** Antibodies to cell surface molecules coupled to paramagnetic beads can be used for quick and easy separation of cells. In this technique cells are mixed with the antibody-coated paramagnetic beads and run through columns containing materials that attract these beads when placed in a strong magnetic field. Cells coated with antibody coupled paramagnetic beads are retained on the column (ie, are positively selected), whereas those not expressing the particular molecule run through (ie, are negatively selected).

☐ **Immunoblotting and Immunoprecipitation.** Immunoblotting allows the detection of one protein in a complex mixture. It also gives information about the molecular size and quantity of the protein. In the most common techniques of separation called SDS-PAGE and Western blot[2], the cells are lysed with non-ionic detergents such as Triton X-100 or NP40 that disrupt the cell membranes but do not interfere with antigen-antibody interactions. The proteins are dissolved in a strong ionic detergent **S**odium **D**odecyl **S**ulphate (SDS). SDS binds to the proteins relatively homogenously and confers a charge that allows their electrophoretic separation. The proteins are loaded on a **p**oly**a**crylamine **ge**l (PAGE) and subjected to an electrical field. The SDS-bound proteins migrate at different rates depending upon their molecular size. The separated protein bands are driven (blotted) into a nitrocellulose membrane by the application of a second electrical field. For unknown reasons, the proteins stick to nitrocellulose and retain their relative positions even when flooded with fluids in the following steps. The blot is then developed using enzyme-linked antibody preparations. The antibodies bind specifically to the protein of interest and upon addition of a colourless substrate yield specific bands of coloured product (fig. A.6).

In immunoprecipitation antibodies linked to solid support such as agarose or sepharose beads are used to isolate a radiolabelled protein from a complex mixture. Protein labelling can be done by two principal methods. All the proteins in a cell can be labelled by growing the cells in medium containing radioactive amino acids. Alternatively, only surface (membrane) proteins can be labelled by radioiodination by a method that does not allow the radioactive iodine to cross the cell membrane. The cells are then lysed and the proteins separated by SDS-PAGE. The size and concentration of the protein can be determined by exposing the gel to an X-ray film. Apart from basic research (eg, to assess the intracellular concentration and distribution of a protein, or to determine whether it undergoes changes in MW as a result of intracellular processing), Western blotting and immunoprecipitation are frequently used to test sera for the presence of antibodies to specific proteins.

B. Cell-based Immunoassays

In order to be able to perform cell-based assays, it is necessary to be able to separate lymphocytes from other cells. Human lymphocytes can be easily isolated from peripheral blood by density gradient centrifugation. Usually a mixture of the carbohydrate polymer Ficoll with a dense compound such as metrizamide or sodium diatrizoate (called Ficoll Hypaque™ or Ficoll-Histopaque™ respectively) is used. Usually 1:1 diluted blood is layered on the gradient. The heavier erythrocytes and granulocytes sediment at the bottom, while a mixture of monocytes and lymphocytes (PBMCs or **P**eripheral **B**lood **M**ononuclear **C**ells) band at the gradient:plasma interface. Unwanted populations of cells can be removed from the mixture by complement-mediated lysis. Alternatively, a population of cells can be positively isolated by the use of antibody-linked magnetic beads (section A.4) or antibodies bound to solid surfaces (panning). Cells can also be differentially eluted from columns containing antibody-coated nylon wool. A 95–99% pure population can be obtained

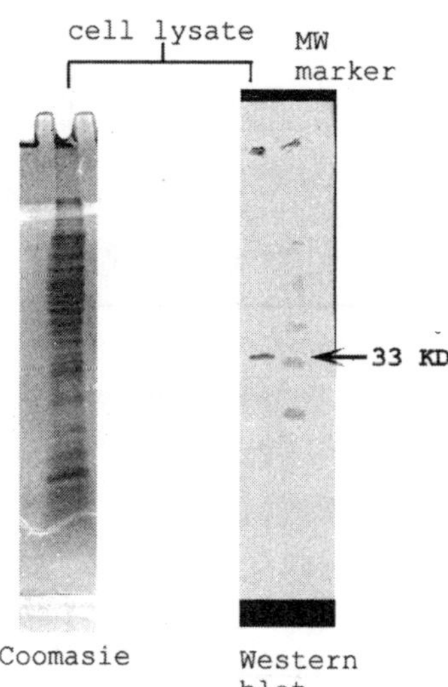

Figure A.6 Western blot. *Western blot allows the detection and quantitation of a protein of interest in the presence of a large number of other proteins. The left panel is Coomasie staining of a reducing SDS-PAGE gel loaded with whole cell lysate of a fibroblast line transfected with HLA-DR4 (human MHC class II molecule). The right panel is a Western blot of a parallel gel which was probed by an anti-HLA-DR4α antibody. Molecular weight markers are normally loaded on the gel to aid in identification of the protein (Courtesy of A.B. Mannan, TIFR, Mumbai, India).*

[2] A comparable technique to detect specific DNA sequences was developed by E.M. Southern and is called the 'Southern blot'. This gave rise to the terms 'Northern blot' for size separation of RNA and 'Western blot' for proteins and proves that scientists do have a sense of humour ☺.

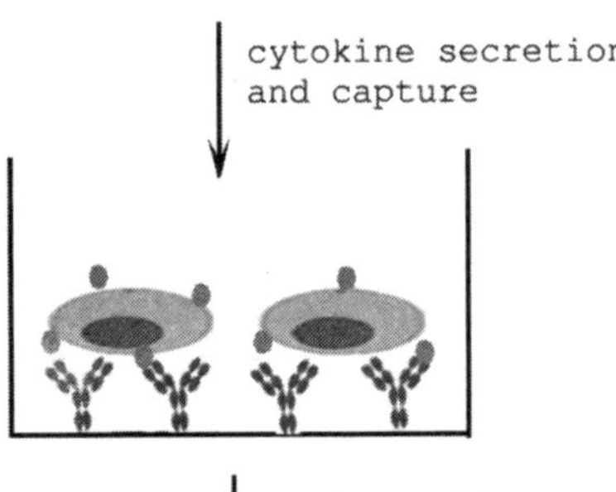

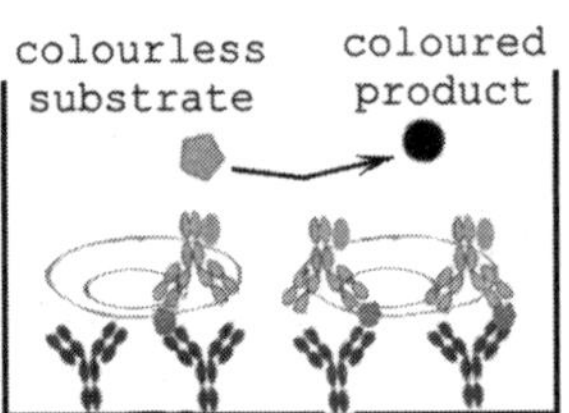

Figure A.7 *Schematic representation of a cytokine ELISPOT assay*

using FACS or magnetic bead cell separation. The isolated populations can then be used to obtain stable cell lines (or clones) for laboratory use.

❑ **ELISPOT**. A modification of ELISA, this technique allows the measuring of frequency of cells secreting a particular cytokine or Ig antibody. In the case of cytokine ELISPOT, T cells stimulated with a mitogen are allowed to settle on a plate coated with anti-cytokine antibody. Any cytokine secreted by a T cell is captured by antibodies in the neighbourhood of that cell. The cells are eventually removed and a second anti-cytokine antibody linked to an enzyme is added to the plate. On addition of substrate, the presence of the cytokine-secreting T cell is revealed by a spot of coloured product (hence the name; fig. A.7). Knowing the number of T cells originally added to the plate, the frequency of T cells secreting that particular cytokine can be easily calculated. The frequency of B cells secreting a particular isotype can similarly be determined by using anti-isotype antibodies. To determine the frequency of antigen-specific B cells, the plate is coated with the antigen and the assay developed using enzyme-linked anti-Ig antibodies.

❑ **Mixed Lymphocyte (or leukocyte) Reaction (MLR).** This technique is used to determine histocompatibility. PBMCs are isolated from the peripheral blood of the individuals who are to be tested for histocompatibility. PBMCs of one of the individual (donor) are either irradiated or treated with Mitomycin C. This ensures that the donor cells will not proliferate, but will be able to present antigen. The donor cells are mixed with PBMCs from the other individual (recipient) and incubated for 5–7 days. The culture is assessed for either T cell proliferation (usually by ^{3}H thymidine incorporation) or CTL response (by ^{51}Cr release). If the two individuals are incompatible, recipient CD4$^+$ T cells will proliferate in response to the irradiated donor MHC class II alleles. By contrast, CD8$^+$ T cells will proliferate and differentiate to effector CTLs in response to MHC class I alleles. These effector CD8$^+$ T cells cause the lysis of ^{51}Cr labelled target cells added to the culture (see below).

❑ **Polyclonal activation assay.** Lymphocytes, whether B or T, proliferate rapidly in response to polyclonal mitogens. These mitogens induce lymphocyte proliferation independent of their antigenic specificity and may be used to test the proliferative ability of human (or animal) lymphocytes, ie, to determine if the individual is immunodeficient or immunosuppressed. Thus, phytohaem-agglutinin obtained from red kidney beans or concanalvin A obtained from Jack beans induce T cell proliferation, whereas LPS is a B cell mitogen. The extent of proliferation is measured by ^{3}H thymidine incorporation into the DNA.

❑ **Assays for CTLs.** Effector CD8$^+$ cytotoxic T cells kill any cells expressing MHC class I:peptide complexes they recognize. CTL assays are therefore designed to determine the lysis of the target cell and use the propensity of live cells to take up, but not spontaneously release, Na$_2$CrO$_3$. The chromate taken up by the cells is released only upon cell death. In the assay, antigen is incubated with autologous (ie, expressing the same haplotype of MHC class I molecules) target cells to allow MHC class I loading. The cells are labelled with radioactive Na$_2$^{51}CrO$_3$ and incubated with CD8$^+$ T cells. The amount of radioactive chromate released in the supernatant is measured (fig. A.8).

❑ **CD4$^+$ T cell assays**. Upon recognition of specific MHC class II:peptide complexes, CD4$^+$ T cells proliferate rapidly and release cytokines such as IL-2 or IFN-γ. Hence the amount of cytokines released can be used to measure the extent of CD4$^+$ T cells activation. In the assay, APCs are incubated with the antigen to allow MHC class II loading. Excess antigen is washed off and the APCs are incubated with autologous CD4$^+$ T cells. The amount of cytokines released in the assay can be determined by ELISAs. Alternatively, a bioassay using an cytokine-dependent cell line can also be used. The supernatant obtained from the CD4⁺ T cell assay is added to the cytokine-dependent cells in a 96 well plate. ^{3}H thymidine is added to wells following incubation. The rapidly proliferating cells incorporate the radioactive thymidine in their DNA. The plate is harvested on glass filter mat and the extent of radioactivity measured with a scintillation counter (fig. A.8).

C. Use of Animal Models

Animal models are required to understand a disease process in its entirety. Samples of tissues taken from the diseased patients (whether human or animal) are not enough to understand the disease process, since tissues and cells are influenced by their environment, and isolated tissues may behave quite differently than when present in the animal. Animal models also allow the testing of new drug candidates and designing novel therapies before undertaking clinical trials involving patients. This is not to say that alternatives do not exist. In fact the law requires that alternatives (mathematical or computer models, tissue culture, etc) be used first before using animal models. Virtually all of our medical advances over the last century have been made using animals. The development of transgenic and KO mice technology has furthered the understanding of a variety of diseases. Examples of the use of transgenic and KO mice include:

❑ Analysis and functioning of genes involved in receptor signalling (eg, T cell receptor signalling).
❑ Understanding cellular development and migration. This is achieved by the introduction of cell markers, such as bacterial β-galactosidase or various versions of the jelly-fish green fluorescent protein (GFP) under the control of ubiquitous or highly specific promoter elements.
❑ Insights in tumour development can be obtained by introducing specific oncogenes under the control of tissue-specific promotors.
❑ The use of KO technology. It is possible to knockout virtually any gene (from cytokines to MHC molecules to RAG genes, you name them we can eliminate them) allowing the study of the importance of those genes in various immune processes.

To obtain transgenic mice, genes responsible for particular traits or disease susceptibility are chosen, extracted, and injected into fertilized mouse eggs. The embryos are harvested and implanted in the uterus of a surrogate mother. Less than one-third of the embryos will develop in healthy pups. DNA from the pups is tested to ensure the presence of a transgene. Even if they have the transgene, the pups will be heterozygous for the gene. They are then mated to obtain the 1:4 pups that will be homozygous for the transgene.

KO mice are obtained by the targeted gene disruption of specific genes by homologous recombination (also called gene targeting). In this technique one gene sequence resident in the mouse genome is replaced by another related, but mutated, sequence. The replacement occurs by homologous recombination. Gene targeting is carried out in mouse embryonic stem cells (ES cells). These cells are derived from a very early (usually male) mouse embryo and can therefore differentiate into all types

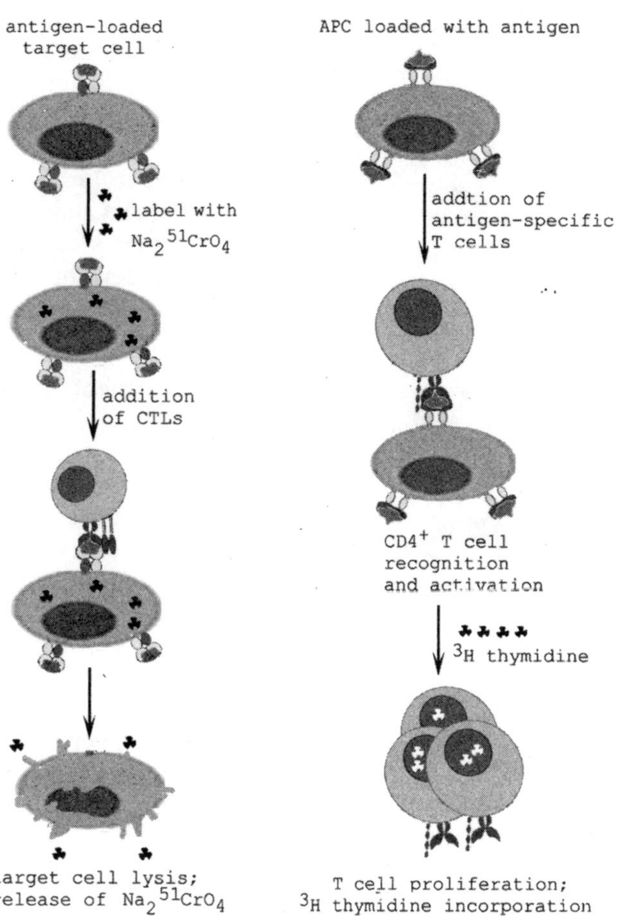

Figure A.8 Schematic representation of CTL assay (left panel) and CD4⁺ T cell assay (right panel).

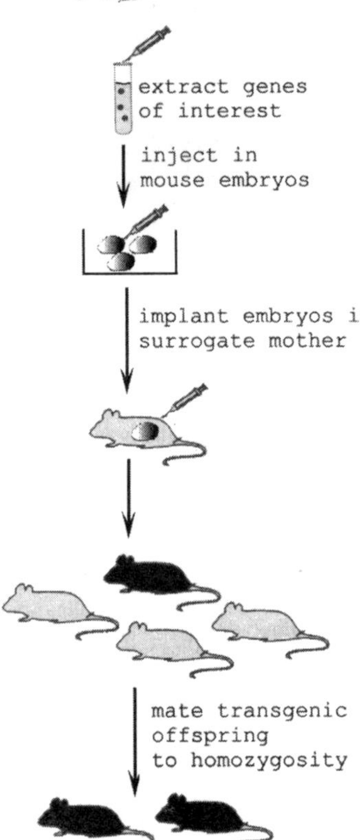

Figure A.9 Major steps in the production of trangenic animals

of cells when introduced into another embryo. The aim is to get the modified ES cells to contribute to the germ line, which gives rise to sperm. Some of the sperms produced will carry the desired mutation and when they fertilize a normal egg the resultant progeny will be heterozygous for that gene, ie, every cell in that mouse will possess one copy of the mutated gene. The mice are mated to obtain homozygous KO mice. In traditional constitutive knockout mice the mutation is present throughout development and in all cells of the adult. Conversely, in conditional knockout mice, other genetic strategies are incorporated that allow mutations to be induced at different stages of development or in selected cell types. Examples of KO mice include the SCID and lpr mice described in chapter 14.

D. Assessment of Immunity

The immune status of an individual can be determined by various means. The simplest is the testing of serum for the presence of specific antibodies by agglutination, ELISA, RIA etc. In the case of autoimmune diseases, patient's serum is allowed to react with tissue sections and the bound antibody examined by immunofluorescence using labelled anti-human Ig antibodies. The presence of activated T cells can be judged by CTL assays or $CD4^+$ T cell assays. Testing serum or cells is sometimes not enough and some test need to be performed directly on the patient. These tests involve injections of minute quantities of the antigen in the patient. The antigen remains localized at the site of injection and elicits a local response, without causing a systemic reaction. Nevertheless there is always the risk of a systemic reaction and the tests need to be used with caution.

❑ **The tuberculin test** or Montoux test is a skin prick test that provides information about previous exposure to the tubercle bacillus. It tests for a DTH response (chapter 15) to a **P**urified **P**rotein **D**erivative (PPD; hence also called the PPD test) obtained from *M. tuberculosis*. A small amount of PPD is injected in the forearm of the individual and the area observed for upto 72 hours. An area of induration and reddening of 10 mm or greater is considered significant. The test is likely to be positive for people living in countries of high incidence of the disease and does not warrant any treatment unless the individual presents with weight loss, low grade fever, persistent coughs, etc.

❑ **The skin test for allergic responses** is used to detect the substance causing an immediate type of hypersensitivity reaction in the patient. A local intracutaneous injection of minute dose of the antigen is given by pricking thc skin with a small test needle through a minute drop of fluid containing the suspected allergen. The test is usually carried out on the forearm. A negative control consists of a drop of saline. A positive test may develop within minutes and consists of a wheal and flare reaction.

Glossary

ABO blood groups – Antigens expressed on red blood cells that are used for typing human blood for transfusion. Individuals who do not express A or B antigens on their erythrocytes can form against them.

Accessory cells – Cells that aid in the immune response but do not directly mediate specific responses. These cells are often involved in antigen presentation to T cells.

Acute lymphoblastic leukaemia – A highly aggressive, undifferentiated form of lymphoid malignancy.

Acute phase proteins – Serum proteins that rapidly increase in concentration following an infection. They are a part of the first line of host defence.

Adaptive (or Acquired) immune response – An immune response generated by antigen-mediated activation of antigen-specific lymphocytes and characterized by the development of immunological memory.

Adaptor proteins – Small proteins that act as linkers between cell surface receptors and downstream members of signalling pathways. All adaptor proteins have a SH2 domain with which they interact with the phosphotyrosine residues generated by receptor-associated tyrosine kinases.

ADCC (Antibody-Dependent Cell-mediated Cytotoxicity) – A cytotoxic reaction mediated by effector cells bearing receptors for the Fc region of IgG antibodies. The antibody links the two cells by binding to epitopes on the target cell via its Fab region and being bound to the effector cell by its Fc region.

Adhesion molecules – Molecules that mediate binding of one cell to another cell or to extracellular matrix proteins. Examples include selectins, integrins, and ICAMs.

Adjuvant – A substance that can non-specifically enhance the immune response to an antigen when administered along with it.

Adoptive immunity – Immunity conferred by transfer of lymphoid cells from an actively immunized donor to a naïve recipient.

Affinity – The measure of the binding strength between an antigenic determinant and antibody-binding site of the Ig molecule.

Affinity maturation – The increase in average affinity (or avidity) of antigen-specific antibodies with respect to time that is observed in an immune response to TD antigens. Affinity maturation is the result of mutations in the rearranged V region genes of the antibodies.

Agglutination – Cross-linking of particulate antigen by antibodies that leads to the separation of the complex (called the agglutinate) from the suspending liquid. Agglutination of RBCs is referred to as haemaglutination.

Agonist peptide – Peptide antigens that activate their specific T cells inducing them to synthesize cytokines and to proliferate.

AICD (Activation-Induced Cell Death) – A phenomenon wherein antigen-activated lymphocytes upregulate the expression of apoptosis-inducing proteins such as Fas or FasL and die unless they receive specific survival signals.

AID (Activation-Induced Deaminase) – A B cell specific enzyme essential for the twin processes of somatic hypermutation and class switch recombination. It increases the diversity of the antibody repertoire by introducing mutations in the rearranged V region genes.

AIDS (Acquired Immune Deficiency Syndrome) – A disease caused by infection with the human immunodeficiency virus (HIV-1 or -2). Although the patient may harbour the virus for years, full blown AIDS occurs only after the loss of most of the CD4$^+$ T cells.

AIRE (Autoimmune Regulator) – A gene that regulates autoimmunity by promoting the expression of tissue-specific genes in the thymus.

Allele – Intraspecies variation observed in a particular gene locus.

Allelic exclusion – Heterozygous individuals express only one allele of the C region of TcR or BcR in spite of the presence of the alternative allele. This is called allelic exclusion.

Allergens – Substances that elicit hypersensitivity type I (or allergic) responses.

Allergy – An exaggerated or inappropriate immune response to innocuous environmental substances that causes tissue damage. Most common forms of allergies such as allergic rhinitis, hay fever, or allergic asthma are caused by the degranulation of mast cells as a result of allergen-mediated cross-linking of FcεRI-bound IgE antibodies.

Alloantigens – Polymorphisms at the MHC locus that stimulate intense reactions to allografted tissues. Individuals who differ in their alloantigens are allogeneic.

Allograft – A graft of tissue from an allogeneic or non-self donor of the same species; allografts are invariably rejected unless the recipient is immunosuppressed.

Alloreactive T cells – T cells that can respond to non-self MHC molecules.

Allotype – The protein product of an allele which may be recognized as an antigen by another individual of the same species.

Altered peptide ligand – A peptide that, when loaded on the appropriate MHC molecule, induces only a partial response from T cells specific for the agonist peptide. It is usually closely related to the agonist peptide in amino acid sequence.

Alternative pathway – One of the pathways of complement activation that is triggered by the binding of complement protein C3b to the surface of a pathogen. Being independent of Ig molecules, it is a feature of innate immunity.

Anamnestic immune responses – See Secondary immune responses.

Anaphylactic shock or systemic anaphylaxis – An allergic reaction to systemically administered antigen that causes circulatory collapse and suffocation because of tracheal swelling. It is the result of degranulation of connective tissue mast cells throughout the body, resulting in the disseminated release of inflammatory mediators. It is caused by the binding of antigen to FcεRI-bound IgE antibodies on mast cells.

Anaphylatoxins – By-products of the complement cascade (C3a and C5a) that cause mast cell degranulation and smooth muscle constriction.

Anaphylaxis – Classical anaphylaxis is an IgE-mediated response resulting in degranulation of mast cells, vasodilation, smooth muscle constriction, etc.

Anergy – A state of unresponsiveness to antigen.

Angiogenesis – New blood vessel formation.

Antagonist peptides – Variants of agonist peptides that deliver a negative signal to specific T cells and inhibit responses to the agonist peptides.

Antibody – A glycoprotein produced by the B lymphocytes in response to an antigen that can specifically and reversibly combine with the molecule that induced its formation. Also see immunoglobulin molecules.

Antibody-Dependent Cell-mediated Cytotoxicity - See ADCC

Antigen – A substance (molecule) capable of stimulating the immune system of an animal and reacting with the product of such stimulation.

Antigen processing – The degradation of proteins or (glyco)lipids to fragments that can be loaded on MHC (like) molecules for presentation to T cells.

Antigenic determinants (epitopes) – The part of the antigen molecule that is recognized by the antibody. Also see Epitope.

Antigen-presentation – The display of antigen fragments loaded on MHC (like) molecules at the cell surface for recognition by T cells.

Anti-Ig antibodies – Antibodies produced against the constant domains of immunoglobulins from a different species.

Antiserum – Serum from an immune individual that contains antibodies against the molecule used for immunization.

APCs (Antigen-Presenting Cells) – Cells that internalize and process antigen, load the antigen-derived fragments on MHC (like) molecules and present them to T cells. Professional APCs trigger an immune response by presenting antigen and delivering costimulatory signals to the T cells (eg, DCs, macrophages, eosinophils and B cells). Non-professional APCs present antigen in the absence of costimulatory signals causing T cell anergy.

Apoptosis – Programmed cell death brought about by the activation of an internal death program. It is characterized by nuclear DNA degradation, nuclear degeneration, and condensation.

Artemis – A protein related to DNA repair enzyme DNA-PKcs, Artemis is thought to be involved in opening of RAG-generated DNA hairpins in the process of $V(D)J$ recombination.

Asthma – A respiratory disorder, usually of allergic origin, characterized by wheezing caused by the constriction of the bronchial tree.

Atopy – The propensity to produce IgE antibodies and develop type I hypersensitivity reactions to innocuous environmental antigens.

Autoantibody – Antibodies specific for self-antigens.

Autografts – Transfer of self-tissues from one site to another.

Autoimmune diseases – Diseases caused by an adaptive immune response to self-antigens.

Autologous – Part of the same individual.

Avidity – The strength with which a multivalent antibody binds to a multivalent antigen.

Azathioprine – A potent immunosuppressive drug that is converted to its active form *in vivo*, which then kills rapidly proliferating cells.

B cell antigen receptor (BcR) – A complex consisting of a membrane immunoglobulin molecule along with associated molecules such as Ig-α-Ig-β heterodimers and the CD19-CD21-CD81complex. The immunoglobulin molecule confers antigen specificity; Ig-α–Ig-β chains are the signalling subunits.

B lymphocyte – A type of lymphocyte that expresses surface immunoglobulin molecules and matures in the bone marrow in mammals. It is the only cell that can produce immunoglobulins.

B1 B cells – A subset of B cells that generally (but not necessarily) express the CD5 molecule. These cells can be activated to proliferate and differentiate independent of T cell help. About 5% of the total B cells are of the B1 type.

B2 B cells – The majority of B cells of the body. These cells do not express CD5, require T cell help for proliferation and differentiation, and can undergo affinity maturation.

BAFF (B cell Activating Factor of the TNF Family) – A pro-survival factor secreted by macrophages and DCs that promotes survival of B cells.

BALT – Bronchus-associated lymphoid tissue.

Bare lymphocyte syndrome – An immunodeficiency disease in which MHC class II molecules are not expressed on cells as a result of one of several different regulatory gene defects.

Basophils – White blood cells containing granules that stain with basic dyes. They are thought to have a function similar to mast cells.

BCG (Bacille of Calmette and Guerin) – An attenuated strain of *Mycobacterium tuberculosis* used in vaccines. It is also used as an adjuvant in animal experiments.

Bcl-2 family of proteins – A group of proteins with pro- and anti-apoptotic functions. Members of this family of proteins affect apoptosis by decreasing (anti-apoptotic) or increasing (pro-apoptotic) mitochondrial permeability.

Bence-Jones Proteins – Free immunoglobulin light chain dimers found in the serum and urine of patients with multiple myelomas.

BLNK (B cell Linker Protein) – An adaptor protein that recruits signalling molecules to lipid rafts.

Blood group antigens – Surface molecules on red blood cells that are detectable with antibodies from other individuals. Antigens routinely tested in blood transfusions are the ABO and Rh antigens.

Blood typing – Determination of blood group (usually ABO and Rh) compatibility of the donor and the recipient.

Bone marrow – The site of haematopoiesis, the source of B and T cell progenitors, and the site of B cell development and antibody generation in mammals.

Bradykinin – A vasoactive peptide that is produced as a result of tissue damage and acts as an inflammatory mediator.

Bruton's X-linked agammaglobulinaemia – See X-linked agammaglobulinaemia.

Btk – Bruton's tyrosine kinase, an enzyme indispensable for B cell receptor signalling.

Bursa of Fabricus – Found at the junction of the hind gut and cloacae, it is a primary lymphoepithelial organ of birds that is the site of B cell maturation.

C regions (Constant regions) – Part of the immunological receptors (B and T cell antigen receptors) that are distal from the ligand binding site and show minimal variability in amino acid sequences amongst different types of immunoglobulins or T cell antigen receptors.

C3a/C5a – See Anaphylatoxins.

C3b – A breakdown product of the complement component C3, C3b is the principal effector molecule of the complement system.

Calnexin – Found in the endoplasmic reticulum, this chaperone protein binds to partly folded members of the immunoglobulin superfamily of proteins and retains them in the endoplasmic reticulum until folding is completed.

CALT – Cutaneous-associated lymphoid tissue.

CAMs (Cell-Adhesion Molecules) – Cell surface proteins involved in binding cells together in tissues as well as in less permanent cell-cell interactions.

Carcinogenesis – The process by which a malignant tumour is formed. Tumour formation requires the accumulation of multiple mutations that allow the growing mass of cells to resist apoptotic signals and survive, proliferate, and eventually invade other tissues.

Carcinoma – A malignant tumour arising from ectodermal or endodermal tissues such as the skin or epithelial lining of internal organs or glands. More than 80% of all tumours are carcinomas.

Carrier – An immunogenic molecule to which other non-immunogenic antigens or haptens can be conjugated to render them immunogenic. The carrier elicits a T cell response, whereas the hapten elicits an antibody response.

Caspases – A family of closely related cysteine proteases that cleave proteins at aspartic acid residues that are important in apoptosis.

Cathelicidins – Anti microbial peptides that are a part of the innate immune system.

CD (Cluster of Differentiation) – A prefix used to identify various markers on cells of the immune system. These are groups of monoclonal antibodies that identify the same cell surface molecule. See Appendix I for a list of some common CDs.

CD3 complex – A multi-component constituent of the T cell antigen receptor that is responsible for signal transduction. It is composed of five chains – γ, δ, ϵ, η, and ζ.

CD4 – A coreceptor expressed on a subset of T cells, CD4 binds the lateral face of the MHC class II molecules. See Appendix I.

CD8 – A coreceptor expressed on a subset of T cells, CD8 binds the lateral face of the MHC class I molecules. See Appendix I.

CDRs (Complementarity Determining Regions, hypervariable regions) – Short segments of about 10 amino acid residues found within variable region of immunological antigen receptors (or free immunoglobulins) that are in contact with the epitope. CDRs are the most variable part of the receptors and determine its specificity.

Cell-mediated immunity – See CMI.

Centroblasts – Large, rapidly dividing cells that arise from antigen-activated B cells in germinal centres.

Centrocytes – Small B cells that arise from centroblasts in germinal centres.

Chemokines – A family of structurally homologous, chemoattractant cytokines that stimulate the migration and activation of cells, especially phagocytic cells and lymphocytes.

Chemotaxis – Increased directional migration of cells in response to concentration gradients of chemotactic substances.

Chimera – An organism consisting of two or more tissues of different genetic composition produced as a result of organ transplant, grafting, or genetic engineering. A chimeric protein is produced by splicing together genetic sequences of two different proteins.

c-Kit (CD117) – See Appendix I.

Class switching (Class Switch Recombination) – See isotype switching.

CLIP (Class II-associated Invariant chain Peptide) – A fragment of invariant chain that remains in the peptide-binding groove of the class II molecule, stabilizes it, and protects premature loading.

Clonal deletion – The elimination of immature lymphocytes that bind self-antigens in the primary lymphoid organs.

Clonal selection theory – A central paradigm of adaptive immunity, the theory states that adaptive immune responses derive from individual, self-tolerant antigen-specific lymphocytes. The specific lymphocytes proliferate in response to antigen and differentiate into antigen-specific effector cells and memory cells.

Clone – Progeny of a single cell that are genetically identical to the parent cell. Clonotypic features are features unique to individual cells or members of a clone.

Cluster of Differentiation – See CD.

CMI (Cell-Mediated Immunity) – Adaptive immunity conferred by presence of cells, and not antibodies.

Coding joint – The joint formed by the imprecise joining of a V gene segment to a D or J gene segment in immunoglobulin or T cell receptor genes.

Codominant alleles – Alleles at one locus that are expressed in roughly equal amounts in heterozygotes.

Cold Agglutinins – Antibodies that agglutinate at temperatures below 37°C.

Collectins – A family of calcium dependent sugar-binding proteins (C-type lectins), containing collagen-like sequences that are important in innate immunity, eg, mannose binding protein.

Combinatorial diversity – Diversity generated by combining separate units of genetic information.

Common lymphoid progenitors – Stem cells that give rise to all lymphocytes. They are derived from pleuripotent haematopoietic stem cells.

Complement – Heat labile serum component consisting of a highly complex group of serum proteins that can attack and bring about the lysis of a variety of pathogens. Complement can be activated by three different pathways – classical, alternative, and MBL.

Complement receptors – Cell surface proteins present on various cells that specifically recognize and bind products of the complement cascade such as C1q, C3a, C3b, C4a, and C5a.

Complementarity Determining Regions – See CDR.

Conformational (discontinuous) epitopes – Epitopes formed from several separate regions in the primary sequence of a protein that are brought together by protein folding.

Constant regions – See C regions.

Contact hypersensitivity – Manifestation of hypersensitivity type IV (delayed-type of hypersensitivity) caused by sensitized T cells responding to antigens that are introduced by contact with the skin.

Continuous (linear) epitopes – Antigenic determinants on proteins that are contiguous in the amino acid sequence.

Coomb's test – A test for antibody binding to red blood cells. See Appendix III.

Coreceptor – A cell surface protein that increases the sensitivity of the binding of the antigen to its receptor, by binding to associated ligands. Eg, CD4/CD8 expressed on T cells and CD19 on B cells.

Corticosteroids – A family of drugs related to steroids that are naturally produced in the adrenal cortex, such as cortisone.

Costimulatory molecules – Molecules expressed on the surface of antigen-presenting cells that bind ligands on T or B cells. Engagement of costimulatory molecules in conjunction with antigen recognition results in activation of the lymphocytes.

CpG nucleotides – Unmethylated cytidine-guanine sequences found in bacterial DNA that have adjuvant effect in mammalian immune systems.

C-reactive protein – An acute phase protein that binds to the phosphatidylcholine moiety of the cell wall polysaccharide of *Streptococcus pneumoniae*.

Cross-matching – A test done in blood typing and histocompatibility testing to ascertain that both the donor and recipient do not have antibodies against each other's cellular antigens.

Cross-presentation – Processing and presentation of exogenous antigens by the MHC class I pathway.

Cross-priming – Activation of cytotoxic T cells by exogenous antigens.

Cross-reactivity – Binding of an antibody to an antigen not used to elicit it.

CTL – See cytotoxic T lymphocytes.

CTLA-4 – CD152; See Appendix I.

Cyclophosphamide – An immunosuppressive drug. It is an alkylating agent that kills all rapidly dividing cells.

Cyclosporin A – Immunosuppressive drug that interferes with T cell antigen receptor signalling. It prevents T cell activation and effector functions.

Cytokines – Small glycoproteins secreted by cells that can affect the activity of other cells. Cytokines exert their effect through specific receptors present on target cells. Cytokines have varied roles in immune responses – they can be pro- or anti-inflammatory, and boost or suppress an immune response. They are the principal mediators of communication between cells of the immune system.

Cytotoxic granules – Lytic vesicles containing perforin and granzymes. They are a defining characteristic of cytotoxic lymphocytes.

Cytotoxic T Lymphocytes (CTLs) – Generally CD8$^+$ MHC class I restricted T cells that can kill infected or transformed host cells.

Cytotoxins – Proteins such as Perforin and Granzymes produced by cytotoxic lymphocytes that cause the destruction of target cells.

***D* (Diversity) gene segments** – Short DNA segments that join *V* and *J* gene segments in the rearranged immunoglobulin heavy chains and T cell receptor β and δ chains.

Death by neglect – A mode of apoptosis induction in lymphocytes, caused by the failure to obtain the necessary survival signals such as growth factors or costimulatory signals. Thymocytes that fail to bind self-MHC molecules undergo death by neglect.

Decay-Accelerating Factor (DAF) – CD55. See Appendix I.

Defensins – Cysteine-rich, cationic, non-enzyme, antimicrobial proteins found on the skin and in neutrophil granules.

Degranulation – In the context of eosinophils or mast cells, it is the release of pharmacological mediators contained in intracytoplasmic vesicles following appropriate stimulus (eg, coligation of Fc receptors on their cell surface).

Delayed-type of hypersensitivity – See DTH.

Dendritic cells (DCs) – Bone marrow derived accessory cells found in the epithelial and lymphoid tissue and characterized by their thin membranous projections. These are the major antigen-presenting cells of the body and are important in initiating an adaptive immune response.

Dermicidin – An antimicrobial protein specifically and constitutively expressed in sweat glands.

Desensitization – The process of exposing an allergic individual to increasing doses of allergen so as to elicit an IgG (instead of IgE) antibody response.

Diacylglycerol (DAG) – An intracellular signalling molecule generated by phospholipase Cγ-mediated hydrolysis of the membrane phospholipid phosphatidylinositol 4,5-bisphosphae (PIP$_2$) during antigen-mediated activation of lymphocytes. It activates cytosolic protein kinase C, which participates in the generation of active transcription factors.

Diapedesis – Movement of blood cells (especially leukocytes) from blood to tissues across the blood vessel walls.

Differentiation antigens – Antigens that are expressed at a particular stage of differentiation of a cell. Many differentiation antigens have important functional roles.

Double Negative thymocytes – Immature thymic T cells that lack both CD4 and CD8 expression; represent ~ 5% of thymocytes.

Double Positive thymocytes – T cells at an intermediate stage of development in the thymus; characterized by expression of both the CD4 and the CD8 molecules. They represent the majority (~ 80%) of thymocytes.

Draining lymph node – Any lymph node that is downstream of a site of infection and thus receives antigens and microbes from the site via the lymphatic system.

DTH (Delayed-Type of Hypersensitivity) – Type IV hypersensitivity mediated by CD4$^+$ T cells. The reaction is elicited hours or days after antigenic challenge.

Effector mechanisms – Processes by which pathogens are destroyed and cleared from the body.

Effector lymphocytes – Formed upon differentiation of naïve lymphocytes, effector cells can mediate the removal of pathogens from the body without the need for further differentiation.

Electrophoresis – Movement of molecules in a charged field.

ELISA (Enzyme-Linked ImmunoSorbent Assay) – An immunoassay in which antigen bound to a solid support is detected by an enzyme linked to an antibody. The enzyme converts a colourless substrate to a coloured product. See Appendix III.

ELISPOT – An adaptation of ELISA that is used to detect cells secreting a particular protein (eg, cytokines or immunoglobulins). See Appendix III.

Embryonic stem cells – Embryonic cells that have the potential to grow continuously in culture and retain the ability to differentiate to all cell lineages.

Endogenous – Originating from the organism.

Endogenous pyrogens – Cytokines that can induce a rise in body temperature. Exogenous pyrogens (eg, LPS) trigger the release of endogenous pyrogens.

Endosomes – Vesicles of the endocytic pathway where antigen internalized by antigen-presenting cells undergoes progressive degradation to peptide fragments.

Endothelium – The inner layer of capillaries, blood vessels, etc.

Enhancers – Sequences within genomic DNA that act as cell specific enhancers of RNA transcription.

Enzyme-Linked ImmunoSorbent Assay – See ELISA.

Eosinophils – Polymorphonuclear leukocytes with azurophilic granules containing pharmacological mediators and vasoactive amines. Cross-linking of FcεRI expressed by these cells leads to their degranulation.

Epithelium – A diverse group of tissues that covers or lines nearly all body surfaces, cavities, and tubes. Epithelial layers provide physical protection and containment; all of the body's internal epithelial organs are lined with epithelium that is coated with mucus.

Epitope spreading – Responses to autoantigens tend to become more diverse as the response persists. This is called epitope or determinant spreading.

Epitopes – Regions on a macromolecule (antigen) recognized by an antigen receptor. A B cell epitope is the part of the antigen recognized by an antibody. A T cell epitope consists of a small fragment of the antigen that is loaded on autologous MHC molecule; the fragment:MHC complex is recognized by the T cell antigen receptor.

Epstein-Barr virus – A herpes virus that selectively infects human B cells by binding to Complement Receptor 2 (CD21). The virus causes Infectious Mononucleosis and can establish a permanent latent infection. It is associated with some B cell malignancies and nasopharyngeal carcinoma.

Equilibrium dialysis – A technique of antibody affinity determination in which the two reactants are separated by semi-permeable membrane. See Appendix III.

ERBB2 – Also called HER2/neu, it is the protein encoded by the gene c-erbB2. ERBB2 is epidermal growth factor receptor tyrosine kinase found on some breast and ovarian cancer tumours.

Erythroblastosis foetalis – Severe haemolytic disease caused in an Rh$^+$ foetus by the crossing over the placenta of maternal anti-Rh IgG antibodies.

Exon – Gene segment that encodes a protein.

Experimental Autoimmune Encephalomyelitis (EAE; Experimental Allergic Encephalomyelitis) – An inflammatory disease of the murine central nervous system. It is the animal model of the human disease Multiple Sclerosis.

Extravasation – The movement of cells or fluid from within blood vessels to the surrounding tissues.

Fab (Fragment, antigen-binding) – A proteolytic fragment of immunoglobulin molecule that contains the antigen-binding site. It consists of one complete light chain and a part of the heavy chain.

FACS (Fluorescence-Activated Cell Sorter) – A machine used to separate cell populations by tagging them with fluorescent antibodies. See Appendix III.

Factor B, D – Serine proteases. The Bb fragment of Factor B triggers the alternative pathway of complement activation by binding C3 and allowing it to be cleaved by Factor D.

Factor H, I – Regulators of the complement cascade.

Fas molecule (CD95) – A member of the TNF receptor family. Ligation of Fas by its ligand can trigger apoptosis in Fas-expressing cells.

Fc (Fragment, crystallizable) – The portion of the immunoglobulin molecule responsible for complement fixation, binding to cells, etc. It consists of the disulphide-linked Carboxy– terminal regions of heavy chains.

Fc receptors (FcRs) – Receptors found on a variety of cell types, eg, macrophages, B and T cells, platelets, eosinophils, mast cells, and basophils that bind the Fc region of immunoglobulin molecules. The cytoplasmic domains of most FcRs have signalling motifs. FcRs mediate many of the cell-dependent effector functions of antibodies.

FcεRI – A type of FcR expressed on eosinophils, basophils, and mast cells that bind IgE antibodies with high affinity. Antigen-mediated coligation of FcεRI-bound IgE antibodies results in the degranulation and release of pharmacological mediators responsible for some of the symptoms of immediate type of hypersensitivity.

FcγR – Types of FcR that bind IgG antibody. FcγRI are high affinity receptors expressed on neutrophils and macrophages that mediate phagocytosis; FcγRII are low affinity receptors that mediate various other functions.

FDCs (Follicualr Dendritic Cells) – Found in the lymphoid follicles, these cells of uncertain origin are characterized by long branching processes that make intimate contact with many different B cells. They are crucial to the process of affinity maturation.

Ficolins – Activators of alternative pathway of complement activation, ficolins are characterized by the presence of both a collagen-like domain and a fibrinogen-like domain.

First set rejection – Allograft rejection by a recipient who has not previously received a graft or has not been exposed to alloantigens from the same donor.

FK506 (Tacrolimus) – An immunosuppressive drug that is similar in activity to cyclosporin A.

FLICE (FADD-like Interleukin-1 beta-Converting Enzyme) – A protease component of the death-inducing signalling complex initiated by the Fas binding.

FLIP (FLICE-Inhibitory Proteins) – Potent inhibitors of Fas-mediated apoptosis expressed in lymphoid tissues. Cells overexpressing viral FLIPs are protected from cell death by apoptosis.

Flow cytometry – A technique of analysis of phenotypes of cell populations using a flow cytometer. See Appendix III.

Freund's adjuvant –An oil-in-water emulsion used as adjuvant in animals. Complete Freund's adjuvant (CFA) contains cells or cell walls of *Mycobaclerium tuberculosis* whereas the incomplete adjuvant is only an oil water emulsion without mycobacterial cell walls.

FRs (Framework regions) – Relatively invariant sequences of the variable regions of the antigen receptors. FRs are responsible for the molecular architecture, while the CDR (hypervariable regions) are responsible for antigen contact.

Fyn – A type of tyrosine kinase.

G proteins – Intracellular proteins that bind GTP and convert it to GDP in the process of cell signal transduction. Heterotrimeric G proteins are receptor-associated, whereas the small G proteins (eg, Ras) act downstream of the transmembrane signalling events.

GALT (Gut-Associated Lymphoid Tissues) – Lymphoid tissues closely associated with the gastrointestinal tract, including the tonsils, Peyer's patches, and intraepithelial lymphocytes.

GATA-3 – TH2-cell specific transcription factor that is the master regulator of TH2 differentiation. GATA-3 induces heritable remodelling of the IL-4 locus and promotes the expression of several TH2 cytokines, thereby committing the cell to TH2 lineage.

Gene therapy – Correction of a genetic defect by the introduction of a normal gene into bone marrow or other cell types.

Germ line hypothesis – A theory of antibody diversity that proposes that all the genes needed for generating the antibody repertoire are present in the fertilized ovum.

Germinal centres – Found in secondary lymphoid tissue during B cell responses to TD antigens, germinal centres are formed around follicular dendritic cell networks when activated B cells migrate into lymphoid tissue. They are the site of B cell isotype switching, somatic hypermutation, antigen-driven selection, and differentiation.

Germline diversity – In context of antigen receptors, germline diversity is receptor diversity caused by the inheritance of multiple gene segments that encode V domains. Antigen receptor diversity generated during gene rearrangement or after receptor gene expression, is termed somatically generated.

Goodpasture's syndrome – Type of autoimmune disease wherein antibodies are produced to type IV collagen of the basement membrane.

Graft – A tissue or organ removed from one site and placed at another. A graft is 'rejected' when the grafted tissue is destroyed by recipient's adaptive immune system.

Graft versus Host Disease – See GVHD.

Granulocyte Macrophage-Colony Stimulating Factor (GM-CSF) – A cytokine involved in the growth and differentiation of myeloid and monocytic lineage cells, including dendritic cells, monocytes and tissue macrophages, and cells of the granulocyte lineage.

Granuloma – Palpable nodules formed at the site of chronic inflammation as a result of delayed-type of hypersensitivity responses. Granulomas can be triggered by persistent infectious agents. They consist of a central area having macrophages fused into multi-nucleate giant cells surrounded by T lymphocytes.

Granulysin – An antimicrobial protein found in cytotoxic granules of cytotoxic T lymphocytes.

Granzymes – Serine esterases found in the granules of cytotoxic T and NK cells. They induce nuclear fragmentation.

Graves' disease – An autoimmune disease in which antibodies against the thyroid-stimulating hormone receptor cause overproduction of thyroid hormone resulting in hyperthyroidism.

Gut-associated lymphoid tissues – See GALT.

GVHD (Graft versus Host Disease) – A disease caused by an attack on recipient tissue by the donor T cells present in the bone marrow graft.

H chain – See Immunoglobulin molecule.

HAART (Highly Active AntiRetroviral Therapy) – A cocktail of chemotherapeutic agents used in HIV treatment. HAART consists of a reverse transcriptase inhibitor and a protease inhibitor.

Haematopoiesis – Generation of cellular elements of blood (erythrocytes, leukocytes, platelets) from haematopoietic stem cells.

Haplotype – A set of genetic determinants located on a single chromosome.

Hapten – A molecule that can bind to an immunoglobulin molecule but not elicit an immune response. Haptens have to be conjugated to a carrier molecule to elicit an immune response.

Helper T cells – See T$_H$ cells.

Heterophile antigens – Antigens or epitopes shared by unrelated (widely divergent) species.

HEV (High Endothelial Venule) – Specialized venules in lymphoid tissues through which lymphocytes migrate. HEV cells express special receptors that allow transmigration of the lymphocytes.

Hinge region – The flexible region of the immunoglobulin molecule that joins the Fab and Fc fragments. The flexibility of this region allows the Fab region of the molecule to adopt a wide range of angles for efficient interaction with the epitopes on the antigen.

Histamine – A vasoactive amine stored in mast cell granules. It causes vasodilation and smooth muscle contraction.

Histocompatibility antigens – MHC molecules expressed on surface of tissue cells. They mediate rejection of allogeneic grafts.

HIV (Human Immunodeficiency Virus) – A retrovirus of the lentivirus family that causes AIDS.

HLA (Human leukocyte antigen) – Genetic designation for human MHC antigens.

HLA-DM and -DO – Human molecules involved in loading peptides onto MHC class II molecules; the murine equivalents are called H2-M and -O.

Hodgkin's lymphoma – An immune system tumour which is derived from mutated B lineage cells.

Homeostasis – A generic term used to describe the status of physiological normality.

HPA (Hypothalamus Pituatary Adrenal) axis – Comprising paraventricular nucleus in the hypothalamus, the anterior pituitary gland, and the adrenal glands, the HPA axis is the classical neuroendocrine system that responds to stress and whose final product, corticosteroids, targets components of the limbic system, particularly the hippocampus. It functions by means of interaction of the nervous and endocrine systems whereby the nervous system regulates the endocrine system and endocrine activity modulates the activity of the central nervous system.

Humanized antibodies – Designer monoclonal antibodies produced by genetic engineering. These are human antibodies containing mouse hypervariable regions of a desired specificity.

Humoral immunity – *Humor* is any fluid of the body. Humoral immunity is the immunity conferred by the presence of antibodies in body fluids.

Hybridomas – *In vitro* cell lines created by fusing two different cell types, one of which is a tumour cell. Fusion of myeloma cell line with plasma cells yields B cell hybridomas, the source of monoclonal antibodies. Fusion of myeloma cells with T cell clones yields T cell hybridomas that are used to detect specific peptide:MHC haplotype complexes.

Hyperacute graft rejection – An immediate (minutes to hours) reaction against allogeneic grafts caused by preformed antibodies that react with antigens on the graft.

Hypereosinophilia – Presence of abnormally large numbers of eosinophils in the blood.

Hypersensitivity – An exaggerated and inappropriate immune response to innocuous antigens, usually detrimental to the health of the individual. Hypersensitivity type I reactions are due to IgE-mediated degranulation of mast cells; type II reactions are due to IgG antibodies binding to tissue antigens; type III reactions are a result of formation of small antigen-antibody complexes; type IV reactions are CD4$^+$ T cell-mediated.

Hypervariable regions – See CDR.

ICAMs (InterCellular Adhesion Molecules) – Cell surface ligands for the leukocyte integrins. ICAMs are crucial in the binding of lymphocytes and other leukocytes to cells, including antigen-presenting cells and endothelial cells.

Iccosomes – Antigen-coated liposome-like particles consisting of antigen, C3b or its fragments, and immunoglobulin derived from membranes of follicular dendritic cells of lymphoid follicles early in a secondary or subsequent antibody response.

ICOS (Inducible T cell Costimulator) – A costimulatory molecule expressed on activated T cells. Binding of ICOS to its ligand known as ICOSL enhances T cell responses.

IDDM (Insulin-Dependent Diabetes Mellitus) – An autoimmune disease caused by the destruction of β cells of pancreatic islets of Langerhans resulting in reduced or total lack of insulin production. IDDM is characterized by an inability to metabolize glucose and increased glucose levels in blood and tissue fluids.

Idiotopes – Antigenic determinants on the variable region, usually the CDRs, of immunoglobulins or T cell receptors. A collection of idiotopes give the idiotype of the antibody.

IFNs – See interferons.

Ii (Invariant chain) – A chaperone molecule synthesized in the endoplasmic reticulum along with MHC class II molecules. Ii promotes folding and assembly of the class II molecules, and helps in its transport to peptide-loading compartments. It also protects the peptide-binding groove of the class II molecule during synthesis and transport.

IL – See interleukins.

Immature B cells – B cells that have rearranged their heavy and light chain V region genes, express surface IgM, but not surface IgD molecules.

Immediate hypersensitivity – See allergy.

Immune complex – A multi-molecular complex of antibody molecules bound to antigen molecules. These can vary greatly in size. Deposition of immune complexes in blood vessel walls or glomeruli can lead to disease.

Immune deviation – A term used to describe the conversion of an immune response from one dominated by T_{H1} to that dominated by T_{H2} type (or *vice versa*).

Immune modulation – A general term encompassing various alterations in an immune response.

Immune privileged sites – Sites of the body where immune responses are limited or constitutively suppressed, eg, the brain, the testes, or the eyes. Immune responses at such sites are often 'deviant', ie, are non-inflammatory as opposed to the pro-inflammatory responses observed at non-privileged sites.

Immune response – The response made by the host to defend itself against a pathogen.

Immune response genes – See Ir genes.

Immune system – Tissues, cells, and molecules involved in adaptive immunity; sometimes used to describe the totality of host defence mechanisms.

Immune tolerance – See tolerance.

Immunity – Ability to resist infections. Derived from Latin *immunis* – exempt from duty to the state.

Immunization (active immunization) – Deliberate provocation of an adaptive immune response by the introduction of an immunogen. By contrast, passive immunization is the injection of immunoglobulins or immune serum.

Immunoblotting (Western blotting) – A technique for protein identification using gel electrophoresis followed by transferring (blotting) the separated proteins to a nitrocellulose membrane, and detection by specific antibodies. See Appendix III.

Immunodeficiencies – A group of inherited or acquired disorders in which some aspect(s) of host defence are absent or functionally defective.

Immunodiffusion – A technique for antigen/antibody detection by allowing them to interact in clear agar gel. See Appendix III.

Immunoelectrophoresis – Identification of antigens by first separating them on the basis of their electrophoretic mobility followed by detection by precipitation in gel.

Immunofluorescence – A technique for detecting molecules expressed by cells using specific antibodies labelled with fluorescent dyes. See Appendix III.

Immunogen – Any molecule that can elicit an adaptive immune response upon introduction (usually by injection) into a person or an animal.

Immunoglobulin (Ig) molecule – Antibody molecule. Each Ig molecule is composed of a pair each of H chains (~ 50 KD) and L chains (~ 25 KD) that associate through disulphide and non-covalent interactions to yield a Y shaped molecule. Each H chain consists of 3 (or 4) constant domains and one variable domain; L chain consists of one each of a constant and a variable domain and is disulphide bonded to the H chain. Each immunoglobulin monomer can combine with two antigenic determinants. The membrane immunoglobulin (mIg) expressed on the surface of B cells, contains an additional transmembrane domain.

Immunoglobulin domain – Three-dimensional protein structure found in many proteins of the immune system. It is about 110 amino acids in length and consists of two layers of β-pleated sheets and an internal disulphide bond.

Immunoglobulin superfamily – Proteins having at least one immunoglobulin or immunoglobulin-like domain.

Immunohistochemistry – A technique for the detection of tissue antigens using antibody-linked enzymes. See Appendix III.

Immunological ignorance – The mechanism of non-responsiveness to a self-antigen even when it is expressed in organs or tissues and T cells capable of responding to the antigen exist in the body. It could be due to levels of antigen expression that are too low for T cell activation or due to the inability of the lymphocytes to gain access to the site of antigen expression.

Immunological memory – A phenomenon in which second or subsequent antigen encounters elicit speedier and more effective protective immune responses.

Immunology – The study of all aspects of host defence against infectious challenge and of adverse consequences thereof.

Immunoprecipitation – Detection of soluble proteins using specific antibodies. See Appendix III.

Immunoreceptor Tyrosine-based Activating/Inhibitory Motifs – See ITAMs/ITIMs.

Immunoregulation – The ability of the immune system to sense and regulate its own responses.

Immunosuppression – Inhibition of one or more components of adaptive or innate system either as a result of disease or because of administration of drugs.

Inflammation – Local accumulation of fluid, plasma proteins, and leukocytes at a site of injury, infection, or local immune response.

Inhibitors of Apoptosis (IAPs) –A family of anti-apoptotic proteins that are conserved across several species. IAPs are the only known endogenous inhibitors of caspases and several of them are regulated via the transcription factor NFκB.

Innate immunity – A form of immune defence that is active in the early phases of host response to an infectious challenge. It is present in all individuals at all times, discriminates between groups of related pathogens, and responds in the same way to repeated exposures to a given pathogen. Unlike the adaptive immune response it is not directed against a particular epitope of the antigen.

Inositol-(1,4,5)-triphosphate (IP$_3$) – One of the cleavage product formed by phospholipase Cγ-mediated hydrolysis of Phosphatidylinositol-(4,5)-bisphosphate (PIP$_2$) during lymphocyte activation. IP$_3$ releases calcium ions from intracellular stores in the endoplasmic reticulum.

Insulin-Dependent Diabetes Mellitus – See IDDM.

Integrins – Heterodimeric cell surface proteins involved in cell-cell and cell-matrix interactions. Some members are also involved in pathogen recognition and phagocyte activation.

Intercellular Adhesion Molecules – See ICAMs.

Interferons (IFNs) – Cytokines produced by the cells of the immune systems of most animals in response to viruses, bacteria, parasites, and tumour cells. They are important in innate and adaptive immune responses.

Interleukins (ILs) – Originally used to describe cytokines that are produced by or act on leukocytes, the term is now used generically irrespective of the source or target.

Introns – Gene segments between exons that do not encode a protein.

Invariant chain – See Ii.

Ir (Immune response) genes – Genes that determine the intensity of the immune response to a particular antigen – genes that encode MHC class II molecules.

ISCOMs – An adjuvant consisting of immune stimulatory complexes of antigen held within a lipid matrix.

Isotype switching – A phenomenon wherein the class of antibodies produced by a B cell in the early phases of the immune response is changed in the later phases of the response (from IgM to IgG/IgA/IgE) without affecting the antigen-binding specificity of the antibodies produced. Class switch recombination is the molecular mechanism that results in isotype switching. In this, the rearranged immunoglobulin V gene segment recombines with one of the downstream C region genes and the intervening C genes are deleted.

Isotypes – Classes of immunoglobulins recognized on the basis of the Constant regions of the heavy or light chains. Five major classes (IgM, IgD, IgG, IgE and IgA) are recognised on the basis of heavy chain constant regions and two (κ and λ) on the basis of the light chain constant region. Each isotype is encoded by a distinct constant region gene.

ITAMs (Immunoreceptor Tyrosine-based Activating Motifs) – A pair of tyrosine-containing motifs (tyrosine-X-X-leucine/isoleucine; where X is any amino acid) found in the cytoplasmic tails of activatory receptors. These are the sites of tyrosine phosphorylation and association of other phosphotyrosine-binding moieties involved in receptor signalling.

ITIMs (Immunoreceptor Tyrosine-based Inhibitory Motifs) – Tyrosine-containing motifs (isoleucine/valine-X-tyrosine-X-X-leucine) found in the cytoplasmic tails of inhibitory receptors. These motifs recruit phosphatases to the receptor site that remove the phosphate groups added by tyrosine kinases.

IVIg (Intravenous Ig) – A pooled immunoglobulin preparation obtained from plasma of donors; used in passive immunization.

J chain – A small, disulphide bonded peptide found in the tail pieces of multimeric immunoglobulins (IgM and IgG).

***J* region** – Short coding sequences between the variable and constant gene segments in all immunoglobulin and T cell receptor loci. They are combined (with or without the *D* segment) to the *V* gene segments during lymphocyte development.

JAK – See Janus kinases.

Janus kinases (JAKs) – A family of intracellular tyrosine kinases involved in the signalling cascade of cytokines. These kinases phosphorylate proteins known as STATs and the signalling pathway is often referred to as JAK-STAT pathway.

Junctional diversity – The diversity created in antigen-specific receptors during the process of joining *V*, *D*, and *J* gene segments.

K cells – A subset of NK cells that express the low affinity receptor for IgG antibodies.

KIRs (Killer cell Ig-like Receptors) – Inhibitory receptors expressed by NK cells that recognize MHC class I molecules.

KO (Knock Out) mice – Mice with targeted disruption of one or more genes created by homologous recombination. The technique enables the study of the function of specific gene product(s).

Kupffer cells – Phagocytic cells that line the hepatic sinusoids.

L chain – See Immunoglobulin molecule.

Lactoferrin – An iron-chelating protein found in milk and mucosal secretions such as tears.

LAK (Lymphokine-Activated Killer) cells – *In vitro* activated NK cells used in cancer therapy. LAK cells are generated by exposing patients' NK cells to high doses of IL-2.

Langerhans cells – Phagocytic immature dendritic cells found in the epidermis.

LAT (Linker of Activation in T cells) – An adaptor protein with several tyrosines that become phosphorylated by the tyrosine kinase ZAP-70. It becomes associated with membrane lipid rafts and co-ordinates downstream signalling events in T cell activation.

Latency – In the context of viral infection, refers to the state in which the virus enters a cell but does not replicate; when reactivated the virus can replicate and cause a disease.

LBP (LPS Binding Protein) – An acute phase protein with the ability to bind and transfer bacterial LPS to CD14.

Lck (Lymphocyte-specific protein tyrosine kinase) – A Src family tyrosine kinase associated with cytoplasmic tails of CD4 and CD8 coreceptors in T cells.

Lentiviruses – A group of retroviruses that include the human immunodeficiency virus, HIV. They cause disease after a long incubation period and the infection can take years to become apparent.

Leukaemia – A malignancy of bone marrow precursors of blood cells in which a large number of malignant cells are found in the bone marrow and also in the blood; can be lymphocytic, myelocytic, or monocytic.

Leukocyte common antigen – See CD45.

Leukocytes – A general term used to describe white blood cells including lymphocytes, polymorphonuclear leukocytes, and monocytes.

Leukocytosis – The presence of increased numbers of leukocytes in the blood; commonly observed in acute infection.

Leukotrienes (LTB4, LTC4, etc) – Lipid inflammatory mediators produced by the lipoxygenase pathway that have powerful pharmacological effects.

LFAs (Leukocyte Functional Antigens) – Cell adhesion molecules; LFA-1 is a β2 integrin, LFA-2 and LFA-3 are members of the immunoglobulin superfamily. LFA-1 is important in T cell adhesion to endothelial cells and antigen presenting cells.

Ligand – Linking or binding molecule.

Lipid rafts – Specialized cell membrane domains enriched in cholesterol and glycosphingolipids; act as assembly points and platforms that facilitate the interaction of particular signalling components.

Lipoxins – Edogenous lipid anti-inflammatory mediators.

LPS (Lipopolysaccharide) – Also called endotoxin, LPS is a component of Gram-negative bacterial cells walls. It stimulates multiple components of the innate immune system and is also a powerful B cell mitogen.

L-selectin – An adhesion molecule of the selectin family found on lymphocytes.

Lymph – The extracellular fluid that accumulates in tissues and is carried by lymphatic vessels back through the lymphatic system to the thoracic duct and into the blood.

Lymph nodes – Secondary lymphoid organs found at locations of lymphatic vessel convergence. They are the sites of initiation of adaptive immune responses.

Lymphatic system – The system of lymphoid channels and tissues that drains extracellular fluid from the periphery via the thoracic duct to the blood. It includes the lymph nodes, Peyer's patches, and other organized lymphoid elements apart from the spleen, which communicates directly with the blood.

Lymphatic vessels or lymphatics – Thin-walled vessels that carry lymph through the lymphatic system. Afferent lymphatics drain fluid from the tissues and help transport antigen and antigen-presenting cells from sites of infection to the lymph nodes. Lymphocytes leave the lymph node through the efferent lymphatic vessel.

Lymphoblast – A lymphocyte that has enlarged and increased its rate of RNA and protein synthesis, usually in preparation of accelerated proliferation.

Lymphocyte homing – Directed migration of subsets of circulating lymphocytes into particular tissue sites regulated by the selective expression of adhesion molecules called homing receptors.

Lymphocytes – A class of white blood cells; consist of T, B, NK and NKT cells. T and B lymphocytes bear variable cell surface receptors for antigen and participate in adaptive immune responses. NK cells express invariant surface receptors and are a part of the innate immune system. NKT cells express NK and T cell receptors.

Lymphoid follicles – B cell rich regions consisting of clusters of B cells organized around follicular dendritic cells. They are the sites of antigen-induced B cell proliferation and differentiation. Primary follicles contain resting B cells and give rise to secondary follicles or germinal centres when they are entered by antigen activated B cells.

Lymphoid organs – Organized tissues characterized by very large numbers of lymphocytes interacting with a non-lymphoid stroma. The central or primary lymphoid organs (the thymus and bone marrow) are the sites of lymphocyte generation. The peripheral or secondary lymphoid organs (lymph nodes, spleen, and mucosal-associated lymphoid tissues such as tonsils and Peyer's patches) are the sites of initiation of adaptive immune responses.

Lymphokines – A term originally used to describe cytokines produced by lymphocytes.

Lymphomas – Tumors of lymphocytes that grow in lymphoid and other tissues. They do not enter the blood in large numbers.

Lymphotoxin – See TNF.

Lysosomes – Acidified organelles of the endocytic pathway that contain many degradative hydrolytic enzymes.

M cells – Delicate membranous cells found in the dome epithelium of Peyer's patches. M cells endocytose and transport antigens without lysosomal degradation.

MAC (Membrane Attack Complex) – A complex formed in the final stages of complement associated lysis. It is composed of terminal components of the complement cascade and multiple molecules of C9. The assembled complex generates a membrane-spanning hydrophilic pore in the target cell membrane causing lethal ionic and osmotic changes in the cell.

Macrophages – Large, mononuclear, phagocytic, and migratory cells found in most tissues of the body; they are derived from blood monocytes and have a critical role in host defence. They are important in innate immunity, as antigen-presenting cells, and as effector cells in humoral and cell-mediated immunity.

MAGE – A family of proteins that is normally expressed only in the testes but is often expressed by melanoma (skin cancer) cells.

MALT – Mucosal-associated lymphoid tissue comprising all lymphoid cells in epithelia and in the lamina propria lying below the body's mucosal surfaces.

Mannan-binding lectin (MBL) or mannose-binding protein (MBP) – A plasma protein that binds to mannose residues found on procaryotic cell walls and opsonizes them. It can activate the complement cascade.

Mannose receptor – An endocytic pattern recognition receptor that binds mannoses and fucoses on microbial cell walls and mediates their phagocytosis.

MAP (Mitogen-Activated Protein) kinases – Present downstream of a variety of receptor-mediated signalling pathways, phosphorylation of MAP kinases results in new gene expression due to the phosphorylation of key transcription factors.

MASP-1 and MASP-2 – Serine proteases that are components of the MBL pathway of complement activation. They cleave C4.

Mast cells – Large cells found in connective tissues throughout the body, but most abundantly in the submucosal tissues and the dermis. They contain granules rich in pharmacological mediators and vasoactive amines, and are the major effectors of immediate type of hypersensitivity. Antigen-mediated cross-linking of FcεRl receptors expressed on mast cells results in their degranulation.

MBP (Major Basic Protein) – An anti-parasitic protein found in the eosinophils. It can also induce tissue injury in allergic and inflammatory diseases and, because it induces injury to the bronchial epithelium, is linked to asthma.

Medulla – Generally the central or collecting point of an organ.

Memory cells – Progeny of antigen-activated naïve lymphocytes that mediate immunological memory. Due to a reprogramming of antigen receptors and signalling molecules, memory cells are more sensitive to antigen and respond more rapidly to it than naïve lymphocytes.

Metastasis – The transfer of pain, function, or disease from one organ to another through contact, blood vessels, or lymphatics. In the context of tumours, it is the formation of secondary tumours at sites away from the primary malignancy.

MHC (Major Histocompatibility Complex) – Cluster of genes that encode the highly polymorphic proteins that serve as peptide display molecules for T cells. MHC class I molecules present processed antigens to CD8$^+$ T cells, whereas MHC class II molecules present processed antigen to CD4$^+$ T cells. The cluster also encodes non-polymorphic MHC class III proteins that have varying roles in host defence.

MHC restriction – A term used to describe the fact that T cells recognize a peptide antigen only when it is bound to a particular MHC allele (usually a self-MHC molecule).

Mindin – A secretory protein that promotes phagocytosis and secretion of pro-inflammatory cytokines.

Minor histocompatibility antigens (minor H antigens) – Polymorphic cellular proteins. Peptides derived from these proteins, when loaded on MHC molecules, can lead to graft rejection.

Mitogen – A substance that can cause cells to divide. B or T cell mitogens can induce B/T cell proliferation irrespective of their antigen specificity and are hence called polyclonal activators.

mlg (membrane immunoglobulin) – See immunoglobulin.

MLR (Mixed Lymphocyte Reaction) – A technique used to test histocompatibility that consists of culturing lymphocytes from two unrelated individuals — the T cells in the culture proliferate in response to the allogeneic MHC molecules on the cells of the other donor. See Appendix III.

Molecular mimicry – A postulated mechanism of autoimmunity induction due to cross-reactivity between the epitopes present on infectious agents and self-antigens.

Monoclonal antibodies (mAbs) – Antibodies of a single specificity produced by a single clone of B cells. See Appendix III.

Monocytes – Bone marrow-derived circulating blood cells that are the precursors of tissue macrophages.

Mucins – Highly glycosylated cell surface proteins that are a major component of mucus.

Mucosa-Associated Lymphoid Tissue – See MALT.

Multiple sclerosis – An autoimmune neurological disease characterized by focal demyelination in the central nervous system, lymphocytic infiltration in the brain, and a chronic, progressive course.

Myasthenia gravis – An autoimmune disease in which autoantibodies against the acetylcholine receptor on skeletal muscle cells cause a block in neuromuscular junctions, leading to progressive muscular weakness and eventual death.

Myeloid progenitors – Bone marrow cells that give rise to the granulocytes and macrophages of the immune system.

Myeloma – A tumour of plasma cells. Myeloma proteins are incomplete or complete immunoglobulins secreted by myeloma tumours.

Myeloperoxidase (MPO) – A critical enzyme in the conversion of hydrogen peroxide (H_2O_2) to hypochlorous acid found in neutrophil granules. Along with H_2O_2 and a halide cofactor, MPO forms the most effective microbicidal and cytotoxic mechanism of leukocytes.

MZ (Marginal Zone) – The lymphoid tissue of the spleen that lies at the border of the white pulp. MZ contains a unique population of B cells, which do not circulate, express a distinct set of surface proteins such as CD5 and CD9, and are a part of the innate immune system.

Naïve lymphocytes – Lymphocytes that have never encountered their specific antigen and are not a progeny of antigen-stimulated mature lymphocyte.

NALT – Nasopharynx-associated lymphoid tissue.

Natural Killer – See NK cells.

Necrosis – Death of cells or tissues due to physical or chemical injury.

Negative selection – The process of removal of self-reactive lymphocytes during their development.

Neonatal FcR (FcRn) – An IgG-specific Fc receptor that mediates the transport of maternal IgG antibodies across the placenta and neonatal intestinal epithelium. It is also thought to regulate plasma IgG antibody catabolism in adults.

Neoplasm – An abnormal mass of tissue, the growth of which exceeds and is uncoordinated with that of normal tissues, and persists in the same excessive manner after cessation of the stimuli that evoked changes.

Neutropaenia – Occurrence of fewer than normal neutrophils in the blood.

Neutrophils – Phagocytic cells having multi-lobed nucleus that are recruited to sites of inflammation.

NFκB – A family of transcription factors important in the transcription of many genes involved in innate and adaptive immune responses.

NK (Natural Killer) cells – Non-T, non-B cytotoxic lymphocytes. They are important in innate and anti tumour responses.

NKT cells – Lymphocytes that express a NK cell receptor and a T cell receptor of limited diversity. NKT cells recognize antigen loaded on CD1 molecules.

Non-homologous DNA End-joining (NHEJ) pathway – A DNA repair pathway that rejoins DNA strand breaks without relying on marked homology.

Nude mouse – A strain of mice having a gene defect that causes hairlessness and a defective formation of thymic stroma. These mice lack mature T cells.

Oedema – Swelling caused by the entry of fluid and cells from the blood into the tissues. It is one of the characteristics of inflammation.

Opsonin – A macromolecule that becomes attached to microbial surfaces and can increase the efficiency of phagocytosis by virtue of being recognized by receptors on phagocytic cells, eg, complement components and immunoglobulin molecules.

Opsonization – Alteration of the surface of a pathogen/particle by deposition of opsonins so that phagocytosis is facilitated.

Oral tolerance – Tolerance induced by oral administration of antigen.

Original antigenic sin – A phenomenon which results in the generation of antibody responses to epitopes shared between the original infecting strain of a virus and subsequent infections by related viruses, while ignoring other highly immunogenic epitopes on the second and subsequent viruses.

PALS (Periarteriolar Lymphoid Sheath) – A part of the inner region of the white pulp of the spleen that contains mainly T cells.

PAMPs (Pathogen-Associated Molecular Patterns) – Molecules present on the cell envelope of micro-organisms that form a unique geometric pattern that is recognized by special receptors on host cells.

Paraproteins – See Bence Jones proteins.

Pattern Recognition Receptors (PRRs) – Receptors of the innate immune system that recognize common molecular patterns on pathogen surfaces. Include molecules such as collections, ficolins, C-reactive proteins, MBP, etc that can recognize distinctive ligands found on the cell walls of certain pathogens. PRRs are an integral part of the innate defence system.

PCA (Passive Cutaneous Anaphylaxis) – A skin test used to detect antigen-specific IgE antibodies.

PD-1 (Programmed Death gene-1) – An inhibitory molecule expressed by activated T cells, B cells, and myeloid cells. Engagement of PD-1 by its ligands is thought to control the proliferation and cytokine expression of these cells.

PECAM-1 – CD31. See Appendix I.

Perforin – A protein found in the granules of cytotoxic T cells and NK cells that polymerizes to form membrane pores in the target cell membrane.

Periarteriolar Lymphoid Sheath – See PALS.

Peripheral tolerance – See tolerance.

Peyer's patches – Organized lymphoid tissue in the lamina propria of the small intestines, especially the ileum.

Phagocytosis – A process by which large particulate matter (>0.5 μm) is internalized by cells. The ingested material is contained in a phagosome, which fuses with one or more lysosomes to form a phagolysosome where the ingested material undergoes degradation.

Phospholipase Cγ (PLCγ) – A key signal transducing enzyme that gets activated upon antigen recognition by the lymphocytes. It catalyzes hydrolysis of phosphatidylinositol 4,5-bisphosphae (PIP_2) to Inositol-(1,4,5)-triphosphate (IP_3) and diacylglycerol (DAG).

pIgR (polymeric Ig receptor) – An Fc receptor expressed by mucosal epithelial cells that mediates transport of polymeric immunoglobulins (IgA and IgM) through the epithelial cells and into the intestinal lumen.

Plasma – The whitish coloured fluid that is left behind after all the cells (leukocytes, erythrocytes and platelets) are removed from blood. It contains water, electrolytes, and plasma proteins.

Plasma cell – Antibody-secreting, terminally differentiated B cell.

Plasmablast – A B cell in a lymph node that is on the path of becoming a plasma cell and shows some of its features.

Platelet Activating Factor (PAF) – A lipid mediator that activates the blood clotting cascade. It can cause bronchoconstriction and vascular dilation.

Platelets – Small, cell-like fragments of bone-marrow derived megakaryocytes, found in the blood, that are crucial for blood clotting.

Pleuripotent stem cells – Cells capable of continuously dividing and differentiating to progenitors of multiple lineages.

Polyclonal antibodies – Antibodies produced by many clones of cells, eg, those found in serum.

Polygenic – Proteins such as MHC molecules that have identical functions, but are encoded by several loci.

Polymorphism – Literally meaning to exist in a variety of different shapes, when used in the context of genes (ie, genetic polymorphism), it means variability at a gene locus in which the variants occur at a frequency of greater than 1%. Each common variant is called a polymorphic gene. The major histocompatibility complex is the most polymorphic gene cluster known in humans.

Polymorphonuclear granulocytes (PMNs) – Leukocytes having a multi-lobed nucleus (Greek *polymorpho* - many shaped) and a large number of granules in the cytoplasm; classified into neutrophils, basophils and eosinophils on the basis of staining reaction.

Positive selection – A thymic process by which only those developing T cells that have receptors recognizing self-MHC molecules are allowed to survive and reach maturity.

Pre-B cell – A developing B cell present only in the haematopoietic tissues; characterized by expression of the μ heavy chain and surrogate light chain.

Precipitation – The separation of the complex of a soluble antigen and its homologous antibody from the suspending fluid. See Appendix III.

Primary immune response – Adaptive immune response to an initial exposure to antigen. Primary immunization generates both the primary immune response and immunological memory.

Pro-B cells – The earliest haematopoietic cells committed to B cell lineage; express B lineage specific markers such as CD19 and CD10.

Progenitors – The more differentiated progeny of stem cells that give rise to distinct subsets of mature blood cells. They lack the capacity for self-renewal possessed by true stem cells.

Promoters – Relatively short nucleotide sequences extending up to 200 base pairs upstream (ie, 5′) from the transcription initiation site where the proteins that initiate transcription bind.

Properdin – A positive regulator of the alternative pathway of complement activation.

Prostaglandins (PG) – Lipid by-products of the arachidonic acid pathway that have a variety of effects on a variety of tissues.

Proteasome – Large multi-protein enzyme complex with a broad range of activity that is the main proteolytic system of all eukaryotic cells. Proteasome-generated peptides are presented by MHC class I molecules.

Protein Kinase C (PKC) – A serine/threonine kinase activated by diacylglycerol. It is crucial to many receptor-mediated signal transduction pathways.

Protein kinases – Enzymes that add phosphate groups to proteins; those adding phosphate groups to tyrosine residues are called protein tyrosine kinases or PTKs.

Proto-oncogenes – Genes involved in regulating cell growth. Mutations in these genes may result in tumours; the mutated genes are called oncogenes.

RAG (Recombination Activating Genes) – Genes encoding RAG-1 and RAG-2 proteins that are critical in T and B cell antigen receptor gene rearrangements.

RANTES – A chemoattractant for peripheral blood monocytes.

Rapamycin (sirolimus) – An immunosuppressive drug that acts on a protein kinase involved in several cell growth and regulation pathways.

Reagins – Old term for IgE antibodies.

Receptor – A cell surface molecule which can specifically bind to particular protein (ligand) in the fluid phase.

Receptor editing – The process of further rearranging light or heavy chains of a self-reactive antigen receptor on immature B cells so as to ablate autoreactivity.

Receptor-mediated endocytosis – The internalization of molecules bound to cell surface receptors.

Recombination Signal Sequences (RSSs) – Flanking gene segments found in V, D, and J gene segments that consist of conserved heptamer and nonamer sequences, separated by non-conserved 12 or 23 nucleotide sequences. RSSs are the targets for the site-specific RAG-1/RAG-2 recombinases that join the gene segments.

Regulatory T cells (TR cells) – T cells that can modulate (usually inhibit) immune responses.

Respiratory burst – A process mediated by phagocyte oxidase by which reactive oxygen intermediates are produced by phagocytes. It is usually triggered by bacterial products or pro-inflammatory mediators.

Rhesus (Rh) antigen – A blood group antigen that is also found on the red blood cells of rhesus monkeys.

Rheumatoid arthritis – An autoimmune inflammatory joint disease.

RIA (Radiommunoassay) – A technique of detection and quantitation of antigen or antibody in which one of the reactant is labelled with a radioactive isotope while the unlabelled reactant is attached to a solid support. See Appendix III.

RNI (reactive nitrogen intermediates) – Potent antimicrobial molecules produced by cells of the immune system and other cells involved in the immune response.

ROI (reactive oxygen intermediates) – Highly reactive metabolites of oxygen, such as superoxide anions and H_2O_2, that are produced by activated phagocytes.

SALT – Skin-associated lymphoid tissue.

Sarcoma – A malignant tumour arising from mesodermal tissue, eg, bone, cartilage, and fat.

Scavenger receptors – Types of pattern recognition receptors found on cells of the innate immune system. They bind to numerous ligands and remove them from the blood.

SCID, *scid* – See Severe Combined Immune Deficiency.

SDS-PAGE – Common abbreviation for polyacrylamide gel electrophoresis. See Appendix III.

Secondary immune response – Immune response induced by a second or subsequent exposure to the antigen.

Secretory component – A fragment of the extracellular domain of polymeric Ig receptor left attached to the IgA antibodies after transport across epithelial cells.

Selectins – A family of carbohydrate-binding cell surface adhesion molecules of leukocytes and endothelial cells that include L-Selectin (CD62L), P-selectin expressed on platelets, and E-selectin found on activated endothelium.

Sensitization – In the context of an allergic reaction, is the prior exposure to the allergen that results in an IgE antibody response.

Sequence motif – A pattern of nucleotides or amino acids shared by different genes or proteins that often have related functions.

Sequestered antigens – Cellular constituents of tissue (eg, lens of the eye) that are hidden or sequestered anatomically from the immune system during embryonic development.

Seroconversion – The phase of an infection when antibodies against the infecting agent are first detectable in the blood.

Serology – The study of serum antibodies and their reaction with antigens. The term is often used to describe diagnosis of infections based on detection of microbe-specific serum antibodies.

Serpins – A family of protease inhibitors.

Serum – The fluid component of clotted blood; a straw coloured liquid obtained after the removal of fibrin from plasma.

Serum sickness – A disease caused by the injection of large doses of proteinic antigens, foreign serum, or serum proteins. Characterized by fever, joint pains, and nephritis, the disease is the result of formation of immune complexes between the injected protein and the antibodies formed against it.

Severe Combined Immune Deficiency (SCID) – An immune deficiency disease in which both antibody- and T cell-mediated immune responses are absent. It is usually the result of T cell deficiencies. The *scid* mutation results in loss of an enzyme needed for DNA-repair (DNA-PK) and such mice are used extensively in immunological research.

Signal joint – A joint formed by the precise joining of recognition signal sequences in the process of somatic recombination that generates lymphocyte antigen receptors.

Signal transduction – The process of converting a signal from one form to another. Binding of a ligand to its receptor causes receptor clustering. This original clustering signal is transduced into chemical signals in the cytoplasm by the activation of receptor-associated protein kinases.

Silencers – Nucleotide sequences that downregulate transcription in both directions over a distance.

Sirolimus – See Rapamycin.

SLE (Systemic Lupus Erythematosus) – An autoimmune disease in which autoantibodies against DNA, RNA, and proteins associated with nucleic acids form immune complexes that damage small blood vessels, especially of the kidney.

Somatic hypermutation – High frequency point mutations in the V region genes of the B cell antigen receptor that occur in germinal centre B cells.

Somatic recombination – A process of DNA recombination occurring in developing lymphocytes by which functional antigen receptor V region genes are assembled from separate *V(D)J* gene segments.

Somatic mutation theory – A theory of antibody diversity that postulates that relatively few genes for the V locus are inherited and that V region of cells destined to be lymphocytes mutates at a rate higher than the rest of the DNA, yielding a large number of clones of immunologically competent cells.

Spleen – An organ in the upper left side of the peritoneal cavity containing a red pulp, involved in removing senescent blood cells, and a white pulp of lymphoid cells. It is the major site of adaptive immune responses to blood borne antigens.

Src-family tyrosine kinases – Receptor-associated protein tyrosine kinases that have several domains, called Src-homology 1, 2, and 3. The SH1 domain contains the active site of the kinase, the SH2 domain can bind to phosphotyrosine residues, and the SH3 domain is involved in interactions with proline-rich regions in other proteins.

STATs (Signal Transducers and Activators of Transcription) – A family of cytoplasmic proteins that function as both signal transducers and transcription activators. They are inactive as monomers and activation involves phosphorylation and dimerization upon which they translocate to the nucleus.

Stem cells – Undifferentiated cells that divide and give rise to additional stem cells and to cells of multiple lineages.

Superantigens – Molecules that stimulate lymphocytes by binding to antigen receptors outside the antigen-binding site. T cell superantigens glue T cell receptors to MHC class II molecules, whereas B cell superantigens coligate adjacent membrane immunoglobulin molecules.

Serotonin (5-hydroxytryptamine) – The principal vasoactive amine released by mast cells. It is also a neurotransmitter synthesized in the central nervous system that is believed to play an important part of the biochemistry of depression, bipolar disorder, and anxiety.

Suppressor T cells – T cells that were postulated to suppress the activity of other T and B cells.

Surfactant Proteins A & D (SP-A and SP-D) – Pattern recognition receptors associated with phospholipids of lung surfactants. They have an important role in the host defence of alveoli and proteins closely resembling them are found in a number of other sites in the body.

Surrogate light chain – A complex of two non-variable proteins, V pre-B and λ5, that associate with the μ heavy chain in pre-B cells to form the pre-B cell antigen receptor.

Syk – A key tyrosine kinase involved in B cell antigen receptor pathways.

Syndrome – Spectrum of symptoms, behaviour, etc that are characteristic of a disease.

Syngraft (syngeneic graft) – A graft between two genetically identical individuals, that is usually not rejected.

Systemic anaphylaxis – The degranulation of mast cells all over the body. It results in widespread vasodilation, tissue fluid accumulation, epiglottal swelling, and may result in death.

Systemic Lupus Erythematosus – See SLE.

T cell antigen Receptor – A clonally distributed, disulphide linked heterodimer consisting of αβ or γδ chains that recognizes peptides (or glycolipds) loaded on MHC (or CD1) molecules. It consists of a membrane proximal constant (C) region and a membrane distal variable (V) region that takes part in antigen-binding and is associated with the CD3 complex that is involved in signal transduction.

T lymphocyte – A subset of lymphocytes defined by their development in the thymus and by their heterodimeric antigen receptors associated with the proteins of the CD3 complex.

TAAs – See Tumour associated antigens.

Tacrolimus – See FK506.

TAP (Transporters associated with Antigen Processing) – A heterodimeric protein involved in transporting short peptides from the cytosol into the lumen of the endoplasmic reticulum to allow their loading on MHC class I molecules.

Tapasin – TAP-associated protein. It is thought to promote the stability and peptide transport activity of TAP and hold the MHC class I molecule in its peptide-receptive conformation.

T-bet – T-box family transcription factor that is expressed in developing and committed T_{H1} cells. It has a central role in T_{H1} lineage development.

TD (Thymus-Dependent) antigens – Antigens that require the involvement of both, antigen-specific B and T cells to elicit a humoral response.

TdT (Terminal deoxynucleotidyl Transferase) – An enzyme expressed in developing lymphocytes that inserts non-templated or N-nucleotides into the junctions between gene segments in T cell receptor and immunoglobulin V region genes.

TGF-β (Transforming Growth Factor-β) – An immunosuppresive cytokine that inhibits the proliferation and differentiation of T cells, activation of macrophages, and counteracts the effects of pro-inflammatory cytokines.

T_H cells (helper T cells) – $CD4^+$ T cells that help the B cells or $CD8^+$ T cells in responding to an antigen. Two subsets of T_H cells are recognized based on their secretory cytokine pattern. T_{H1} cells are mainly involved in activating macrophages and cytotoxic T lymphocytes whereas T_{H2} cells stimulate B cells.

Thymocytes – A precursor of T lymphocyte found in the thymus.

Thymus – A bilobed lymphoepithelial organ overlying the heart that is the site of T cell maturation.

TI (Thymus-Independent) antigens – Antigens that can mediate activation and proliferation of antigen-specific B cells without the involvement of antigen-specific T cells.

Tingible body macrophages – Phagocytic cells in the germinal centres that engulf apoptotic B cells.

TNF (Tumour Necrosis Factor) – Pro-inflammatory cytokines. TNF-α is produced by macrophages and T cells and has multiple functions in immunity. TNF-β, also called lymphotoxin, is cytotoxic. It is also critical for the development of lymphoid organs.

TNFR (Tumour Necrosis Factor Receptor) – Trimeric cell surface proteins having a varied role in immunity.

Tolerance – Antigen-specific unresponsiveness of the immune system induced by a previous exposure to the antigen. Substances that induce tolerance are called tolerogens. Central tolerance is established in lymphocytes developing in central lymphoid organs. Peripheral tolerance is acquired by mature lymphocytes in the peripheral tissues.

Toll-like Receptors (TLRs) – Members of a family of pattern recognition receptors that are important in innate immunity. All the members are homologues of the Toll originally described in *Drosophila*.

Tonsils – Lymphoepithelial structures found at the openings of the respiratory and digestive tract.

Toxoids – Inactivated toxins that have lost their toxicity but retained their immunogenicity.

Transcytosis – Active transport of molecules across epithelial cells.

Transplantation – Grafting or transfer of tissue or cells from one individual to another.

Transfusion – Transfer of blood or blood products from one individual to another. An immunological reaction to such transfused products is called transfusion reaction.

Transgenic animals – Animals that express an exogenous gene. See Appendix III.

TSAs – See Tumour specific antigens.

TSS (Toxic Shock Syndrome) – A systemic toxic reaction caused by the massive production of cytokines by $CD4^+$ T cells activated by the bacterial superantigen Toxic Shock Syndrome Toxin-1 (TSST-1).

Tumour – A swelling caused by a mass of cells. Benign tumours are normally slow-growing, circumscribed, encapsulated, with well-defined edges, and do not invade surrounding tissue. Malignant tumours are often rapidly growing, aggressive, invasive masses of cells.

Tumour Associated Antigens (TAAs) – Antigens found on both normal and cancerous cells.

Tumour Specific Antigens (TSAs) – Antigens expressed exclusively by tumour cells and are not found on normal body cells.

Tyrosine kinases (Protein Tyrosine Kinases or PTKs) – Enzymes that specifically phosphorylate tyrosine residues in proteins. Tyrosine kinases critical for B cell activation are Blk, Fyn, Lyn, and Syk, whereas those critical for T cell activation are Lck, Fyn, and ZAP-70.

Urticaria – Red itchy skin welts (hives) that are the result of an allergic reaction.

V (Variable) region – The N-terminal domain of the light or heavy chain of T cell receptor or immunoglobulin molecule.

V(D)J recombination – A process found exclusively in vertebrate lymphocytes that allows the recombination of different gene segments into sequences encoding complete protein chains of immunoglobulins and T cell receptors.

Vaccination – The deliberate introduction of a dead or attenuated (non-pathogenic) form of the pathogen or its products in an individual with the intention of eliciting an adaptive immune response.

Valency – In the context of an antibody or antigen, it is the number of different molecules of the ligand that the antigen or antibody can combine with at one time.

Vasoactive amines – Histamine, 5-hydroxytryptamine, serotonin, etc that are present in granules of basophils, mast cells, platelets, eosinophils. They act on the endothelium of smooth muscles causing its retraction.

Vesicles – Small membrane-bound compartments within the cytosol.

Western blot – A technique of protein detection. It involves separation of proteins by gel electrophoresis, followed by transferring (blotting) to a nitrocellulose membrane, and probing with specific antibodies. See Appendix III.

Wheal and flare reaction – Local swelling and redness of the skin at a site of an immediate hypersensitivity reaction.

Xenotransplantation – The transfer of cells, tissues, or organs between disparate species.

X-linked agammaglobulinaemia (Bruton's agammaglobulinaemia) – A genetic disorder in which B cell development is arrested at the pre-B-cell stage and mature B cells or antibodies are not formed. The disease is due to a defect in the gene encoding the protein tyrosine kinase Btk.

X-linked hyper IgM syndrome – A disease characterized by high serum IgM levels but deficient IgG, IgE, or IgA antibody formation. It is due to a defect in the gene encoding the CD40 ligand (CD154).

ZAP-70 – A tyrosine kinase indispensable for T cell receptor signalling.

Zymogen – Is a pro-enzyme, which needs to be activated before it can act.

Zymosan – An insoluble preparation from yeast cell wall. It is a mixture of glucans, mannans, proteins and lipids.

β_2-microglobulin – A polypeptide that is a constituent of some membrane proteins. It is non-covalently associated with, and is an integral part of, MHC class I molecules.

$\alpha\beta$ T cells – T cells expressing an antigen receptor made of α and β subunits. These are the conventional T cells.

$\gamma\delta$ T cells – T cells bearing antigen receptor consisting of the γ and δ chains. They recognize antigen independent of MHC molecules.

Bibliography

This bibliography lists some of the recent review articles which were used as reference material while writing this book. It is not meant to be exhaustive, rather it should serve as a starting point for those interested in further reading. While compiling the list, we have also kept in mind the accessibility of the journals, either in print or on the net.Internet sites of possible interest to teachers and students alike are listed at the end.

Chapter 1

Matzinger, P. (2002). The danger model: a renewed sense of self. *Science,* 296:301.

Medzhitov, R. and Janeway, C.A. Jr (2002). Decoding the patterns of self and nonself by the innate immune system. *Science,* 296:298.

Sun, P.D. (2003). Structure and function of natural-killer-cell receptors. *Immunology Research,* 27:539.

Chapter 2

Abraham, S.N. and Arock, M. (1998). Mast cells and basophils in innate immunity. *Seminars in Immunology,*10:373.

Akira, S. (2003). Mammalian toll-like receptors. *Current Opinion in Immunology,* 5:5.

Belardelli, F. and Ferrantini, M. (2002). Cytokines as a link between innate and adaptive antitumor immunity. *Trends in Immunology,* 23:201.

Bogdan, C. (2001). Nitric oxide and the immune response. *Nature Immunology,* 2(10):907.

Chandra, R.K. (2002). Nutrition and the immune system from birth to old age. *European Journal of Clinical Nutrition,* 56 Suppl 3:S73.

Colucci, F., Caligiuri, M.A. and Di Santo, J.P. (2003). What does it take to make a natural killer? *Nature Reviews Immunology,* 3:413.

Gabay, C. and Kushner, I. (1999). Acute-phase proteins and other systemic responses to inflammation. *New England Journal of Medicine,* 340:448.

Gordon, S. (2002). Pattern recognition receptors: doubling up for the innate immune response. *Cell,* 111:927.

Greenberg, S. and Grinstein, S. (2002). Phagocytosis and innate immunity. *Current Opinion in Immunology,* 14:136.

Hacker, G., Redecke, V. and Hacker, H. (2002). Activation of immune system by bacterial CpG DNA. *Immuology,* 105:245.

Holmskov, U., Thiel, S. and Jensenius, J.C. (2003). Collectins and ficolins: humoral lectins of the innate immune defense. *Annual Review of Immunology,* 21:547.

Janeway, C.A. Jr. and Medzhitov, R. (2002). Innate immune recognition. *Annual Review of Immunology,* 20:197.

Lipscomb, M.F. and Masten, B.J. (2002). Dendritic cells: Immune regulators in health and disease. *Physiology Reviews,* 82:97.

Marshall, J.S. and Jawdat, D.M. (2004). Mast cells in innate immunity. *Journal of Allergy and Clinical Immunology,* 114:21.

McDonald, C. and Nunez, G. (2004). Minding the fort. *Nature Immunology,* 5:16.

Mortensen, R.F. (2001). C-reactive protein, inflammation, and innate immunity. *Immunological Research,* 24:163.

Nathan, C. (2002). Points of control in inflammation. *Nature,* 420:846.

Natarajan, K., Dimasi, N., Wang, J., Mariuzza, R.A. and Margulies, D.H. (2002). Structure and function of natural killer cell receptors: Multiple molecular solutions to self, nonself discrimination. *Annual Review of Immunology,* 20:853.

Netea, M.G., Van der Graaf, C., Van der Meer, J.W. and Kullberg, B.J. (2004). Toll-like receptors and the host defense against microbial pathogens: bringing specificity to the innate-immune system. *Journal of Leukocyte Biology,* 75:749.

Nizet, V. and Gallo, R.L. (2003). Cathelicidins and innate defense against invasive bacterial infection. *Scandinavian Journal of Infectious Diseases,* 35:670.

Peiser, L., Mukhopadhyay, S. and Gordon, S. (2002). Scavenger receptors in innate immunity. *Current Opinion in Immunology,* 14:123.

Schittek, B., Hipfel, R., Sauer, B., Bauer, J., Kalbacher, H., Stevanovic, S., Schirle, S., Schroeder, K., Blin, N., Meier, F., Rassner, G. and Garbe, C. (2001). Dermcidin: a novel human antibiotic peptide secreted by sweat glands. *Nature Immunology,* 2:1133.

Sopori, M. (2002). Effects of cigarette smoke on the immune system. *Nature Reviews Immunology,* 2:372.

Suffredini, A.F., Fantuzzi, G., Badolato, R., Oppenheim, J.J. and O'Grady, N.P. (1999). New insights into the biology of the acute phase response. *Journal of Clinical Immunology,* 19:203.

Underhill, D.M. and Ozinsky, A. (2002). Phagocytosis of microbes: complexity in action. *Annual Review of Immunology,* 20:825.

Webster, J.I., Tonelli, L. and Sternberg, E.M. (2002). Neuroendocrine regulation of immunity. *Annual Review of Immunology,* 20:125.

Yang, D., Biragyn, A., Kwak, L.W. and Oppenheim, J.J. (2002). Mammalian defensins in immunity: more than just microbicidal. *Trends in Immunology,* 23:291.

Chapter 3

Blom, A.M., Villoutreix, B.O. and Dahlback, B. (2004). Complement inhibitor C4b-binding protein-friend or foe in the innate immune system? *Molecular Immunology,* 40:1333.
Chan, R.K., Ibrahim, S.I., Verna, N., Carroll, M., Moore, F.D. Jr and Hechtman H.B. (2003). Ischaemia-reperfusion is an event triggered by immune complexes and complement. *British Journal of Surgery,* 90:1470.
Gadjeva, M., Takahashi K. and Thiel S. (2004). Mannan-binding lectin — a soluble pattern recognition molecule. *Molecular Immunology,* 41:113.
Gadjeva, M., Thiel S. and Jensenius, J.C. (2001). The mannan-binding-lectin pathway of the innate immune response. *Current Opinion in Immunology,* 13:74.
Kohl, J. (2001). Anaphylatoxins and infectious and non-infectious inflammatory diseases. *Molecular Immunology,* 38:175.
Mastellos, D. and Lambris, J.D. (2002). Complement: more than a 'guard' against invading pathogens? *Trends in Immunology,* 23:485.
Roos, A., Xu, W., Castellano, G., Nauta, A.J., Garred, P., Daha, M.R. and Van Kooten, C. (2004). A pivotal role for innate immunity in the clearance of apoptotic cells. *European Journal of Immunology,* 34:921.
Rus, H.G., Niculescu, F.I. and Shin, M.L. (2001). Role of the C5b-9 complement complex in cell cycle and apoptosis. *Immunological Reviews,* 180:49.
Sahu, A. and Lambris, J.D. (2001). Structure and biology of complement protein C3, a connecting link between innate and acquired immunity. *Immunological Reviews,* 180:35.
Smith, G.P. and Smith, R.A. (2001). Membrane-targeted complement inhibitors. *Molecular Immunology,* 38:249.
Turner, M.W. (2003). The role of mannose-binding lectin in health and disease. *Molecular Immunology,* 40:423.

Chapter 4

Lesinski, G.B. and Westerink, M.A. (2001). Novel vaccine strategies to T-independent antigens. *Journal of Microbiological Methods,* 47:135.
Schijns, V.E. (2000). Immunological concepts of vaccine adjuvant activity. *Current Opinion in Immunology,* 12:456.
Silverman, G.J. and Goodyear C.S. (2002). A model B-cell superantigen and the immunobiology of B lymphocytes. *Clinical Immunology,* 102:117.
Snapper, C.M. and Mond, J.J. (1996). A model for induction of T cell-independent humoral immunity in response to polysaccharide antigens. *Journal of Immunology,* 157:2229.
Torres, B.A., Kominsky, S., Perrin, G.Q., Hobeika, A.C. and Johnson, H.M. (2001). Superantigens: the good, the bad, and the ugly. *Experimental Biological Medicine* (Maywood), 226:164.
Zinkernagel, R.M. (2000). Localization dose and time of antigens determine immune reactivity. *Seminars in Immunology,* 12:163.

Chapter 5

Crivellato, E., Vacca, A. and Ribatti, D. (2004). Setting the stage: an anatomist's view of the immune system. *Trends in Immunology,* 25:210.
Fu, Y.X. and Chaplin, D.D. (1999). Development and maturation of secondary lymphoid tissues. *Annual Reviews of Immunology,* 17:399.
Nagler-Anderson, C. (2001). Man the barrier! Strategic defences in the intestinal mucosa. *Nature Reviews Immunology,* 1:59.
Perry, M. and Whyte, A. (1998). Immunology of the tonsils. *Immunology Today,* 19:41.
Shortman, K. and Liu, Y. (2002). Mouse and human dendritic cell subtypes. *Nature Reviews Immunology,* 2:454.
Von Andrian, U.H. and Mempel, T.R. (2003). Homing and cellular traffic in lymph nodes. *Nature Reviews Immunology,* 3:867.

Chapter 6

Allison, T.J. and Garboczi, D.N. (2002). Structure of gammadelta T cell receptors and their recognition of non-peptide antigens. *Molecular Immunology,* 38:1051.
Cantrell, D.A. (2003). Regulation and function of serine kinase networks in lymphocytes. *Current Opinion in Immunology,* 15:294.
Jordan, M.S., Singer, A.L. and Koretzky, G.A. (2003). Adaptors as central mediators of signal transduction in immune cells. *Nature Immunology,* 4:110.
Niiro, H. and Clark, E.A. (2002). Regulation of B-cell fate by antigen-receptor signals. *Nature Reviews Immunology,* 2:945.
Penninger, J.M., Irie-Sasaki, J., Sasaki, T. and Oliveira-dos-Santos, A.J. (2001). CD45: new jobs for an old acquaintance. *Nature Immunology,* 2:389.
Tsubata, T. (1999). Co-receptors on B lymphocytes. *Current Opinion in Immunology,* 11:249.
Van der Merwe, P.A. and Davis, S.J. (2003). Molecular interactions mediating T cell antigen recognition. *Annual Reviews of Immunology,* 21:659.
Werlen, G. and Palmer, E. (2002). The T-cell receptor signalosome: a dynamic structure with expanding complexity. *Current Opinion in Immunology,* 14:299.

Chapter 7

Ackerman, A.L. and Cresswell, P. (2004). Cellular mechanisms governing cross-presentation of exogenous antigens. *Nature Immunology,* 5:678.

Antoniou, A.N., Powis, S.J. and Elliott, T. (2003). Assembly and export of MHC class I peptide ligands. *Current Opinion in Immunology,* 15:75.

Brigl, M. and Brenner, M.B. (2004). CD1: antigen presentation and T cell function. *Annual Reviews of Immunology,* 22:817.

Bryant, P. and Ploegh, H. (2004). Class II MHC peptide loading by the professionals. *Current Opinion in Immunology,* 16:96.

Hewitt, E.W. (2003). The MHC class I antigen presentation pathway: strategies for viral immune evasion. *Immunology,* 110:163.

Hudrisier, D. and Bongrand, P. (2002). Intercellular transfer of antigen-presenting cell determinants onto T cells: molecular mechanisms and biological significance. *FASEB Journal,* 16:477.

Jacob, S., McClintock, M.K., Zelano, B. and Ober, C. (2002). Paternally inherited HLA alleles are associated with women's choice of male odor. *Nature Genetics,* 30:175.

Klein, J. and Sato, A. (2000). The HLA system. Second of two parts. *New England Journal of Medicine,* 343:782.

Shastri, N., Schwab S. and Serwold, T. (2002). Producing nature's gene-chips: the generation of peptides for display by MHC class I molecules. *Annual Reviews of Immunology,* 20:463.

Villadangos, J.A. (2001). Presentation of antigens by MHC class II molecules: getting the most out of them. *Molecular Immunology,* 38:329.

Yung, Yu C., Yang, Z., Blanchong, C.A. and Miller, W. The human and mouse MHC class III region: a parade of 21 genes at the centromeric segment. *Immunology Today,* 21:320.

Chapter 8

Alcami, A. (2003). Viral mimicry of cytokines, chemokines and their receptors. *Nature Reviews Immunology,* 3:36.

Bishop, G.A. and Hostager, B.S. (2001). B lymphocyte activation by contact-mediated interactions with T lymphocytes. *Current Opinion in Immunology,* 13:278.

Buckley, R.H. (2000). Primary immunodeficiency diseases due to defects in lymphocytes. *New England Journal of Medicine,* 343:1313.

Carding, S.R. and Egan, P.J. (2002). Gammadelta T cells: functional plasticity and heterogeneity. *Nature Reviews Immunology,* 2:336.

Chan, K.F., Siegel, M.R. and Lenardo, J.M. (2000). Signaling by the TNF receptor superfamily and T cell homeostasis. *Immunity,* 13:419.

Germain, R.N. (2002). T-cell development and the CD4-CD8 lineage decision. *Nature Reviews Immunology,* 2:309.

Godfrey, D.I., Hammond, K.J., Poulton, L.D., Smyth, M.J. and Baxter, A.G. (2000). NKT cells: facts, functions and fallacies. *Immunology Today,* 11:573.

Hardy, R.R. and Hayakawa, K. (2001). B cell development pathways. *Annual Reviews of Immunology,* 19:595.

Hayakawa, K. and Hardy, R.R. (2000). Development and function of B-1 cells. *Current Opinion in Immunology,* 12:346.

Hildeman, D.J., Zhu, Y., Mitchell, T.C., Kappler, J. and Marrack, P. (2002). Molecular mechanisms of activated T cell death *in vivo. Current Opinion in Immunology,* 14:354.

Hogquist, K.A. (2001). Signal strength in thymic selection and lineage commitment. *Current Opinion in Immunology,* 13:225.

Jenkins, M.K., Khoruts, A., Ingulli, E., Mueller, D.L., McSorley, S.J., Reinhardt, R.L., Itano, A. and Pape, K.A. (2001). In vivo activation of antigen-specific CD4 T cells. *Annual Reviews of Immunology,* 19:23.

Kaech, S.M., Wherry, E.J. and Ahmed, R. (2002). Effector and memory T-cell differentiation: implications for vaccine development. *Nature Reviews Immunology,* 2:251.

Kurosaki, T. (2002). Regulation of B cell fates by BCR signaling components. *Current Opinion in Immunology,* 14:341.

Lanzavecchia, A. and Sallusto, F. (2002). Progressive differentiation and selection of the fittest in the immune response. *Nature Reviews Immunology,* 2:982.

Mackay, C.R. (2002). Chemokines: immunology's high impact factors. *Nature Immunology,* 2:95.

Martin, F. and Kearney, J.F. (2001). B1 cells: similarities and differences with other B cell subsets. *Current Opinion in Immunology,* 13:195.

Martin, F. and Kearney, J.F. (2002). Marginal-zone B cells. *Nature Reviews Immunology,* 2:323.

McHeyzer-Williams, M.G. (2003). B cells as effectors. *Current Opinion in Immunology,* 15:354.

Meffre, E., Casellas, R. and Nussenzweig, M.C. (2000). Antibody regulation of B cell development. *Nature Immunology,* 1:379.

Mills, D.M. and Cambier, J.C. (2003). B lymphocyte activation during cognate interactions with CD4+ T lymphocytes: molecular dynamics and immunologic consequences. *Seminars in Immunology,* 15:325.

Murphy, K.M. and Reiner, S.L. (2002). The lineage decisions of helper T cells. *Nature Reviews Immunology,* 2:933.

Reiner, S.L. (2001). Helper T cell differentiation, inside and out. *Current Opinion in Immunology,* 13:351.

Savino, W., Mendes-da-Cruz, D.A., Silva, J.S., Dardenne, M. and Cotta-de-Almeida, V. (2002). Intrathymic T-cell migration: a combinatorial interplay of extracellular matrix and chemokines? *Trends in Immunology,* 23:305.

Seder, R.A. and Ahmed, R. (2003). Similarities and differences in CD4+ and CD8+ effector and memory T cell generation. *Nature Immunology,* 4:835.

Sharpe, A.H. and Freeman, G.J. (2002). The B7-CD28 superfamily. *Nature Reviews Immunology,* 2:116.

Shevach, E.M. (2002). CD4+ CD25+ suppressor T cells: more questions than answers. *Nature Reviews Immunology,* 2:389.

Smith, S.A. and Kotwal, G.J. (2001). Virokines: novel immunomodulatory agents. *Expert Opinion in Biological Therapy,* 1:343.

Wang, L.D. and Clark, M.R. (2003). B-cell antigen-receptor signalling in lymphocyte development. *Immunology,* 110:411.

Chapter 9

Aalberse, R.C. and Schuurman, J. (2002). IgG4 breaking the rules. *Immunology,* 105:9.

Breedveld, F.C. (2000). Therapeutic monoclonal antibodies. *Lancet,* 355:735.

Heyman, B. (2000). Regulation of antibody responses via antibodies, complement, and Fc receptors *Annual Reviews of Immunology,* 18:709.

Johansen, F.E., Braathen, R. and Brandtzaeg, P. (2000). Role of J Chain in Secretory Immunoglobulin Formation *Scandinavian Journal of Immunology,* 52:240.

Muyldermans, S., Cambillau, C. and Wyns, L. (2001). Recognition of antigens by single domain antibody fragments: the superfluous luxury of paired domains. *Trends in Biochemical Sciences,* 26:230.

Novak, N., Kraft, S. and Bieber, T. (2001). IgE receptors. *Current Opinion in Immunology,* 13:721.

Ober, R.J., Martinez, C., Lai, X., Zhou, J. and Ward, E.S. (2004). Exocytosis of IgG as mediated by the receptor, FcRn: an analysis at the single-molecule level. *Proceedings of the National Academy of Science of the USA,* 101:11076.

Phalipon, A. and Corthesy, B. (2003). Novel functions of the polymeric Ig receptor: well beyond transport of immunoglobulins. *Trends in Immunology,* 24:55.

Pre'homme, J., Petit, I., Barra, A., Morel, F., Lecron, J. and Lelie'vre, E. (2000). Structural and functional properties of membrane and secreted IgD. *Molecular Immunology,* 37:871.

Sewell, W.A.C. and Jolles, S. (2002). Immunomodulatory action of intravenous immunoglobulin. *Immunology,* 107:387.

Takai, T. (2002). Roles of Fc receptors in autoimmunity *Nature Reviews Immunology,* 2:580.

Woof, J.M. and Burton, D.R. (2004). Human antibody-Fc receptor interactions illuminated by crystal structures. *Nature Reviews Immunology,* 4:89.

Chapter 10

Besmer, E., Gourzi, P. and Papavasiliou, F.N. (2004). The regulation of somatic hypermutation. *Current Opinion in Immunology,* 16:241.

Chaudhuri, J. and Alt, F.W. (2004). Class-switch recombination: interplay of transcription, DNA deamination and DNA repair. *Nature Reviews Immunology,* 4:541.

Durandy, A. (2003). Activation-induced cytidine deaminase: a dual role in class-switch recombination and somatic hypermutation. *European Journal of Immunology,* 33:2069.

Feeney, A.J. (2000). Factors that influence formation of B cell repertoire. *Immunology Research,* 21:195.

Gearhart, P.J. (2002). Immunology: the roots of antibody diversity. *Nature,* 419:29.

Gearhart, P.J. and Wood, R.D. (2001). Emerging links between hypermutation of antibody genes and DNA polymerases. *Nature Reviews Immunology,* 1:187.

Gellert, M. (2002). V(D)J recombination: RAG proteins, repair factors, and regulation. *Annual Reviews of Biochemistry,* 71:101.

Guzman-rojas, L., Sims-mourtada, J.C., Rangel, R. and Martinez-valdez, H. (2002). Life and death within germinal centres: a double-edged sword. *Immunology,* 107:167.

Honjo, T., Kinoshita, K. and Muramatsu M. (2002). Molecular mechanism of class switch recombination: linkage with somatic hypermutation. *Annual Reviews of Immunology,* 20:165.

Honjo, T., Muramatsu, M. and Fagarasan, S. (2004). AID: how does it aid antibody diversity? *Immunity,* 20:659.

Jung, D. and Alt, F.W. (2004). Unraveling V(D)J recombination; insights into gene regulation. *Cell,* 116:299.

Kenter, A.L. (2003). Class-switch recombination: after the dawn of AID. *Current Opinion in Immunology,* 15:190.

Kouskoff, V. and Nemazee, D. (2001). Role of receptor editing and revision in shaping the B and T lymphocyte repertoire. *Life Sciences,* 69:1105.

Lieber, M.R., Ma, Y., Pannicke, U. and Schwarz, K. (2003). Mechanism and regulation of human non-homologous DNA end-joining. *Nature Reviews Molecular Cell Biology,* 4:712.

Manis, J.P., Tian, M. and Alt, F.W. (2002). Mechanism and control of class-switch recombination. *Trends in Immunology,* 23:31.

Martin, A. and Scharff, M.D., (2002). AID and mismatch repair in antibody diversification. *Nature Reviews Immunology,* 2:605.

Roth, D.B. (2003). Restraining the V(D)J recombinase. *Nature Reviews Immunology,* 3:656.

Schlissel, M.S. (2002). Does artemis end the hunt for the hairpin-opening activity in V(D)J recombination? *Cell,* 109:1.

Schlissel, M.S. (2003). Regulating antigen-receptor gene assembly. *Nature Reviews Immunology,* 3:890.

Tew, J.G., Wu, J., Fakher, M., Szakal, A.K. and Qin, D. (2001). Follicular dendritic cells: beyond the necessity of T cell help. *Trends in Immunology,* 22:361.

Van Eijk, M., Defrance, T., Hennino, A. and de Groot, C. (2001). Death-receptor contribution to the germinal-center reaction. *Trends in Immunology,* 22:677.

Chapter 11

Barry, M. and Bleackley, R.C. (2002). Cytotoxic T lymphocytes: all roads lead to death. *Nature Reviews Immunology,* 2:401.

Berzofsky, J.A., Ahlers, J.D. and Belyakov, I.M. (2001). Strategies for designing and optimizing new generation vaccines. *Nature Reviews Immunology,* 1:209.

Clayberger, C. and Krensky, A.M. (2003). Granulysin. *Current Opinion in Immunology,* 15:560.

Lieberman, J. (2003). The ABCs of granule-mediated cytotoxicity: new weapons in the arsenal. *Nature Reviews Immunology,* 3:61.

Raja, S.M., Metkar, S.S. and Froelich, C.J. (2003). Cytotoxic granule-mediated apoptosis: unraveling the complex mechanism. *Current Opinion in Immunology,* 15:528.

Russell, J.H. and Ley, T.J. (2002). Lymphocyte-mediated cytotoxicity. *Annual Reviews of Immunology,* 20:323.

Trapani, J.A. and Smyth, M.J. (2002). Functional significance of the perforin/granzyme cell death pathway. *Nature Reviews Immunology,* 2:735.

Chapter 12

Garside, P. and Mowat, A.M. (2001). Oral tolerance. *Seminars in Immunology,* 13:177.

Green, D.R. and Ferguson, T.A. (2001). The role of Fas ligand in immune privilege. *Nature Reviews Molecular Cell Biology,* 2:917.

Hori, S., Takahashi, T. and Sakaguchi, S. (2003). Control of autoimmunity by naturally arising regulatory CD4+ T cells. *Advances in Immunology,* 81:331.

Lechler, R., Chai, J.G., Marelli-Berg, F. and Lombardi, G. (2001). The contributions of T-cell anergy to peripheral T-cell tolerance. *Immunology,* 103:262.

Mahnke, K., Knop, J. and Enk, A.H. (2003). Induction of tolerogenic DCs: 'you are what you eat' *Trends in Immunology,* 24:646.

Mathis, D. and Benoist, C. (2004). Back to central tolerance. *Immunity,* 20:509.

Mowat, A.M. (2003). Anatomical basis of tolerance and immunity to intestinal antigens. *Nature Reviews Immunology,* 3:331.

Ohashi, P.S. and DeFranco, A.L. (2002). Making and breaking tolerance. *Current Opinion in Immunology,* 6:744.

Roncarolo, M.G. and Levings, M.K. (2000). The role of different subsets of T regulatory cells in controlling autoimmunity. *Current Opinion in Immunology,* 12:676.

Sprent, J. and Kishimoto, H. (2001). The thymus and central tolerance. *Philosophical Transactions of Royal Society of London Series B Biological. Sciences,* 356:609.

Steinman, R.M. and Nussenzweig, M.C. (2002). Avoiding horror autotoxicus: the importance of dendritic cells in peripheral T cell tolerance. *Proceedings of the National Academy of Science of the USA,* 99:351.

Streilein, J.W. (2003). Ocular immune privilege: the eye takes a dim but practical view of immunity and inflammation. *Journal of Leukocyte Biology,* 74:179.

't Hart, B.A. and van Kooyk, Y. (2004). Yin-Yang regulation of autoimmunity by DCs. *Trends in Immunology,* 25:353.

Walker, L.S. and Abbas, A.K. (2002). The enemy within: keeping self-reactive T cells at bay in the periphery. *Nature Reviews Immunology,* 2:11.

Zouali, M. (2001). Immunological Tolerance: Mechanisms. *Encyclopaedia of Life Sciences,* 1.

Chapter 13

Cascalho, M. and Platt, J.L. (2001). The immunological barrier to xenotransplantation. *Immunity,* 14:437.

Daniels, G. (2001). A century of human blood groups. *Weiner Klinische Wochenschrift,* 113:781.

Erlebacher, A. (2001). Why isn't the fetus rejected? *Current Opinion in Immunology,* 13:590.

Goodnough, L.T., Shander, A. and Brecher, M.E. (2003). Transfusion medicine: looking to the future. *Lancet,* 361:161.

Gorantla, V.S., Barker, J.H., Jones, J.W. Jr, Prabhune, K., Maldonado, C. and Granger, D.K. (2000). Immunosuppressive agents in transplantation: mechanisms of action and current anti-rejection strategies. *Microsurgery,* 20:420.

Kansu, E. (2004). The pathophysiology of chronic graft-versus-host disease. *International Journal of Hematology,* 79:209.

Lechler, R.I., Garden, O.A. and Turka, L.A. (2003). The complementary roles of deletion and regulation in transplantation tolerance. *Nature Reviews Immunology,* 3:147.

Rogers, N.J. and Lechler, R.I. (2001). Allorecognition. *American Journal of Transplantation,* 1:97.

Shapiro, A.M., Nanji, S.A. and Lakey, J.R. (2003). Clinical islet transplant: current and future directions towards tolerance. *Immunological Reviews,* 196:219.

Chapter 14

Bach, J.F. (2002). The effect of infections on susceptibility to autoimmune and allergic diseases. *New England Journal of Medicine,* 347:911.

Caton, A.J. (2003). Mechanisms, manifestations, and failures of self-tolerance. *Immunology Research,* 27:161.

Cline, A.M. and Radic, M.Z. (2004). Apoptosis, subcellular particles, and autoimmunity. *Clinical Immunology,* 112:175.

Firestein, G.S. (2004). The T cell cometh: interplay between adaptive immunity and cytokine networks in rheumatoid arthritis. *Journal of Clinical Investigations,* 114:471.

Fujinami, R.S. (2001). Viruses and autoimmune disease—two sides of the same coin? *Trends in Microbiology,* 9:377.

Harrison, L.C. and Hafler, D.A. (2000). Antigen-specific therapy for autoimmune disease. *Current Opinion in Immunology,* 12:704.

Illei, G.G. and Lipsky, P.E. (2000). Novel, non-antigen-specific therapeutic approaches to autoimmune/inflammatory diseases. *Current Opinion in Immunology,* 12:712.

Miller, S.D. and Vanderlugt, C.L. (2002). Epitope spreading in immune mediated diseases: implications for immunotherapy. *Nature Reviews Immunology,* 2:85.

Nepom, G.T. (2002). Therapy of autoimmune diseases: clinical trials and new biologics. *Current Opinion in Immunology,* 14:812.

Notkins, A.L. (2002). Immunologic and genetic factors in type 1 diabetes. *Journal of Biological Chemistry,* 277:43545.

O'Shea, J.J., Ma, A. and Lipsky, P. (2002). Cytokines and autoimmunity. *Nature Reviews Immunology,* 2:37.

Chapter 15

Blank, U. and Rivera, J. (2004). The ins and outs of IgE-dependent mast-cell exocytosis. *Trends in Immunology,* 25:266.

Gould, H.J., Sutton, B.J., Beavil, A.J., Beavil, R.L., McCloskey, N., Coker, H.A., Fear, D. and Smurthwaite, L. (2003). The biology of IgE and the basis of allergic disease. *Annual Review of Immunology,* 21:579.

Herrick, C.A. and Bottomly, K. (2003). To respond or not to respond: T cells in allergic asthma. *Nature Reviews Immunology,* 3:405.

Kawakami, T. and Galli, S.J. (2002). Regulation of mast-cell and basophil function and survival by IgE *Nature Reviews Immunology,* 2:773.

Pichler, W.J. (2004). Immune mechanism of drug hypersensitivity. *Immunology and allergy clinics of North America*, 24:373.

Ring, J., Krämer, U., Schäfer, T. and Behrendt, H. (2001). Why are allergies increasing? *Current Opinion in Immunology*, 13:701.

Robbie-Ryan, M. and Brown, M.A. (2002). The role of mast cells in allergy and autoimmunity. *Current Opinion in Immunology*, 14:728.

Saini, S.S. and MacGlashan, D. (2002). How IgE upregulates the allergic response. *Current Opinion in Immunology*, 14:694.

Sandor, M., Weinstock, J.V. and Wynn, T.A. (2003). Granulomas in schistosome and mycobacterial infections: a model of local immune responses. *Trends in Immunology*, 24:44.

Valenta, R. (2002). The future of antigen-specific immunotherapy of allergy. *Nature Reviews Immunology*, 2:446.

Valenta, R., Ball, T., Focke, M., Linhart, B., Mothes, N., Niederberger, V., Spitzauer, S., Swoboda, I., Vrtala, S., Westritschnig, K. and Kraft, D. (2004). Immunotherapy of allergic disease. *Advances in Immunology*, 82:105.

Yazdanbakhsh, M., Kremsner, P.G. and van Ree, R. (2002). Allergy, Parasites, and the Hygiene Hypothesis. *Science*, 296:490.

Chapter 16

Allen, T.M. (2003). Ligand-targeted therapeutics in anticancer therapy. *Nature Reviews Cancer*, 2:750.

Ames, B.N. and Wakimoto, P. (2002). Are vitamin and mineral deficiencies a major cancer risk? *Nature Reviews Cancer*, 2:694.

Blattman, J.N. and Greenberg, P.D. (2004). Cancer immunotherapy: a treatment for the masses. *Science*, 305:200.

Carter, P. (2001). Improving the efficacy of antibody-based cancer therapies. *Nature Reviews Cancer*, 1:118.

Igney, F.H. and Krammer, P.H. (2002). Death and anti-death: Tumour resistance to apoptosis. *Nature Reviews Cancer*, 2:277.

Smyth, M.J., Hayakawa, Y., Takeda, K. and Yagita, H. (2002). Newaspects of natural-killer-cell surveillance and therapy of cancer. *Nature Reviews Cancer*, 2:850.

Schuler, G., Schuler-Thurner, B. and Steinman, R.M. (2003). The use of dendritic cells in cancer immunotherapy. *Current Opinion in Immunology*, 15:138.

Smyth, M.J., Godfrey, D.I. and Trapani, J.A. (2001). A fresh look at tumor immunosurveillance and immunotherapy. *Nature Immunology*, 2:293.

Todryk, S. (2002). A sense of tumour for the immune system. *Immunology*, 107:1.

Vousden, K.H. and Lu, X. (2002). Live or let die: The cell's response to p53. *Nature Reviews Cancer*, 2:594.

Chapter 17

Burton, G.F., Keele, B.F., Estes, J.D., Thacker, T.C. and Gartner, S. (2002). Follicular dendritic cell contributions to HIV pathogenesis. *Seminars in Immunology*, 14:275.

Fackler, O.T. and Baur, A.S. (2002). Live and Let Die: Nef Functions beyond HIV Replication. *Immunity*, 16:493.

Greene, W.C. and Matija, Peterlin B. (2002). Charting HIV's remarkable voyage through the cell: Basic science as a passport to future therapy. *Nature Medicine*, 8:673.

Lehner, T. (2002). The role of CCR5 chemokine ligands and antibodies to CCR5 coreceptors in preventing HIV Infection. *Trends in Immunology*, 7:347.

Lieberman, J., Manjunath, N. and Shankar, P. (2002). Avoiding the kiss of death: how HIV and other chronic viruses survive. *Current Opinion in Immunology*, 14:478.

Matija, Peterlin B. and Trono, D. (2003). Hide, shield and strike back: How HIV-infected cells avoid immune eradication. *Nature Reviews Immunology*, 3:97.

Internet Links

http://www.lupus.org/
http://www.nlm.nih.gov/medlineplus/rheumatoidarthritis.html
www.britannica.com
http://www.unaids.org
http://pir.georgetown.edu/pirwww/aboutpir
http://users.rcn.com/jkimball.ma.ultranet
http://www.belmont.edu/Science/Biology
http://www.tulane.edu/~biochem
http://www.immunology.klimov.tom.ru/3-2-4.html#IGSF
http://pps98 colorado.edu/courses/4300.cryst.bbk.ac.uk
http://mcdb. /
http://www.lclark.edu/~reiness/immuno
http://www.kcom.edu/faculty/chamberlain/Website/MSTUART
http://www.els.net/
www.copewithcytokines.de
www.microbiology.adelaide.edu.au/immunol/
http://pages2.inrete.it/mbiomed/immu.html
http://www.med.sc.edu:85/links/immunol-link.htm
http://encyclopedia.thefreedictionary.com/
http://ocw.mit.edu/OcwWeb/index.htm
http://www.ncbi.nlm.nih.gov/prow/

Index